Neurobiology of Epilepsy: From Genes to Networks

Neurobiology of Epilepsy: From Genes to Networks

Editor: Karl Smith

AMERICAN
MEDICAL PUBLISHERS
www.americanmedicalpublishers.com

AMERICAN
MEDICAL PUBLISHERS
www.americanmedicalpublishers.com

Cataloging-in-Publication Data

Neurobiology of epilepsy : from genes to networks / edited by Karl Smith.
p. cm.
Includes bibliographical references and index.
ISBN 979-8-88740-301-4
1. Epilepsy. 2. Neurobiology. 3. Epilepsy--Genetic aspects. 4. Epileptics. 5. Neurology. I. Smith, Karl.
RC372 .N48 2023
616.853--dc23

American Medical Publishers,
41 Flatbush Avenue,
1st Floor, New York,
NY 11217, USA

ISBN 979-8-88740-301-4 (Hardback)

Contents

Preface

Epilepsy refers to a group of non-communicable neurological disorders characterized by recurrent epileptic seizures. Due to abnormal electrical activity in the brain, epileptic seizures can range from brief and nearly undetectable periods to long periods of vigorous shaking. Physical injuries can occur as a result of these episodes, either directly such as broken bones or through causing accidents. Excessive and abnormal neuronal activity in the cortex of the brain, which may be seen in the electroencephalogram (EEG) of an individual, is the underlying mechanism of epileptic seizures. Epilepsy can be caused by both genetic and acquired factors. Serious brain trauma, stroke, tumors, and brain problems originating from a previous infection are the acquired causes. Epilepsy is normally managed with daily medication, in patients who have suffered a second seizure. However, medication may be taken after the first seizure in patients at high risk for subsequent seizures. This book is compiled in such a manner, that it will provide in-depth knowledge about neurobiology of epilepsy. It will help the readers in keeping pace with the rapid changes in this field.

After months of intensive research and writing, this book is the end result of all who devoted their time and efforts in the initiation and progress of this book. It will surely be a source of reference in enhancing the required knowledge of the new developments in the area. During the course of developing this book, certain measures such as accuracy, authenticity and research focused analytical studies were given preference in order to produce a comprehensive book in the area of study.

This book would not have been possible without the efforts of the authors and the publisher. I extend my sincere thanks to them. Secondly, I express my gratitude to my family and well-wishers. And most importantly, I thank my students for constantly expressing their willingness and curiosity in enhancing their knowledge in the field, which encourages me to take up further research projects for the advancement of the area.

Editor

1

Insights into the mechanisms of absence seizure generation provided by EEG with functional MRI

Patrick W. Carney[1,2,3] **and Graeme D. Jackson**[1,2,3] *

[1] The Florey Institute for Neuroscience and Mental Health, Heidelberg, VIC, Australia
[2] The University of Melbourne, Parkville, VIC, Australia
[3] Austin Health, Heidelberg, VIC, Australia

***Correspondence:**
Graeme D. Jackson, Melbourne Brain Centre, 245 Burgundy Street, Heidelberg, VIC 3084, Australia
e-mail: g.jackson@brain.org.au

Absence seizures (AS) are brief epileptic events characterized by loss of awareness with subtle motor features. They may be very frequent, and impact on attention, learning, and memory. A number of pathophysiological models have been developed to explain the mechanism of absence seizure generation, which relies heavily on observations from animal studies. Studying the structural and functional relationships between large-scale brain networks in humans is only practical with non-invasive whole brain techniques. EEG with functional MRI (EEG-fMRI) is one such technique that provides an opportunity to explore the interactions between brain structures involved in AS generation. A number of fMRI techniques including event-related analysis, time-course analysis, and functional connectivity (FC) have identified a common network of structures involved in AS. This network comprises the thalamus, midline, and lateral parietal cortex [the default mode network (DMN)], caudate nuclei, and the reticular structures of the pons. The main component displaying an increase in blood oxygen level dependent (BOLD) signal relative to the resting state, in group studies, is the thalamus while the most consistent cortical change is reduced BOLD signal in the DMN. Time-course analysis shows that, rather than some structures being activated or inactivated during AS, there appears to be increase in activity across components of the network preceding or following the electro-clinical onset of the seizure. The earliest change in BOLD signal occurs in the DMN, prior to the onset of epileptiform events. This region also shows altered FC in patients with AS. Hence, it appears that engagement of this network is central to AS. In this review, we will explore the insights of EEG-fMRI studies into the mechanisms of AS and consider how the DMN is likely to be the major large-scale brain network central to both seizure generation and seizure manifestations.

Keywords: epilepsy, absence seizures, functional MRI, default mode network, functional connectivity

CLINICAL

TYPICAL ABSENCE SEIZURES AND ABSENCE SEIZURE SYNDROMES

Genetic generalized epilepsy (GGE) is common and accounts for approximately 20% of epilepsy diagnoses (1). Initially referred to as idiopathic generalized epilepsy, this syndrome was defined by the ILAE Commission on Classification in 1985 (2). This referred to "forms of generalized epilepsies in which all seizures are initially generalized, and their EEG expression is a generalized, bilateral, synchronous, symmetrical discharge." Furthermore, this syndrome was seen in individuals "presenting a normal interictal state without neurological or neuroradiolgical signs." In the most recent classification commission document (3), the term genetic replaced idiopathic given the clear genetic origins of this condition. Furthermore, in the current classification, "Generalized epileptic seizures are conceptualized as originating at some point within, and rapidly engaging, bilaterally distributed networks. Such bilateral networks can include cortical and sub-cortical structures, but do not necessarily include the entire cortex" (3). This reflects current views on seizure generation in generalized epilepsies highlighting that a seizure "focus" may initiate a generalized seizure.

A number of generalized seizure types are seen in GGE (1981). These included absence seizures (AS), myoclonic seizures (MS), and generalized tonic–clonic seizures (GTCS). Using a combination of seizure type, seizure frequency, and the age at seizure onset, GGE can be further sub-classified into sub-syndromes (1989). It is uncertain to what extent sub-syndrome classification identifies true physiological differences between the disorders in people with "GGE" (4). The sub-classification is useful for defining groups for study and provides information that assists in predicting outcome and response to therapy, although there can be considerable clinical heterogeneity within sub-groups.

Different types of AS have also been defined (3, 5, 6). The major distinction exists between typical and atypical AS, which were first defined by the ILAE in 1981 (6). Typical AS were defined according to clinical features, and ictal and interictal features. Although not stated in this classification, individuals with atypical AS usually have a slow EEG background and the presence of this seizure type is generally associated with intellectual disability, multiple other seizure types, poorer response to medical therapy, and a poorer outcome (7). Atypical absence is a feature of the Lennox–Gastaut syndrome (LGS) (2). In the more recent classification, documents include a third category: absence with special features. This group includes myoclonic absence seizures (MAS) in which AS are commonly associated with persistent rhythmic axial myoclonus (8) and eyelid myoclonia during which there is regular rhythmic eyelid myoclonus with or without loss of awareness (9).

As outlined above, AS may be seen in a number of epilepsy syndromes with the relative frequency and pattern of the AS helping to define the syndrome classification. **Table 1** shows the typical syndromes and the common seizure types.

Childhood absence epilepsy (CAE) and juvenile absence epilepsy (JAE) are the archetypal absence epilepsy syndromes with typical AS being the defining seizure type in each of these syndromes. The ILAE (2, 10) syndrome classification of CAE involved the following criteria:

1. Occurring in children of school age (peak manifestation age 6–7 years).
2. Very frequent (several to many per day) absences.
3. The EEG reveals bilateral, synchronous symmetrical spike waves, usually 3 Hz, on a normal background activity.
4. During adolescence, generalized tonic–clonic seizures often develop. Otherwise, absences may remit or, more rarely, persist as the only seizure type.

Juvenile absence epilepsy is defined by a later onset and lower frequency of AS when compared to CAE.

> "Manifestation occurs around puberty. Seizure frequency is lower than in pyknolepsy (CAE), with absences occurring less frequently than every day, mostly sporadically. Association with GTCS is frequent, and GTCS precede the absence manifestations more often than in CAE, often occurring on awakening. Not infrequently, the patients also have myoclonic seizures." (10)

Table 1 | ILAE-defined syndromes in which absence seizures are commonly observed.

Syndrome	AS type	Other seizure types
GGE SUB-SYNDROMES		
Childhood absence epilepsy	Typical AS	GTCS
Juvenile absence epilepsy	Typical AS	GTCS, myoclonus, absence status
Juvenile myoclonic epilepsy	Typical AS	Myoclonus, GTCS
Eyelid myoclonia with absence (Jeavon's syndrome)	Eyelid myoclonia Typical AS	GTCS, myoclonus
Epilepsy with myoclonic absence seizures	Myoclonic AS	GTCS
OTHER SYNDROMES		
Lennox–Gastaut syndrome	Atypical AS	Tonic seizures, GTCS, myoclonus, focal seizures
Genetic epilepsy with febrile seizures plus (GEFS+)	Typical AS	GTCS, myoclonus, other

AS, absence seizure; GTCS, generalized tonic–clonic seizure.

COGNITIVE IMPACT OF ABSENCE SEIZURES

Absence seizures clearly have an impact on short-term cognitive function. However, despite their brief and relatively benign appearance, the presence of AS appears to have more significant long-term cognitive consequences. AS themselves can have a variable effect on consciousness both within and between seizures in an individual (11, 12). Furthermore, variable aspects of a patient's cognition may be impaired suggesting that selective brain networks may be involved during AS (11, 13). Exactly what the mechanism involved in the disruption of cognition is unclear; however, it has been speculated that focal involvement of bilateral frontal association cortex disrupts normal processing leading to impairment of specific cognitive functions (11).

There is some discrepancy in the types of cognitive deficits seen in GGE and children with AS; however, it is clear that the generalized epilepsies have a significant and pervasive neuro-cognitive impact, and that AS themselves may contribute unequally to this morbidity. A number of studies have attempted to more clearly elaborate the cognitive and psychiatric impacts of generalized epilepsies and absence epilepsy in childhood (14–18). It appears that children with CAE have significantly lower IQs, linguistic deficits, and attentional inefficiencies, as well as social and thought problems when compared to matched controls, and this appears to be related to duration of illness, seizure frequency, and medications (18). The commonalities between psychiatric and epilepsy diagnoses may reflect a common involvement of the mesial, ventral, and dorso-lateral pre-frontal cortex (18). Cognitive deficits may be more marked in children when seizures begin before 4 years of age (15). Furthermore, when comparing children with GGE, with and without AS, it was found that children with AS had more pronounced deficits in verbal performance measures when compared to those with convulsions and controls (16). In JME, it has been noted that there is impaired deactivation of the default mode network (DMN) and abnormal coupling of cognitive and motor systems, which is felt to explain the interaction between cognitive effort and myoclonus (19). Similarly, in CAE, it may be that abnormal network connectivity contributes to long-term learning risk despite good seizure control and that these deficits are potentially greater in children with AS as a result of the nature of the network disturbance.

PATHOPHYSIOLOGICAL MODELS OF GSW IN AS

To understand the mechanisms of AS generation, one needs to consider both the cellular networks involved in seizure generation, as well as the large-scale functional networks involved. At a cellular level, thalamo-cortical networks appear to be the major seizure generating apparatus (20, 21). The thalamo-cortical circuitry has been studied extensively in the generation of sleep spindles, and this circuitry informs our understanding of GSW (22). A central role of the thalamus in the generation of seizures and epileptiform discharges seems intuitive. The thalamus displays rhythmic firing and has extensive reciprocal connections to the cortex, with excitatory neurons (glutamatergic) arising from the dorsal thalamus conveying information to the cortex and excitatory cortical neurons projecting back to the thalamus (21, 23). Inhibition of this circuit is provided by cortical and thalamic projections to the reticular nucleus of the thalamus. Reticular neurons release gamma-aminobutyric acid (GABA), which in turn inhibits the excitatory stimuli from cortex and thalamus (21). This cyclical excitatory (spike) and inhibitory (wave) activity is mediated by voltage-gated calcium channels (24).

The physiological role of thalamo-cortical networks is well established in the maintenance of the sleep–wake cycle, awareness, and cognition (20, 21, 25), and these pathways were felt to be the underlying network substrate for generalized discharges (20, 21). More recently, a number of authors have challenged this assertion (25–27). Importantly, the clinical validation for a relationship between AS and spindles has been questioned. AS occur in wakefulness or while drowsing and although fragmentary GSW may be seen in NREM sleep, at times related to spindle activity, AS otherwise are observed when physiological sleep oscillations are inactivated (25). In rodent genetic absence models, oscillations of thalamo-cortical circuits tend to involve the sensori-motor cortex and do not resemble sleep spindles as closely (25). These observations inform newer ideas of network models of AS, which challenge longstanding views of generalized discharges.

Early experimental models of spike-and-wave activity gave rise to the *centrencephalic theory* of epilepsy, which implicated the thalamus as the likely central driver of epileptiform activity (28). An opposing view held that the role of seizure generation lay diffusely in the cortex and directly contradicted the need for a central driver (29). These contrasting theories were united by research carried out by Gloor, which lead to the proposal of the *generalized cortico-reticular theory* in which spike-and-wave arose from interactions between ascending inputs from the thalamus and a diffusely hyper-excitable cortex (30). More recently, it has been suggested that a cortical focus is required to initiate generalized activity (26). The *cortical focus theory* is strongly influenced by data derived from newer rodent models of epilepsy, particularly absence epilepsy (25, 31–33). An apparent cortical focus at the onset of a seizure was then followed by oscillation within the thalamo-cortical network without a specific driver. This view is encompassed in the most recent classification commission document, which refers to generalized seizures originating "at some point within, and rapidly engaging, bilaterally distributed networks" (3).

In vitro and *in vivo* animal studies of thalamo-cortical circuitry have clearly established the underlying cellular mechanisms of spike-and-wave generation. Furthermore, animal models have led to important observations as to the potential networks involved. What is lacking is the translation of these models to the human condition. Non-invasive functional imaging studies provide this opportunity.

FUNCTIONAL IMAGING IN ABSENCE EPILEPSY

A number of imaging techniques have been employed, which provide the ability to explore structures involved in the generation of AS. Although EEG with functional MRI (EEG-fMRI) has become a dominant means of studying the functional consequences of AS on the human brain, a number of other techniques have also been used to study blood flow (34–36) and metabolic changes (37–39) associated with AS. Doppler ultrasonography of the middle cerebral artery (MCA) has demonstrated a reduction in blood flow as a result of AS (34, 40), whereas single photon emission tomography (SPECT) identified decreases in cerebral blood flow (CBF) in the frontal and parieto-occipital areas during the ictal phase and generalized blood flow increases during the postictal phase without an increase metabolic demand (35). The use of positron emission tomography (PET) with fluorinated glucose (FDG) provides information about changes in metabolic activity but over a much longer time scale. In children with AS, there was a diffuse increase in cerebral glucose metabolism compared to baseline during seizures (37); however, the same finding has not been observed in adults with IGE during GSW (38, 39). The use of $H_2{}^{15}O$ with PET provides a functional marker for blood flow rather than glucose metabolism and has demonstrated that during AS, there is a global increase in CBF, seen greatest in the thalamus (41). Although these studies provide somewhat conflicting evidence as to the metabolic changes, we may expect to see during AS and GSW, the overall impression is that AS require greater energy use and thus promotes increased blood flow.

FUNCTIONAL MRI

Functional MRI relies on a series of assumptions about the relationship between neuronal activity, neuronal metabolic demand, CBF, and oxygen delivery and utilization [for review see Ref. (42)]. fMRI utilizes the blood oxygen level dependent (BOLD) response as a surrogate for neuronal metabolic activity to enable visualization of brain regions in response to both physiological and pathological paradigms.

The physiological parameters that influence BOLD signal are cerebral metabolic rate of oxygen consumption ($CMRO_2$), the CBF, and the cerebral blood volume (CBV). Following a physiological stimulus, there is an increase in $CMRO_2$, which leads to an increase in CBF. As a result, CBV also increases. A number of experiments have been performed to define what the normal BOLD response to a brief physiological stimulus is likely to be (43–45) (**Figure 1**). Although there is general agreement about the normal physiological BOLD response, it is not clear whether the canonical hemodynamic response function (HRF) is also observed during pathological activation of neuronal regions. An assumption is made that the BOLD response is canonical during statistical analysis using the general linear model. However, a number of studies have highlighted that BOLD change in the pathological state, particularly in epilepsy, may not be canonical (46–48). As a result, more robust statistical results may be achieved with HRFs tailored to suit the patient population being studied (48).

FMRI studies of patients with AS have been used with great success to understand the functional and structural mechanisms of seizure generation. EEG with fMRI enables the identification of BOLD change associated with AS by either acquiring fMRI data with the onset of an epileptiform discharge (early spike-triggered EEG-fMRI studies) or continuously recording EEG whilst acquiring fMRI data (continuous EEG-fMRI). Continuous EEG-fMRI, now commercially available, has many advantages, including the ability to mark up events offline facilitating careful identification of events for analysis. Both methods demonstrate regions of both increased BOLD and decreased BOLD. It is important to note that negative BOLD is most likely a reflection of a relative reduction in neuronal activity compared to the resting state rather than an aberration of neuronal coupling or a vascular steal phenomenon (49–51).

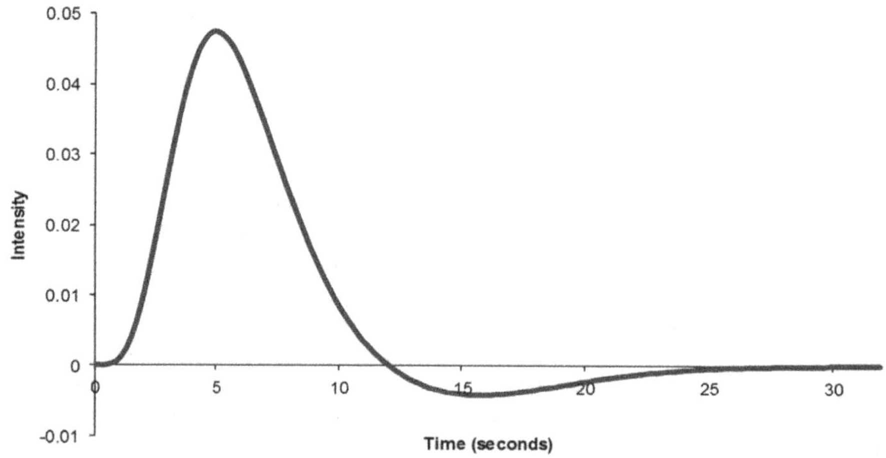

FIGURE 1 | Typical BOLD impulse response model generated using SPM8.

Event-related fMRI, with acquisition of continuous BOLD data, also allows the study of functional connectivity (FC), the other major technique applied to the study of AS. Continuous BOLD data can be gathered without concurrent EEG; however, the advantage of performing a BOLD free run with EEG is the ability to insure that there is no epileptiform activity during the period of recording. FC can be estimated non-invasively with fMRI by measuring the correlation between spontaneous low-frequency hemodynamic fluctuations in different brain regions (52), which have been linked to the synchronization of slow fluctuations in underlying neuronal networks (53). FC demonstrates a temporal correlation in BOLD change across remote regions of the brain, suggesting that these regions may exist as a network of structures performing a complimentary function. The combination of EEG-fMRI and FC has provided an important bridge between animal models and the human condition.

EEG-fMRI AND ABSENCE NETWORKS

The "core" absence network

A number of studies have identified consistent cortical and sub-cortical structures involved in the generation of AS and GSW in both group analyses of patients with CAE (54–57), JAE (58), and in patients with mixed, often refractory, GGE syndromes, and phenotypes (59–65). In our study of a tightly defined group of untreated patients with CAE, we dubbed this the "core" network to suggest that it is crucial to the generation spike-and-wave. This network may be insufficient in itself to generate seizures, and it is likely that the influence of other structures on the network may influence the seizure manifestations (57). It would appear that this network reflects structures, which are consistently involved in, or influenced by the generation of generalized epileptiform activity regardless of phenotype. Furthermore, this supports the notion that a consistent network of regions is likely to exist within GGE despite different syndrome diagnosis, duration of disease, medication use, and genetic heterogeneity.

The core network comprises the thalamus, midline, and lateral parietal cortex (the DMN) and the striatum (predominantly the caudate nuclei) (**Figure 2**). Other sub-cortical structures have been identified in different studies including the reticular structures of the pons (57) and cerebellum (56, 65). Cortical BOLD change outside of the DMN has also been observed including increased BOLD in the occipital lobe (56), anterior cingulate (65), anterior and lateral temporal lobes, and insula cortex (56, 62). Decreased cortical BOLD has also been seen in the medial pre-frontal cortex (56, 65, 66), the temporal poles (66), and sub-group differences in BOLD change in the dorso-lateral pre-frontal cortex (66). Using canonical HRF analysis, the main component consistently displaying an increase in BOLD signal relative to the resting state is the thalamus. The other structures show relative decreases in BOLD signal compared to the resting state.

The thalamus

As stated above, the thalamus has retained a central role in models of absence generation given its role as a relay station for information transfer in the brain with strong reciprocal connection to the cortex. A robust positive thalamic BOLD response has been consistently observed associated with AS (54–58, 66) and interictal GSW (59–63, 65). It has been suggested that the spatial extent of thalamic involvement extends beyond the thalamus into the nearby striatal structures (67). Using event-related independent components analysis (eICA), it has been possible to identify two thalamic components, one located in the midline, which may reflect the local venous drainage into thalamostriate veins, while the other component involves the lateral thalamic nuclei and lentiform nuclei bilaterally (**Figure 3**). The spatial extent of thalamic involvement as identified using EEG-fMRI, however, is uncertain. Given requirements for spatial smoothing in the analysis, functional imaging may simplify more complex BOLD change within discrete thalamic nuclei.

Although EEG-fMRI lacks the temporal information of EEG alone, nonetheless important information about the timing of BOLD signal change can be gathered. The time course of the thalamic BOLD change associated with AS has been studied in a number of papers using varied techniques including shifting

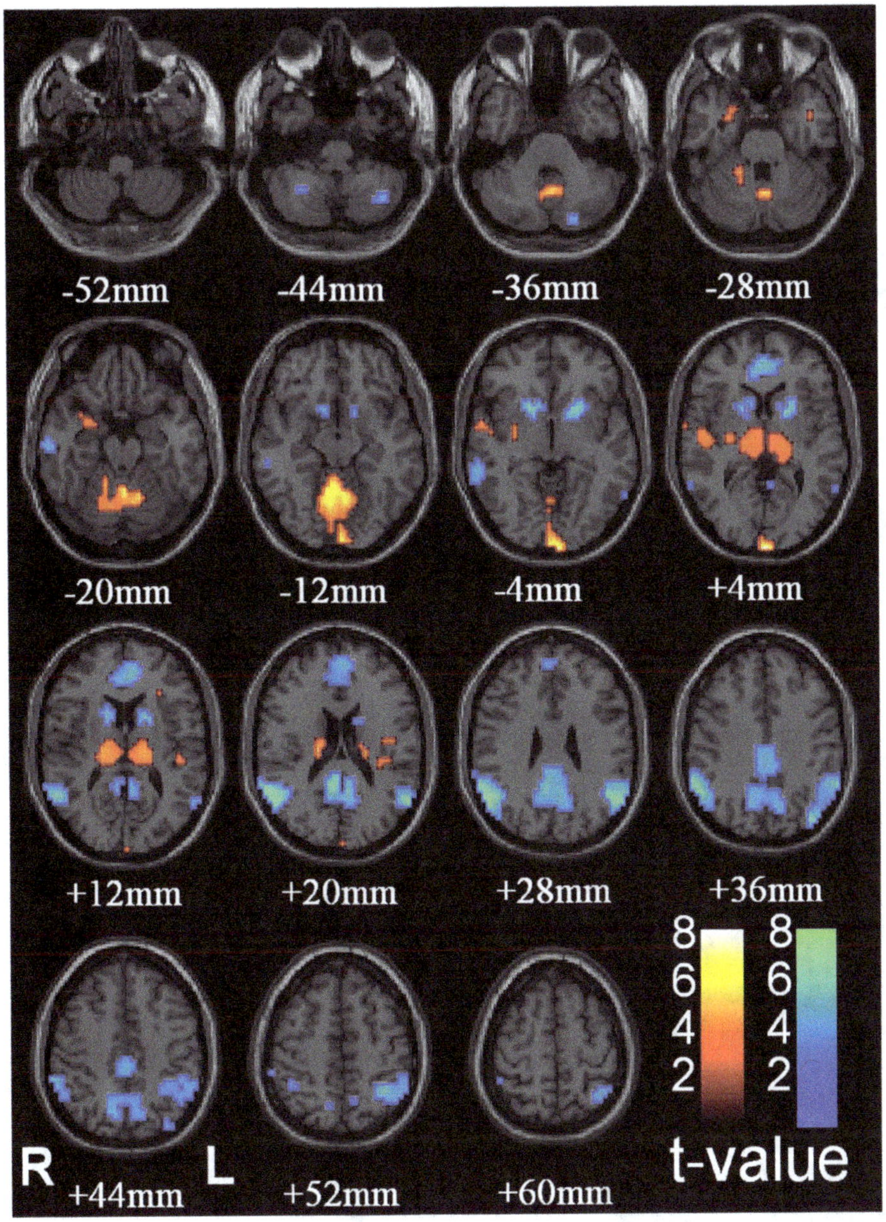

FIGURE 2 | Thalamic increases and "default mode" cortical decreases are the most prominent changes seen with conventional HRF modeling in SPM. fMRI increases (warm colors) and decreases (cool colors) are shown resulting from group analysis with second-level random-effects analysis, FDR-corrected height threshold *p*_0.05, and extent threshold *k*_3 voxels (voxel dimensions_ 2 _ 2 _ 2 mm). Functional data are superimposed on the Montreal Neurological Institute brain template "colin27" (single_subj_T1 in SPM2) displayed in radiological right–left convention. In total, 54 seizures in nine patients (40 in 8 patients during CPT or RTT; 14 in 4 patients during VFT, 3 patients with both CPT/RTT and VFT runs) were analyzed using GLM with canonical HRF in SPM2. The dataset in this analysis was the same as Figure 1. fMRI increases were seen in bilateral thalamus, occipital (calcarine) cortex, and to a lesser extent in the midline cerebellum, anterior and lateral temporal lobes, insula, and adjacent to the lateral ventricles. fMRI decreases were seen in the bilateral lateral parietal, medial parietal, and cingulate cortex and basal ganglia (46) (published with permission from the Journal of Neuroscience, SFN).

the event-related time course relative to event onset (64, 68), brain-wide analysis of mean percentage BOLD change without *a priori* presumption of the HRF (56) and region of interest analysis of relative BOLD signal change (55, 57, 66). To summarize these different approaches, it has generally been observed that an increase in thalamic BOLD signal is closely associated with the onset of the epileptiform event (AS or GSW), although initial BOLD change may precede event onset (64), occur congruent with event onset (55, 57, 65, 66), or follow event onset (56). There is some debate whether the time course is canonical or that it deviates significantly from the canonical response. Our observation has been that the BOLD response is canonical, in contrast to

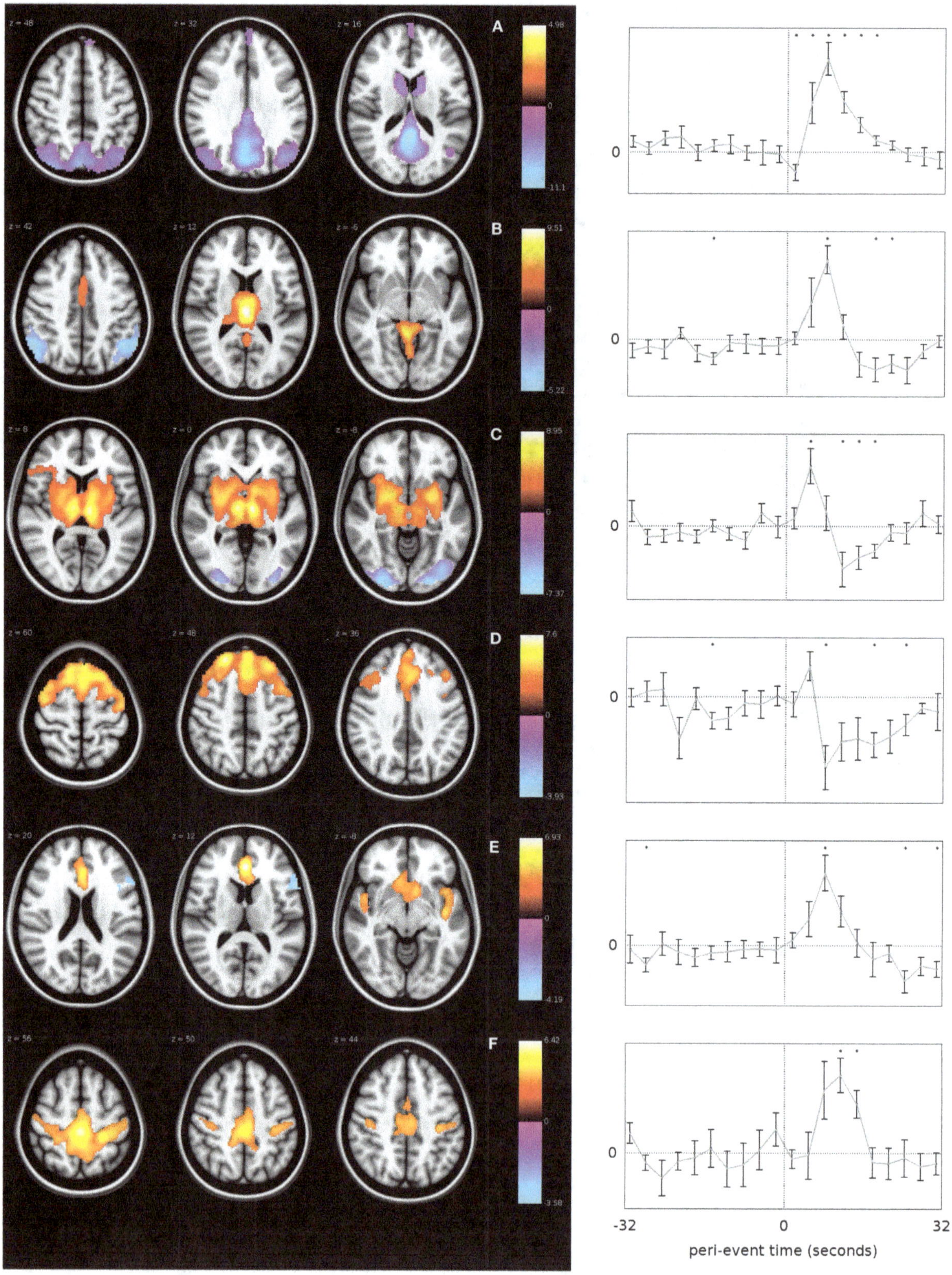

FIGURE 3 | GSW-related networks identified using event-related ICA. Each row represents a different network, labeled from **(A–F)**. The plots on the right show the mean time course of fMRI signal change within each network with error bars indicating the standard error, over the time period from −32 to +32 s relative to the GSW onset. The vertical dotted line in each plot

(Continued)

FIGURE 3 | Continued
represents the time of GSW onset, and the horizontal dotted line represents the baseline fMRI signal level. Asterisks indicate where the BOLD signal is significantly different to baseline ($p < 0.05$, uncorrected). The images on the left are *z*-statistic maps, thresholded to show significant ($p < 0.05$) clusters of voxels, overlaid upon a reference anatomical image. The hot and cool colors in the images indicate whether the brain region shows a positive or negative modulation with respect to the network time course, i.e., they are analogous to activations and deactivations except with respect to the network-specific time course instead of a canonical HRF (67) (published with permission from Epilepsia, ILAE/Willey Blackwell).

the other elements of the "core" network, and we have speculated that the thalamus therefore appears to behave physiologically and reactively to the onset of epileptiform activity, although it may be critical to sustaining the seizure (66).

Cortical BOLD changes in EEG-fMRI

Cortical BOLD change can be seen in a number of locations in individual studies of AS and GSW; however, the most consistent and reproducible cortical BOLD change in group event-related analysis of AS is in the mesial parietal cortex (precuneus and posterior cingulate) and lateral parietal cortex (angular gyrus and supramarginal gyrus). These cortical regions are the major components of the DMN, which is an important cognitive attentional network involved in non-task directed, internal processing (69, 70). There is much speculation as to the functional implications of parietal/DMN change, and this will be discussed in detail in "The Role of Default Mode Network in the Occurrence of Absence Seizures" section.

The fact that BOLD change is only seen consistently in the parietal lobe at a group level, and that there is an apparent reduction in metabolic activity sits in contrast to the published literature. Observations from other functional imaging techniques described in "Functional Imaging in Absence Epilepsy" section lead us to expect generalized increases in BOLD signal in the cortex. There is also ample evidence to suggest that we might see focal BOLD increase in cortical regions. A number of animal studies have suggested that focal cortical regions, particularly in the sensorimotor area, may be involved in the onset of GSW. Multi-site EEG recordings in WAG/Rij rats (26, 31) and in GAERS rats (25) have demonstrated onset of AS focally in the peri-oral region. Similar observations have been made using fMRI in these animal models of AS (71–73). A number of human electrophysiology studies of GGE have also identified the possibility of a focal driver of AS, particularly involving the mesial and orbitofrontal cortex (74–77). Taken together, this animal and human electrophysiology data suggest that although the electrographic and clinical manifestations of GGE are generalized, a focal trigger may exist and this would be expected to be the cause of an increase in cortical BOLD activity. This trigger is likely to vary cross individuals and GGE syndromes and is likely to be highly connected to the DMN.

Changes in the mesial and lateral parietal cortex associated with AS was first identified by Archer *et al.* (59) using spike-triggered fMRI. In this paper, the authors speculated that the parietal cortex may be involved in the initiation of epileptiform discharges although providing alternative views that this may reflect the disruptive effect of GSW on cortical function or is merely "a marker of the epilepsy syndrome's intermittent neurophysiological abnormality." Negative BOLD change in the parietal cortex has been detected reproducibly both in AS (54, 56–58, 66) and during interictal discharges in a range of GGE syndromes (55, 59–65, 78). The time-course analysis of BOLD change in parietal cortex had a more complex (non-canonical) hemodynamic response than is reflected in the statistical maps. A number of studies have shown BOLD change in the parietal cortex occurs prior to the onset of the epileptiform event, and certainly before changes in the thalamus, with sustained increases in BOLD starting several seconds prior to the electrographic onset and the subsequent negative BOLD change (56, 57, 63–65). These responses were identified only as a decrease in BOLD signal in the statistical maps and hence simplify important temporal fluctuations in regional metabolic activity, particularly at event onset. The multimodal parietal association cortices are the major structure in the DMN, which has been demonstrated to play a role in a number of physiological and pathophysiological processes. To better understand the implications of the fluctuations of BOLD in the parietal cortex for the occurrence of AS and GSW, we must first consider the normal function of the DMN.

The importance of frontal cortical BOLD change

As discussed above, it would be expected that BOLD signal change would be seen in the frontal cortex as a consistent finding, given the observations made in animal models, as well as observations from electrophysiology. Negative BOLD change has been identified in the mesial frontal and anterior cingulate cortex in several studies (55, 56, 65, 66), which is not surprising given this region is a component of the DMN. Focal cortical BOLD change may be seen in individual cases (55, 65, 68), and it has been suggested that there may be subject specific changes in BOLD signal, which are consistent within individuals but vary from subject to subject (68). Another possibility is that frontal cortical BOLD change may reflect differences in sub-groups of patients with absence epilepsy (66). What is clear is that BOLD signal in the frontal lobe is influenced by AS (see **Figure 4** for individual case results). When using a standardized event-related analysis of a group or individual, this may appear as increases, decreases, or no change. However, in group and individual analyses of BOLD time course, there are clear increases in BOLD signal in frontal cortical networks occurring prior to, co-incident with, or following the event onset. This is highlighted in our paper on sub-group differences in frontal cortical BOLD in which the division into frontal negative or frontal positive was dependent on the timing of the BOLD signal increase relative to the event onset, not whether BOLD signal increased or decreased (66). Given the wealth of clinical, electrophysiological, and functional data highlighting the importance of frontal lobe activity in seizure generation, it is important for fMRI techniques to better explore the contribution of frontal lobes to seizure generation.

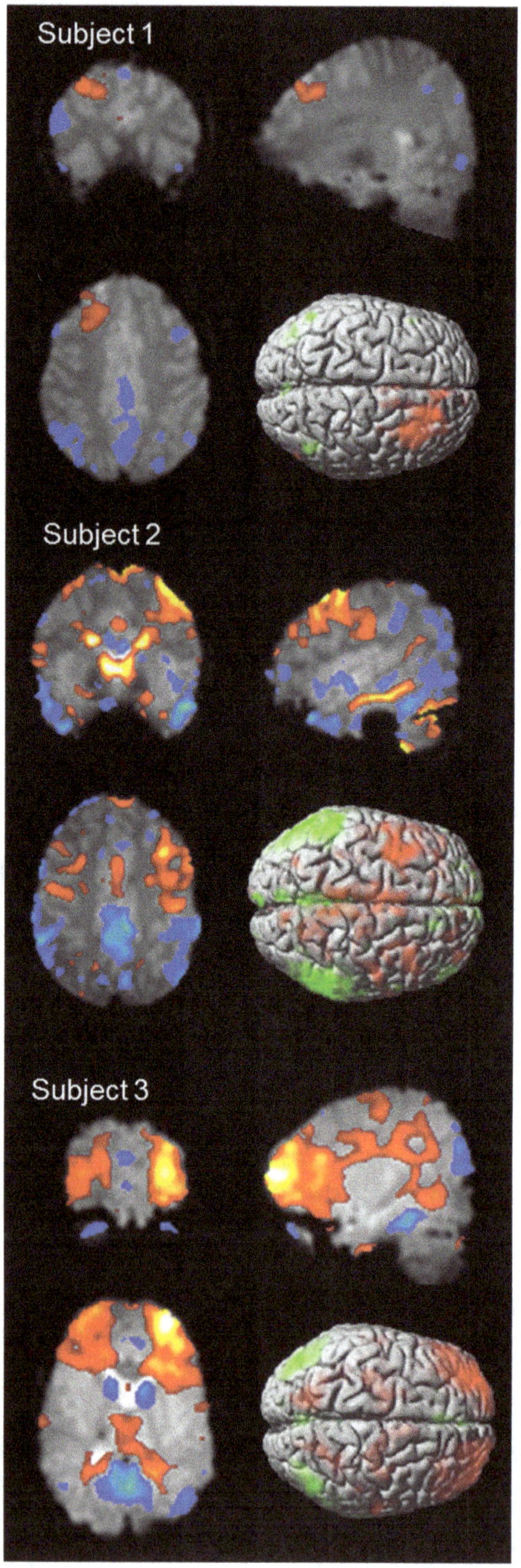

FIGURE 4 | Continued

FIGURE 4 | Continued
BOLD signal change for three subjects showing variability of cortical BOLD change (figure previously unpublished). Color maps of positive BOLD (red to white: 0 to +10) and negative BOLD (blue to green: 0 to −10) change superimposed on subjects mean EPI image are displayed in three plains ($p < 0.001$). A single surface rendered image is also displayed demonstrating the cortical surface involved. Subject 1: 16 years female with onset of AS at age 5 who developed refractory AS and GTCS. EEG-fMRI of 6 (14 s) bursts of interictal activity. Subject 2: 13 years male with onset of AS at age 8 who achieved seizure control on mono-therapy. EEG-fMRI of 11 AS (105 s). Subject 3: 5 years female with AS since 4 who achieved seizure control on mono-therapy. EEG-fMRI of 6 AS (83 s).

Is there a difference between an absence and an interictal discharge?

It is clear that not all burst of spike-and-wave, even when prolonged, will cause a clinically evident absence seizure (11). Patients with AS may demonstrate fragmentary interictal discharges or even prolonged bursts of spike-and-wave without clear impairment of consciousness or impairment of task performance. It appears that there may be differences in the spatial distribution of BOLD change depending on discharge type, as well as the timing of the BOLD signal change.

A number of elegant studies performed in the Blumenfeld lab have specifically looked at this issue by performing simultaneous EEG-fMRI whilst performing cognitive and motor tasks (56, 79, 80). In one study, they observed that if there was no impairment of performance during a cognitive task, despite typical EEG changes of an AS, there was no significant cortical BOLD change during these events (79). Similar observations about the spatial extent of cortical BOLD change have been made when GSW are compared directly to AS within a patient group with the extent and magnitude of BOLD change being higher in the parietal cortex during AS (81). Given these observations, it may be that the basis for cognitive impairment does relate directly to the extent of cortical involvement and not the appearance of the epileptiform activity, which may not arise due to cortical BOLD change itself. In contrast, a single case report of a patient with prolonged bursts of spike-and-wave (up to 5 s during fMRI) who did not demonstrate cognitive impairment showed a typical bilateral deactivation of the default mode (82). These authors concluded that BOLD change in this region is not sufficient to explain cognitive impairment.

We have also studied this issue of the timing of BOLD change. We defined interictal discharges and AS according to the cognitive effect observed during the subjects routine EEG (66, 83). We were able to study the time course of BOLD change within subjects according to whether the discharge was interictal or ictal (83). We found the overall pattern of the BOLD signal change to be similar between event categories, although there was a trend suggesting that the BOLD signal change was more prolonged and of greater magnitude in AS compared to GSW. Interestingly, we observed a delay in onset of BOLD signal change in the thalamus in AS when compared to asymptomatic GSW. Previous studies have suggested a difference in BOLD time course between different events (AS and polyspike-and-wave) (55, 63, 65) but these differences have not been directly compared within a single cohort. A potential difference in the timing of BOLD signal change dependent on event type is interesting in that it may reflect differences in the underlying pathophysiology of brief interictal events that self-terminate without clinical symptoms, compared to AS. Our data suggest that an early thalamic response correlates with asymptomatic termination of the spike-wave event. Whether this reflects a true physiological difference has not been established.

Is there a difference between typical and atypical absence?

The possibility that typical and atypical AS may be different has never been directly addressed using functional MRI. Although considered separately in the ILAE classification, there is evidence that these two event types may form a continuum (84). Slow spike-and-wave (SSW) and paroxysmal fast activity (PFA) have been studied in LGS, and there are important differences when compared to GGE (85–87). Epileptiform activity (SSW and PFA) in LGS gives significant positive activation in the brainstem and thalamus (86). More recently, in a study of patients with LGS, SSW led to a more variable pattern of BOLD change with less consistent thalamic activation and deactivation in primary cortical regions when compared to the reported literature on GSW (87). Importantly, this SSW pattern was in stark contrast to the pattern of activation seen in PFA. Although it is not possible to say whether the BOLD response to typical AS is likely to differ to atypical AS, the evidence relating to SSW and GSW certainly suggests major differences in the behavior of the networks involved.

Connectivity

A number of studies have employed resting-state connectivity measures to identify whether disturbance of connectivity relationships are present, independent of epileptiform events, in CAE, as well as other GGE syndromes (88). There has been some inconsistency in these findings, which may be explained by differing GGE sub-syndromes, influences of age and medications, and physiological changes, as well as errors introduced by certain pre-processing steps (88–90). Decreases in resting-state functional connectivity (rFC) have been demonstrated bilaterally in the medial pre-frontal cortex, angular gyrus, and inferior parietal lobule in patients with CAE compared to controls, without evidence of areas of increased connectivity (91). Furthermore, these changes appear to be increased with increased duration of epilepsy. Attentional processing is also disrupted in CAE (92). This study used an attention task to define a frontal lobe network and assessed its FC to other brain regions. They demonstrated that children with AS had impaired rFC compared to controls. This provides an alternative anatomical and functional basis for cognitive dysfunction in CAE (92). In a related study (80), an abnormal increase in rFC was identified between orbitofrontal cortex in CAE also indicating altered network performance, which may contribute to cognitive inefficiencies. Using whole brain rFC, reduction in whole brain connectivity between the thalamus and cortex has also been shown (93). Although patients with CAE showed a similar pattern of thalamic FC to controls, this was diminished in both the spatial extent and the magnitude of the correlation. Taken together, these studies suggest a fundamental change in the interaction between thalamus and cortex in CAE in the "baseline" or resting state with alterations in the normal relationships with connected brain networks.

THE ROLE OF DEFAULT MODE NETWORK IN THE OCCURRENCE OF ABSENCE SEIZURES

THE DEFAULT MODE NETWORK

The observation of task-induced activity decreases in parietal and frontal cortical regions was first made during a meta-analysis of PET studies of visual processing (94). This network of regions was later termed the DMN (95) and was confirmed by several other studies (70, 96). The DMN is involved in internalized cognitive activity including random thoughts and free associations of ideas and memories (69, 70). Functions in the DMN are likely to be integrated with physiological information such as body position and sensation. The term REST network, meaning "random episodic silent thinking," to reflect the importance of increase in activity in this network at times when goal-directed tasks are not being performed (70). The contrasting network is the attentional network, which during goal-directed attentional tasks, demonstrates activation in the dorsal fronto-parietal regions (97). The brain appears to switch between states of DMN activation and deactivation associated with task attention and concentration. This switching between cognitive states reflects an important phenomenon of presumed functional coherence throughout the brain (98).

The DMN includes the midline and lateral parietal structures and the midline and lateral frontal cortex superiorly. Studies of the DMN over differing developmental ages show important changes within the network (99). Local or regional correlations weaken and more distant correlations strengthen, due to a range of developmental processes including synaptic pruning and myelination (100, 101). These changes occur between portions of the brain that are functionally related in adults (102). However, pediatric networks have a fundamentally different structure and are not just simple precursors to the adult form (99). The complex development of DMN interactions reflects its intrinsic importance to a range of brain functions and possible varying role throughout neural development. The DMN is also known to function in sleep and even in the anesthetized state, and much of the brains resting-state energy demands are consumed by activity in the DMN (98, 103).

The observation that much of the low-frequency "noise" in BOLD signal displays striking patterns of coherence lead to the concept of FC (52). Perhaps not surprisingly, when this technique was applied to the DMN, the presence of resting-state coherence of these functional regions was confirmed (104). In a recent review, Raichle (103) has argued for a new way to consider task-related BOLD signal change, particularly in the DMN. He has suggested that the evidence does not support BOLD signal change as reflecting immediate response to task, particularly as BOLD change tends to be sluggish, but rather that BOLD changes in regions like the DMN are a "reflection of changes in the slow components of the brain's intrinsic activity in response to changing environmental contingencies." Although it is clear that there is relative inactivation of the DMN during epileptiform events and AS, precisely why we consistently see this pattern is not well understood.

THE DMN AT REST IN ABSENCE EPILEPSY

There appears to be a fundamental change in network connectivity in the resting-state functional networks in the brains of children with AS, and most likely in all forms of GGE (88, 91–93). It does appear that the relationships within normal attentional networks are likely to be abnormal in the resting state in absence epilepsy. There is ample evidence of cognitive inefficiencies seen in CAE and other GGE syndromes (14–18). Although these observations may be influenced by the effects of seizures and medications, it is likely that there is fundamental abnormality in the function of these networks beyond these effects as demonstrated in JME (19). It would seem intuitive that, given the likely brain-wide effects of genetic abnormalities that cause GGE, this would predispose to alterations in normal connectivity relationships in the resting state. Given we know that development of the DMN is dynamic throughout childhood (99), we can hypothesize that it is the very dynamic nature of these changes that can contribute to the onset and offset of AS at differing developmental ages with the expression of different genes during development. Studying the development of FC changes over time in patients compared to controls may help to answer this question.

THE PARIETAL CORTEX "PERMITS" EPILEPTIFORM EVENTS

Two views have been taken as to the role of the DMN in AS. One view argues that the DMN is "switched off" during spike-and-wave discharges leading to the clinical features of reduced awareness associated with GSW and AS (62), while the other view suggests that a causal relationship exists between this region and epileptiform activity (59, 105). The first view holds that the switching from "active" resting brain activity in the DMN to a reduction in DMN activity reflects inactivation of internal self-reflective processes and therefore loss of awareness. Blumenfeld and Taylor (106) proposed a network inhibition hypothesis for loss of awareness during seizures. They suggested that seizure inhibition of sub-cortical activating systems lead to impairment of awareness by disrupting their interaction with the DMN. Certainly this hypothesis fits nicely with event-related analysis during AS showing negative BOLD in both the pons and DMN. However, there is evidence that DMN change is not secondary and is more directly involved in genesis of the absence events:

1. Default mode network negative BOLD change is seen independent of event type. We have observed that negative BOLD in the DMN occurs regardless of whether the event is an interictal discharge or an AS. Hence, DMN negative BOLD is seen even when awareness is maintained.
2. The DMN time course shows that BOLD changes occur before an absence occurs and awareness becomes impaired.
3. Evidence of DMN change associated with a huge range of tasks and the observations of functional coherence, suggesting this is not reactive but pro-active neural network.

The evidence of early change in the BOLD signal in the DMN suggests that either activity in the DMN initiates the generation of GSW and AS, or the DMN must be in a certain state to "permit" or facilitate the occurrence of epileptiform events (105). One can speculate that the level of activity in the DMN has a permissive effect on the occurrence of AS, which is to say that fluctuating states of awareness contribute to an environment conducive to the generation of epileptiform activity. Within that "conducive" environment, a further "trigger" is required to initiate an epileptiform event. Following this, there is engagement of thalamo-cortical systems, and dependent on the timing of this engagement (perhaps relating to the onset of thalamic activity as discussed above), an interictal or ictal event may occur. The observation that AS often occur at times of fatigue or rest, when the DMN is engaged, would support the notion of a permissive environment.

CONCLUSION

The use of functional MRI to study AS has provided invaluable insights into the mechanism of this common seizure type. fMRI techniques have enabled the translation of animal models of seizure generation to the human condition, provided a map of the neural networks needed for seizure generation, and demonstrated ictal and interictal disturbance of normal physiological networks. What is clear from the temporal information regarding BOLD change is that there are important increases in neuronal activity, which occur prior to, co-incident with, and following the onset of AS in a range of important cortical and sub-cortical networks. Time and again, the DMN has been identified as a core network with changed activity central to AS and interictal epileptiform discharges. What cannot be established is to what extent BOLD change in this region is a consequence of an absence, or, perhaps more likely, facilitating its occurrence. Furthermore, fMRI has provided important observations regarding the potential cognitive and phenotypic importance of the frontal lobe in absence epilepsy syndromes, consistent with the clinical and animal data. As fMRI techniques continue to develop enabling more sophisticated techniques of acquisition and analysis in individual patients, this valuable research and clinical tool is likely to further facilitate our understanding of the mechanisms of absence seizure generation.

AUTHOR CONTRIBUTIONS

The manuscript was drafted by Patrick W. Carney who organized the structure, content, and focus of the review article. Graeme D. Jackson reviewed the manuscript and provided critical commentary on the ideas and concepts discussed. The ideas expressed in the article reflect the collaborative work of both authors. Both authors agree on the final manuscript and are accountable for the ideas expressed.

ACKNOWLEDGMENTS

The authors acknowledge NHMRC Program Grant in Epilepsy, Operational Infrastructure Support Program of the State Government of Victoria, and Pfizer Inc., Neuroscience Research Grant. Patrick W. Carney has been supported by The Dowd Foundation, The Brain Foundation, and The Royal Australian College of Physicians. Graeme D. Jackson is supported by an NHMRC Fellowship Grant. They thank Shawna Farquharson and the radiography team at the Florey; Dr. David Abbott, Dr. Richard Masterton, and Dr. Danny Flanagan for methods development and analysis; Dr. John Archer for critical commentary and assistance with developing the ideas in the manuscript; the neurologists at Austin Health; and the patients and subjects who have participated in this research.

REFERENCES

1. Jallon P, Latour P. Epidemiology of idiopathic generalized epilepsies. *Epilepsia* (2005) **46**(Suppl 9):10–4. doi:10.1111/j.1528-1167.2005.00309.x

2. ILAE. Proposal for classification of epilepsies and epileptic syndromes. Commission on classification and terminology of the international league against epilepsy. *Epilepsia* (1985) **26**:268–78. doi:10.1111/j.1528-1157.1985.tb05417.x
3. Berg AT, Berkovic SF, Brodie MJ, Buchhalter J, Cross JH, Van Emde Boas W, et al. Revised terminology and concepts for organization of seizures and epilepsies: report of the ILAE Commission on classification and terminology, 2005-2009. *Epilepsia* (2010) **51**:676–85. doi:10.1111/j.1528-1167.2010.02522.x
4. Luders HO, Acharya J, Alexopoulos A, Baumgartner C, Bautista J, Burgess R, et al. Are epilepsy classifications based on epileptic syndromes and seizure types outdated? *Epileptic Disord* (2006) **8**:81–5.
5. Gastaut H. Clinical and electroencephalographical classification of epileptic seizures. *Epilepsia* (1970) **11**:102–13. doi:10.1111/j.1528-1157.1970.tb03871.x
6. ILAE. Proposal for revised clinical and electroencephalographic classification of epileptic seizures. From the commission on classification and terminology of the international league against epilepsy. *Epilepsia* (1981) **22**:489–501. doi:10.1111/j.1528-1157.1981.tb06159.x
7. Stefan H, Snead OC III, Eeg-Olofsson O. Typical and atypical absence seizures, myoclonic absences and eyelid myoclonia. 2nd ed. In: Engel J, Pedley TA, editors. *Epielpsy: A Comprehensive Textbook*. Philadelphia, PA: Lippincott, Williams and Wilkins (2008). p. 573–84.
8. Engel J Jr; International League Against Epilepsy. A proposed diagnostic scheme for people with epileptic seizures and with epilepsy: report of the ILAE Task Force on classification and terminology. *Epilepsia* (2001) **42**:796–803. doi:10.1046/j.1528-1157.2001.10401.x
9. Appleton RE, Panayiotopoulos CP, Acomb BA, Beirne M. Eyelid myoclonia with typical absences: an epilepsy syndrome. *J Neurol Neurosurg Psychiatry* (1993) **56**:1312–6. doi:10.1136/jnnp.56.12.1312
10. ILAE. Proposal for revised classification of epilepsies and epileptic syndromes. Commission on classification and terminology of the international league against epilepsy. *Epilepsia* (1989) **30**:389–99. doi:10.1111/j.1528-1157.1989.tb05316.x
11. Blumenfeld H. Consciousness and epilepsy: why are patients with absence seizures absent? *Prog Brain Res* (2005) **150**:271–86. doi:10.1016/S0079-6123(05)50020-7
12. Sadleir LG, Scheffer IE, Smith S, Carstensen B, Carlin J, Connolly MB, et al. Factors influencing clinical features of absence seizures. *Epilepsia* (2008) **49**:2100–7. doi:10.1111/j.1528-1167.2008.01708.x
13. Goldie L, Green JM. Spike and wave discharges and alterations of conscious awareness. *Nature* (1961) **191**:200–1. doi:10.1038/191200a0
14. Bailet LL, Turk WR. The impact of childhood epilepsy on neurocognitive and behavioral performance: a prospective longitudinal study. *Epilepsia* (2000) **41**:426–31. doi:10.1111/j.1528-1157.2000.tb00184.x
15. Pavone P, Bianchini R, Trifiletti RR, Incorpora G, Pavone A, Parano E. Neuropsychological assessment in children with absence epilepsy. *Neurology* (2001) **56**:1047–51. doi:10.1212/WNL.56.8.1047
16. Henkin Y, Sadeh M, Kivity S, Shabtai E, Kishon-Rabin L, Gadoth N. Cognitive function in idiopathic generalized epilepsy of childhood. *Dev Med Child Neurol* (2005) **47**:126–32. doi:10.1017/S0012162205000228
17. Jones JE, Watson R, Sheth R, Caplan R, Koehn M, Seidenberg M, et al. Psychiatric comorbidity in children with new onset epilepsy. *Dev Med Child Neurol* (2007) **49**:493–7. doi:10.1111/j.1469-8749.2007.00493.x
18. Caplan R, Siddarth P, Stahl L, Lanphier E, Vona P, Gurbani S, et al. Childhood absence epilepsy: behavioral, cognitive, and linguistic comorbidities. *Epilepsia* (2008) **49**:1838–46. doi:10.1111/j.1528-1167.2008.01680.x
19. Vollmar C, O'Muircheartaigh J, Barker GJ, Symms MR, Thompson P, Kumari V, et al. Motor system hyperconnectivity in juvenile myoclonic epilepsy: a cognitive functional magnetic resonance imaging study. *Brain* (2011) **134**:1710–9. doi:10.1093/brain/awr098
20. Kostopoulos GK. Spike-and-wave discharges of absence seizures as a transformation of sleep spindles: the continuing development of a hypothesis. *Clin Neurophysiol* (2000) **111**(Suppl 2):S27–38. doi:10.1016/S1388-2457(00)00399-0
21. Steriade M. Sleep, epilepsy and thalamic reticular inhibitory neurons. *Trends Neurosci* (2005) **28**:317–24. doi:10.1016/j.tins.2005.03.007
22. Steriade M, McCormick DA, Sejnowski TJ. Thalamocortical oscillations in the sleeping and aroused brain. *Science* (1993) **262**:679–85. doi:10.1126/science.8235588
23. Blumenfeld H. The thalamus and seizures. *Arch Neurol* (2002) **59**:135–7. doi:10.1001/archneur.59.1.135
24. Blumenfeld H. Cellular and network mechanisms of spike-wave seizures. *Epilepsia* (2005) **46**(Suppl 9):21–33. doi:10.1111/j.1528-1167.2005.00311.x
25. Pinault D, O'Brien TJ. Cellular and network mechanisms of genetically-determined absence seizures. *Thalamus Relat Syst* (2005) **3**:181–203. doi:10.1017/S1472928807000209
26. Meeren H, Van Luijtelaar G, Lopes Da Silva F, Coenen A. Evolving concepts on the pathophysiology of absence seizures: the cortical focus theory. *Arch Neurol* (2005) **62**:371–6. doi:10.1001/archneur.62.3.371
27. Halasz P, Kelemen A. New vistas and views in the concept of generalized epilepsies. *Ideggyogy Sz* (2009) **62**:366–80.
28. Penfield W, Jasper H. *Epilepsy and the Functional Anatomy of the Human Brain*. Oxford: Little, brown & Co (1954).
29. Gibbs FA, Gibbs EL. *Atlas of Electroencephalography*. Cambridge, MA: Addison-Wesley (1952).
30. Gloor P. Generalized cortico-reticular epilepsies. Some considerations on the pathophysiology of generalized bilaterally synchronous spike and wave discharge. *Epilepsia* (1968) **9**:249–63. doi:10.1111/j.1528-1157.1968.tb04624.x
31. Meeren HK, Pijn JP, Van Luijtelaar EL, Coenen AM, Lopes Da Silva FH. Cortical focus drives widespread corticothalamic networks during spontaneous absence seizures in rats. *J Neurosci* (2002) **22**:1480–95.
32. Pinault D. Cellular interactions in the rat somatosensory thalamocortical system during normal and epileptic 5-9 Hz oscillations. *J Physiol* (2003) **552**:881–905. doi:10.1113/jphysiol.2003.046573
33. Meeren HK, Veening JG, Moderscheim TA, Coenen AM, Van Luijtelaar G. Thalamic lesions in a genetic rat model of absence epilepsy: dissociation between spike-wave discharges and sleep spindles. *Exp Neurol* (2009) **217**:25–37. doi:10.1016/j.expneurol.2009.01.009
34. Nehlig A, Vergnes M, Waydelich R, Hirsch E, Charbonne R, Marescaux C, et al. Absence seizures induce a decrease in cerebral blood flow: human and animal data. *J Cereb Blood Flow Metab* (1996) **16**:147–55. doi:10.1097/00004647-199601000-00017
35. Nehlig A, Valenti MP, Thiriaux A, Hirsch E, Marescaux C, Namer IJ. Ictal and interictal perfusion variations measured by SISCOM analysis in typical childhood absence seizures. *Epileptic Disord* (2004) **6**:247–53.
36. Roche-Labarbe N, Zaaimi B, Berquin P, Nehlig A, Grebe R, Wallois F. NIRS-measured oxy- and deoxyhemoglobin changes associated with EEG spike-and-wave discharges in children. *Epilepsia* (2008) **49**:1871–80. doi:10.1111/j.1528-1167.2008.01711.x
37. Engel J Jr, Kuhl DE, Phelps ME. Patterns of human local cerebral glucose metabolism during epileptic seizures. *Science* (1982) **218**:64–6. doi:10.1126/science.6981843
38. Theodore WH, Brooks R, Margolin R, Patronas N, Sato S, Porter RJ, et al. Positron emission tomography in generalized seizures. *Neurology* (1985) **35**:684–90. doi:10.1212/WNL.35.5.684
39. Ochs RF, Gloor P, Tyler JL, Wolfson T, Worsley K, Andermann F, et al. Effect of generalized spike-and-wave discharge on glucose metabolism measured by positron emission tomography. *Ann Neurol* (1987) **21**:458–64. doi:10.1002/ana.410210508
40. Bode H. Intracranial blood flow velocities during seizures and generalized epileptic discharges. *Eur J Pediatr* (1992) **151**:706–9. doi:10.1007/BF01957579
41. Prevett MC, Duncan JS, Jones TD, Fish DR, Brooks DJ. Demonstration of thalamic activation during typical absence seizures using H215 O and PET. *Neurology* (1995) **45**:1396–402. doi:10.1212/WNL.45.7.1396
42. Logothetis NK. The ins and outs of fMRI signals. *Nat Neurosci* (2007) **10**:1230–2. doi:10.1038/nn1007-1230
43. Boynton GM, Engel SA, Glover GH, Heeger DJ. Linear systems analysis of functional magnetic resonance imaging in human V1. *J Neurosci* (1996) **16**:4207–21.
44. Friston KJ, Fletcher P, Josephs O, Holmes A, Rugg MD, Turner R. Event-related fMRI: characterizing differential responses. *Neuroimage* (1998) **7**:30–40. doi:10.1006/nimg.1997.0306
45. Glover GH. Deconvolution of impulse response in event-related BOLD fMRI. *Neuroimage* (1999) **9**:416–29. doi:10.1006/nimg.1998.0419
46. Bai X, Berman R, Negishi M, Novotny EJ, Constable RT, Blumenfeld H. Timing and correlation of fMRI network changes in typical childhood absence seizures. In: *Neurosciences*. Washington: Society for Neuroscience (2008).

47. Lemieux L, Laufs H, Carmichael D, Paul JS, Walker MC, Duncan JS. Noncanonical spike-related BOLD responses in focal epilepsy. *Hum Brain Mapp* (2008) **29**:329–45. doi:10.1002/hbm.20389
48. Masterton RA, Harvey AS, Archer JS, Lillywhite LM, Abbott DF, Scheffer IE, et al. Focal epileptiform spikes do not show a canonical BOLD response in patients with benign rolandic epilepsy (BECTS). *Neuroimage* (2010) **51**:252–60. doi:10.1016/j.neuroimage.2010.01.109
49. Gotman J, Benar CG, Dubeau F. Combining EEG and fMRI in epilepsy: methodological challenges and clinical results. *J Clin Neurophysiol* (2004) **21**:229–40. doi:10.1097/01.WNP.0000139658.92878.2A
50. Shmuel A, Augath M, Oeltermann A, Logothetis NK. Negative functional MRI response correlates with decreases in neuronal activity in monkey visual area V1. *Nat Neurosci* (2006) **9**:569–77. doi:10.1038/nn1675
51. Hamandi K, Laufs H, Noth U, Carmichael DW, Duncan JS, Lemieux L. BOLD and perfusion changes during epileptic generalised spike wave activity. *Neuroimage* (2008) **39**:608–18. doi:10.1016/j.neuroimage.2007.07.009
52. Biswal B, Yetkin FZ, Haughton VM, Hyde JS. Functional connectivity in the motor cortex of resting human brain using echo-planar MRI. *Magn Reson Med* (1995) **34**:537–41. doi:10.1002/mrm.1910340409
53. Shmuel A, Leopold DA. Neuronal correlates of spontaneous fluctuations in fMRI signals in monkey visual cortex: implications for functional connectivity at rest. *Hum Brain Mapp* (2008) **29**:751–61. doi:10.1002/hbm.20580
54. Labate A, Briellmann RS, Abbott DF, Waites AB, Jackson GD. Typical childhood absence seizures are associated with thalamic activation. *Epileptic Disord* (2005) **7**:373–7.
55. Moeller F, Siebner HR, Wolff S, Muhle H, Granert O, Jansen O, et al. Simultaneous EEG-fMRI in drug-naive children with newly diagnosed absence epilepsy. *Epilepsia* (2008) **49**:1510–9. doi:10.1111/j.1528-1167.2008.01626.x
56. Bai X, Vestal M, Berman R, Negishi M, Spann M, Vega C, et al. Dynamic time course of typical childhood absence seizures: EEG, behavior, and functional magnetic resonance imaging. *J Neurosci* (2010) **30**:5884–93. doi:10.1523/JNEUROSCI.5101-09.2010
57. Carney PW, Masterton RA, Harvey AS, Scheffer IE, Berkovic SF, Jackson GD. The core network in absence epilepsy. Differences in cortical and thalamic BOLD response. *Neurology* (2010) **75**:904–11. doi:10.1212/WNL.0b013e3181f11c06
58. Laufs H, Lengler U, Hamandi K, Kleinschmidt A, Krakow K. Linking generalized spike-and-wave discharges and resting state brain activity by using EEG/fMRI in a patient with absence seizures. *Epilepsia* (2006) **47**:444–8. doi:10.1111/j.1528-1167.2006.00443.x
59. Archer JS, Abbott DF, Waites AB, Jackson GD. fMRI "deactivation" of the posterior cingulate during generalized spike and wave. *Neuroimage* (2003) **20**:1915–22. doi:10.1016/S1053-8119(03)00294-5
60. Aghakhani Y, Bagshaw AP, Benar CG, Hawco C, Andermann F, Dubeau F, et al. fMRI activation during spike and wave discharges in idiopathic generalized epilepsy. *Brain* (2004) **127**:1127–44. doi:10.1093/brain/awh136
61. Hamandi K, Salek-Haddadi A, Fish DR, Lemieux L. EEG/functional MRI in epilepsy: the queen square experience. *J Clin Neurophysiol* (2004) **21**:241–8. doi:10.1097/00004691-200407000-00002
62. Gotman J, Grova C, Bagshaw A, Kobayashi E, Aghakhani Y, Dubeau F, et al. Generalized epileptic discharges show thalamocortical activation and suspension of the default state of the brain. *Proc Natl Acad Sci U S A* (2005) **102**:15236–40. doi:10.1073/pnas.0504935102
63. Moeller F, Siebner HR, Wolff S, Muhle H, Boor R, Granert O, et al. Changes in activity of striato-thalamo-cortical network precede generalized spike wave discharges. *Neuroimage* (2008) **39**:1839–49. doi:10.1016/j.neuroimage.2007.10.058
64. Szaflarski JP, Lindsell CJ, Zakaria T, Banks C, Privitera MD. Seizure control in patients with idiopathic generalized epilepsies: EEG determinants of medication response. *Epilepsy Behav* (2010) **17**:525–30. doi:10.1016/j.yebeh.2010.02.005
65. Benuzzi F, Mirandola L, Pugnaghi M, Farinelli V, Tassinari CA, Capovilla G, et al. Increased cortical BOLD signal anticipates generalized spike and wave discharges in adolescents and adults with idiopathic generalized epilepsies. *Epilepsia* (2012) **53**:622–30. doi:10.1111/j.1528-1167.2011.03385.x
66. Carney PW, Masterton RA, Flanagan D, Berkovic SF, Jackson GD. The frontal lobe in absence epilepsy: EEG-fMRI findings. *Neurology* (2012) **78**:1157–65. doi:10.1212/WNL.0b013e31824f801d
67. Masterton RA, Carney PW, Abbott DF, Jackson GD. Absence epilepsy subnetworks revealed by event-related independent components analysis of functional magnetic resonance imaging. *Epilepsia* (2013) **54**:801–8. doi:10.1111/epi.12163
68. Moeller F, Levan P, Muhle H, Stephani U, Dubeau F, Siniatchkin M, et al. Absence seizures: individual patterns revealed by EEG-fMRI. *Epilepsia* (2010) **51**:11. doi:10.1111/j.1528-1167.2010.02698.x
69. Andreasen NC, O'Leary DS, Cizadlo T, Arndt S, Rezai K, Watkins GL, et al. Remembering the past: two facets of episodic memory explored with positron emission tomography. *Am J Psychiatry* (1995) **152**:1576–85.
70. Mazoyer B, Zago L, Mellet E, Bricogne S, Etard O, Houde O, et al. Cortical networks for working memory and executive functions sustain the conscious resting state in man. *Brain Res Bull* (2001) **54**:287–98. doi:10.1016/S0361-9230(00)00437-8
71. Tenney JR, Duong TQ, King JA, Ludwig R, Ferris CF. Corticothalamic modulation during absence seizures in rats: a functional MRI assessment. *Epilepsia* (2003) **44**:1133–40. doi:10.1046/j.1528-1157.2003.61002.x
72. Nersesyan H, Hyder F, Rothman DL, Blumenfeld H. Dynamic fMRI and EEG recordings during spike-wave seizures and generalized tonic-clonic seizures in WAG/Rij rats. *J Cereb Blood Flow Metab* (2004) **24**:589–99. doi:10.1097/01.WCB.0000117688.98763.23
73. Tenney JR, Marshall PC, King JA, Ferris CF. fMRI of generalized absence status epilepticus in conscious marmoset monkeys reveals corticothalamic activation. *Epilepsia* (2004) **45**:1240–7. doi:10.1111/j.0013-9580.2004.21504.x
74. Lombroso CT. Consistent EEG focalities detected in subjects with primary generalized epilepsies monitored for two decades. *Epilepsia* (1997) **38**:797–812. doi:10.1111/j.1528-1157.1997.tb01467.x
75. Lagae L, Pauwels J, Monte CP, Verhelle B, Vervisch I. Frontal absences in children. *Eur J Paediatr Neurol* (2001) **5**:243–51.
76. Holmes MD, Brown M, Tucker DM, Holmes MD, Brown M, Tucker DM. Are "generalized" seizures truly generalized? Evidence of localized mesial frontal and frontopolar discharges in absence. *Epilepsia* (2004) **45**:1568–79. doi:10.1111/j.0013-9580.2004.23204.x
77. Amor F, Baillet S, Navarro V, Adam C, Martinerie J, Quyen Mle V. Cortical local and long-range synchronization interplay in human absence seizure initiation. *Neuroimage* (2009) **45**:950–62. doi:10.1016/j.neuroimage.2008.12.011
78. Moeller F, Siebner HR, Ahlgrimm N, Wolff S, Muhle H, Granert O, et al. fMRI activation during spike and wave discharges evoked by photic stimulation. *Neuroimage* (2009) **48**:682–95. doi:10.1016/j.neuroimage.2009.07.019
79. Berman R, Negishi M, Vestal M, Spann M, Chung MH, Bai X, et al. Simultaneous EEG, fMRI, and behavior in typical childhood absence seizures. *Epilepsia* (2010) **51**(10):2011–22. doi:10.1111/j.1528-1167.2010.02652.x
80. Bai A, Guo J, Killory B, Vestal M, Berman R, Negishi M, et al. Resting functional connectivity between the hemispheres in childhood absence epilepsy. *Neurology* (2011) **76**:1960–7. doi:10.1212/WNL.0b013e31821e54de
81. Li Q, Luo C, Yang T, Yao Z, He L, Liu L, et al. EEG-fMRI study on the interictal and ictal generalized spike-wave discharges in patients with childhood absence epilepsy. *Epilepsy Res* (2009) **87**:160–8. doi:10.1016/j.eplepsyres.2009.08.018
82. Moeller F, Muhle H, Wiegand G, Wolff S, Stephani U, Siniatchkin M. EEG-fMRI study of generalized spike and wave discharges without transitory cognitive impairment. *Epilepsy Behav* (2010) **18**:313–6. doi:10.1016/j.yebeh.2010.02.013
83. Carney PW, Jackson GD. EEG-fMRI in patients with generalised epilepsy. 1st ed. In: Mulert C, Lemieux L, editors. *EEG-fMRI: Physiological Basis, Technique and Applications.* Berlin: Springer (2010). p. 333–48.
84. Holmes GL, McKeever M, Adamson M. Absence seizures in children: clinical and electroencephalographic features. *Ann Neurol* (1987) **21**:268–73. doi:10.1002/ana.410210308
85. Hamandi K, Salek-Haddadi A, Laufs H, Liston A, Friston K, Fish DR, et al. EEG-fMRI of idiopathic and secondarily generalized epilepsies. *Neuroimage* (2006) **31**:1700–10. doi:10.1016/j.neuroimage.2006.02.016
86. Siniatchkin M, Coropceanu D, Moeller F, Boor R, Stephani U. EEG-fMRI reveals activation of brainstem and thalamus in patients with Lennox-Gastaut syndrome. *Epilepsia* (2011) **52**:766–74. doi:10.1111/j.1528-1167.2010.02948.x
87. Pillay N, Archer JS, Badawy RA, Flanagan DF, Berkovic SF, Jackson G. Networks underlying paroxysmal fast activity and slow spike and wave in Lennox-Gastaut syndrome. *Neurology* (2013) **81**:665–73. doi:10.1212/WNL.0b013e3182a08f6a
88. Moeller F, Maneshi M, Pittau F, Gholipour T, Bellec P, Dubeau F, et al. Functional connectivity in patients with idiopathic generalized epilepsy. *Epilepsia* (2011) **52**:515–22. doi:10.1111/j.1528-1167.2010.02938.x

89. Weissenbacher A, Kasess C, Gerstl F, Lanzenberger R, Moser E, Windischberger C. Correlations and anticorrelations in resting-state functional connectivity MRI: a quantitative comparison of preprocessing strategies. *Neuroimage* (2009) **47**:1408–16. doi:10.1016/j.neuroimage.2009.05.005
90. Saad ZS, Gotts SJ, Murphy K, Chen G, Jo HJ, Martin A, et al. Trouble at rest: how correlation patterns and group differences become distorted after global signal regression. *Brain Connect* (2012) **2**:25–32. doi:10.1089/brain.2012.0080
91. Luo C, Li Q, Lai Y, Xia Y, Qin Y, Liao W, et al. Altered functional connectivity in default mode network in absence epilepsy: a resting-state fMRI study. *Hum Brain Mapp* (2011) **32**:438–49. doi:10.1002/hbm.21034
92. Killory BD, Bai X, Negishi M, Vega C, Spann MN, Vestal M, et al. Impaired attention and network connectivity in childhood absence epilepsy. *Neuroimage* (2011) **56**:2209–17. doi:10.1016/j.neuroimage.2011.03.036
93. Masterton RA, Carney PW, Jackson GD. Cortical and thalamic resting-state functional connectivity is altered in childhood absence epilepsy. *Epilepsy Res* (2012) **99**:327–34. doi:10.1016/j.eplepsyres.2011.12.014
94. Shulman GI, Fiez JA. Common blood flow changes across visual tasks: II. Decreases in cerebral cortex. *J Cogn Neurosci* (1997) **9**:5. doi:10.1162/jocn.1997.9.5.648
95. Raichle ME, Macleod AM, Snyder AZ, Powers WJ, Gusnard DA, Shulman GL. A default mode of brain function. *Proc Natl Acad Sci U S A* (2001) **98**:676–82. doi:10.1073/pnas.98.2.676
96. Binder JR, Frost JA, Hammeke TA, Bellgowan PS, Rao SM, Cox RW. Conceptual processing during the conscious resting state. A functional MRI study. *J Cogn Neurosci* (1999) **11**:80–95. doi:10.1162/089892999563265
97. Fox MD, Snyder AZ, Vincent JL, Corbetta M, Van Essen DC, Raichle ME. The human brain is intrinsically organized into dynamic, anticorrelated functional networks. *Proc Natl Acad Sci U S A* (2005) **102**:9673–8. doi:10.1073/pnas.0504136102
98. Fox MD, Raichle ME. Spontaneous fluctuations in brain activity observed with functional magnetic resonance imaging. *Nat Rev Neurosci* (2007) **8**:700–11. doi:10.1038/nrn2201
99. Power JD, Fair DA, Schlaggar BL, Petersen SE. The development of human functional brain networks. *Neuron* (2010) **67**:735–48. doi:10.1016/j.neuron.2010.08.017
100. Lin W, Zhu Q, Gao W, Chen Y, Toh CH, Styner M, et al. Functional connectivity MR imaging reveals cortical functional connectivity in the developing brain. *AJNR Am J Neuroradiol* (2008) **29**:1883–9. doi:10.3174/ajnr.A1256
101. Smyser CD, Inder TE, Shimony JS, Hill JE, Degnan AJ, Snyder AZ, et al. Longitudinal analysis of neural network development in preterm infants. *Cereb Cortex* (2010) **20**:2852–62. doi:10.1093/cercor/bhq035
102. Fair DA, Cohen AL, Power JD, Dosenbach NU, Church JA, Miezin FM, et al. Functional brain networks develop from a "local to distributed" organization. *PLoS Comput Biol* (2009) **5**:e1000381. doi:10.1371/journal.pcbi.1000381
103. Raichle ME. Two views of brain function. *Trends Cogn Sci* (2010) **14**:180–90. doi:10.1016/j.tics.2010.01.008
104. Greicius MD, Krasnow B, Reiss AL, Menon V. Functional connectivity in the resting brain: a network analysis of the default mode hypothesis. *Proc Natl Acad Sci U S A* (2003) **100**:253–8. doi:10.1073/pnas.0135058100
105. Vaudano AE, Laufs H, Kiebel SJ, Carmichael DW, Hamandi K, Guye M, et al. Causal hierarchy within the thalamo-cortical network in spike and wave discharges. *PLoS One* (2009) **4**(8):e6475. doi:10.1371/journal.pone.0006475
106. Blumenfeld H, Taylor J. Why do seizures cause loss of consciousness? *Neuroscientist* (2003) **9**:301–10. doi:10.1177/1073858403255624

2

Study on the relationships between intrinsic functional connectivity of the default mode network and transient epileptic activity

Renaud Lopes[1,2], Friederike Moeller[3], Pierre Besson[1,4], François Ogez[1], William Szurhaj[1,4], Xavier Leclerc[1,2], Michael Siniatchkin[3], Mathilde Chipaux[5], Philippe Derambure[1,4] and Louise Tyvaert[1,4]*

[1] UMR 1046, University of Lille 2, Lille, France
[2] In vivo Imaging Core Facility, IMPRT-IFR114, Lille University Medical Center, Lille, France
[3] Department of Neuropaediatrics, Christian-Albrechts-University, Kiel, Germany
[4] Department of Clinical Neurophysiology, Lille University Medical Center, Lille, France
[5] Department of Pediatric Neurosurgery, Fondation Ophtalmologique A. de Rothschild, Paris, France

***Correspondence:**
Louise Tyvaert, UMR 1046, Department of Clinical Neurophysiology, Lille University Medical Center, rue Emile Laine, Lille 59037, France
e-mail: louise.tyvaert@chru-lille.fr

Rationale: Simultaneous recording of electroencephalogram and functional MRI (EEG–fMRI) is a powerful tool for localizing epileptic networks via the detection of hemodynamic changes correlated with interictal epileptic discharges (IEDs). fMRI can be used to study the long-lasting effect of epileptic activity by assessing stationary functional connectivity during the resting-state period [especially, the connectivity of the default mode network (DMN)]. Temporal lobe epilepsy (TLE) and idiopathic generalized epilepsy (IGE) are associated with low responsiveness and disruption of DMN activity. A dynamic functional connectivity approach might enable us to determine the effect of IEDs on DMN connectivity and to better understand the correlation between DMN connectivity changes and altered consciousness.

Method: We studied dynamic changes in DMN intrinsic connectivity and their relation to IEDs. Six IGE patients (with generalized spike and slow-waves) and 6 TLE patients (with unilateral left temporal spikes) were included. Functional connectivity before, during, and after IEDs was estimated using a sliding window approach and compared with the baseline period.

Results: No dependence on window size was observed. The baseline DMN connectivity was decreased in the left hemisphere (ipsilateral to the epileptic focus) in TLEs and was less strong but remained bilateral in IGEs. We observed an overall increase in DMN intrinsic connectivity prior to the onset of IEDs in both IGEs and TLEs. After IEDs in TLEs, we found that DMN connectivity increased before it returned to baseline values. Most of the DMN regions with increased connectivity before and after IEDs were lateralized to the left hemisphere in TLE (i.e., ipsilateral to the epileptic focus).

Conclusion: Results suggest that DMN connectivity may facilitate IED generation and may be affected at the time of the IED. However, these results need to be confirmed in a larger independent cohort.

Keywords: default mode network, functional connectivity, dynamic, epileptic interictal event, temporal lobe epilepsy, idiopathic generalized epilepsy, posterior cingulate gyrus, precuneus

INTRODUCTION

Epilepsy is a common neurological disease defined by the occurrence of electrically and clinically measurable epileptic seizures. Cognitive and behavioral functions may be altered, leading to severe social and professional handicap. By definition, the patient's clinical state is altered at the time of the ictal event and during the immediate postictal period. However, functional brain impairments can also be observed during the interictal state. These cognitive impairments may be due to factors such as structural lesions, medication effects, the underlying cause of epilepsy, and/or the occurrence of interictal epileptic discharges (IEDs) observed in electroencephalography (EEG). The repetition of IEDs may be responsible for long-lasting effects on the brain's functional plasticity and may thus lead to cognitive disturbances (1). However, a

---

Abbreviations: BOLD, blood oxygen level dependent; DMN, default mode network; dMPFC, dorsal medial prefrontal cortex; EEG, electroencephalogram; fMRI, functional magnetic resonance imaging; HRF, hemodynamic response function; ICA, independent component analysis; IED, interictal epileptic discharge; IGE, idiopathic generalized epilepsy; IPL, inferior parietal lobule; MFG, middle frontal gyrus; MTG, middle temporal gyrus; NBS, network-based statistics; PCC, precuneus/posterior cingulate cortex; PHG, parahippocampal gyrus; RSN, resting-state network; TLE, temporal lobe epilepsy; TP, temporal pole; WOI, window of interest.

transient cognitive impairment has also been observed at the time of each IED (2–5). This effect has been noticed for both generalized spike and wave bursts and focal epileptic events.

Simultaneous recording of the EEG and functional magnetic resonance imaging (fMRI) has provided new insights into the effect of IEDs on brain function. Event-related analyses have shown that at the time of the IED, the blood-oxygen-level-dependent (BOLD) signal increases at the epileptic focus (corresponding to activation). Furthermore, the BOLD signal may decrease to a variable extent at some distance from the epileptic focus (i.e., deactivation). In group analyses, this deactivation appears to involve a specific brain functional network – the default mode network (DMN) (6–9). The DMN involves several cortical areas (such as the posterior cingulate, the precuneus, the bilateral inferior parietal lobule, and the mesial prefrontal cortex) (10–13). This network is usually activated during wakefulness at rest and deactivated during sleep or during a task that requires great attention (14). The alteration in DMN activity observed at the time of an IED suggests that epileptic activity has a direct effect on awareness and cognitive performance. Deactivation within the DMN has been observed in patients with idiopathic generalized epilepsy (IGE) (6, 15, 16) and patients with temporal lobe epilepsy (TLE) (7, 8). However, the exact pattern of DMN deactivation has not been studied with respect to the side of the focus or the exact type of IED (17).

The long-lasting effect of epileptic activity on the brain's functional organization during a prolonged resting-state period (classically 10 min) has been investigated in network functional connectivity studies. Based on the analysis of coherent low-frequency BOLD fluctuations, several local spatial patterns [defined as resting-state networks (RSNs)] have been identified and thus constitute a new functional map of the brain (12). The DMN is one of these distinct RSNs; in healthy subjects, its intrinsic connectivity is characterized by low intra- and inter-individual variability (18). Moreover, structural imaging analysis suggests that RSNs (such as the DMN) reflect anatomic connectivity (19, 20). DMN connectivity is low in IGE patients, relative to healthy controls (21–24). Similar patterns of low DMN connectivity have been observed in TLE patients (25–28). Pittau et al. (29) also demonstrated that the mesial structures in TLE patients were less connected to the DMN.

Studies of DMN connectivity and epilepsy have been performed on 10-min resting-state blocks (based on the assumption that DMN connectivity is stable over 10 min). However, there is increasing evidence to suggest that the intrinsic connectivity and spatial extent of the RSNs fluctuates in a periodic manner (30–35). Furthermore, epileptic activity may affect these fluctuations (36). Characterization of these influences is crucial for better understanding the epileptic discharge and its relationship with cognitive disturbances in patients with epilepsy.

In the present study, we assessed the dynamic changes in DMN intrinsic connectivity and its relation to epileptic activity. We hypothesized that DMN connectivity is affected by the occurrence of IEDs (i.e., connectivity differs before, during, and after IEDs). However, these changes may depend on the type of IED. To better characterize these effects, we chose to evaluate two different types of IEDs: (i) generalized spike and slow-wave bursts and (ii) left focal temporal epileptic spikes. A generalized spike and wave burst might affect the connectivity of the DMN on both sides of the brain, whereas, focal IED might lead to more lateralized changes in the DMN. Our objective was to better understand the relationship between the occurrence of IEDs and the disturbance of RSNs.

MATERIALS AND METHODS

SUBJECTS

We retrospectively selected patients registered in the EEG–fMRI databases in the Department of Clinical Neurophysiology at Lille University Medical Center (Lille, France) (from April 2011 to December 2013) and the Department of Neuropaediatrics at the University Hospital of Kiel (Kiel, Germany) (from May 2006 to December 2009).

The inclusion criteria were related to the number and type of IEDs. We first selected IGE patients with isolated or short generalized spike and wave events recorded during the EEG–fMRI session. Secondly, we selected focal epilepsy patients with unilateral temporal IEDs. Patients were suffering from epilepsy with temporal lobe involvement (TLE). In order to perform a group analysis of our data, we chose patients with IEDs from the temporal lobe on the same side of the brain (the left). Patients had to present no more than two types of IED, and only the predominant IED-related to the epileptic focus was studied. Absence or focal seizures were not considered and patients with seizures during the fMRI session were excluded from the study. Furthermore, patients selected for this study had to present at least 10 separate IEDs during the EEG–fMRI session. And, due to our constraints of the analysis explained in Section "Dynamical Functional Connectivity," an interval of at least 80 s between each IED was required for completion of the analysis. All patients were right-handed. Data from EEG–fMRI sessions with high-amplitude movement artifacts (>1 mm in each direction) were excluded from the analysis. Hence, patients were included in one of two groups: (i) IGE patients with typical, generalized slow-wave spikes, or short bursts on the EEG, and (ii) TLE patients with unilateral (left) temporal spikes.

All patients were receiving antiepileptic medication at the time of the study (**Table 1**). The patients (and their parents in minors) gave their written informed consent to participation. The study was performed according to the Declaration of Helsinki and the protocol was approved by the institutional research ethics boards.

EEG–fMRI ACQUISITION

In Lille, the EEG signal was recorded using 25 separate scalp MRI-compatible electrodes placed according to the international 10–20 system. In Kiel, a 30-electrodes Easycap system (Falk-Minow Services, Herrsching-Breitbrunn, Germany) was used. In both cases, FCz was the reference. To improve patient comfort and reduce movement artifacts, the head was maintained in position with foam cushions. Data were transmitted via an optic fiber cable from a Micromed amplifier (Micromed, Italy, 5 kHz sampling rate) in Lille and from a BrainAmp-MR amplifier (Brain Products Co., Munich, Germany, 5 kHz sampling rate) in Kiel to the EEG monitor located outside the scanner room. The EEG was recorded with a 1024 Hz sampling rate.

In both centers, functional imaging was performed with a 3 T MRI scanner (Achieva Philips, Best, The Netherlands) and

Table 1 | Clinical and EEG characteristics of the patients in the IGE and TLE groups.

Pt	Group center	Sex	Age (years)	Disease duration (years)	AEDs	Epilepsy type	Struct. MRI	IEDs			
								Nb	Mean duration (s)	Side	Type and location
1	IGE Lille	M	13	9	LMG, VPA	Childhood absence epilepsy	N	20	1.8	–	GSW
2	IGE Lille	F	23	18	TPM, BZD	Juvenile myoclonic epilepsy	N	14	2.5	–	GSW
3	IGE Kiel	F	13	10	VPA, LTG, LEV	Myoclonic absence epilepsy	N	12	<1	–	GSW
4	IGE Kiel	M	6	1	VPA, TPM, LEV	Myoclonic absence epilepsy	N	12	<1	–	GSW
5	IGE Kiel	M	10	6	LTG, ESM	Childhood absence epilepsy	N	16	<1	–	GSW
6	IGE Kiel	M	5	1	LTG, ESM	Childhood absence epilepsy	N	17	2.5	–	GSW
7	TLE Lille	F	14	10	OXCBZ, TPM, VPA	Temporo-occipital	Temporo-occipital DNET	14	<1	Left	Temporo-occipital spikes
8	TLE Lille	F	20	17	LCM, BZD	Fronto-temporal	N	22	<1	Left	Fronto-temporal spikes
9	TLE Lille	F	45	15	OXCBZ, TPM, BZD	Temporo-perisylvian	N	14	<1	Left	Temporo-perisylvian rhythmic theta bursts
10	TLE Lille	F	33	14	LMG, TPM, LCM	Temporo-perisylvian	Temporo-insular dysplasia	14	<1	Left	Temporo-perisylvian spike and waves
11	TLE Lille	F	22	9	CBZ, LCM, ZNS, BZD	Temporo-occipital	N	12	2.4	left	Temporo-occipital polyspikes
12	TLE Lille	F	18	9	LMG, LVT, BZD	Temporal	N	10	<1	Left	Temporal spikes
Mean ± SD			18.5 ± 11.4	9.9 ± 5.5							

Pt, patient; AEDs, antiepileptic drugs; OXCBZ, oxcarbazepine; TPM, topiramate; LMG, lamotrigine; VPA, valproate; LCM, lacosamide; LVT, levetiracetam; ZNS, zonisamide; BZD, benzodiazepin; ETSM, ethosuximide; IEDs, interictal epiletiform discharges; N, normal; GSW, generalized spike and waves; Nb, number; M, male; F, female; DNET, dysembryoplastic neuroepithelial tumor; Struc., structural.

a standard, 8-channel SENSE head coil. A T1-weighted structural image (voxel dimensions: 0.8 mm × 0.8 mm × 1.3 mm; slices: 130; matrix: 288 × 288; TE: 2 ms; TR: 20 ms; flip angle: 30°) was used for superposition on the functional images. For functional data, six or seven 10-min runs were acquired with a T2*-weighted EPI sequence (voxel dimensions: 4 mm × 4 mm × 4 mm; slices: 34; matrix: 64 × 64; TE: 35 ms; TR: 2000 ms; flip angle: 90°; volumes: 300) in Lille and with a 15-min T2*-weighted EPI sequence (voxel dimensions: 3.125 mm × 3.125 mm × 3.79 mm; slices: 30; matrix: 64 × 64; TE: 45 ms; TR: 2250 ms; flip angle: 90°; volumes: 540) in Kiel.

The patients were recorded at rest for up to 2 h inside the MRI. They were instructed to rest and to keep their eyes closed throughout the whole MRI session. The EEG signal was used by a neurologist to monitor the patient during the entire recording. In order to display a clear EEG, the gradient artifact was corrected online using an adaptive filtering algorithm (Brain Products, Munich, Germany). Only the raw EEG was recorded. No specific drug dose step-down, sleep deprivation, or seizure induction methods were used. Patients received chloral hydrate before the MRI session.

EEG ANALYSIS

The EEG signal was processed off-line using Brain Vision Analyzer software (Brain Products, Munich, Germany), with correction of the gradient artifact and filtering of the EEG signal (37). A 50 Hz low-pass filter was applied to remove any remaining artifacts. Independent component analysis (ICA) was used to extract the ballistocardiogram artifact (38). After correction of the EEG, a neurologist reviewed the signal. Epileptiform events were marked according to their type, location, and duration. The predominant IED type was selected according to its frequency of occurrence and to its relevance to the suspected epileptic focus.

fMRI PREPROCESSING

Structural data were preprocessed by Freesurfer software (v.5.1)[1]. Each subject's structural data underwent non-uniformity and intensity correction, skull stripping, and automatic tissue classification. Preprocessing and analysis of fMRI data were performed using a combination of Statistical Parametric Mapping software (SPM12[2]; Wellcome Department of Cognitive Neurology, University College London, UK), and in-house software implemented in MATLAB v7.11 (Mathworks Inc., Natick, MA, USA). Functional image preprocessing included the removal of the first three image volumes (to avoid T1 equilibration effects), realignment, slice-timing correction (using the middle slice as the reference frame), and registration against the structural data. Nuisance signals were removed using a two-step linear regression. The first regression removed linear/quadratic trends (to account for scanner drift) and six motion parameters. The second regression removed five "nuisance signals" obtained by means of a principal component analysis of white matter and ventricle signals using the component-based noise correction (CompCor) approach (39, 40). Residual data were corrected for high temporal frequencies (low-pass filtering with a 0.1 Hz cut-off).

Lastly, structural and functional preprocessed data were spatially normalized to match the Montreal Neurological Institute (MNI) template. For that, a non-linear registration was applied to match the preprocessed T1-weighted data to the MNI template, using SPM software. Then, the transformation was applied to preprocessed fMRI data and resampled by spline interpolation into a final voxel size of 3 mm × 3 mm × 3 mm.

THE DMN MASK

Connectivity-based methods have been used to detect functionally connected brain networks with high consistency and reproducibility across subjects and sessions (41). Graph theory has been recently used to study the topological organization of these brain networks, by modeling the brain as a collection of nodes (e.g., brain regions) and edges (e.g., connectivity) [see Ref. (42), for an excellent review]. In this study, we are interested in the topological organization of DMN using a graph theory-based approach.

To study DMN intrinsic connectivity, we had first to identify the network. In view of the small number of study participants and the "double dipping" issue (43), the DMN was identified using data from healthy volunteers (part of the 1000 Functional Connectome Project, a publicly available collection of resting-state fMRI datasets from a number of laboratories around the world).[3] The corresponding institutional review boards have approved or provided waivers for the submission of anonymized data, which were obtained after provision of written, informed consent by each participant. We selected 198 healthy volunteers (76 males and 122 females, aged 18–26) from the Beijing dataset. The DMN was then identified using group-level spatial ICA, as implemented in the GIFT toolbox.[4] We used a low-order model (20 components) to extract the DMN into one component using the infomax ICA algorithm repeated 10 times. After thresholding to z-score >2, seven clusters (or regions of interest) per hemisphere were identified by selecting 30 voxels around the peak of each cluster. Thus seven regions per hemisphere were defined in MNI space: the precuneus/posterior cingulate cortex (PCC) (MNI coordinate: 8, −53, 15 and −8, −55, 18), inferior parietal lobule (IPL) (MNI coordinate: 48, −64, 31 and −45, −69, 32), middle temporal gyrus (MTG) (MNI coordinate: 56, −2, −25 and −57, −6, −22), parahippocampal gyrus (PHG) (MNI coordinate: 27, −21, −23 and −26, −26, −20), temporal pole (TP) (MNI coordinate: 40, 21, −37 and −41, 19, -37), middle frontal gyrus (MFG) (MNI coordinate: 6, 54, −9 and −7, 51, −11) and dorsal medial prefrontal cortex (dMPFC) (MNI coordinate: 20, 39, 46 and −21, 32, 47).

DYNAMICAL FUNCTIONAL CONNECTIVITY

Functional connectivity is commonly computed by estimating the covariance between regions. However, estimation of the covariance matrix can be a difficult statistical problem for two reasons: (i) the positive definite constraint on the matrix and (ii) the fact that there are more connections than samples. Connectivity can also be measured by estimating the inverse covariance matrix (the precision matrix) between regions under sparsity constraints. The zero entries in this matrix correspond to conditional independence between regions if the data are normally distributed. This procedure amounts to limit the number of edges in graphical models. The graphical least absolute shrinkage and selection operator (GLASSO) (44) is an extension of the least absolute shrinkage and selection operator (45) for estimating a sparse precision matrix with l1-constraint. This approach was recently applied to estimate brain region functional connectivity in a small number of samples (46–48).

The mean BOLD time courses were extracted from the $N = 14$ defined DMN regions. The functional connectivity was estimated for four conditions, corresponding to windowed segments of the time courses [referred to as "before," "during," "after," and "baseline" windows of interest (WOIs)]. **Figure 1** shows the selection of a WOI of length L. We used a tapered window created by convolving a rectangle (length: L TRs) with a Gaussian ($\sigma = 2$ TRs). Assuming that an event occurred at time t, the "before" WOI corresponded to a window from t–L TRs to t TRs, with a "during" WOI from t TRs to $t + \text{L}$ TRs, an "after" WOI from $t + 2\text{L}$ TRs to $t + 3\text{L}$ TRs, and a "baseline" WOI from $t + 4\text{L}$ TRs to $t + 5\text{L}$ TRs. No other events occurred during these periods or after 2L TRs from the end of "baseline" period. In the experiments, we varied the length L from 6 to 10. In view of our constraints, use of broader WOIs generated too few events.

[1] http://surfer.nmr.mgh.harvard.edu/
[2] http://www.fil.ion.ucl.ac.uk/spm/software/spm12/
[3] http://fcon_1000.projects.nitrc.org/
[4] http://mialab.mrn.org/software/gift/index.html

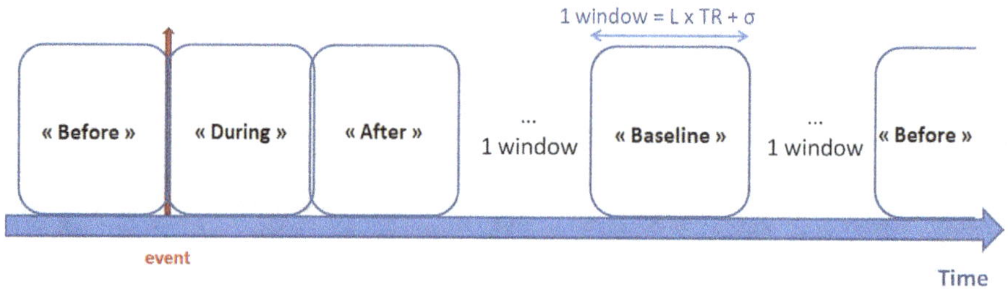

FIGURE 1 | Definition of the WOIs. The red arrow represents the timing of the epileptic event (according to EEG data). Four types of window were defined: "before," "during," and "after" the epileptic event, together with the "baseline" period (i.e., with no epileptic events LTR seconds before and after the window). Tapered windows were used by convolving a rectangle (length: L TRs) with a Gaussian ($\sigma = 2$ TRs).

According to the literature (49–51), early BOLD response can precede the IEDs observed on scalp EEG. Supplementary analyses were conducted to check this effect. We performed additional EEG–fMRI analyses using different timings of hemodynamic response function (HRF) preceding the IEDs (−9s, −7s, −5s, −3s, and 0) [for method see Ref. (49, 50)]. None of our subjects had significant BOLD changes according to these early convolved HRFs.

Next, for each condition, the functional connectivities between each region were computed using the windowed time series from corresponding WOI of length L. The covariance matrix was estimated from the regularized precision matrix using the GLASSO approach (i.e., the Ω that maximizes the penalized Gaussian log-likelihood) by using a coordinate descent optimization procedure (44):

$$\log\det(\Omega) - \operatorname{tr}\left(\sum \Omega\right) - \lambda\|\Omega\|_1 \quad (1)$$

where "det" means the determinant of Ω and λ is the regularization parameter optimized for each subject after evaluating the log-likelihood of unseen data (windowed covariance matrices from the same subject) in a cross-validation framework. For each condition, the regularized covariance matrix W was Fisher-transformed to improve normality.

For each subject, we applied a general linear model on the covariance matrices estimated for each condition in the previous step, in order to investigate its contrast effect size. Thus, four "mean regularized covariance matrices" M (corresponding to contrast effect results from each condition) were obtained for each subject. These matrices will be subjected to later inter-condition analyses. This step was repeated for different lengths of window [i.e., Ref. (6, 8, 10)].

STATISTICAL ANALYSIS OF STATIC CONNECTIVITY

Although the direct comparison of the static connectivity between TLE and IGE groups was not the main aim of this study, we performed a common graph theory-based approach using static functional connectivity. We wished to see if such an analysis of our patient groups would be consistent with previous results in the literature.

We compared DMN intrinsic functional connectivity in the TLE and IGE groups by considering whole time series. For each subject, the average whole time series of each DMN regions (see The DMN Mask) was computed and we measured the degree of DMN integration, as described in Marrelec et al. (52). A Bayesian numerical sampling scheme was used for the inference of integration measures in a group analysis. The integration was approximated from 1000 samples.

STATISTICAL ANALYSIS OF DYNAMIC CONNECTIVITY

In this section, we were interested in DMN intrinsic connectivity for TLE and IGE groups, separately. We compared the four conditions for each group of patients. The statistical comparison of connectivity between conditions was performed using graph theory. The mean covariance matrices M were represented as a graph $G = (V, E)$, where $V = \{V_i\}_{i=1,\ldots,N}$ are the nodes (brain regions) and $E = \{E_i\}_{i=1,\ldots,N;\, j=1,\ldots,N}$ are the elements of the matrix corresponding to edge weights (or connections). We used a multiscale approach to investigate the differences between the four conditions ("before" vs. "during" vs. "after" vs. "baseline" WOIs) at the network, node, and edge levels.

At the network level, the DMN integration I for each condition and a given subject s was computed to capture the overall level of statistical dependence within the network:

$$I_{i,s} = \frac{1}{2}\log\left(\det\left(M_{i,s}\right)\right),\ i = 1, \ldots, 4 \quad (2)$$

where $M_{i,s}$ is the covariance matrix estimated for condition i and subject s, and "det" means the determinant of the matrix.

A non-parametric paired difference test (Wilcoxon's signed-rank test) was applied on integration measures. The resulting p-values were corrected at $p < 0.05$ using false discovery rate (FDR), yielding increased and decreased integrations between two conditions.

At the node-level, two topology measures were used: the node strength (i.e., the sum of weights of links connected to a node i, also known as weighted node degree):

$$k_i = \sum_{j=1}^{N} E_{i,j} \quad (3)$$

and the clustering coefficient of node i, which is the average "intensity" of triangles around a node and reflects the prevalence of clustered connectivity around a node:

$$C_i = \frac{\sum_{j,h=1}^{N} \left(w_{ij} w_{ih} w_{jh}\right)^{1/3}}{k_i \left(k_i - 1\right)} \quad (4)$$

The clustering coefficient was computed according to the Brain Connectivity toolbox.[5]

A Wilcoxon signed-rank test was applied to these measurements and the resulting p-values were FDR-corrected at $p < 0.05$ (indicating differences in inter-node connectivity values when comparing two conditions).

At the edge level, we focused on comparing DMN intrinsic connectivity at a pairwise level. A network-based statistics (NBS) approach (53) was used to identify pairs of regions between which the strength of connectivity was altered in the conditions of one group. NBS approach has already been used to show altered structural connectivity in absence epilepsy (54) and TLE (55). For the comparison of two conditions for S subjects, a primary threshold ($p = 0.05$) was first applied to a t-statistic computed from the matrices $\{M_s\}_{s=1\,\ldots\,S}$. This t-statistic was computed for each graph edge, in order to determine any connected components and their size. A family wise error-corrected p-value was then assigned to each network using permutation testing. The condition label on each covariance matrix was permuted (10,000 permutations) constrained for repeated (within-subject) measures to assess statistical significance between two conditions. Lastly, only statistically significant networks (with a p-value of 0.05 corrected for multiple comparisons) were selected.

The brain networks were visualized with BrainNet Viewer software[6] (56).

RESULTS

SUBJECTS

In view of the restrictive inclusion criteria, only 12 patients were eligible for inclusion (6 IGE patients and 6 TLE patients). Details on all subjects included in the study are listed in **Table 1**. Indeed, in Lille and Kiel databases patients' recruitment was based on IEDs frequency. Then only active epileptic patients were recorded in order to maximize the chance to observe IEDs during the MRI session. In our study, to perform our analysis an interval of at least 80 s between each IED was required. This criterion was rarely obtained. In the IGE group, we included four males and two females (mean ± SD age: 11.5 ± 6.5 years; mean epilepsy duration: 7.5 ± 6.4 years). Based on the International League against Epilepsy criteria (57), three of them were suffering from childhood absence seizure, two were suffering from myoclonic absence epilepsy, and one was suffering from juvenile myoclonic epilepsy (**Table 1**). The structural MRI datasets were normal in all patients. The TLE group comprised six females (mean ± SD age: 25.3 ± 11 years; mean epilepsy duration: 12.3 ± 3.4 years). All six were suffering from epilepsy involving the left temporal lobe with left temporal IEDs. The structural MRI datasets were normal in four cases (patients 8, 9, 11, and 12). Patient 10 had a left temporo-insular dysplasia and patient 7 presented a left temporo-occipital dysembryoplastic neuroepithelial tumor.

DMN CONNECTIVITY AT THE NETWORK LEVEL

We first compared DMN intrinsic functional connectivity in the TLE and IGE groups by considering whole time series. **Figure 2** shows that DMN integration in the TLE group was significantly lower than in the IGE group. The error bars indicated the standard deviation of the 1000 samples. This result was confirmed by inspection of the DMN maps for the two groups (thresholded for a z-score >2) using the GroupICA approach (the same method as used for healthy volunteers in Section "The DMN Mask") (**Figure 2**). In the TLE group, the DMN was composed of the PCC and the right IPL. In the IGE group, it was composed of the PCC and the bilateral IPL, MTG, PHG, and dMPFC regions. Furthermore, we observed negative connections between the DMN and the left superior frontal and inferior frontal gyri for the TLE group. DMN anti-correlated network was larger in the IGE group (with the occipital pole and the bilateral inferior frontal and superior insula gyri) than in the TLE group.

We then studied DMN intrinsic functional connectivity in the four WOIs. Functional connectivity was estimated using a window size of eight TRs (from 16s to 18s). When varying the window size from 6 to 10 TRs, we did not find any significant differences between the respective results. Hence, a window size of eight TRs was chosen because it provided a good trade-off between the ability to resolve dynamic changes and the ease of computing regularized covariance matrices. **Table 2** shows the inter-condition differences in DMN integration. In the TLE group, significantly stronger integrations were found in the "before" and "after" WOIs than in the "during" and "baseline" WOIs. There were no significant differences between "during" and "baseline" WOIs. These data indicate that the most significant changes occur before and after an epileptic event. However, the DMN intrinsic connectivity was similar during an IED and during the "baseline" period. In the IGE group, we did not observe any significant inter-conditions difference in DMN integration. Although we found greater DMN integration in the "before," "during," and "after" WOIs than in the "baseline" WOI, the differences were not significant (with p-values of 0.08, 0.16, and 0.18, respectively).

DMN CONNECTIVITY AT THE NODE LEVEL

After studying connectivity at the network level, we sought to determine which nodes (or brain regions) were most involved in the inter-condition differences described above. Two topological measures were used to quantify the nodes' function: node strength and the clustering coefficient. **Figure 3** summarizes the results obtained for the TLE group; no significant differences between "during" and "baseline" WOIs were observed for either measure. The "before" and "during" WOIs differed most in terms of numbers of nodes (4), and differed significantly in terms of node strength and the clustering coefficient. According to both measures, the PCC and left MFG regions had greater connectivity before an IED than during an IED. Likewise, the right IPL region had greater connectivity with its neighborhood. Intrinsic hyperconnectivity of the DMN was also observed in the "before" WOI comparing with

[5]http://sites.google.com/site/bctnet/

[6]http://www.nitrc.org/projects/bnv/

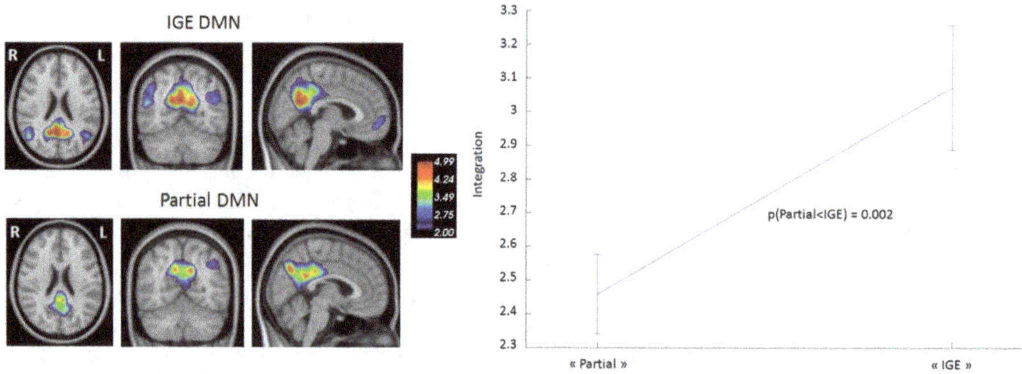

FIGURE 2 | DMN functional connectivity in TLE vs. IGE groups. The DMN integration (dimensionless) was computed for each subject of the two groups. A Bayesian numerical sampling scheme was used for the inference of integration measures in a group analysis. The integration was approximated from 1000 samples. The error bars indicated the standard deviation of the 1000 samples. There was significantly less integration in the TLE group than in the IGE group (right panel). To illustrate this difference, DMN was estimated for each group using the same groupICA approach than the Section "DMN mask" (left panel). Maps were thresholded (z-score > 2).

Table 2 | Mean integration of the DMN network for the TLE and IGE groups under different conditions and for a window size of eight TR.

	Before events	During events	After events	Baseline
TLE patients	1.09 ± 0.14	$0.89 \pm 0.13^{(+)(x)}$	1.06 ± 0.09	$0.90 \pm 0.10^{(+)(x)}$
IGE patients	1.15 ± 0.18	1.08 ± 0.20	1.09 ± 0.23	1.01 ± 0.20

(+) and (x) indicate significantly different (p < 0.05) means in a paired Wilcoxon signed-rank test when comparing the designated column with the "before" and "after" columns, respectively.

the "baseline" WOI but this phenomenon involved different brain regions. Only regions from the left hemisphere (PCC–PHG–TP) differed in terms of clustering coefficient. Lastly, hyperconnectivity was also observed for regions when comparing the "after" condition on one hand with the "during" and "baseline" conditions on the other. However, the hyperconnectivity in the "after" condition was less intense than for "before" condition. We observed that the left and right PCC regions were hubs of hyperconnectivity after (but not before) the IED.

In the IGE group, there were no significant inter-condition differences in node-level intrinsic connectivity of the DMN (**Figure 4**).

DMN CONNECTIVITY AT THE EDGE LEVEL

Our last analysis focused on DMN intrinsic connectivity at the edge (connection) level. In a first step, a one-sample t-test was performed on each condition using NBS. For one condition, we compared the mean regularized covariance matrices from all subjects. **Figures 5** and **6** show pairs of regions that were significantly connected ($p < 0.05$, corrected) during each condition in both epilepsy groups. For TLE and IGE groups, the DMN intrinsic connectivity was relatively high for all conditions. We did not see a condition with very few connected regions. For TLE group, it seemed that the temporal regions (TP–MTG and PHG) showed greater connectivity in the "before" and "during" WOIs than in the "after" and "baseline" WOIs. For IGE group, it seemed that the DMN intrinsic connectivity was higher in the "before," "during," and "after" WOIs than in the "baseline" WOI.

In a second step, the conditions were compared in a paired t-test to statistically validate these observations (again using NBS). The only statistically significant difference was that between the "before" WOI and all other WOIs in the TLE group (**Figure 7**). A larger difference between "before" and "during" WOIs than "after" or "baseline" WOIs was observed (especially for the left PCC node). The PCC was more strongly connected with the parietal, frontal, and temporal regions in the "before" WOI than in the other WOIs. Although differences were observed in the two hemispheres, the number of significant connections was higher in the left hemisphere than in the right hemisphere. This difference was especially marked for connections between extra-temporal and temporal regions. Only connections between the left PHG and the right PCC and right IPL were significantly stronger in the "before" WOI than in the "after" WOI. Lastly, the "before" WOI had greater connectivity between temporal and extra-temporal regions than the "baseline" WOI. Indeed, differences were observed for connections involving the left and right TPs and the left PHG. The "after" WOI did not differ significantly from the "during" and "baseline" WOIs at this level of connectivity.

DISCUSSION

The present study focused on two different types of epilepsy (TLE and IGE) with a common clinical feature: reduced responsiveness at the time of the epileptic discharge. In both types of epilepsy, the DMN is known to be affected by IEDs (5–7, 13–15). We first compared DMN connectivity (based on a standard analysis) in TLE and IGE patients. The decrease in DMN functional connectivity was lateralized (on the focus-side) in TLE patients and was diffuse in IGE patients. By performing a time-resolved analysis of changes in DMN intrinsic connectivity, we found that the overall level of connectivity increased before the onset of the IED in both IGE and TLE patients. This effect was more marked in the TLE group with recovery of a spatially bilateral DMN connectivity pattern prior

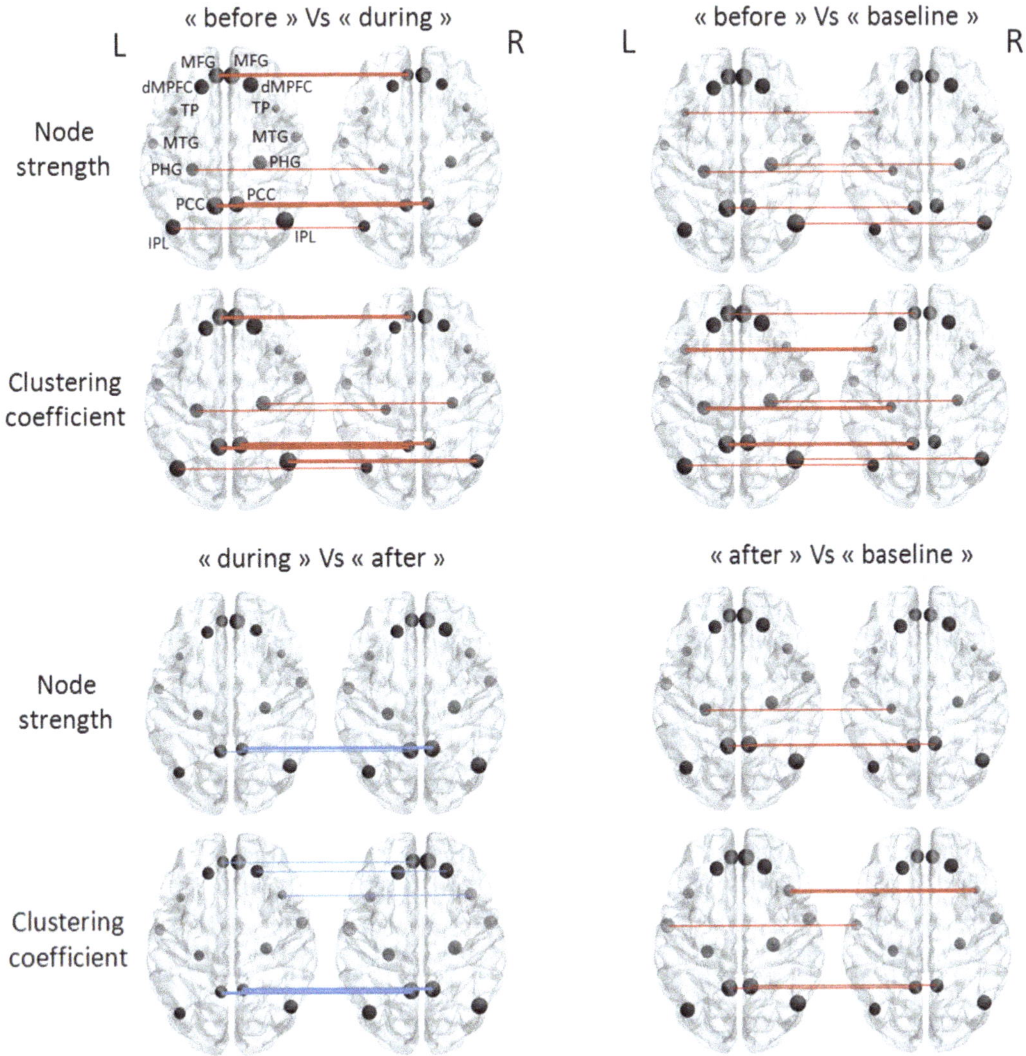

FIGURE 3 | Pairwise comparisons of node strength and the clustering coefficient in the TLE group (in a Wilcoxon signed-rank test). The node sizes correspond to the mean network measure being tested. Colors indicated the direction of change (the red lines mean a decrease, and the blue lines an increase, from the first condition to the second). Different line style indicated significance (thin for FDR-corrected *p*-values <0.1 and thick for FDR-corrected *p*-values <0.05).

to the IED. In TLE patients, the DMN connectivity increased after the IED (predominantly in the PCC) and then returned to baseline values (baseline DMN configuration).

BASELINE DMN CONNECTIVITY AND EPILEPSY

Before studying the time course of change in the DMN connectivity, we wished to confirm the literature reports of alterations in DMN connectivity in IGE and TLE patients by analyzing the resting-state (i.e., the period free of IEDs). We also sought to determine whether the DMN connectivity pattern differed as a function of the type of epilepsy. Firstly, we observed that the DMN connectivity pattern remained bilateral in IGE patients. In the TLE group, the level of DMN connectivity was clearly lower than in the IGE group (**Figure 2**); it involved all the nodes but had a right predominance pattern: the left IPL, MTG, and PHG did not form part of the DMN. These results agree with literature data on both types of epilepsy. In TLE patients, only one study failed to observe an asymmetric pattern with lower functional connectivity on the focus-side (26). However, the authors in the latter study did not monitor the resting-state period; residual IEDs (or even seizures) may have occurred and thus affected the analysis. Zhang et al. (28) and Luo et al. (22) observed low connectivity in the dMPFC and very low or even no connectivity in the mesial temporal lobe and the superior temporal gyrus ipsilateral to the epileptic focus-side. These researchers observed this pattern in right and left TLE patients. Although the right TLE patients showed low functional connectivity in right and left mesial temporal lobes, the left TLE patients had only low functional connectivity in the left mesial temporal lobe. Greater functional connectivity in the posterior cingulate gyrus was only observed in patients with right

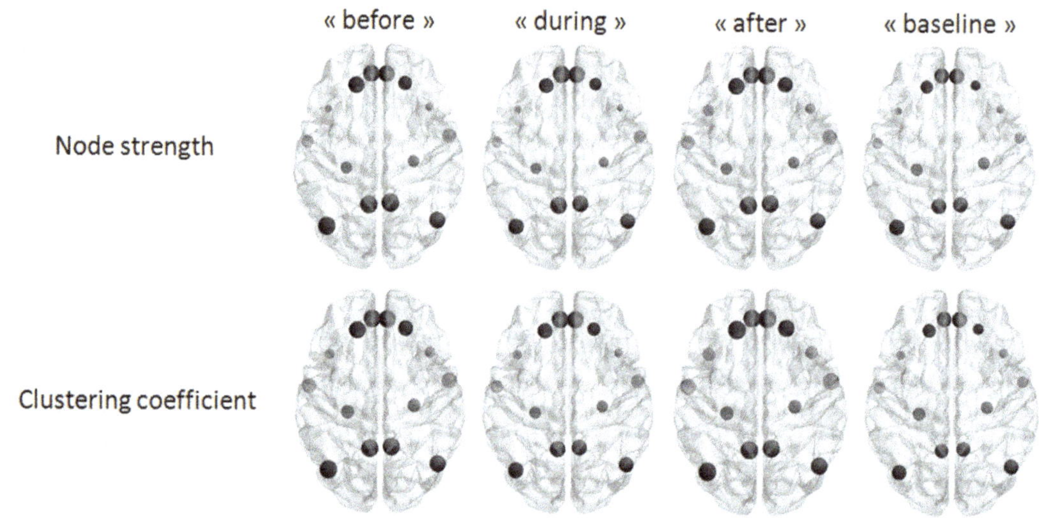

FIGURE 4 | Pairwise comparisons of node strength and the clustering coefficient in the IGE group (in a Wilcoxon signed-rank test) thresholded at FDR-corrected *p*-values <0.05. The node sizes correspond to the mean network measure being tested.

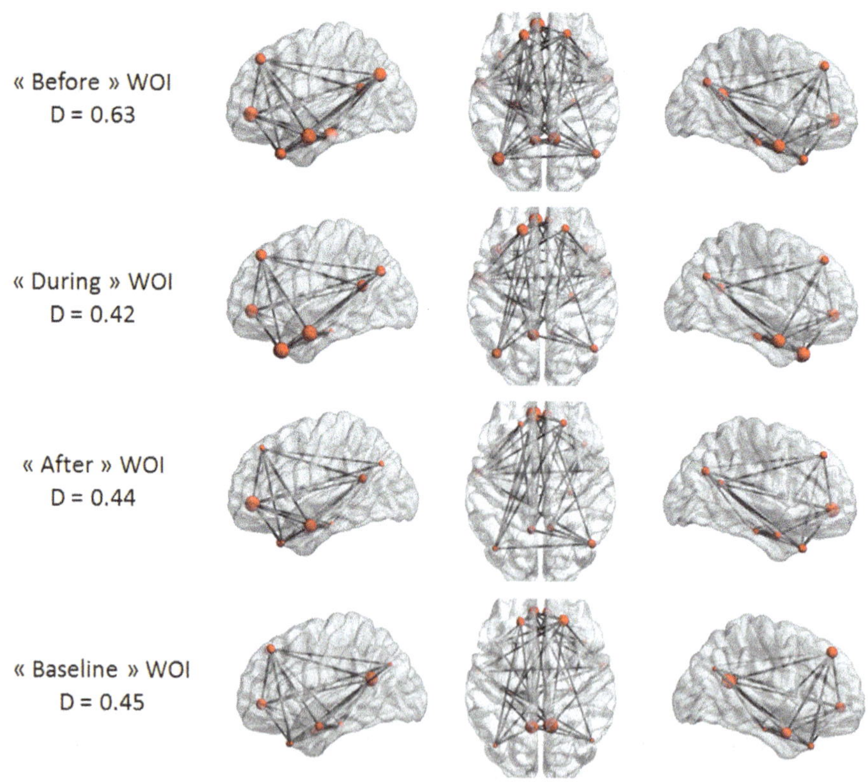

FIGURE 5 | Maps of DMN intrinsic connectivity in the TLE group. The node sizes correspond to the number of connections for a node and the gray lines show significant connections between pairs of regions (FDR-corrected $p < 0.05$). The variable D represents the network density (i.e., the number of significant connections divided by the total number of connections).

TLE. Frings et al. (25) confirmed the presence of an asymmetric DMN disconnection after observing low functional connectivity between the precuneus and temporal structures in left TLE patients. In studies using region of interest methods, the overall DMN connectivity in IGE patients is found to be lower than in controls (22–24). Using ICA, Wang et al. (58) observed low

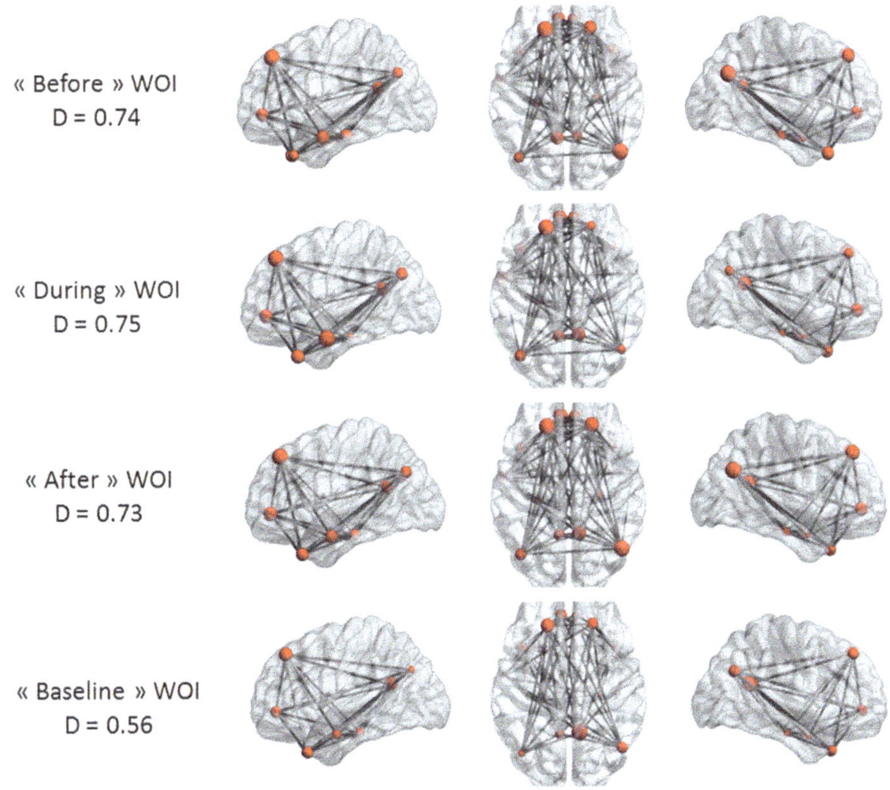

FIGURE 6 | Maps of DMN intrinsic connectivity in the IGE group. The node sizes correspond to the number of connections for a node and the gray lines show significant connections between pairs of regions (FDR-corrected $p < 0.05$). The variable D represents the network density (i.e., the number of significant connections divided by the total number of connections).

functional connectivity in the dMPFC, precuneus and right angular gyrus, and high connectivity in the PCC. These MRI studies did not monitor the EEG. As mentioned above, the epileptic event might directly interfere with overall DMN connectivity. Recently, Kay et al. 's (21) EEG–fMRI study focused on IED-free periods and observed low overall connectivity in the posterior part of the DMN (the PCC, the left and right inferior parietal areas and, to a lesser extent, the left and right prefrontal gyri). Our present results are similar to the literature findings, even though we had small numbers of patients in each group. In TLE and IGE patients, our present results and the literature data emphasize the effect of chronic epileptic discharges on the overall functional connectivity of the brain. During clinical epileptic events in IGE and TLE, cognitive impairment is associated with changes in the DMN configuration. Recurrent IEDs and/or seizures may account for the observed reorganization of DMN connectivity in both types of epilepsy. One can speculate that low functional connectivity in the DMN in IGE and TLE patients may result in cognitive impairment during the interictal period. Although we observed abnormally low DMN connectivity in both types of epilepsy, TLE was further characterized by a marked lower temporal connectivity in the left hemisphere (the left PHG, MTG, IPL, and PCC). This clear, focus-side decrease in DMN connectivity in TLE (relative to IGE) rules out the hypothesis whereby differences in DMN connectivity are due to differences in the mean age of IGE and TLE groups. The mechanisms underlying the changes in the DMN may vary according to the type of epilepsy. In IGE, seizures and IEDs involve widespread, bilateral subcortical, and cortical areas at the same time via thalamo-cortical and cortico-cortical networks (6, 51, 59–65), even though focal onset can sometimes be observed (66, 67). DMN connectivity could be affected by recurrent activation of these thalamo-cortical and cortico-cortical networks on both sides of the brain. TLE is defined by the emergence of an aberrant epileptic network in the temporal lobe, which involves unilateral, local anatomical, and functional reorganization. This local epileptic activity can affect distant areas of the brain (such as the DMN), suggesting that focal epileptic discharge has a widespread asymmetric effect (predominantly on the focus-side).

IEDs AND THE INTRINSIC DYNAMIC CONNECTIVITY OF THE DMN

The main aim of this study was to evaluate the changes in intrinsic DMN connectivity before, during, and after the IED. Indeed, the standard method for measuring DMN connectivity is based on observing the resting-state period for around 10 min. It is assumed that brain activity and RSN connectivity are stable during this time. However, it is known that brain states cannot necessarily be controlled during the resting-state; subjects are submitted to variable external and internal stimuli that will affect their brain processes in different ways. The assumption made in many studies (that ongoing activity is sufficiently random to be averaged)

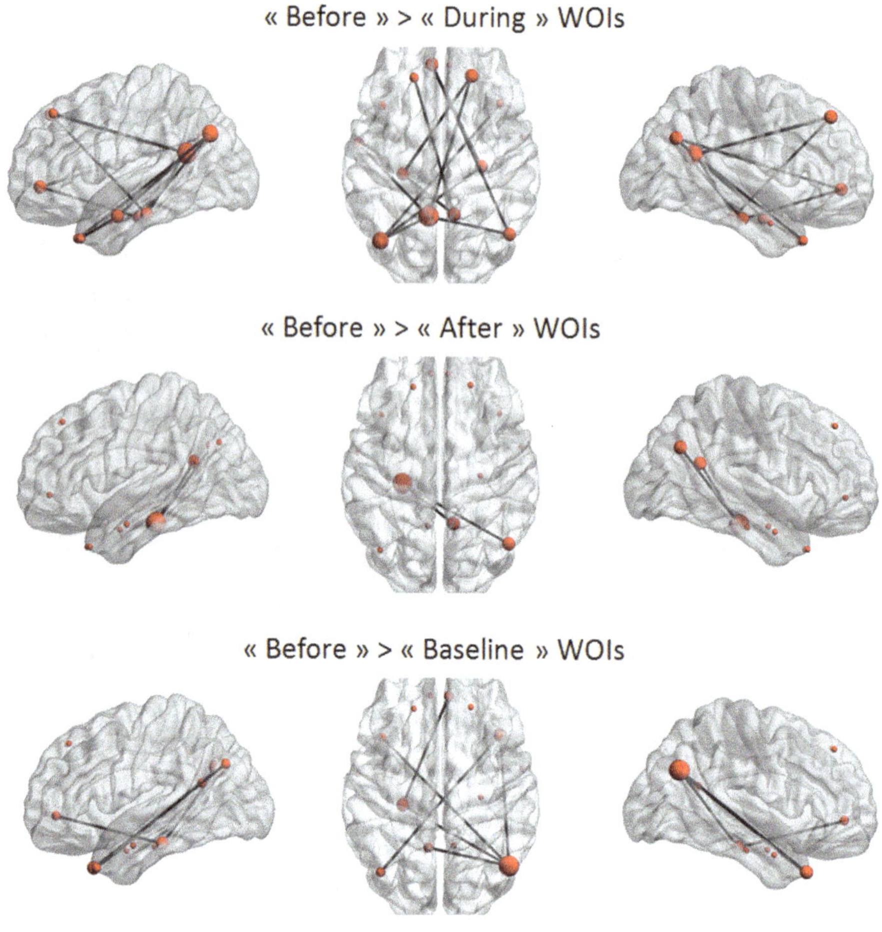

FIGURE 7 | Significant differences between two WOIs in the TLE group. The node sizes correspond to the number of connections for a node and the gray lines show significant connections between pairs of regions (FDR-corrected $p < 0.05$).

induces a bias. It is clear that brain activity displays specific features that are not random over time (68). Recent research has demonstrated that RSN connectivity also changes over time, with periodic fluctuations reflecting different brain states (30–34). This time course is random. Conventionally defined RSNs correspond to the sum of the brain's different network configurations. Over long time scales, RSNs may reflect anatomic connectivity (19, 20). Over short time scales, different configurations of each RSN can be observed but they are always based on the brain's underlying functional structure. Based on this concept of dynamic changes in RSN connectivity, it is possible to evaluate the effect of the IED or seizure on the RSNs' respective time courses. Liao et al. (36) were the first to explore this concept with a view to better understanding the network properties involved in the onset and offset of absence seizures. The researchers particularly studied the dynamic interactions between DMN and the thalamic network at and around the time of the epileptic event. They found a negative correlation between the two networks at the time of the absence seizure and a positive correlation during the baseline period. These results confirmed previous EEG–fMRI studies (based on event-related analysis) that reported an anti-correlated BOLD signal pattern in the DMN and in the thalami (overall DMN deactivation and activation of the thalami) at the time of the absence seizure. In our present work, we chose to evaluate the effect of the epileptic event on DMN intrinsic connectivity during different time windows (before, during, and after the IED and at baseline). Although our initial analysis showed that overall DMN connectivity is affected during IED-free periods, it did not provide information on the specific effect of the IED on connectivity.

DMN connectivity changes during the IED

At the time of the IED, RSN connectivity is necessarily affected by the epileptic event itself. Indeed, we hypothesized that structures displaying a significant increase or decrease in the BOLD (i.e., a hemodynamic response) at the time of the IED are highly connected. Previous event-related EEG–fMRI studies revealed a transient decrease in the BOLD signal in DMN areas at the time of generalized spike and slow-wave discharges and the focal TLE spikes (6–8, 15, 16). We assumed that the intrinsic connectivity of the DMN would be affected, with greater connectivity in the nodes in deactivated brain areas and decreased connectivity in nodes in non-deactivated areas. In fact, we did not find any difference in DMN connectivity when comparing the "during" period and the baseline period. This means that in IGE patients, the DMN connectivity remained stable and uniform including all the usual DMN nodes. This result is consistent with the findings of event-related EEG–fMRI studies, i.e., bilateral, symmetric DMN deactivation at the time of generalized spike and slow-wave bursts. In TLE, DMN connectivity was low and asymmetric during IEDs. The left temporal and parietal DMN nodes (the PHG, IPL, and MTG) were disconnected from the usual DMN components. These nodes are probably affected by the specific temporal lobe epileptic network involved in IED generation. The similar connectivity configurations in the "during" and "baseline" conditions suggest that the baseline DMN reflects functional (and probably structural) alterations caused by recurrent epileptic discharges.

DMN connectivity changes before the IED

In both TLE and IGE, we always observed greater DMN connectivity several seconds before the onset of the IED (in the −8 TR to 0 s WOI). In the TLE group, the DMN configuration "before" the IED was characterized by an increase in DMN connectivity in the left PCC and dMPFC (relative to the "during" configuration). When compared with the "baseline" connectivity pattern, DMN connectivity was particularly enhanced in the PCC, left MTG, left PHG, and left TP. In the IGE group, this effect was not statistically significant. However, we observed a trend toward greater DMN connectivity during the "before" window than during other time windows ($p = 0.008$). In view of the lack of statistical power, we were not able to identify specific structures that may be particularly affected by this increase in connectivity. This statistical issue may be due to the small size of the study population and the small differences between a normal DMN configuration and the IGE configuration.

Changes in DMN connectivity observed before the electrical epileptic event at the scalp is consistent with previous observations of metabolic changes before EEG events. Indeed, several studies have demonstrated that oxygenation and BOLD changes may occur several seconds before the generalized spike and slow-waves or before focal spikes (49–51, 69, 70). Early BOLD changes could be observed up to 9 s before the EEG event. This long delay suggests that mechanisms other than "invisible" electrical changes may precede scalp IED changes, i.e., primary hemodynamic and metabolic events may occur before the electrical changes. Likewise, Zhao et al. (71, 72) used optical imaging of the cortical surface to observe isolated oxygenation changes before the seizure onset. If focal IEDs and seizures can indeed be triggered or conditioned by an early hemodynamic and/or metabolic event, the latter appears to only affect a small, focal, cortical area (50, 71). More recently, a dynamic time course study (66) reported a significant BOLD signal increase in DMN structures (the orbitofrontal, cingulate gyrus, lateral parietal, and precuneus areas) more than 5 s before IEDs in absence seizures. In contrast, the thalami were only involved later on in the absence seizures. Our observation of increased connectivity in DMN agrees with these findings. However, the early change in DMN connectivity suggests the presence of a more complex process, with involvement of brain areas far from the epileptic focus. We observed increased DMN connectivity over a broad time window [−8 TRs (−18/−16 s) to 0 s], suggesting that this process may occur earlier than the early BOLD changes described in the literature (observed up to 9 s before the EEG event). Vaudano et al. has suggested that the DMN is involved in IED generation, with a causal link between early BOLD changes in DMN structures and the occurrence of IEDs (73). The latter researchers used dynamic causal modeling to investigate the involvement of the precuneus, thalamus, and prefrontal cortex in the spike and slow-wave discharges in IGE. They found that the onset of a generalized spike and slow-waves was linked to early activity in the posterior cingulate gyrus. This had already been suspected by Archer et al. (74) in five IGE patients, in whom only an negative BOLD response of the posterior cingulate gyrus was observed at the time of the IEDs. In the present study, we observed changes in the configuration of the DMN, with greater connectivity between the various DMN structures (including the posterior cingulate gyrus). This result corroborates Vaudano et al.'s finding. However, our study was not restricted to the PCC area and we further demonstrated that this early process affected other DMN nodes. Moreover, we found that this early process occurred in TLE patients and (albeit as a non-significant trend) in IGE patients. This implies that a specific configuration of the DMN is present before IEDs in both types of epilepsy. We suggest that in IGE, higher intrinsic connectivity in the DMN could activate the thalami and stimulate specific cortico-subcortical interactions required for generalized IEDs. We suggest that a similar process occurs in TLE: the change in DMN connectivity several seconds before the IED is characterized by a switch from the usual right predominance DMN pattern to a bilateral pattern (i.e., increased DMN connectivity in left TP, PHG, MTG, PCC, and dMPFC). This would mean that structures on the focus-side are transiently reconnected to other DMN nodes. This may increase the level of interaction between the DMN and the epileptic network. The IEDs in IGE and TLE may result from a particular interaction between a highly connected DMN and the epileptic network (a focalized, temporal network in TLE and a cortico-subcortical network in IGE).

This early switch in DMN configuration is not random and probably reflects a specific change in brain state. We speculate that the early DMN configuration reflects a physiologic fluctuation in brain state as a function of external or internal stimuli. This specific state may facilitate the occurrence of epileptic discharge. As mentioned above, the DMN is related to the consciousness state and is modulated by attention-demanding tasks. Interestingly, it has been firmly established that the occurrence of seizures and IEDs depends on the level of awareness (2). Although IEDs are responsible for disrupting normal function (leading to transient cognitive impairment at the time of the event) (75, 76), there is also evidence to suggest that cognitive tasks can directly affect the occurrence of IEDs (3). The level of attention also seems be related to the frequency of IEDs (2, 77, 78). Aart et al. (2) reported that the IED frequency in generalized and focal epileptic patients changed during cognitive testing. More recently, Matsumoto et al. (78) used a visual memory task to show that the IED rate fell as the gamma power preceding the IED onset increased. This high-frequency oscillation modulation was related to a memory-encoding task. Moreover, Fahoum et al. (17) demonstrated that DMN BOLD activity fell in parallel with the gamma band power in DMN components. Taken as a whole, these findings suggest that specific cognitive tasks (leading to gamma power fluctuations) or awareness fluctuations may change DMN connectivity and thus facilitate IED generation.

DMN connectivity changes after the IED time window

Compared with the "during IED" configuration, we observed greater connectivity of the right and left PCCs in TLE patients. There was no clear difference between the "after" and "baseline" periods. In the "during" period, we found that the PCC and the left-side temporal and parietal nodes were partly disconnected from the standard DMN nodes. Recovery of a baseline configuration means that the PCC has to be transiently hyperconnected to other DMN nodes (since the left-side temporal and parietal nodes are still disconnected). The PCC is less extensively connected to other DMN nodes during the IED, and this configuration is corrected after the IED. The role of the PCC in consciousness mechanisms has been studied; it appears to be the primary substrate for conscious awareness (79). Alteration of the PCC's function during cingulate gyrus epilepsy or absence epilepsy is associated with loss of consciousness. Transient cognitive impairment is observed during focal and generalized IEDs (75, 76). A change in PCC function may be one explanation. Our results show that the PCC's connectivity with other parts of the DMN may also be crucial for change in awareness during IEDs. As Laureys et al. (79) mentioned, the PCC has a pivotal role in consciousness/awareness regulation because of its anatomic position (with strong links to the anterior thalamus nucleus and the brainstem's arousal system in the thalamus). In the present study, we failed to reproduce this effect in the IGE group. It would be interesting to investigate the involvement of the PCC in a larger number of IGE patients.

METHODOLOGICAL CONSIDERATIONS AND PERSPECTIVES

Our study focused on the relationship between the IED and the DMN connectivity changes. This work was based on the recent observation that RSNs fluctuates over time (30–34) and the hypothesis that the epileptic activity may affect these fluctuations. For this purpose, dynamic connectivity was estimated using a sliding window approach described and validated by Chang et al. (31). If this methodological approach was suitable for our research hypothesis, it also raised several methodological issues.

Firstly, the main limitation of the present study was the small number of patients ($n = 6$) in each group. This was explained by the severe selection criteria (at least 10 isolated IEDs with an interval of at least 80 s between each IED were required). To perform relevant statistical analysis on these small size groups, non-parametric statistical analyses were used. This study is a preliminary work and it would be useful to increase the sample size for further analyses (especially to evaluate effect of disease duration, effect of antiepileptic drugs...) and to confirm our hypotheses. Secondly, the regions of interest of the DMN were chosen using a group-level spatial ICA of 198 healthy volunteers (76 males and 122 females) aged 18–26. The IGE patients were younger than the TLE patients and the healthy volunteers. This high range of ages is related to the different types of epilepsy. Indeed, if IGE is affecting mostly infants and adolescents, TLE is affecting young adults and adults. Previous studies of difference in DMN intrinsic connectivity between children and young adults (80, 81) found similar spatial patterns, with only weaker DMN connectivity and decreased spatial extent in the dMPFC in the children. As described in Section "DMN Connectivity at the Network Level," we found weaker DMN connectivity in the TLE group than in the IGE group. We performed the DMN integration comparisons between IGE and TLE patients using whole time series without the dMPFC node. This analysis yielded similar result. Hence, differences in mean age are unlikely to have biased our data on DMN functional connectivity changes. The wide range of the subject's ages could also be an issue for spatial normalization of fMRI data. Visual inspection of spatial normalization results was performed to detect abrupt differences in quality of registration between children and adults and no relation was found between this spatial normalization and age of subjects. Even if the effect of brain maturation cannot be totally ruled out on our results, the difference observed between IGEs and TLEs in term of DMN functional connectivity changes is likely to be due to the type of epileptic disorders and events. The two groups also exhibit a difference in gender (six females in TLE group and two females in IGE group). Our results are unlikely to be affected by this difference as the DMN connectivity has been shown to be robust and similar between sexes (82, 83). Thirdly, to define the different windows ("baseline," "before," "during," and "after") we used the IED timing. If the "during" and "after" windows are easy to define based on the timing and the short duration of each IED, the "baseline" and the "before" window may raise more difficulties. The epileptic activity in our work is defined by the occurrence of IEDs observed on scalp EEG. Scalp EEG can be blind to deeper epileptic activities especially in TLE patients. This point is a common limitation of the literature on EEG–fMRI studies. Facing this difficulty, authors focusing on functional resting-states networks used also the period of EEG without IEDs as the baseline to avoid interferences with epileptic activity (19). In our study, we can suggest that if this deeper epileptic activity had interfered on our results, because the occurrence of this specific activity would have been random, our results would have been statistically irrelevant. We showed that especially in TLEs our results on DMN intrinsic connectivity are statistically consistent. We suggest then that deeper epileptic activity is possible but is unlikely to affect our analysis. Intracerebral EEG (iEEG) recording simultaneously with fMRI may be one way to control this "deeper" epileptic activity. However, the spatial sample of intracerebral electrodes is also limited and can provide other bias. To go further, we checked that no BOLD change can be observed before the scalp IEDs timing. Indeed previous works showed that in IGE patients and in some cases of focal epilepsy (49, 50) an early BOLD change can be observed. This early BOLD change would affect the signal during the "before" window and provide heterogeneity between patients.

The dynamic connectivity was estimated using a sliding window approach. Thus, the length (L) of the windows was an important degree of freedom. The dependency of the window of length L were investigated in the present study, but the range ($L = \{6$ TRs, $\ldots$, 10 TRs$\}$) was limited due to the need of at least 4L between each IED. In fact, windows larger than $L = 10$ TRs (20 s/22.5 s) did not contain enough IEDs per subject. We varied the window size from 6 TRs to 10 TRs and did not find any statistically significant differences between the respective results (Figure S1 in Supplementary Material). We chose to report results with windows of length $L = 8$TRs because it provided a good trade-off between time resolution and the ability to compute regularized covariance matrices with a low standard deviation. Furthermore, the TR values in Kiel and in Lille were slightly different (2 s and 2.25 s, respectively). Although, a variation in TR can impact the quality of the BOLD signal, the slight overall difference (2 s for an 8 TR window) is unlikely to be significant. Moreover, we showed that larger windows (10 TRs) yielded the same results. The next step in the procedure was the estimation of DMN functional connectivity within the WOIs. Due to the relatively small window length, we decided to estimate the precision matrix (the inverse covariance matrix) rather than the covariance matrix. Use of the precision matrix is suitable when the number of connections is greater than the number of samples (as in the present study). However, different approaches could be used to study the dynamic functional connectivity of the DMN or other brain regions. In this study, the window length was a degree of freedom of our method. Other approaches to investigate the dynamic functional connectivity could be used to avoid the need of defining a window length. Previous studies were interested in dynamic functional connectivity without the need of defining WOIs. Two kinds of approaches have been used: (i) in looking for spatial patterns of dynamic connectivity and (ii) in investigating the temporal pattern of dynamic connectivity. Li et al. (84) showed that the time course of functional connectivity can be divided into quasi-stable segments via a sliding time window approach. These time segments were used to differentiate between healthy volunteers and patients with post-traumatic stress disorder. Ma et al. (85) used independent vector analysis to identify dynamic changes in spatial functional connectivity. The researchers found significantly more fluctuations and more variable patterns of spatial network concordance in schizophrenia patients than in healthy volunteers.

In the validation part of the present study, a graph analysis was used to compare the "before," "during," "after," and "baseline" WOIs in both the TLE and IGE groups. A multiscale network, node and edge analysis was applied. At the network and node-levels, many different network measures can be computed by calculating measures of integration and segregation (86). We chose to limit our analysis by measuring only DMN network integration at the network level and node strength and the clustering coefficient at the node-level. We selected these criteria because they are easier to interpret. Our results revealed inter-conditions differences in DMN intrinsic connectivity in both the TLE and IGE groups.

Small window lengths were used in this study (6, 8, and 10 TRs), which causes methodological issues in the estimation of the covariance matrix. Recently developed fMRI sequences could be used to increase the time resolution (i.e., by decreasing the TR). Significant shortening of TR has been achieved using "slice" multiplexing, in which multiple slices are excited and acquired simultaneously. This approach significantly increases statistical power in functional connectivity analyses (87).

Lastly, our previous research (88) showed that a wavelet-based approach can be used to detect epileptic activity in BOLD signals alone (i.e., without the need to record the EEG). Although this method was able to detect much the same spatial patterns of epileptic activity as EEG–fMRI, only a few IEDs were detected. The dynamic changes in DMN functional connectivity could be used to improve the sensitivity and specificity of this type of approach. In the future, we intend to combine both dynamic functional connectivity and the wavelet-based approach, with a view to improve the robustness of IEDs detection in the BOLD signal.

CONCLUSION

In the present study, we investigated dynamic changes in DMN intrinsic connectivity and their relation to epileptic activity. We showed that DMN connectivity is specifically affected by the IED occurrence. The greatest changes in DMN connectivity were observed before IEDs. These changes may be caused by specific brain states that facilitate IED generation. During and after IEDs, the observed change in DMN connectivity emphasized the pivotal role of the PCC in IED-related awareness fluctuations. Due to the low number of subjects, the results found in this study need to be confirmed in a larger independent cohort. Future research should investigate more precisely the relationship between the occurrence of IEDs and states of awareness/consciousness in epilepsy. The dynamic approach of the RSNs connectivity will provide a powerful tool to investigate IEDs and seizure physiopathological mechanisms.

REFERENCES

1. Van Bogaert P, Urbain C, Galer S, Ligot N, Peigneux P, De Tiege X. Impact of focal interictal epileptiform discharges on behaviour and cognition in children. *Neurophysiol Clin* (2012) **42**(1–2):53–8. doi:10.1016/j.neucli.2011.11.004
2. Aarts JH, Binnie CD, Smit AM, Wilkins AJ. Selective cognitive impairment during focal and generalized epileptiform EEG activity. *Brain* (1984) **107**(Pt 1):293–308. doi:10.1093/brain/107.1.293
3. Binnie CD, Marston D. Cognitive correlates of interictal discharges. *Epilepsia* (1992) **33**(Suppl 6):S11–7.
4. Kleen JK, Scott RC, Holmes GL, Roberts DW, Rundle MM, Testorf M, et al. Hippocampal interictal epileptiform activity disrupts cognition in humans. *Neurology* (2013) **81**(1):18–24. doi:10.1212/WNL.0b013e318297ee50
5. Blumenfeld H. Impaired consciousness in epilepsy. *Lancet Neurol* (2012) **11**(9):814–26. doi:10.1016/S1474-4422(12)70188-6
6. Gotman J, Grova C, Bagshaw A, Kobayashi E, Aghakhani Y, Dubeau F. Generalized epileptic discharges show thalamocortical activation and suspension of the default state of the brain. *Proc Natl Acad Sci U S A* (2005) **102**(42):15236–40. doi:10.1073/pnas.0504935102
7. Laufs H, Hamandi K, Salek-Haddadi A, Kleinschmidt AK, Duncan JS, Lemieux L. Temporal lobe interictal epileptic discharges affect cerebral activity in "default mode" brain regions. *Hum Brain Mapp* (2007) **28**(10):1023–32. doi:10.1002/hbm.20323
8. Morgan VL, Gore JC, Abou-Khalil B. Functional epileptic network in left mesial temporal lobe epilepsy detected using resting fMRI. *Epilepsy Res* (2010) **88**(2–3):168–78. doi:10.1016/j.eplepsyres.2009.10.018
9. Kobayashi E, Grova C, Tyvaert L, Dubeau F, Gotman J. Structures involved at the time of temporal lobe spikes revealed by interindividual group analysis of EEG/fMRI data. *Epilepsia* (2009) **50**(12):2549–56. doi:10.1111/j.1528-1167.2009.02180.x
10. Buckner RL, Andrews-Hanna JR, Schacter DL. The brain's default network: anatomy, function, and relevance to disease. *Ann N Y Acad Sci* (2008) **1124**:1–38. doi:10.1196/annals.1440.011
11. Fox MD, Snyder AZ, Vincent JL, Corbetta M, Van Essen DC, Raichle ME. The human brain is intrinsically organized into dynamic, anticorrelated functional networks. *Proc Natl Acad Sci U S A* (2005) **102**(27):9673–8. doi:10.1073/pnas.0504136102

12. Greicius MD, Krasnow B, Reiss AL, Menon V. Functional connectivity in the resting brain: a network analysis of the default mode hypothesis. *Proc Natl Acad Sci U S A* (2003) **100**(1):253–8. doi:10.1073/pnas.0135058100
13. Raichle ME, MacLeod AM, Snyder AZ, Powers WJ, Gusnard DA, Shulman GL. A default mode of brain function. *Proc Natl Acad Sci U S A* (2001) **98**(2):676–82. doi:10.1073/pnas.98.2.676
14. Shulman GL, Fiez JA, Corbetta M, Buckner RL, Miezin FM, Raichle ME, et al. Common blood flow changes across visual tasks: II. Decreases in cerebral cortex. *J Cogn Neurosci* (1997) **9**(5):648–63. doi:10.1162/jocn.1997.9.5.648
15. Blumenfeld H. Consciousness and epilepsy: why are patients with absence seizures absent? *Prog Brain Res* (2005) **150**:271–86. doi:10.1016/S0079-6123(05)50020-7
16. Hamandi K, Salek-Haddadi A, Laufs H, Liston A, Friston K, Fish DR, et al. EEG-fMRI of idiopathic and secondarily generalized epilepsies. *Neuroimage* (2006) **31**(4):1700–10. doi:10.1016/j.neuroimage.2006.02.016
17. Fahoum F, Zelmann R, Tyvaert L, Dubeau F, Gotman J. Epileptic discharges affect the default mode network – fMRI and intracerebral EEG evidence. *PLoS One* (2013) **8**(6):e68038. doi:10.1371/journal.pone.0068038
18. Jeong B, Choi J, Kim JW. MRI study on the functional and spatial consistency of resting state-related independent components of the brain network. *Korean J Radiol* (2012) **13**(3):265–74. doi:10.3348/kjr.2012.13.3.265
19. Greicius MD, Supekar K, Menon V, Dougherty RF. Resting-state functional connectivity reflects structural connectivity in the default mode network. *Cereb Cortex* (2009) **19**(1):72–8. doi:10.1093/cercor/bhn059
20. Skudlarski P, Jagannathan K, Calhoun VD, Hampson M, Skudlarska BA, Pearlson G. Measuring brain connectivity: diffusion tensor imaging validates resting state temporal correlations. *Neuroimage* (2008) **43**(3):554–61. doi:10.1016/j.neuroimage.2008.07.063
21. Kay BP, DiFrancesco MW, Privitera MD, Gotman J, Holland SK, Szaflarski JP. Reduced default mode network connectivity in treatment-resistant idiopathic generalized epilepsy. *Epilepsia* (2013) **54**(3):461–70. doi:10.1111/epi.12057
22. Luo C, Li Q, Lai Y, Xia Y, Qin Y, Liao W, et al. Altered functional connectivity in default mode network in absence epilepsy: a resting-state fMRI study. *Hum Brain Mapp* (2011) **32**(3):438–49. doi:10.1002/hbm.21034
23. McGill ML, Devinsky O, Kelly C, Milham M, Castellanos FX, Quinn BT, et al. Default mode network abnormalities in idiopathic generalized epilepsy. *Epilepsy Behav* (2012) **23**(3):353–9. doi:10.1016/j.yebeh.2012.01.013
24. Song M, Du H, Wu N, Hou B, Wu G, Wang J, et al. Impaired resting-state functional integrations within default mode network of generalized tonic-clonic seizures epilepsy. *PLoS One* (2011) **6**(2):e17294. doi:10.1371/journal.pone.0017294
25. Frings L, Schulze-Bonhage A, Spreer J, Wagner K. Remote effects of hippocampal damage on default network connectivity in the human brain. *J Neurol* (2009) **256**(12):2021–9. doi:10.1007/s00415-009-5233-0
26. Haneef Z, Lenartowicz A, Yeh HJ, Engel J Jr, Stern JM. Effect of lateralized temporal lobe epilepsy on the default mode network. *Epilepsy Behav* (2012) **25**(3):350–7. doi:10.1016/j.yebeh.2012.07.019
27. Liao W, Zhang Z, Pan Z, Mantini D, Ding J, Duan X, et al. Altered functional connectivity and small-world in mesial temporal lobe epilepsy. *PLoS One* (2010) **5**(1):e8525. doi:10.1371/journal.pone.0008525
28. Zhang Z, Lu G, Zhong Y, Tan Q, Liao W, Wang Z, et al. Altered spontaneous neuronal activity of the default-mode network in mesial temporal lobe epilepsy. *Brain Res* (2010) **1323**:152–60. doi:10.1016/j.brainres.2010.01.042
29. Pittau F, Grova C, Moeller F, Dubeau F, Gotman J. Patterns of altered functional connectivity in mesial temporal lobe epilepsy. *Epilepsia* (2012) **53**(6):1013–23. doi:10.1111/j.1528-1167.2012.03464.x
30. Allen EA, Damaraju E, Plis SM, Erhardt EB, Eichele T, Calhoun VD. Tracking whole-brain connectivity dynamics in the resting state. *Cereb Cortex* (2014) **24**(3):663–76. doi:10.1093/cercor/bhs352
31. Chang C, Glover GH. Time-frequency dynamics of resting-state brain connectivity measured with fMRI. *Neuroimage* (2010) **50**(1):81–98. doi:10.1016/j.neuroimage.2009.12.011
32. Di X, Biswal BB. Dynamic brain functional connectivity modulated by resting-state networks. *Brain Struct Funct* (2013). doi:10.1007/s00429-013-0634-3
33. Handwerker DA, Roopchansingh V, Gonzalez-Castillo J, Bandettini PA. Periodic changes in fMRI connectivity. *Neuroimage* (2012) **63**(3):1712–9. doi:10.1016/j.neuroimage.2012.06.078
34. Kang J, Wang L, Yan C, Wang J, Liang X, He Y. Characterizing dynamic functional connectivity in the resting brain using variable parameter regression and Kalman filtering approaches. *Neuroimage* (2011) **56**(3):1222–34. doi:10.1016/j.neuroimage.2011.03.033
35. Tagliazucchi E, von Wegner F, Morzelewski A, Brodbeck V, Laufs H. Dynamic BOLD functional connectivity in humans and its electrophysiological correlates. *Front Hum Neurosci* (2012) **6**:339. doi:10.3389/fnhum.2012.00339
36. Liao W, Zhang Z, Mantini D, Xu Q, Ji GJ, Zhang H, et al. Dynamical intrinsic functional architecture of the brain during absence seizures. *Brain Struct Funct* (2013). doi:10.1007/s00429-013-0619-2
37. Allen PJ, Josephs O, Turner R. A method for removing imaging artifact from continuous EEG recorded during functional MRI. *Neuroimage* (2000) **12**(2):230–9. doi:10.1006/nimg.2000.0599
38. Benar C, Aghakhani Y, Wang Y, Izenberg A, Al-Asmi A, Dubeau F, et al. Quality of EEG in simultaneous EEG-fMRI for epilepsy. *Clin Neurophysiol* (2003) **114**(3):569–80. doi:10.1016/S1388-2457(02)00383-8
39. Behzadi Y, Restom K, Liau J, Liu TT. A component based noise correction method (CompCor) for BOLD and perfusion based fMRI. *Neuroimage* (2007) **37**(1):90–101. doi:10.1016/j.neuroimage.2007.04.042
40. Chai XJ, Castanon AN, Ongur D, Whitfield-Gabrieli S. Anticorrelations in resting state networks without global signal regression. *Neuroimage* (2012) **59**(2):1420–8. doi:10.1016/j.neuroimage.2011.08.048
41. Damoiseaux JS, Rombouts SA, Barkhof F, Scheltens P, Stam CJ, Smith SM, et al. Consistent resting-state networks across healthy subjects. *Proc Natl Acad Sci U S A* (2006) **103**(37):13848–53. doi:10.1073/pnas.0601417103
42. Wang J, Zuo X, He Y. Graph-based network analysis of resting-state functional MRI. *Front Syst Neurosci* (2010) **4**:16. doi:10.3389/fnsys.2010.00016
43. Kriegeskorte N, Simmons WK, Bellgowan PS, Baker CI. Circular analysis in systems neuroscience: the dangers of double dipping. *Nat Neurosci* (2009) **12**(5):535–40. doi:10.1038/nn.2303
44. Friedman J, Hastie T, Tibshirani R. Sparse inverse covariance estimation with the graphical lasso. *Biostatistics* (2008) **9**(3):432–41. doi:10.1093/biostatistics/kxm045
45. Tibshirani R. Regression shrinkage and selection via the Lasso. *J R Stat Soc Series B Stat Methodol* (1996) **58**(1):267–88.
46. Allen EA, Erhardt EB, Damaraju E, Gruner W, Segall JM, Silva RF, et al. A baseline for the multivariate comparison of resting-state networks. *Front Syst Neurosci* (2011) **5**:2. doi:10.3389/fnsys.2011.00002
47. Cribben I, Haraldsdottir R, Atlas LY, Wager TD, Lindquist MA. Dynamic connectivity regression: determining state-related changes in brain connectivity. *Neuroimage* (2012) **61**(4):907–20. doi:10.1016/j.neuroimage.2012.03.070
48. Varoquaux G, Baronnet F, Kleinschmidt A, Fillard P, Thirion B. Detection of brain functional-connectivity difference in post-stroke patients using group-level covariance modeling. *Med Image Comput Comput Assist Interv* (2010) **6361**:200–8. doi:10.1007/978-3-642-15705-9_25
49. Hawco CS, Bagshaw AP, Lu Y, Dubeau F, Gotman J. BOLD changes occur prior to epileptic spikes seen on scalp EEG. *Neuroimage* (2007) **35**(4):1450–8. doi:10.1016/j.neuroimage.2006.12.042
50. Jacobs J, Levan P, Moeller F, Boor R, Stephani U, Gotman J, et al. Hemodynamic changes preceding the interictal EEG spike in patients with focal epilepsy investigated using simultaneous EEG-fMRI. *Neuroimage* (2009) **45**(4):1220–31. doi:10.1016/j.neuroimage.2009.01.014
51. Moeller F, Siebner HR, Wolff S, Muhle H, Granert O, Jansen O, et al. Simultaneous EEG-fMRI in drug-naive children with newly diagnosed absence epilepsy. *Epilepsia* (2008) **49**(9):1510–9. doi:10.1111/j.1528-1167.2008.01626.x
52. Marrelec G, Bellec P, Krainik A, Duffau H, Pelegrini-Issac M, Lehericy S, et al. Regions, systems, and the brain: hierarchical measures of functional integration in fMRI. *Med Image Anal* (2008) **12**(4):484–96. doi:10.1016/j.media.2008.02.002
53. Zalesky A, Fornito A, Bullmore ET. Network-based statistic: identifying differences in brain networks. *Neuroimage* (2010) **53**(4):1197–207. doi:10.1016/j.neuroimage.2010.06.041
54. Xue K, Luo C, Zhang D, Yang T, Li J, Gong D, et al. Diffusion tensor tractography reveals disrupted structural connectivity in childhood absence epilepsy. *Epilepsy Res* (2014) **108**(1):125–38. doi:10.1016/j.eplepsyres.2013.10.002
55. Besson P, Dinkelacker V, Valabregue R, Thivard L, Leclerc X, Baulac M, et al. Structural connectivity differences in left and right temporal lobe epilepsy. *Neuroimage* (2014) **100**:135–44. doi:10.1016/j.neuroimage.2014.04.071

56. Xia M, Wang J, He Y. BrainNet Viewer: a network visualization tool for human brain connectomics. *PLoS One* (2013) **8**(7):e68910. doi:10.1371/journal.pone.0068910
57. Engel J Jr. International League Against Epilepsy (ILAE). A proposed diagnostic scheme for people with epileptic seizures and with epilepsy: report of the ILAE Task Force on Classification and Terminology. *Epilepsia* (2001) **42**(6):796–803. doi:10.1046/j.1528-1157.2001.10401.x
58. Wang Z, Lu G, Zhang Z, Zhong Y, Jiao Q, Zhang Z, et al. Altered resting state networks in epileptic patients with generalized tonic-clonic seizures. *Brain Res* (2011) **1374**:134–41. doi:10.1016/j.brainres.2010.12.034
59. Aghakhani Y, Bagshaw AP, Benar CG, Hawco C, Andermann F, Dubeau F, et al. fMRI activation during spike and wave discharges in idiopathic generalized epilepsy. *Brain* (2004) **127**(Pt 5):1127–44. doi:10.1093/brain/awh136
60. Berg AT, Berkovic SF, Brodie MJ, Buchhalter J, Cross JH, van Emde Boas W, et al. Revised terminology and concepts for organization of seizures and epilepsies: report of the ILAE commission on classification and terminology, 2005-2009. *Epilepsia* (2010) **51**(4):676–85. doi:10.1111/j.1528-1167.2010.02522.x
61. Bernhardt BC, Rozen DA, Worsley KJ, Evans AC, Bernasconi N, Bernasconi A. Thalamo-cortical network pathology in idiopathic generalized epilepsy: insights from MRI-based morphometric correlation analysis. *Neuroimage* (2009) **46**(2):373–81. doi:10.1016/j.neuroimage.2009.01.055
62. Blumenfeld H. From molecules to networks: cortical/subcortical interactions in the pathophysiology of idiopathic generalized epilepsy. *Epilepsia* (2003) **44**(Suppl 2):7–15. doi:10.1046/j.1528-1157.44.s.2.2.x
63. Blumenfeld H. Cellular and network mechanisms of spike-wave seizures. *Epilepsia* (2005) **46**(Suppl 9):21–33. doi:10.1111/j.1528-1167.2005.00311.x
64. Blumenfeld H, Taylor J. Why do seizures cause loss of consciousness? *Neuroscientist* (2003) **9**(5):301–10. doi:10.1177/1073858403255624
65. Cavanna AE, Monaco F. Brain mechanisms of altered conscious states during epileptic seizures. *Nat Rev Neurol* (2009) **5**(5):267–76. doi:10.1038/nrneurol.2009.38
66. Bai X, Vestal M, Berman R, Negishi M, Spann M, Vega C, et al. Dynamic time course of typical childhood absence seizures: EEG, behavior, and functional magnetic resonance imaging. *J Neurosci* (2010) **30**(17):5884–93. doi:10.1523/JNEUROSCI.5101-09.2010
67. Moeller F, LeVan P, Muhle H, Stephani U, Dubeau F, Siniatchkin M, et al. Absence seizures: individual patterns revealed by EEG-fMRI. *Epilepsia* (2010) **51**(10):2000–10. doi:10.1111/j.1528-1167.2010.02698.x
68. Deco G, Jirsa VK, McIntosh AR. Emerging concepts for the dynamical organization of resting-state activity in the brain. *Nat Rev Neurosci* (2011) **12**(1):43–56. doi:10.1038/nrn2961
69. Roche-Labarbe N, Zaaimi B, Berquin P, Nehlig A, Grebe R, Wallois F. NIRS-measured oxy- and deoxy-hemoglobin changes associated with EEG spike-and-wave discharges in children. *Epilepsia* (2008) **49**(11):1871–80. doi:10.1111/j.1528-1167.2008.01711.x
70. Tyvaert L, LeVan P, Dubeau F, Gotman J. Noninvasive dynamic imaging of seizures in epileptic patients. *Hum Brain Mapp* (2009) **30**(12):3993–4011. doi:10.1002/hbm.20824
71. Zhao M, Nguyen J, Ma H, Nishimura N, Schaffer CB, Schwartz TH. Preictal and ictal neurovascular and metabolic coupling surrounding a seizure focus. *J Neurosci* (2011) **31**(37):13292–300. doi:10.1523/JNEUROSCI.2597-11.2011
72. Zhao M, Suh M, Ma H, Perry C, Geneslaw A, Schwartz TH. Focal increases in perfusion and decreases in hemoglobin oxygenation precede seizure onset in spontaneous human epilepsy. *Epilepsia* (2007) **48**(11):2059–67. doi:10.1111/j.1528-1167.2007.01229.x
73. Vaudano AE, Laufs H, Kiebel SJ, Carmichael DW, Hamandi K, Guye M, et al. Causal hierarchy within the thalamo-cortical network in spike and wave discharges. *PLoS One* (2009) **4**(8):e6475. doi:10.1371/journal.pone.0006475
74. Archer JS, Abbott DF, Waites AB, Jackson GD. fMRI "deactivation" of the posterior cingulate during generalized spike and wave. *Neuroimage* (2003) **20**(4):1915–22. doi:10.1016/S1053-8119(03)00294-5
75. Holmes GL, Lenck-Santini PP. Role of interictal epileptiform abnormalities in cognitive impairment. *Epilepsy Behav* (2006) **8**(3):504–15. doi:10.1016/j.yebeh.2005.11.014
76. Kleen JK, Scott RC, Holmes GL, Lenck-Santini PP. Hippocampal interictal spikes disrupt cognition in rats. *Ann Neurol* (2010) **67**(2):250–7. doi:10.1002/ana.21896
77. Guey J, Bureau M, Dravet C, Roger J. A study of the rhythm of petit mal absences in children in relation to prevailing situations. The use of EEG telemetry during psychological examinations, school exercises and periods of inactivity. *Epilepsia* (1969) **10**(4):441–51.
78. Matsumoto JY, Stead M, Kucewicz MT, Matsumoto AJ, Peters PA, Brinkmann BH, et al. Network oscillations modulate interictal epileptiform spike rate during human memory. *Brain* (2013) **136**(Pt 8):2444–56. doi:10.1093/brain/awt159
79. Laureys S, Owen A, Schiff N. Coma science: clinical and ethical implications. Preface. *Prog Brain Res* (2009) **177**:13–4. doi:10.1016/S0079-6123(09)17736-1
80. Supekar K, Uddin LQ, Prater K, Amin H, Greicius MD, Menon V. Development of functional and structural connectivity within the default mode network in young children. *Neuroimage* (2010) **52**(1):290–301. doi:10.1016/j.neuroimage.2010.04.009
81. Thomason ME, Chang CE, Glover GH, Gabrieli JD, Greicius MD, Gotlib IH. Default-mode function and task-induced deactivation have overlapping brain substrates in children. *Neuroimage* (2008) **41**(4):1493–503. doi:10.1016/j.neuroimage.2008.03.029
82. Bluhm RL, Osuch EA, Lanius RA, Boksman K, Neufeld RW, Theberge J, et al. Default mode network connectivity: effects of age, sex, and analytic approach. *Neuroreport* (2008) **19**(8):887–91. doi:10.1097/WNR.0b013e328300ebbf
83. Weissman-Fogel I, Moayedi M, Taylor KS, Pope G, Davis KD. Cognitive and default-mode resting state networks: do male and female brains "rest" differently? *Hum Brain Mapp* (2010) **31**(11):1713–26. doi:10.1002/hbm.20968
84. Li X, Zhu D, Jiang X, Jin C, Zhang X, Guo L, et al. Dynamic functional connectomics signatures for characterization and differentiation of PTSD patients. *Hum Brain Mapp* (2014) **35**(4):1761–78. doi:10.1002/hbm.22290
85. Ma S, Calhoun VD, Phlypo R, Adali T. Dynamic changes of spatial functional network connectivity in healthy individuals and schizophrenia patients using independent vector analysis. *Neuroimage* (2014) **90**:196–206. doi:10.1016/j.neuroimage.2013.12.063
86. Rubinov M, Sporns O. Complex network measures of brain connectivity: uses and interpretations. *Neuroimage* (2010) **52**(3):1059–69. doi:10.1016/j.neuroimage.2009.10.003
87. Feinberg DA, Moeller S, Smith SM, Auerbach E, Ramanna S, Gunther M, et al. Multiplexed echo planar imaging for sub-second whole brain fMRI and fast diffusion imaging. *PLoS One* (2010) **5**(12):e15710. doi:10.1371/journal.pone.0015710
88. Lopes R, Lina JM, Fahoum F, Gotman J. Detection of epileptic activity in fMRI without recording the EEG. *Neuroimage* (2012) **60**(3):1867–79. doi:10.1016/j.neuroimage.2011.12.083

3

Identification of pre-spike network in patients with mesial temporal lobe epilepsy

Nahla L. Faizo[1], Hana Burianová[1,2], Marcus Gray[1], Julia Hocking[1,3], Graham Galloway[1] and David Reutens[1,4]*

[1] Centre for Advanced Imaging, University of Queensland, Brisbane, QLD, Australia
[2] ARC Centre of Excellence in Cognition and its Disorders, Macquarie University, Sydney, NSW, Australia
[3] School of Psychology and Counseling, Queensland University of Technology, Brisbane, QLD, Australia
[4] Royal Brisbane and Women's Hospital, Brisbane, QLD, Australia

***Correspondence:**
David Reutens, Centre for Advanced Imaging, The University of Queensland, Brisbane, QLD 4072, Australia
e-mail: d.reutens@uq.edu.au

Background: Seizures and interictal spikes in mesial temporal lobe epilepsy (MTLE) affect a network of brain regions rather than a single epileptic focus. Simultaneous electroencephalography and functional magnetic resonance imaging (EEG-fMRI) studies have demonstrated a functional network in which hemodynamic changes are time-locked to spikes. However, whether this reflects the propagation of neuronal activity from a focus, or conversely the activation of a network linked to spike generation remains unknown. The functional connectivity (FC) changes prior to spikes may provide information about the connectivity changes that lead to the generation of spikes. We used EEG-fMRI to investigate FC changes immediately prior to the appearance of interictal spikes on EEG in patients with MTLE.

Methods/principal findings: Fifteen patients with MTLE underwent continuous EEG-fMRI during rest. Spikes were identified on EEG and three 10 s epochs were defined relative to spike onset: spike (0–10 s), pre-spike (−10 to 0 s), and rest (−20 to −10 s, with no previous spikes in the preceding 45s). Significant spike-related activation in the hippocampus ipsilateral to the seizure focus was found compared to the pre-spike and rest epochs. The peak voxel within the hippocampus ipsilateral to the seizure focus was used as a seed region for FC analysis in the three conditions. A significant change in FC patterns was observed before the appearance of electrographic spikes. Specifically, there was significant loss of coherence between both hippocampi during the pre-spike period compared to spike and rest states.

Conclusion/significance: In keeping with previous findings of abnormal inter-hemispheric hippocampal connectivity in MTLE, our findings specifically link reduced connectivity to the period immediately before spikes. This brief decoupling is consistent with a deficit in mutual (inter-hemispheric) hippocampal inhibition that may predispose to spike generation.

Keywords: interictal spikes, hippocampus, mesial temporal lobe epilepsy, EEG-fMRI, functional connectivity, network

INTRODUCTION

Mesial temporal lobe epilepsy (MTLE) is the most common symptomatic focal epilepsy and is frequently associated with hippocampal sclerosis (HS), i.e., neuronal cell loss and gliosis of the hippocampus (1, 2). While HS has been understood to represent a focal neuro-pathological alteration linked to the generation of seizures (i.e., the epileptogenic focus) (3), not all patients become seizure free after surgical resection of the hippocampus (4). Hence, the concept of the epileptogenic focus has been revised to incorporate the involvement of an "epileptogenic network" of brain regions, in which the hippocampus is a key component (5).

Epileptogenic networks have been explored via single photon emission computed tomography (SPECT) (6), positron emission tomography (PET) (7), and simultaneous electroencephalography (EEG) and functional magnetic resonance imaging (EEG-fMRI) (8). Of these, EEG-fMRI has the potential to be the most informative, as it is able to provide highly spatially resolved three-dimensional maps of brain activation (fMRI), which can be linked to interictal electrical discharges seen on EEG. EEG-fMRI studies in patients with MTLE have demonstrated widespread activation and deactivation in temporal lobe structures, particularly in the hippocampus ipsilateral to scalp recorded interictal spikes, as well as in extra-temporal regions (9, 10). Perhaps more importantly, EEG-fMRI findings have also demonstrated hemodynamic alterations that occur immediately prior to interictal spikes (11, 12). These pre-spike BOLD changes were reported by Jacobs et al. (13) to be more focal than spike-triggered alterations reported by Kobayashi et al. (8) and Salek-Haddadi et al. (14), suggesting that hemodynamic alterations preceding interictal spikes may provide better localization of regions involved in spike generation (8, 13, 14).

A common way to identify functional brain networks is to assess functional connectivity (FC) between spatially separated regions. FC measures the degree of covariance between the activity in a specific brain region and other areas across the whole brain. In MTLE, decreased FC in ipsilateral mesial temporal lobe networks and increased contralateral compensatory connectivity during the interictal state have been reported (15, 16). Delineation of FC patterns related to interictal spikes may be useful in shedding light on the mechanisms that underlie these changes, and potentially MTLE seizures. Although the exact physiologic relationship between interictal spikes and seizures are not fully understood (17, 18), there is a growing evidence that the neural network involved in generating interictal spikes is a reliable estimator of the network that generates seizures (19–21). The aim of this study was to use EEG-fMRI to investigate FC changes immediately prior to the appearance of interictal spikes on EEG in patients with MTLE.

MATERIALS AND METHODS

PARTICIPANTS

Fifteen patients (9 females, mean age: 38 years; 6 males, mean age: 42 years) with MTLE (10 left and 5 right lateralized) and 15 age-matched healthy controls participated in the study. Patients were recruited from the Royal Brisbane and Women's Hospital Epilepsy clinic, whereas healthy participants were recruited via the University of Queensland Human Research volunteer scheme. All patients underwent comprehensive clinical assessment and the diagnosis of MTLE was based on the following: (a) seizure semiology consistent with MTLE; (b) interictal spikes confirmed during in-patient video-EEG monitoring performed within the last year, and (c) MRI scan consistent with a temporal lobe focus (no lesion or ipsilateral HS). Patient exclusion criteria included absence of interictal spikes during monitoring, recurrent unprovoked seizures, and the presence of metal implants. Patients' clinical details and spike distributions are summarized in **Table 1**. Only one patient had been free of seizures for 6 months and recurrent seizures occurred in the remainder. All EEG-fMRI recordings were acquired during the interictal state. Healthy controls were screened for current or previous brain injury, neurological, or psychiatric disorders. All participants provided written informed consent prior to enrollment, and the study was approved by the Human Research Ethics Committee (HREC) at the Royal Brisbane Women's Hospital (RBWH) and the Centre for Advanced Imaging, the University of Queensland.

PROCEDURE

The study was conducted at the Centre for Advanced Imaging, the University of Queensland. An MRI compatible 64-channel electrode cap was positioned on patients' heads according to the international 10:20 system and prepared with a conductive non-abrasive gel (chloride 10%). All electrodes, including the ground (AFz) and reference electrodes (FCz) impedances, were below 5 kΩ. One additional electrode recorded ECG from the chest. Patients then underwent a 40-min simultaneous EEG-fMRI recording, having been instructed to remain still, awake, and relaxed with their eyes closed. Healthy control participants underwent only resting state fMRI without the EEG recording.

EEG DATA ACQUISITION AND PREPROCESSING

Electroencephalography was acquired with an MR-compatible Brain Products EEG System (Brain Products, Gilching, Germany), using a 64-channels cap with silver silver/chloride (Ag/AgCl) electrodes. EEG data were recorded using Brain Vision Recorder software version 1.20.0001 (Brainproducts Co., Munich,

Table 1 | Summary of the patients' clinical details and spike distribution

Patients	Lateralization of epilepsy	Age of epilepsy onset	Duration of the disease (years)	Clinical MRI	Total number of spikes across 6 runs	AEDs
1	R	21	12	HS	47	Levetiracetam, gabapentin, clobazam
2	L	20	25	N	None	Levetiracetam
3	R	14	7	N	None	Levetiracetam, clobazam, valproate
4	R	21	26	HS	52	Levetiracetam, carbamazepine, valproate
5	R	21	2	N	None	Lamotrigine, carbamazepine, valproate
6	L	30	25	N	50	Levetiracetam, lamotrigine
7	L	17	6	N	24	Lamotrigine
8	R	16	14	HS	None	Levetiracetam, oxacarbazepine, clobazam
9	L	20	24	N	49	Levetiracetam, lamotrigine, phenytoin
10	L	17	3	N	35	Pregabalin, cabamazepine
11	L	25	7	N	32	Lamotrigine, oxacarbazepine, topiramate
12	L	23	21	N	54	Levetiracetam, lacosamide, valproate
13	R	35	2	N	37	Lacosamide
14	L	4	55	N	32	Carbamazepine, phenytoin, clonazepam
15	L	25	8	N	34	Carbamazepine, levetiracetam, lamotrigine, valproate

R, right; L, left; HS, hippocampal sclerosis; N, normal; none, no spikes have been identified during EEG-fMRI; AEDs, anti-epileptic drugs.

Germany). After recording, EEG datasets were preprocessed using EEGLAB software (22). Gradient artifacts introduced by MRI scanning were corrected with the Artifact Slice Template Removal (FASTR) algorithm (23, 24). Low pass (70 Hz), high pass (1 Hz), and notch (50–60 Hz) filtering were then used to remove frequency movement artifacts. An optimal basis set was formed to define the variations in the pulse artifact and create a template, which was then subtracted from the EEG data. Residual artifacts were removed using independent component analysis (ICA). An expert neurologist then reviewed the preprocessed EEG records to identify interictal spikes. Three out of the 15 patients did not show any spikes throughout the recording, and the EEG of one other patient contained movement artifacts. These data were not included in further analysis.

fMRI DATA ACQUISITION AND PREPROCESSING

Structural and functional MR data were acquired using a 3 T Siemens Magnetom Trio scanner, with a 12-channel head coil. fMRI-BOLD weighted images with full brain coverage were acquired with a single-shot gradient-echo planar image sequence (36 slices, TR = 2500 ms, TE = 30 ms, flip angle = 90°, matrix = 64 × 64, 3.3 mm isotropic voxels). T1-weighted (MP-RAGE) anatomical images were acquired (192 slices, TR = 1900 ms, TE = 2.13 ms, flip angle = 9°, matrix = 192 × 256 × 256, 0.9 mm isotropic voxels). EEG-fMRI data were collected in six runs, with each EPI run lasting 5:05 min, and the anatomical images 4:35 min.

MRI preprocessing was conducted using SPM8 (Wellcome Trust Centre for Neuroimaging, London, UK), in Matlab (Mathworks, Sherborne, MA, USA) (http://www.fil.ion.ucl.ac.uk/spm/software/spm8/). Functional images were slice time corrected, realigned, and normalized via the SPM8 Segment routine prior to spatial smoothing with an 8 mm FWHM isotropic Gaussian kernel.

fMRI ANALYSIS

Functional magnetic resonance imaging analysis was conducted in four steps, using *Partial Least Square* (PLS) software (25, 26). First, event-related analysis was used to identify activation in mesial temporal lobe, and, in particular, in the hippocampus ipsilateral to the seizure focus. Second, we examined the time course of activity within the hippocampal region. Third, we examined the FC of the peak voxel in this cluster to delineate large-scale networks during the spike, pre-spike, and rest periods. Finally, we tested whether the FC maps from the previous analysis were correlated with seizure recency, i.e., time from the last seizure. The three 10 s periods were defined relative to spike onset on EEG: spike (0–10 s), pre-spike (−10 to 0 s), and rest (i.e., baseline) (−20 to −10 s, with no previous spikes in the preceding 45 s). This time window was chosen because the hemodynamic response function returns to baseline 25 s after a single burst of neural activity (i.e., the interictal spike). Our study was designed to examine short-term changes in connectivity, and was based on previous findings that pre-spike BOLD signal alterations are evident up to 9 s before interictal spikes (13, 27). On this basis, we selected the interval between 25 s after a spike and 10 s before the next spike as baseline. A total of 186 spike onsets were included in the analysis. Images from patients with right TLE were flipped along the antero–posterior axis, so that in all patients the seizure focus was on the left. Therefore, all results were expressed as ipsilateral or contralateral, referring to the spikes recognized on the EEG.

Partial Least Square is a multivariate tool that enables delineation of distributed brain regions in relation to task demands (task PLS), behavioral performance (behavior PLS), or activity in a given seed region (seed PLS). Briefly, PLS uses singular value decomposition (SVD) of a single matrix that contains all participants' data to identify latent variables (LVs) that explain the covariance in the data. Each LV consists of three components: singular image of brain saliences (the brain image that best reflects the correlation of the task or behavior changes across conditions), design saliences (a set of weights that indicate the relationship between brain activity in a singular brain image and each of the assigned conditions), and singular value (the amount of covariance captured by the LV). For each LV in each condition, brain scores are calculated by multiplying each voxel's salience by the normalized BOLD signal value in the voxel, and summing across all brain voxels for each subject. Conceptually, brain scores represent the weighted average of the contribution each voxel makes to the specific pattern of connectivity. The statistical assessment is determined using a permutation test and bootstrap estimation of standard errors for the brain (voxel) saliences. Permutation tests assess the significance of the LV by resampling the singular value with participants being randomly reassigned (without replacement) to different conditions. Bootstrap resampling is independent of permutation, assessing by resampling the voxel saliences with replacement of subjects but maintained assignment of participants to conditions. Resampling with 100 bootstrap steps was satisfactory to estimate standard error of the voxel weights/saliences (bootstrap ratio or BSR) for each LV. Peak voxels above BSR of 3 (i.e., $p < 0.002$) were considered reliable. Corrections for multiple comparisons were not required because the extractions of brain saliences are calculated in a single mathematical step on the whole brain.

Event-related task PLS was conducted to identify spike-related activation. Then, the peak voxel time course within the activated region in the ipsilateral hippocampus was tested across the three epochs with four TRs per epoch, each TR being 2500 ms. PLS connectivity analysis was conducted using the peak voxel activated by spikes in the ipsilateral hippocampus as the seed voxel. BOLD signal intensities in that voxel were extracted and correlated with every other voxel in the brain in each condition across all subjects. The correlation of brain activity between the seed voxel and every other voxel in the brain across different conditions and subjects was calculated and stacked into a single combined matrix of correlations called the behavior matrix. The behavior matrix was then decomposed with SVD into a set of LVs that describe the network/regions (FC pattern) that correlated with the ipsilateral hippocampal activity in different conditions. Finally, to examine the relation between FC patterns in the three states (spike, pre-spike, and rest) and seizure recency, we conducted seed/behavior analysis by adding the time from last seizure (in weeks) as a variable in the subsequent PLS connectivity analysis. We were thus able to assess whether spike, pre-spike, or resting FC maps, defined in relation to the ipsilateral hippocampus, were related to interval from last seizure.

RESULTS

WHOLE BRAIN ANALYSIS

Event-related task PLS analysis of spike, pre-spike, and rest states yielded significant activity in the ipsilateral mesial temporal structures. As hypothesized, spike-related activation was seen in the ipsilateral hippocampus (relative to pre-spike) and was accompanied by increased activity in the ipsilateral parahippocampal gyrus, middle temporal gyrus, precuneus, contralateral middle temporal gyrus, and insula (**Figure 1**; **Table 2**). Additionally, activity in the ipsilateral medial frontal gyrus and the right inferior and superior frontal gyri were decreased during interictal spikes, relative to the pre-spike period.

Analysis of the time course and degree of activation in the peak voxel within the ipsilateral hippocampal cluster (MNI coordinates; −21, −27, −12) revealed a decrease in ipsilateral hippocampal activity during the 10 s pre-spike period when compared to rest and spike conditions (**Figure 2**). Paired t-tests showed that spike and pre-spike time courses differed significantly between TR1′, TR2′ during pre-spike and TR2″,TR3″ during spike ($p = 0.002$, $p = 0.005$, respectively).

FUNCTIONAL CONNECTIVITY ANALYSIS

During the rest epoch, the ipsilateral hippocampus was functionally connected with the contralateral hippocampus, and the parahippocampal gyri, fusiform gyri, amygdala, and cerebellar cortex bilaterally (**Figures 3Aa1,Bb1**; **Table 3**). Activity in the ipsilateral hippocampus was also correlated with structures of the default mode network including the precuneus, bilateral superior frontal, medial temporal, and cingulate gyri. The strongest connectivity, however, was demonstrated with the contralateral hippocampus and the parahippocampal gyri, amygdala, and cerebellar cortices bilaterally.

During the pre-spike period, the ipsilateral hippocampus showed connectivity to the ipsilateral parahippocampal gyrus, bilateral cerebellar cortices, ipsilateral insula, bilateral lentiform nuclei, and contralateral caudate nucleus (**Figures 3Aa2,Bb2**; **Table 4**).

At the time of spikes, the ipsilateral hippocampus showed a connectivity pattern similar to the pattern of connectivity during rest, except for increased connectivity to the contralateral insula (**Figures 3Aa3,Bb3**; **Table 5**). Also, in the spike epoch, negative correlations were observed with both superior frontal gyri. The main differences between pre-spike and spike conditions were that during pre-spike, the connectivity of the ipsilateral hippocampus to the contralateral hippocampus, both parahippocampal gyri and cerebellar cortex were significantly reduced, whereas negative correlation in activity was observed with insula, lentiform nuclei, and cingulate gyri bilaterally.

Seed/behavior correlation analysis revealed similar maps to those seen in the previous FC analysis (**Figure 3C**). Importantly, this additional analysis showed that seizure recency was strongly correlated with the pre-spike (a negative correlation of $r = -0.64$) (**Figure 3, c2**) and rest conditions (a positive correlation $r = 0.4$) (**Figure 3, c1**), but not with the spike condition (**Figure 3, c3**).

DISCUSSION

We used EEG-fMRI to investigate FC changes immediately prior to the appearance of interictal spikes on EEG in patients with MTLE.

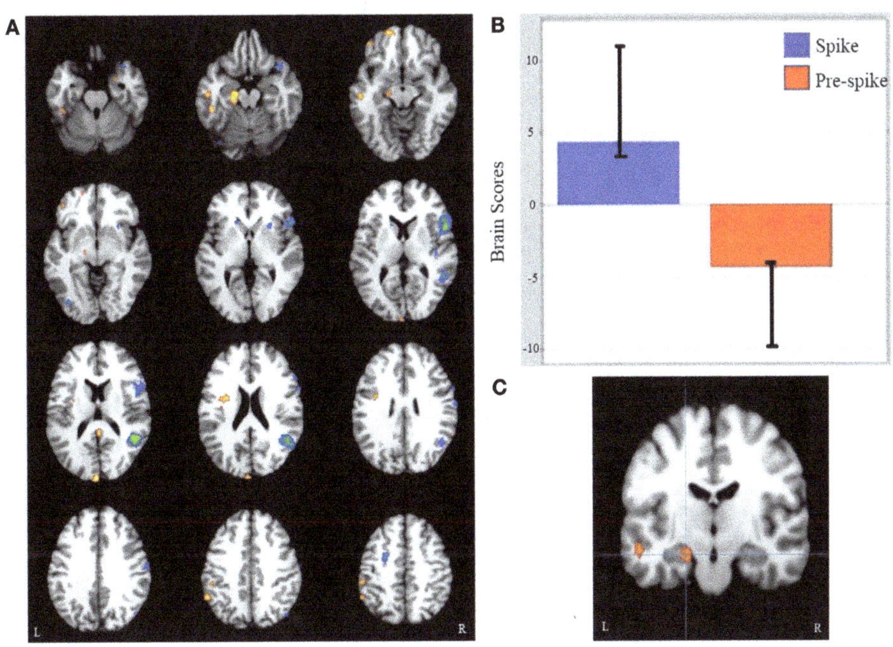

FIGURE 1 | Task PLS results. **(A)** A pattern of whole brain activity in spikes versus pre-spike. **(B)** Brain scores related to the pattern seen in **(A)**. **(C)** L hippocampus activation cluster, from which the peak voxel was used for functional connectivity analysis.

Our findings showed spike-related activation in the ipsilateral hippocampus. In addition, we demonstrated the significantly reduced ipsilateral hippocampal activity, and the loss of bilateral hippocampal FC immediately before the appearance of electrographic spikes. Moreover, we showed that the pre-spike connectivity pattern is related to seizure recency, suggesting that the altered FC changes prior to spikes was influenced by the time from last seizure. Spike-related activation in the ipsilateral hippocampus is consistent with previous EEG-fMRI studies on patients with MTLE (8, 28, 29).

In the FC analysis, the most striking finding was the significant loss of connectivity between the hippocampi several seconds before the appearance of spikes on EEG. During rest and spiking, there was a coupled coherence between the two hippocampi. However, this coherence decreased dramatically a few seconds prior to the onset of interictal spikes and are in keeping with a role for altered inter-hippocampal interaction in the initiation of spikes.

Table 2 | Whole brain analysis, spike versus pre-spike.

Region	Side	Peak MNI coordinates			Ratio[a]
		x	*y*	*z*	
Positive correlations					
HP, para HP, amygdale	L	−15	−15	−12	4.34
Middle temporal gyrus	R	69	6	−21	4.62
Precuneus	R	3	−42	69	4.11
	L	−3	−40	71	4.08
Middle temporal gyrus	L	−52	−20	−10	4.04
Insula	R	−30	−12	−18	3.49
Negative correlations					
Inferior frontal gyrus	R	51	15	6	−6.99
Superior frontal gyrus	R	48	−48	15	−6.28
Medial frontal gyrus	L	−12	−18	66	−4.24

HP, hippocampus; L, left; R, right; MNI, Montreal Neurological Institute; SE, standard error.

[a] *Salience/SE ratio in bootstrap analysis.*

The hippocampi are anatomically and functionally connected by the fornix (30), a major input and output pathway for the hippocampus (31, 32). Previously, it was thought that seizure and epileptiform discharges are initiated in one hippocampus and propagate to the contralateral hippocampus through the fornix. However, the short delay (20 ms) between activity in right and left hippocampi raises the possibility that the hippocampi are functionally synchronized (33). Studies of inter-hippocampal synchronization using intracranial EEG in animals and human beings have shown that normally, there is electrophysiological coherence between the hippocampi in the delta wave frequency range during wakefulness (0.5–2 Hz) (34, 35) and rapid eye movement sleep (36). Functional synchronization may involve the input that both hippocampi receive from each other via commissural fibers in the fornix. In animal models of MTLE, there is significant loss of synchronization at high frequencies between the hippocampi prior to the onset of epileptiform discharges (37). Our results support and translate these findings into human beings using EEG-fMRI FC analysis. We found that the loss of coherent synchronization between the two hippocampi occurred a few seconds before the appearance of interictal spikes.

Previous studies on animal models of focal epilepsy have shown hemodynamic changes prior to spikes (38, 39). These pre-spike changes have been related to early synchronization of a population of neurons before interictal discharges. In human beings, EEG-fMRI has also demonstrated early BOLD changes in the pre-spike period. Both positive and negative pre-spike BOLD changes have been described and have been found to be more focal than the spike-related BOLD signals. Correlation of early BOLD changes with findings from invasive EEG recording has revealed pre-spike synchronized neural discharges from areas exhibiting early BOLD changes (27). These pre-spike EEG discharges were observed on the intracranial EEG but not detected with scalp EEG.

Interictal inter-hemispheric hippocampal FC (40) has been investigated using resting state fMRI in MTLE. Decreased FC within the ipsilateral temporal lobe and between temporal lobe

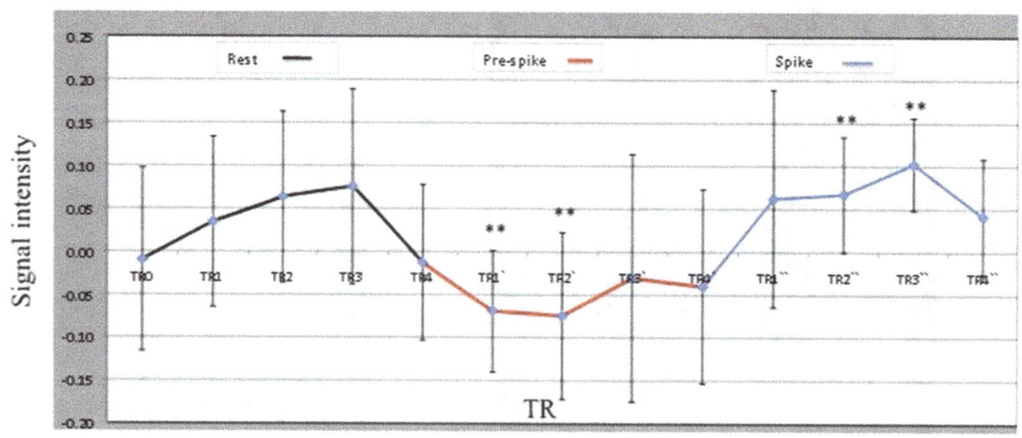

FIGURE 2 | Peak voxel (−21, −27, −12) BOLD signal intensities within the ipsilateral hippocampal activation across three conditions: rest, pre-spike, and spike. TRs, TRs′, and TRs″ represent the 4TRs for rest, pre-spike, and spike, respectively. Each TR is 2.5 s.

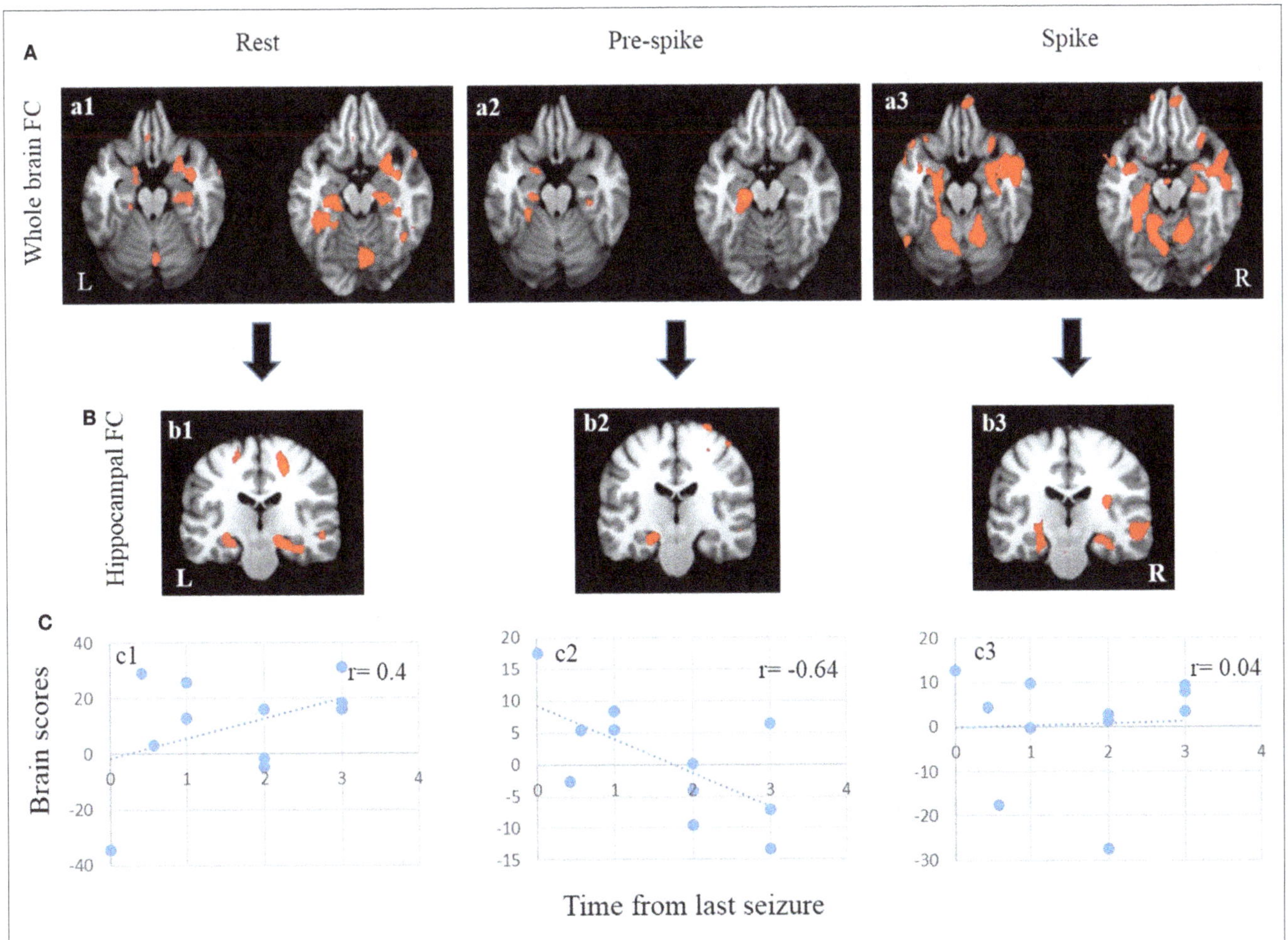

FIGURE 3 | FC and seed/behavior results. **(A)** From left to right, patterns of whole brain FC during rest (a1), pre-spike (a2), and spike (a3). **(B)** From left to right, patterns of bilateral hippocampal FC during rest (b1), pre-spike (b2), and spike (b3). **(C)** From left to right, seed/behavior correlation between FC maps in a1 (c1), a2 (c2), and a3 (c3).

structures in both hemispheres has been reported. EEG-fMRI has been used to examine the relationship between connectivity and brain states related to interictal spikes. In these studies, reduced FC between the hippocampus ipsilateral to the seizure focus with the contralateral hippocampus has been reported in relation to interictal activity in patients with unilateral MTLE, when compared to controls (41). Pereira et al. (42) has demonstrated that healthy subjects exhibit high FC between the hippocampi, whereas in patients with MTLE, the basal connectivity between the hippocampi is disrupted. Our findings support and extend the knowledge from previous reports of reduced bilateral hippocampal activity. Specifically, we showed that the loss of connectivity between the hippocampi is linked to the pre-spike period. Our approach in defining different brain states (i.e., background, pre-spike, and spike) facilitated the identification of altered FC during the transition from rest to spike states. It remains to be determined whether these changes in FC are due principally to changes in firing patterns in the ipsilateral (abnormal) hippocampus, the contralateral hippocampus, or to a complex desynchronized pattern of firing in both hippocampi. It is possible that decreased connectivity reflects a reduction in inter-hemispheric inhibition from the contralateral hippocampus, which plays a role in the emergence of interictal spikes. Further research is needed to differentiate between these alternatives. Seizure recency influenced short-term connectivity patterns. The shorter the interval from the last seizure, the greater the recruitment of the pre-spike network, whereas the rest network was more strongly recruited with longer intervals from the last seizure.

This study and others have emphasized the usefulness of EEG-fMRI and FC in examining brain connectivity in disease, but conclusions from these studies should take into account their limitations. In our study, the possibility that not all interictal spikes were visible in scalp recorded EEG (43) may limit the accuracy and specificity of our analysis. Additionally, we report findings in a small sample of patients, which is likely to have reduced statistical power (44). Each subject was scanned only once, and the FC patterns were derived from the average of all pre-spike periods across all subjects. Each patient had a differing number of spikes, as reported in **Table 1**, and our estimates of FC were based on the average of all pre-spike periods available. The variability

Table 3 | Functional connectivity pattern during rest.

Region	Side	Peak MNI coordinates			Ratio[a]
		x	y	z	
Para HP, amygdale	L	−21	−12	−15	47.09
HP, para HP, amygdale	R	24	−15	−4	13.5
Cerebellum	L	−24	−51	−9	29.32
	R	31	−53	−15	15.22
Fusiform	L	−36	−42	−14	4.51
	R	37	−40	−15	4.00
Precuneus	R	2	−72	47	4.03
	L	−2	−72	51	4.59
Cingulate gyrus	R	16	−29	42	4.007
	L	−21	−26	42	4.32
Superior frontal gyrus	R	30	51	51	7.68
	L	−5	19	58	3.48
Medial frontal gyrus	L	−20	−2	42	6.20
Medial temporal gyrus	R	50	−4	−20	6.85
	L	−50	−2	−23	6.08
Brainstem		0	−23	−23	6.85

HP, hippocampus; L, left; R, right; MNI, Montreal Neurological Institute; SE, standard error.

[a]Salience/SE ratio in bootstrap analysis.

Table 4 | Functional connectivity pattern during pre-spike.

Region	Side	Peak MNI coordinates			Ratio[a]
		x	y	z	
Para HP, amygdale	L	−18	−15	−11	16.92
Middle temporal gyrus	L	−61	−28	−11	5.04
Caudate	R	20	25	−10	7.95
Lentiform nucleus	L	−13	6	−13	7.2
	R	17	6	−11	8.12
Cingulate gyrus	L	−7	22	30	−9.2
	R	8	21	33	−6.05
Insula	L	−43	−15	−10	4.55
	R	44	−13	−10	4.55

HP, hippocampus; L, left; R, right; MNI, Montreal Neurological Institute; SE, standard error.

[a]Salience/SE ratio in bootstrap analysis.

in connectivity across epochs and subjects is taken into account in the statistical inference insofar as significant voxels represent the consistent features of the connectivity maps. Furthermore, the large range of AEDs prescribed and the relatively low number of subjects precluded the analysis of the influence of specific drug classes on connectivity patterns. Finally, we concede there may be a degree of temporal blurring in examining connectivity time linked to interictal spikes in a dataset with a temporal resolution of 2.5 s. However, if it were possible to remove this effect, the focal pattern of connectivity that we observed during the pre-spike period might be expected to be even stronger.

Table 5 | Functional connectivity pattern during spike.

Region	Side	Peak MNI coordinates			Ratio[a]
		x	y	z	
Para HP, amygdale	L	−25	−15	−15	23.05
HP, para HP, amygdale	R	29	−15	−13	5.01
Cerebellum	L	−23	−53	−10	29.32
	R	31	−52	−15	15.22
Fusiform	R	38	−65	−3	4.60
Insula	R	44	−42	25	9.11
	L	−2	−72	51	4.59
Lentiform nucleus	L	−20	−15	−8	13.75
Red nucleus		0	−15	−7	6.05
Superior frontal gyrus	L	−18	21	58	−4.68
	R	24	20	58	−5.6
Middle frontal gyrus	L	−36	5	44	−6.72

HP, hippocampus; L, left; R, right; MNI, Montreal Neurological Institute; SE, standard error.

[a]Salience/SE ratio in bootstrap analysis.

To conclude, our main findings indicate that ipsilateral hippocampal activity and FC are reduced during the period immediately prior to the appearance of interictal spikes. These findings may provide insights about the patho-physiological state of mesial temporal lobe structures underlying the genesis of spikes.

ACKNOWLEDGMENTS

The authors thank Associate Professor Cecilie Lander, Dr. Lata Vadlamudi, Dr. Jia Tho, Dr. James Pelekanos, and Fred Tremayne, from the Department of Neurology at the RBWH, for their help in the recruitment of patients. This work was supported by the National Health and Medical Research Council (NHMRC) program grant.

REFERENCES

1. Serrano-Castro PJ, Sanchez-Alvarez JC, Garcia-Gomez T. [Mesial temporal sclerosis (II): clinical features and complementary studies]. *Rev Neurol* (1998) **26**(152):592–7.
2. Blumcke I. Neuropathology of focal epilepsies: a critical review. *Epilepsy Behav* (2009) **15**(1):34–9. doi:10.1016/j.yebeh.2009.02.033
3. Jackson GD, Briellmann RS, Kuzniecky RI. In: Jackson GD, Briellmann RS, Kuzniecky RI, editors. *Magnetic Resonance in Epilepsy in Temporal Lobe Epilepsy.* Amsterdam: Elsevier Inc (2004).
4. Janszky J, Pannek HW, Janszky I, Schulz R, Behne F, Hoppe M, et al. Failed surgery for temporal lobe epilepsy: predictors of long-term seizure-free course. *Epilepsy Res* (2005) **64**(1–2):35–44. doi:10.1016/j.eplepsyres.2005.02.004
5. Wendling F, Chauvel P, Biraben A, Bartolomei F. From intracerebral EEG signals to brain connectivity: identification of epileptogenic networks in partial epilepsy. *Front Syst Neurosci* (2010) **4**:154. doi:10.3389/fnsys.2010.00154
6. Andersen AR, Gram L, Kjaer L, Fuglsang-Frederiksen A, Herning M, Lassen NA, et al. SPECT in partial epilepsy: identifying side of the focus. *Acta Neurol Scand Suppl* (1988) **117**:90–5. doi:10.1111/j.1600-0404.1988.tb08009.x
7. Carne RP, O'Brien TJ, Kilpatrick CJ, MacGregor LR, Hicks RJ, Murphy MA, et al. MRI-negative PET-positive temporal lobe epilepsy: a distinct surgically remediable syndrome. *Brain* (2004) **127**(Pt 10):2276–85. doi:10.1093/brain/awh257
8. Kobayashi E, Bagshaw AP, Benar CG, Aghakhani Y, Andermann F, Dubeau F, et al. Temporal and extratemporal BOLD responses to temporal lobe interictal spikes. *Epilepsia* (2006) **47**(2):343–54. doi:10.1111/j.1528-1167.2006.00427.x

9. Kobayashi E, Grova C, Tyvaert L, Dubeau F, Gotman J. Structures involved at the time of temporal lobe spikes revealed by interindividual group analysis of EEG/fMRI data. *Epilepsia* (2009) **50**(12):2549–56. doi:10.1111/j.1528-1167.2009.02180.x
10. Laufs H, Hamandi K, Salek-Haddadi A, Kleinschmidt AK, Duncan JS, Lemieux L. Temporal lobe interictal epileptic discharges affect cerebral activity in "default mode" brain regions. *Hum Brain Mapp* (2007) **28**(10):1023–32. doi:10.1002/hbm.20323
11. Hawco CS, Bagshaw AP, Lu Y, Dubeau F, Gotman J. BOLD changes occur prior to epileptic spikes seen on scalp EEG. *Neuroimage* (2007) **35**(4):1450–8. doi:10.1016/j.neuroimage.2006.12.042
12. Rathakrishnan R, Moeller F, Levan P, Dubeau F, Gotman J. BOLD signal changes preceding negative responses in EEG-fMRI in patients with focal epilepsy. *Epilepsia* (2010) **51**(9):1837–45. doi:10.1111/j.1528-1167.2010.02643.x
13. Jacobs J, Levan P, Moeller F, Boor R, Stephani U, Gotman J, et al. Hemodynamic changes preceding the interictal EEG spike in patients with focal epilepsy investigated using simultaneous EEG-fMRI. *Neuroimage* (2009) **45**(4):1220–31. doi:10.1016/j.neuroimage.2009.01.014
14. Salek-Haddadi A, Diehl B, Hamandi K, Merschhemke M, Liston A, Friston K, et al. Hemodynamic correlates of epileptiform discharges: an EEG-fMRI study of 63 patients with focal epilepsy. *Brain Res* (2006) **1088**(1):148–66. doi:10.1016/j.brainres.2006.02.098
15. Morgan VL, Gore JC, Abou-Khalil B. Functional epileptic network in left mesial temporal lobe epilepsy detected using resting fMRI. *Epilepsy Res* (2010) **88**(2–3):168–78. doi:10.1016/j.eplepsyres.2009.10.018
16. Waites AB, Briellmann RS, Saling MM, Abbott DF, Jackson GD. Functional connectivity networks are disrupted in left temporal lobe epilepsy. *Ann Neurol* (2006) **59**(2):335–43. doi:10.1002/ana.20733
17. Gotman J. Relationships between interictal spiking and seizures: human and experimental evidence. *Can J Neurol Sci* (1991) **18**(Suppl):573–6.
18. Avoli M, Biagini G, de Curtis M. Do interictal spikes sustain seizures and epileptogenesis? *Epilepsy Curr* (2006) **6**(6):203–7. doi:10.1111/j.1535-7511.2006.00146.x
19. Janszky J, Fogarasi A, Jokeit H, Schulz R, Hoppe M, Ebner A. Spatiotemporal relationship between seizure activity and interictal spikes in temporal lobe epilepsy. *Epilepsy Res* (2001) **47**(3):179–88. doi:10.1016/S0920-1211(01)00307-2
20. Hufnagel A, Dumpelmann M, Zentner J, Schijns O, Elger CE. Clinical relevance of quantified intracranial interictal spike activity in presurgical evaluation of epilepsy. *Epilepsia* (2000) **41**(4):467–78. doi:10.1111/j.1528-1157.2000.tb00191.x
21. Marsh ED, Peltzer B, Brown MW III, Wusthoff C, Storm PB Jr, Litt B, et al. Interictal EEG spikes identify the region of electrographic seizure onset in some, but not all, pediatric epilepsy patients. *Epilepsia* (2010) **51**(4):592–601. doi:10.1111/j.1528-1167.2009.02306.x
22. Delorme A, Makeig S. EEGLAB: an open source toolbox for analysis of single-trial EEG dynamics including independent component analysis. *J Neurosci Methods* (2004) **134**(1):9–21. doi:10.1016/j.jneumeth.2003.10.009
23. Niazy RK, Beckmann CF, Iannetti GD, Brady JM, Smith SM. Removal of FMRI environment artifacts from EEG data using optimal basis sets. *Neuroimage* (2005) **28**(3):720–37. doi:10.1016/j.neuroimage.2005.06.067
24. Negishi M, Abildgaard M, Nixon T, Constable RT. Removal of time-varying gradient artifacts from EEG data acquired during continuous fMRI. *Clin Neurophysiol* (2004) **115**(9):2181–92. doi:10.1016/j.clinph.2004.04.005
25. McIntosh AR, Lobaugh NJ. Partial least squares analysis of neuroimaging data: applications and advances. *Neuroimage* (2004) **23**(Suppl 1):S250–63. doi:10.1016/j.neuroimage.2004.07.020
26. Krishnan A, Williams LJ, McIntosh AR, Abdi H. Partial least squares (PLS) methods for neuroimaging: a tutorial and review. *Neuroimage* (2011) **56**(2):455–75. doi:10.1016/j.neuroimage.2010.07.034
27. Pittau F, Levan P, Moeller F, Gholipour T, Haegelen C, Zelmann R, et al. Changes preceding interictal epileptic EEG abnormalities: comparison between EEG/fMRI and intracerebral EEG. *Epilepsia* (2011) **52**(6):1120–9. doi:10.1111/j.1528-1167.2011.03072.x
28. Aghakhani Y, Kobayashi E, Bagshaw AP, Hawco C, Benar CG, Dubeau F, et al. Cortical and thalamic fMRI responses in partial epilepsy with focal and bilateral synchronous spikes. *Clin Neurophysiol* (2006) **117**(1):177–91. doi:10.1016/j.clinph.2005.08.028
29. Morgan VL, Gore JC, Abou-Khalil B. Cluster analysis detection of functional MRI activity in temporal lobe epilepsy. *Epilepsy Res* (2007) **76**(1):22–33. doi:10.1016/j.eplepsyres.2007.06.008
30. Wyllie E. Epileptic Seizures and Syndromes. In: Gupta DKLA, editor. *The Treatment of Epilepsy: Principles and Practice*. 4th ed. Philadelphia: Lippincott Williams & Wilkins (2006).
31. Duvernoy HM, Cattin F, Risold P-Y. In: Duvernoy HM, editor. The human hippocampus: functional anatomy, vascularization and serial sections with MRI. *Structure, Functions, and Connections*. Besançon: Springer (2013).
32. Andersen P, Morris R, Amaral D, Bliss T, O'Keefe J. *The Hippocampus Book*. New York: Oxford University Press (2007).
33. Wang Y, Toprani S, Tang Y, Vrabec T, Durand DM. Mechanism of highly synchronized bilateral hippocampal activity. *Exp Neurol* (2014) **251**:101–11. doi:10.1016/j.expneurol.2013.11.014
34. Moroni F, Nobili L, De Carli F, Massimini M, Francione S, Marzano C, et al. Slow EEG rhythms and inter-hemispheric synchronization across sleep and wakefulness in the human hippocampus. *Neuroimage* (2012) **60**(1):497–504. doi:10.1016/j.neuroimage.2011.11.093
35. Green JD, Arduini AA. Hippocampal electrical activity in arousal. *J Neurophysiol* (1954) **17**(6):533–57.
36. Buzsaki G, Buhl DL, Harris KD, Csicsvari J, Czeh B, Morozov A. Hippocampal network patterns of activity in the mouse. *Neuroscience* (2003) **116**(1):201–11. doi:10.1016/S0306-4522(02)00669-3
37. Meier R, Haussler U, Aertsen A, Deransart C, Depaulis A, Egert U. Short-term changes in bilateral hippocampal coherence precede epileptiform events. *Neuroimage* (2007) **38**(1):138–49. doi:10.1016/j.neuroimage.2007.07.016
38. Makiranta M, Ruohonen J, Suominen K, Niinimaki J, Sonkajarvi E, Kiviniemi V, et al. BOLD signal increase preceeds EEG spike activity – a dynamic penicillin induced focal epilepsy in deep anesthesia. *Neuroimage* (2005) **27**(4):715–24. doi:10.1016/j.neuroimage.2005.05.025
39. Zwiener U, Eiselt M, Giessler F, Nowak H. Relations between early prespike magnetic field changes, interictal discharges, and return to basal activity in the neocortex of rabbits. *Neurosci Lett* (2000) **289**(2):103–6. doi:10.1016/S0304-3940(00)01271-4
40. Morgan VL, Rogers BP, Sonmezturk HH, Gore JC, Abou-Khalil B. Cross hippocampal influence in mesial temporal lobe epilepsy measured with high temporal resolution functional magnetic resonance imaging. *Epilepsia* (2011) **52**(9):1741–9. doi:10.1111/j.1528-1167.2011.03196.x
41. Pittau F, Grova C, Moeller F, Dubeau F, Gotman J. Patterns of altered functional connectivity in mesial temporal lobe epilepsy. *Epilepsia* (2012) **53**(6):1013–23. doi:10.1111/j.1528-1167.2012.03464.x
42. Pereira FR, Alessio A, Sercheli MS, Pedro T, Bilevicius E, Rondina JM, et al. Asymmetrical hippocampal connectivity in mesial temporal lobe epilepsy: evidence from resting state fMRI. *BMC Neurosci* (2010) **11**:66. doi:10.1186/1471-2202-11-661471-2202-11-66
43. Tao JX, Ray A, Hawes-Ebersole S, Ebersole JS. Intracranial EEG substrates of scalp EEG interictal spikes. *Epilepsia* (2005) **46**(5):669–76. doi:10.1111/j.1528-1167.2005.11404.x
44. Handwerker DA, Ollinger JM, D'Esposito M. Variation of BOLD hemodynamic responses across subjects and brain regions and their effects on statistical analyses. *Neuroimage* (2004) **21**(4):1639–51. doi:10.1016/j.neuroimage.2003.11.029

4

Mapping epileptic activity: Sources or networks for the clinicians?

Francesca Pittau[1], Pierre Mégevand[2], Laurent Sheybani[3], Eugenio Abela[4], Frédéric Grouiller[5], Laurent Spinelli[1], Christoph M. Michel[3], Margitta Seeck[1] and Serge Vulliemoz[1]*

[1] EEG and Epilepsy Unit, Neurology Department, University Hospitals and Faculty of Medicine of Geneva, Geneva, Switzerland
[2] Laboratory for Multimodal Human Brain Mapping, Hofstra North Shore LIJ School of Medicine, Manhasset, NY, USA
[3] Functional Brain Mapping Laboratory, Department of Fundamental Neurosciences, University of Geneva, Geneva, Switzerland
[4] Support Center of Advanced Neuroimaging (SCAN), Institute for Diagnostic and Interventional Neuroradiology, University Hospital Inselspital, Bern, Switzerland
[5] Radiology Department, University Hospitals and Faculty of Medicine of Geneva, Geneva, Switzerland

***Correspondence:**
Serge Vulliemoz, EEG and Epilepsy Unit, Neurology Department, University Hospitals of Geneva, 4 rue Gabrielle-Perret-Gentil, Geneva 4 1211, Switzerland
e-mail: serge.vulliemoz@hcuge.ch

Epileptic seizures of focal origin are classically considered to arise from a focal epileptogenic zone and then spread to other brain regions. This is a key concept for semiological electro-clinical correlations, localization of relevant structural lesions, and selection of patients for epilepsy surgery. Recent development in neuro-imaging and electro-physiology and combinations, thereof, have been validated as contributory tools for focus localization. In parallel, these techniques have revealed that widespread networks of brain regions, rather than a single epileptogenic region, are implicated in focal epileptic activity. Sophisticated multimodal imaging and analysis strategies of brain connectivity patterns have been developed to characterize the spatio-temporal relationships within these networks by combining the strength of both techniques to optimize spatial and temporal resolution with whole-brain coverage and directional connectivity. In this paper, we review the potential clinical contribution of these functional mapping techniques as well as invasive electrophysiology in human beings and animal models for characterizing network connectivity.

Keywords: connectivity, resting-state network, epilepsy, animal model, EEG, fMRI, MEG, intracranial EEG

INTRODUCTION

Epilepsy is one of the most frequent chronic neurological disorder, with an incidence of 50/100,000/year and a prevalence of 0.5–1% (1, 2). One third of these patients are drug resistant (3). Focal seizures are classically considered to be caused by an abnormal neuro-electrical activity of a focal epileptogenic zone and a subsequent spreading to other brain regions. This concept is intimately linked to the correlation between ictal signs and symptoms, electro-physiological activity, and structural lesion [anatomo-electro-clinical correlation (4)]. Furthermore, this hypothesis is crucial to select drug-resistant focal epilepsy patients for surgery, a widely accepted effective therapy (5, 6). The aim of epilepsy surgery is to remove the epileptogenic zone with the preservation of the eloquent areas (7).

Recent progress in neuro-imaging and electro-physiology suggests that focal seizures and focal epilepsies are actually related to an abnormal function of a network of cortical and subcortical brain structures rather than to a single epileptogenic region (8–14). The occurrence of epileptic activity is due to the abnormal neuronal activity of these connected regions and abnormal interactions between them (epileptic network). This conceptual shift is reflected in the new terminology proposal for seizures and epilepsies of the International League against Epilepsy, which proposes "*focal*" as indicating seizures arising primarily "within networks limited to one hemisphere and that may be discrete or more widely distributed" (15). Generalized seizures are considered as "originating within and rapidly engaging, bilaterally distributed networks" of cortical and subcortical regions. Inside these networks, some brain regions are responsible for seizure initiation and propagation, whereas other nodes are more remotely involved, their activity modulating, or being modulated by the epileptic discharge.

There is increasing evidence that epileptic activity strongly interacts with physiological brain networks, notably the so-called "resting-state networks" (RSNs) (8, 16). A RSN is a set of brain regions that shows temporal correlations in their activity (as measured by hemodynamic or electrical signals) and that are functionally related. They are observed during rest but correspond to the networks revealed in different behavioral and cognitive task (e.g., attention, vision, etc.). This has led to the new concept that the apparently resting spontaneous brain activity shows continuous interaction among brain networks responsible for various classes of sensory/behavioral functions (17). RSNs are highly organized in space, reproducible from subject to subject, and differ with aging and between genders (18).

In this paper, we review the converging evidence from different brain mapping techniques in human and animal models that epilepsy is related to the dysfunction of a large-scale brain networks, with alterations of physiological brain networks. We will particularly focus on the clinical impact of this new view of epilepsy as a network disease.

METHODS

An electronic literature search was conducted for articles on this topic regarding human and animal subjects. Sources searched included PubMed and relevant books. Words used in the search included the text words and subject headings of epilep*, functional connect*, resting-state functional network*, temporal epilepsy, extra-temporal epilepsy, electroencephalogram (or EEG), simultaneous functional MRI (fMRI) and EEG (or EEG-fMRI), electric and magnetic source imaging (or MSI, ESI), intracranial EEG (or iEEG or sEEG), cortico-cortical evoked potential, and single-pulse electrical stimulation. The words were searched independently and in combination. For each citation considered, the abstract was read (when available), and articles were excluded if they were outside the scope of the review. Studies published only in abstract form, letters, and technical reports were excluded. The bibliography of each of the retrieved papers was examined to identify relevant references that could have been missed by electronic search. The findings were described taking into account the limit of words and the critical insight of the authors.

HOW TO MEASURE RESTING-STATE NETWORKS? FUNCTIONAL CONNECTIVITY

Functional interactions between brain regions activity, can be characterized in several ways. On the one hand, functional connectivity (FC), the most widely used metrics, measures the statistical dependency between different signals obtained by correlation analysis. However, such strategy does not account for the direction of the information flow and cannot therefore infer causality relationships. On the other hand, effective or directed connectivity investigates directional relationships and aims at describing causal influences. Effective connectivity can be investigated using model-driven techniques such as structural equation modeling (19) and dynamic causal modeling (DCM) (20), data-driven techniques such as Granger-causal modeling (21), or by recording the response of remote areas to focal stimulation of a given brain region [cortico-cortical evoked potentials (22)]. Connectivity studies can be applied among a set of predefined relevant brain regions selected by the investigator, between one seed region and the rest of the brain or at the whole-brain scale, using the spatial resolution of the recording technique. A detailed description of the various approaches used for measuring connectivity is beyond the scope of this review and the reader is referred to studies comparing various approaches to better understand the specific limitations of each technique (23–25). The results obtained by such connectivity analysis between all pairs of brain regions can be represented in so-called connectivity matrices. Graph topological analysis is then increasingly applied to reduce the complexity of the data and extract meaningful characteristics of the networks (26).

BLOOD OXYGEN LEVEL DEPENDENT SIGNAL AND PHYSIOLOGICAL RESTING-STATE NETWORKS

The concept of brain networks originated, and has largely benefited, from the use of resting-state fMRI. fMRI detects blood oxygen level dependent (BOLD) signal change reflecting metabolically active brain areas not only in relation to a specific physiologic or pathologic event (27) but also in resting-state (RS) condition (resting-state-fMRI or RS-fMRI).

Biswal and colleagues demonstrated for the first time (1995) that brain regions that are functionally related, show temporal correlations in the low frequency component of the BOLD signal. In other words, fMRI FC detects zones that exhibit correlated BOLD fluctuations and, as a result, belong to the same functional network (28). Studies in monkeys (29) and in human beings (30) suggest that FC is related to neuronal processes.

Functional connectivity can be measured while the subject is performing a behavioral and cognitive task (task-related FC), or while the subject is not performing any specific task (RS-FC). The RSN that is mainly activated in condition of resting wakefulness and deactivated in task performing is called default-mode network (DMN) (31). This physiological RSN is involved in self-referential thoughts and consciousness (32, 33). The concept of "resting" is debatable. Usually, subjects are instructed to lie down in the scanner with the eyes closed, and are invited to not sleep.

Different methods have been developed to extract RSNs, some requiring an "*a priori* hypothesis," like seed-based approach (34), other do not [i.e., independent component analysis (35), or bootstrap analysis (36)]. The description of the methodological aspects is outside the scope of this review. Other papers can be consulted (14, 37, 38).

EEG/MEG AND PHYSIOLOGICAL RESTING-STATE NETWORKS

Functional connectivity algorithms similar to those used for fMRI BOLD signals can be applied to MEG or EEG current-density estimations in the source space, revealing brain areas that are synchronized in specific frequency bands. As with fMRI, such analysis can be applied to task-related (39), as well as to spontaneous resting-state activity (40, 41). The unique advantage of EEG/MEG connectivity analysis is the high temporal resolution that allows studying fast fluctuations within large-scale network interactions and fast switches between resting-state networks.

FC analysis of EEG/MEG considers the time-course of electromagnetic signals and looks at correlations of oscillating networks (42). Beyond this view of temporal oscillations, EEG recordings can be considered as time-series of scalp potential maps that vary across time with the temporal resolution in the order of milliseconds (43). Several studies have shown that spontaneous EEG signals can be explained by the alternation of periods of stable topography, lasting almost 100 ms, very reproducible across subjects, and modifiable by neurological (44) or psychiatric impairment (45). These periods are called microstates and can be identified throughout an individual's life (46) suggesting that they might be mediated by predetermined anatomical connections. During rest, four different microstates are consistently observed, and they can be considered as "basic building blocks" of spontaneous mental activities (47). A recent review on this topic is available (48).

It has been shown (49) that the temporal dynamic of EEG microstates have hemodynamic correlates that can be measured with EEG-fMRI and that each physiological microstate map corresponds to one of the well-described BOLD RS network. Such clear correlates between EEG and BOLD are less well found when looking at classical power fluctuations in specific EEG frequency bands (50). This finding strongly suggests that the EEG microstates can be the candidates for the electro-physiological signatures of fMRI RSNs. Scale-invariance of the alternation between microstates has been demonstrated to be the base of this coupling over such a wide temporal scale (51).

EVIDENCE FOR BRAIN NETWORKS INVOLVED IN EPILEPTIC ACTIVITY

As described above, FC at the whole-brain level can be studied with EEG, MEG, fMRI, iEEG, or the combination of these techniques. They have been applied to patients with focal or generalized epilepsy to characterize spatial and temporal properties of epileptic networks.

EEG AND MEG-BASED CONNECTIVITY IN EPILEPSY

EEG and MEG are appealing non-invasive techniques for estimating brain connectivity in epilepsy because they measure neuroelectrical activity more directly than fMRI and can potentially offer a higher temporal resolution.

Several studies using concordance with intracranial recordings or post-operative outcome have established that electric and magnetic source imaging (ESI, MSI) are reliable techniques for estimating the localization of the cortical generators of epileptic activity (52–55) and these techniques now offer a much more convincing strategy to investigate connectivity directly between the activity of cortical regions. Therefore, both ESI and MSI studies will be discussed together hereunder. Studies using connectivity analysis in the sensor space are not discussed here because of their severe limitations of interpretation due to important caveats related to sensor cross-talk, volume conduction, and reference choice of the electromagnetic signals (56). The projection of the signal in source space requires the selection of a head model describing the propagation of the electromagnetic signal (forward problem) and an inverse solution (estimating the cortical activity from the EEG/MEG recording, inverse problem) (48, 57, 58). A variety of head models exists, from template averaged normal brain to highly sophisticated realistic models based on individual anatomy, and they have been used in epilepsy imaging and cognitive neurosciences. Validation in patients with invasive EEG or surgical resection showed that the individual anatomy was important for the localization accuracy (54), but that the performance of highly sophisticated models did not outperform less computer-intensive models also based on individual anatomy, as these were disturbed by the presence of brain lesions in patients with epilepsy (59). Regarding inverse solutions, dipole models consider a single or a few equivalent dipole(s) as sources of the EEG/MEG signals of sources distributed in the whole cortex (48). While both approaches might yield complimentary results for localizing epileptic sources (60), distributed sources are best suited to the study of connectivity between cortical patches at a large brain scale.

The analysis of interictal epileptic discharges has principally aimed at localizing epileptic generators in the context of pre-surgical evaluations rather than studying large brain networks. Case reports or small MEG series showed promising results for the localizing value of the regions with high information outflow, estimated by connectivity analysis (61–63). In addition, based on development in cognitive neurosciences, the background activity measured by MEG and EEG in the classical frequency bands has also been used as a substrate to estimate abnormal connectivity in patients with epilepsy and correlate it with clinical variables. In patients with brain tumors, increased theta-band connectivity and more profound network alterations were associated with a higher number of epileptic seizures (64) and there is higher post-operative network improvement in patients who become seizure free (65).

In generalized epilepsies, connectivity studies have highlighted a network of hyperconnected anterior regions in photosensitive patients (66). Network analysis using graph theory in five patients with absence epilepsy showed a build-up of connectivity changes occurring before the onset of generalized spike-wave discharges (67). This shows the potential of such a technique for our understanding of the large-scale brain networks underlying hyperexcitability and interictal to ictal transition. A similar approach has been applied to iEEG recordings of interictal to ictal transition in patients with focal cortical dysplasia (12).

Another study used co-occurrence of MEG interictal spikes to build graphs of connectivity between the estimated sources of these spikes. In seven patients also investigated with stereotactic iEEG, the connections revealed by MEG were confirmed by iEEG (68).

Similarly to fMRI studies, future work will need to distinguish between transient connectivity alterations related to interictal discharges, that are known to be associated with subtle cognitive impairment (69), and deeper connectivity changes based on background activity alterations. The tools are now available to benefit from the high temporal resolution of EEG/MEG to further investigate these issues and this field has recently attracted an intense interest. While MEG offers advantages over EEG for longitudinal studies of post-operative cases, due to its insensitivity to skull defects, the development of long-term high-density EEG system, its greater versatility compared to MEG and its potential combination with fMRI will be precious for recording seizures and exploring network changes leading to their initiation, spread, and termination.

EEG-fMRI CONNECTIVITY IN EPILEPSY

Simultaneous EEG and fMRI (EEG-fMRI) detects hemodynamic changes in the brain related to events of interest identified in the EEG (70). Combining high temporal resolution of EEG signal with high spatial resolution of BOLD images, EEG-fMRI has been shown to be useful to characterize various forms of focal and generalized epileptic abnormalities (hereunder called "spikes" for practical reasons) (71). EEG-fMRI helps to localize epileptic focus in patients with drug-resistant focal epilepsy candidate for surgery (72, 73). From the first publications (74, 75), EEG-fMRI has demonstrated that BOLD responses to a focal spike can be multifocal, also present at a distance from the presumed focus (**Figure 1**), corroborating the concept of epileptic network (9). Studying such networks can inform about patients' prognosis after surgery. While focal responses predict a good post-operative outcome, diffuse results are associated with a poor outcome, probably reflecting that a larger network is involved in the epileptogenic zone (76, 77). Epileptic activity can also be detected in the absence of spikes and fMRI analysis based on EEG topography can reveal epileptogenic networks (78).

BOLD responses to a neural event are usually detected with a delay of 4–6 s (79). Nevertheless, hemodynamic changes to spikes can have different peak times (80), and can occur before the spike is visible on the scalp (81). Dynamic analysis of BOLD response (82, 83) can tell us which brain areas are first activated,

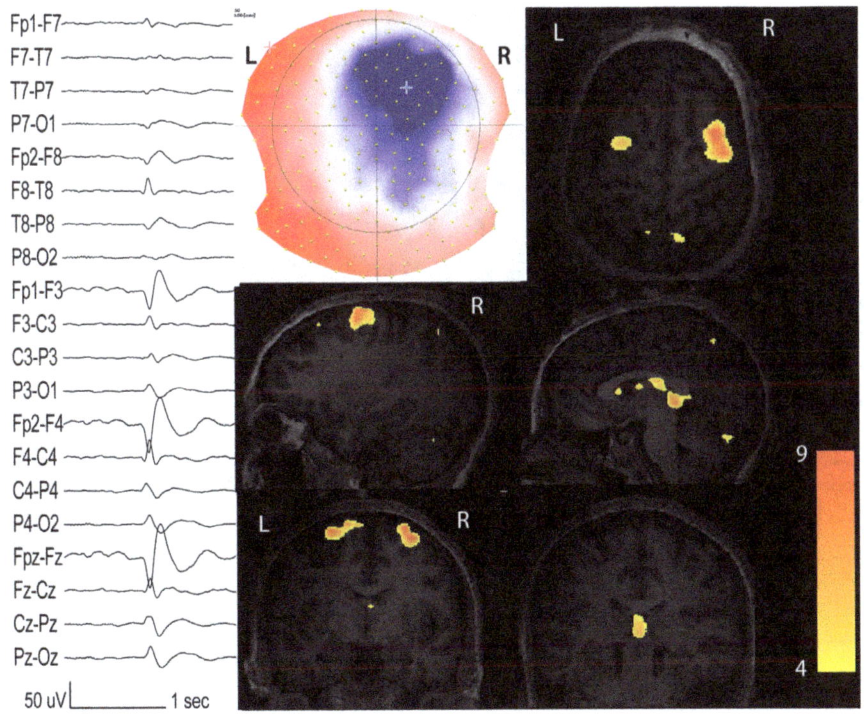

FIGURE 1 | Interictal network revealed by EEG-fMRI. Patients with non-lesional right frontal epilepsy. Marked events inside the EEG-fMRI session: right frontal spikes with phase reversal at F4 (on the left: longitudinal bipolar montage from 204 channels EEG). On the middle: scalp voltage map of the spike (204 electrodes, viewed from the top) with the maximal right frontal negativity (blue). BOLD response (t-value = 4; $p < 0.05$ corrected for family-wise-error) has maximal activation in the spike topography but other clusters with inferior statistical values are present in the contra-lateral homologous region and in the thalamus.

by comparing early BOLD response vs. late BOLD response. However, this analysis does not address the concept of causality and the sluggishness and variability of BOLD responses prevent a more accurate investigation into the temporal dynamics and directionality of the connections (24). Causality within epileptic network can be addressed by effective connectivity approaches like Dynamic Causal Modeling (DCM) (37, 84).

The combination of ESI with EEG-fMRI can offer complementary information for improving each single technique (**Figure 2**). Although EEG-fMRI and ESI measure different signals (hemodynamic the first, electrical the second), the concordance between ESI performed during fMRI recordings can allow distinguishing between hemodynamic changes related to spike onset vs. propagation, adding important temporal information to the limited fMRI temporal resolution (85, 86).

EEG-fMRI studies can give insights about epileptogenesis. Interictal spikes of different types of epilepsy (frontal, temporal, and posterior quadrant), are associated with deactivation in the precuneus and posterior cingulate cortex (10), regions involved in the DMN (**Figure 3**). Other physiological RSNs could be affected by spikes: this interaction and its clinical consequences need to be clarified in future studies. A common involvement of the cingulate gyri in temporal lobe and frontal lobe epilepsy was reported (10), probably resulting from rapid spread of epileptic activity originating from the temporal and frontal areas, which both involve the limbic system.

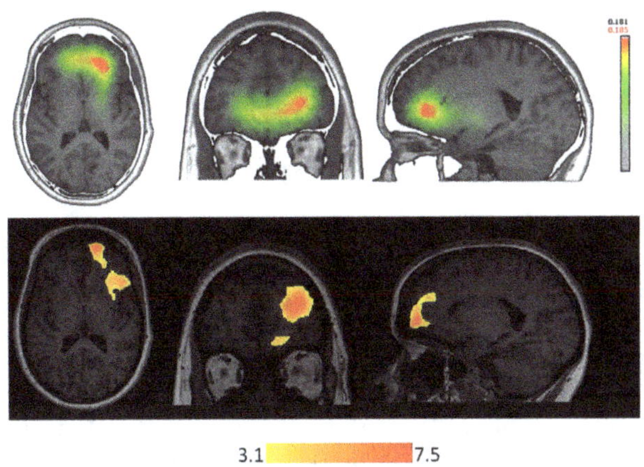

FIGURE 2 | Techniques using different types of signal are concordant in localizing the epileptic focus in a patient with right orbito-frontal focal cortical dysplasia. On the top-line: ESI (256 electrodes, simplified realistic head model ISMAC, distributed inverse solution LORETA) performed on right frontal spikes (FP2-F8). On the bottom-line: EEG-fMRI performed on the same type of events recorded inside the scanner.

A specific area, localized in the medial orbito-frontal gyrus (piriform cortex), called "area tempestas", seems to be involved in the genesis or propagation of epileptic activity (87, 88) in focal

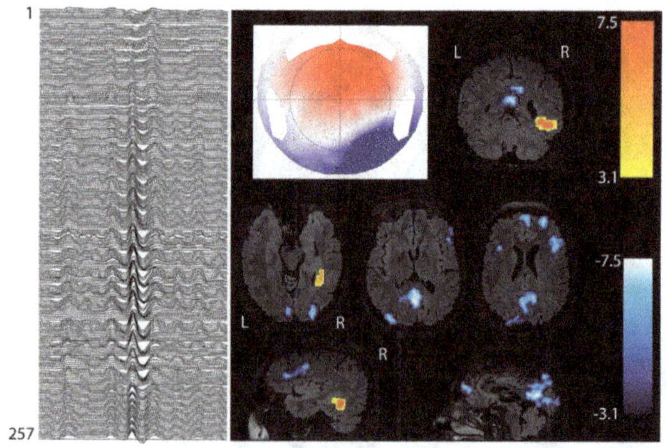

FIGURE 3 | Interictal involvement of DMN in focal epilepsy. Patients with right hemispheric extended periventricular nodular heterotopia. Marked epileptic events inside the scanner: right posterior temporal spikes with phase reversal at P8 (on the left: 256 channel EEG; referential montage Fz-Cz). BOLD increase is concordant with the spike topography (topographic map on the middle), whereas BOLD decrease is present in the regions of default-mode network (DMN).

epilepsies. A DCM study supported the hypothesis of a causal link between hemodynamic changes in this structure and a specific type of reflex epilepsy, although in a single patient (89). Several other findings seem to corroborate the important role of the area tempestas: (i) its decrease in benzodiazepine receptor (87), (ii) its epileptogenic role in animal kindling models of temporal lobe epilepsy (TLE) (90–92), and (iii) its increase in gray matter volume in patient with frontal lobe epilepsy when compared to controls (93).

From a methodological point of view, multimodal combination between EEG/ESI, fMRI, and diffusion imaging tractography will allow exploring functional and structural connectivity at a finer spatio-temporal scale. Some initial small studies have highlighted the potential of these combinations (94–96).

fMRI and EEG-fMRI studies in focal epilepsy

Unfortunately, only few of the many studies on RS-FC have been done with the simultaneous recording of EEG. Spikes cause a transient cognitive impairment, by affecting, e.g., memory retrieval in rats (97), and memory maintenance and retrieval in human beings (69). Therefore, a more consistent use of simultaneous EEG while performing fMRI for RS or task-related studies in epileptic patients is needed to determine the influence of spikes on the determined BOLD networks. Indeed a study where EEG activity was monitored during a working memory-fMRI session (98) has shown that the task-related BOLD dramatically changes when spikes occur. Another advantage of the simultaneous recording of EEG in the scanner is that it allows monitoring the transition between different alertness states in order to assure that the subject is in RS and not in drowsiness/sleep state. A very recent review (99) has accurately discussed this issue and summarized the relevant studies.

Temporal lobe epilepsy. The majority of RS-fMRI studies in focal epilepsies have focused on TLE, which is the most common form of focal epilepsy in adults and offers the advantage of being one of the most homogeneous groups within the focal epilepsy syndromes.

Temporal lobe epilepsy has been the first epileptic syndrome to be considered as epileptogenic network (100) with relatively well characterized components encompassing different structures in the mesial temporal lobe (amygdala and hippocampus), adjacent cortex including enthorhinal cortex and lateral temporal cortex, and extra-temporal structures (i.e., thalamus and orbito-frontal cortex). fMRI connectivity studies (some with simultaneous EEG recording, others without) conducted by seeding the principal nodes of the mesial temporal network showed impaired connectivity with the other nodes of the network (101–103). Decreased connectivity is the most common finding among those studies. Nevertheless, there are reports of increased function of the unaffected hippocampus in patients with unilateral MTLE, both in the RS (104) and during task-related (105, 106) acquisitions. Morgan et al. (107) have shown that RS cross-hippocampal FC is disrupted at the beginning of the disease and then increases linearly with epilepsy duration after 10 years, suggesting that length of disease influences FC patterns. Bettus et al. (108) studied the electro-physiological correlates of BOLD signal fluctuations in structures exhibiting epileptiform discharges, by measuring correlations between intracerebral EEG and resting-state fMRI in five patients with TLE. They found an increase in connectivity measured from the intracerebral EEG but a decrease of connectivity measured from the BOLD signal in regions with epileptiform abnormalities relative to non-affected areas. This discrepancy, obtained by measuring connectivity of two signals of different nature (electrical and hemodynamic), demonstrates the challenge in interpreting connectivity changes. It could also suggest an alteration of neurovascular coupling in TLE.

In unilateral mesial TLE (MTLE), the affected amygdala and hippocampus (and to a lesser extent on the contra-lateral side) are less connected between them and also with other consistent RSNs, such as the mesolimbic and the DMN, suggesting that these functional interictal changes explain cognitive and psychiatric impairments often found in patients with this type of epilepsy (109). Several fMRI studies, with and without EEG, have shown an abnormal FC between physiological consistent RSNs [i.e., language (110)] and MTL structures.

Default-mode network. Laufs and colleagues (8) have shown that deactivation in DMN, involved in consciousness, is more frequent for spikes in patients with TLE than extra-TLE. Deactivation in the same regions in response to temporal spikes was also demonstrated by Kobayashi et al. (111) and by Fahoum et al. (10). Frings et al. (112) showed decreased DMN-hippocampus FC in MTLE patients compared to controls during an object-location memory task, underlying the importance of the intact connection between these structures to preserve memory. This concept was validated in post-surgical follow-up studies (see below). An impairment of the connections between DMN and MTL structures has been demonstrated also in RS with a seed-based fMRI analysis (113). The same group (114) combined fMRI RS-FC and diffusion tensor imaging, and showed that the decreased FC within the DMN in MTLE is correlated to abnormal structural connectivity. Although functional DMN connectivity is generally decreased in MTLE, few nodes can be hyperconnected and this may play a compensatory role for the loss of functional connections in other regions of the network (115). The same study, performed with an independent component analysis, has also shown distinct patterns of FC impairment with DMN between the left and right MTLE. The same difference has been further reported (116), suggesting that impaired cognition and memory in TLE may be different in right vs. left TLE. Morgan and colleagues (117) have identified a region in the ventral lateral nucleus of the right thalamus whose connectivity to the hippocampi separates left from right TLE subjects, suggesting that quantifying resting-state FC across this network may be a potential indicator of lateralization of TLE (useful step in the pre-surgical assessments).

Functional connectivity findings are related with clinical data: McCormick et al. (118) shows that MTLE patients with respect to controls have reduced connectivity from the posterior DMN to the epileptogenic hippocampus and increased DMN connectivity to the contra-lateral hippocampus. Stronger DMN connectivity to the epileptogenic hippocampus was associated with better pre-surgical memory and with greater postsurgical memory decline, whereas stronger DMN connectivity to the contra-lateral hippocampus was associated with less postsurgical memory decline. Following surgery, DMN connectivity to the remaining hippocampus increased from pre-surgical values and showed enhanced correlation with postsurgical memory function.

Hippocampi are considered by some authors as nodes of the DMN (119), but there is not unanimity on this interpretation (32, 120, 121). It is important to remember that all the regions of the brain can be functionally connected: a region belonging to a specific network (like the mesial temporal network) can belong also to a less specific network encompassing the previous one. This classification depends on how many different physiological RSNs are extracted from specific analyses: for instance, by extracting four physiological RSNs, the probability that the mesial temporal regions will be included in the DMN is higher than if the number of extracted network is higher (122).

Mesolimbic network. Patients with unilateral MTLE have important decreases of FC with the ventromesial limbic prefrontal regions and with the nucleus accumbens (109). These regions belong to a dopaminergic mesolimbic network, involved in long-term memory for novel events and reward (123). Hippocampus and amygdala have been often described as part of this network (124, 125), and several findings suggest that this network is affected in MTLE. The preferential seizure spread from mesial temporal lobes to mesial frontal lobes, especially the orbito-frontal cortex, has been demonstrated by ictal iEEG in patients with MTLE, suggesting that mesial orbito-frontal cortex is strongly affected by mesial temporal activity (126). On the other hand, dopaminergic alterations have been demonstrated in the pathophysiology of major depression, and dysfunctional activity of the mesolimbic dopaminergic system plays a crucial role in depressive behavior (127, 128). Structures belonging to mesolimbic network are functionally (129) and structurally (130) impaired in MTLE patients who have psychiatric impairments, such as anxiety/depression. A recent study (131) showed that the subgenual anterior cingulate cortex (mesolimbic network key-node) is affected only in MTLE patients that have primary affective disorders and not in those without such disorders and neither in controls. The same study confirms these FC findings with voxel-based morphometry and diffusion tensor imaging, corroborating the concept that the affective psychopathology often diagnosed in patients with MTLE has a neurobiological correlate. Antidepressant drugs, when effective, could modulate these connectivity impairments.

The amygdala has often been described as part of mesolimbic network and it is also involved in emotional processing of stimuli. Facial emotion recognition, particularly for "fear," is impaired in patients with TLE, especially on the right hemisphere (132–135). Broicher and colleagues (136) showed through fearful-face fMRI-paradigm that the altered amygdala FC in TLE patients is strongly related to the poor performance in behavioral tests evaluating the theory of mind abilities (ability of decoding thoughts and behavior of other human beings). Another study with the same paradigm showed that, in right TLE patients, pre-operative right amygdala activation correlates with post-operative change of anxiety and depression scores [i.e., greater increases in anxiety and depression in patients with greater preoperative activation (137)]. This confirms that pre-surgical study of FC between TLE and other brain structures can help to predict post-surgery neuropsychological consequences.

Attention network. Several studies have shown that dorsal and ventral attention networks are functionally altered in MTLE, explaining why patients with this type of epilepsy have often worse performances than healthy controls (HC) in attention tasks. Cataldi et al. (138) have recently reviewed this topic.

Extra-temporal lobe epilepsy. Extra-temporal lobe epilepsies are characterized by a wide range of focus localization and etiology. For this reason, group studies with homogeneous clinical phenotype are difficult to achieve. This contrasts with the large body of group studies in MTLE, which take advantage from the frequent uniform pathology of atrophy and cell-loss in amygdala-hippocampus structures. A group-analysis EEG-fMRI study in different types of epilepsy (frontal, temporal, and posterior quadrant) showed that focal spikes are associated with networks of widespread metabolic changes, specific for each type of epilepsy (10).

Negishi et al. (139) revealed higher lateral pre-surgery FC maps in drug-resistant patients with good surgical outcome (seizure-free at 1-year) compared to those with poor outcome. A recent study on 23 patients with frontal lobe epilepsy used the same seed-FC approach (seed at maximal BOLD value of the spike-related activation map) (140), finding an increased FC in the neighborhood of the seed and a decrease in regions remote to the seed compared to controls. Patient-specific connectivity pattern was not significantly changed when comparing fMRI runs with spikes vs. fMRI without any spike detectable on the simultaneous EEG. Patients with drug-resistant frontal lobe epilepsy (141) recruit wider areas compared to controls when performing an fMRI memory encoding task paradigm, particularly in the contra-lateral frontal lobe, suggesting the presence of compensatory mechanisms to maintain memory function.

Generalized epilepsy

Different theories have been proposed about the patho-physiology of "generalized seizures". Meeren et al. (142) reviewed this topic. All these theories consider cortex and thalamus as being involved in the generation of the typical 2.5–4 Hz generalized spike-wave discharges (GSWD) detected on scalp EEG, but it is still unclear, which of them is the "primum movens" (143). As discussed below, animal studies in genetic models of absence epilepsy are crucial to gain understanding of these conditions because no invasive validation can be contemplated in human beings. These animal studies suggest that GSWDs are triggered in a restricted cortical region (144–147).

Several EEG-fMRI studies showed that during short GSWD (16, 148–150) and absence (151–154), there is a characteristic pattern of subcortical (medio-dorsal thalamic and striatus) activation and cortical deactivation, especially in areas of the DMN. It has been hypothesized that the DMN deactivation is linked to reduced consciousness (i.e., absences) (16, 155, 156). A dynamic analysis study on 17 absences from nine patients with absence epilepsy and classical pattern of 3–4 Hz GSWDs (83) showed that BOLD responses were remarkably consistent in space and time across different absences of one patient, but were different from patient to patient. Furthermore, this study shows early frontal BOLD activations (specific for each patient), supporting the cortical focus theory. Another EEG-fMRI study on 11 children with absence seizures (157) revealed that the first brain zone showing BOLD increase was the parietal cortex, this activity starting 10 s before the onset of the discharge. Additionally, this study demonstrated the hemodynamic involvement of subcortical structures in GSWD, including the reticular structures of the brainstem. Focal cortical involvement before the onset of GSWD has been demonstrated also by a magnetoencephalography study in human beings (158) and a near-infrared spectroscopy study applied on the frontal cortex (159). An exhaustive review on focal abnormalities in idiopathic generalized epilepsy (IGE) has been recently published (160). All these findings support the conceptual transition from "primarily generalized epilepsy," (implying that all brain regions simultaneously would generate GSWD) to seizures "originating within and rapidly engaging, bilaterally distributed networks" of cortical and subcortical regions (15).

Concerning the role of subcortical structures, in patients with IGE, it has been shown that both the anterior nucleus of thalamus (ANT) and the centromedian/parafascicular (Cm/Pf) nucleus (which provides diffuse inputs to the cortex) are activated during GSWD; the activity of the cortico-reticular Cm/Pf preceded that of the ANT, suggesting that the Cm/Pf is involved in GSWD initiation or early propagation, while the ANT in its maintenance (161).

Recent studies have used fMRI to investigate whether resting-state FC between thalamus, basal ganglia, and DMN areas is altered in patients with IGE, even during GSWD-free periods of brain activity (**Figure 4**). Wang et al. (162) used ICA to map RSNs in 16 patients with IGE and 16 HC. They found that the DMN had simultaneously reduced FC within the anterior cingulate cortex, but increased connectivity in the precuneus. Moreover, they found widespread connectivity reductions in prefrontal, sensorimotor, and even auditory cortices (162). Reduced resting-state FC

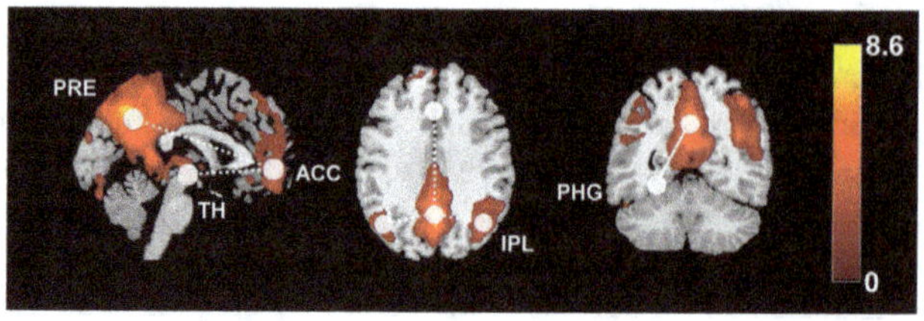

FIGURE 4 | This diagram summarizes the functional connectivity (FC) changes in patients with idiopathic generalized epilepsy compared to healthy controls. The color map shows the default-mode network (z-scores) derived from independent component analysis or RS-fMRI data overlaid on a standard single-subject anatomy (Montreal Neurological Institute space). Widespread FC reductions were found within the DMN (dashed lines), as well as between anterior DMN and the thalamus. Increased FC related to increased disease duration has been observed between posterior DMN regions and the parahippocampal gyrus (solid line). ACC, anterior cingulate cortex, IPL, inferior parietal lobule, PRE, precuneus, PHG, parahippocampal gyrus, TH, thalamus.

between frontal areas and the rest of the DMN was later confirmed (163). An important question is whether these changes in DMN connectivity are meaningfully related to clinical information, e.g., disease duration or responsiveness to medication. Of note, in both aforementioned studies, there were significant correlations between RS-FC and disease duration: the reduction in connectivity was inversely correlated to disease duration, indicating that long-standing epilepsy leads to progressive disruption of DMN integration. Interestingly, a study of structural and FC in 26 IGE patients and HC, showed that the degree of coupling between functional and structural connectivity networks is decreased, and exhibited a negative correlation with epilepsy duration in patients (164).

Other RSNs can be affected in patients with IGE, reflecting specific cognitive impairment when compared to controls. A seed-based RS-FC study in 14 patients with IGE showed that attention network is impaired even in interictal periods, and that this impairment is related with the disease duration (165).

One study in 60 IGE patients specifically addressed the question whether pharmacoresistance was correlated with RS-FC changes in the DMN (166). DMN connectivity was reduced in the IGE group compared to HC, and the strongest decrease was found in those patients that were resistant to valproate. Finally, a recent study directly addressed RS-FC within the thalamo-cortical system (167), finding decreased RS-FC between thalamus and anterior DMN. Collectively, these studies suggest that there is a loss of functional integration in the thalamocortical and default-mode system of the brain in IGE, even outside the GSWD. Although small sample size and heterogeneous methodology limit "generalization," the abnormal RS-FC patterns found in IGE so far could serve as endophenotypes of different IGE syndromes, and thus inform clinical diagnostics. Importantly, the confounding effect of anti-epileptic drug on dysconnectivity needs to be further elucidated.

The most frequent IGE syndrome is juvenile myoclonic epilepsy (JME), where seizures are characterized by myoclonic jerks of the upper limbs, often triggered by cognitive inputs. Several RS and task-related functional studies have shown an impairment of connectivity among supplementary motor area and the rest of the brain (168–170), suggesting that this structure may represent the anatomic basis for triggering motor seizures in JME. JME patients have often personality characteristics suggestive of a frontal lobe dysfunction (e.g., risk-taking behavior, dysexecutive syndrome). A task-related FC study in JME patients (171) shows that patients with ongoing seizures learn less from previous experiences compared to seizure-free patients and to controls.

Pediatric syndromes

Numerous EEG-fMRI studies have been conducted on pediatric syndromes [for review, see in Ref. (172)]. Several studies in Lennox–Gastaut syndrome (173–175) have shown hemodynamic involvement of brainstem, thalamus, and basal ganglia during paroxysmal fast activity and slow spike-and-wave discharges, underlying the importance of cortical–subcortical networks in Lennox–Gastaut syndrome. A group-analysis study in patients with myoclonic-astatic-epilepsy (176) showed that GSWD are related not only to a thalamo-cortical network (commonly found in IGE), but also to brain areas associated with motor function, suggesting that the involvement of these structures may predispose to the typical myoclonic jerks observed in this syndrome.

Concerning idiopathic focal epilepsies of childhood, these comprise a broad spectrum of phenotypes showing an overlap with each other, from benign childhood epilepsy with centro-temporal spikes (BECTS) to more severe seizure and cognitive disorders, like atypical benign partial epilepsy (ABPE), continuous spikes and waves during slow sleep (CSWS), and Landau-Kleffner syndrome. In patients with BECTS, EEG-fMRI studies have revealed focal spike-associated BOLD signal changes in the sensorimotor cortex, well corresponding to spikes localization, and typical seizure semiology (177–180). In patients with CSWS, a consistent neuronal network including both cortical and subcortical structures was described with positive BOLD signal changes in the perisylvian region, insula, cingulated cortex, and thalamus, and negative BOLD signal changes in the DMN areas and caudate nucleus (181). Source analysis of the simultaneously recorded EEG in these patients allowed differentiating initiation from propagation of epileptic activity in these common networks. The importance of assessing sleep state when studying networks is given by the report of a patient, whose centro-temporal spikes were recorded during wakefulness and sleep. BOLD response during wakefulness showed a focal activation concordant with the spike topography, whereas BOLD response to the same event during sleep showed the involvement of a thalamic–perisylvian neural network similar to the one previously observed in patients with CSWS, suggesting a common sleep-related network dysfunction even in cases with milder phenotypes (182).

A single-subject and group-analysis study (183) on patients with ABPE demonstrated that this syndrome is characterized by patterns similar to studies in rolandic epilepsy (focal BOLD signal changes in the spike field) as well as patterns observed in CSWS (distant BOLD signal changes in cortical and subcortical structures), thereby corroborating the concept that idiopathic focal epilepsies of childhood form a spectrum of overlapping syndromes.

An EEG-fMRI study in thirteen patients with ring 20 chromosome syndrome (184) shows specific networks involved by different interictal and ictal events of interest, suggesting that some hemodynamic networks are the expression of epilepsy-related cognitive and behavioral deficits typical of ring 20 chromosome syndrome, whereas others can be common to other syndromes with neurobehavioral regression.

INTRACRANIAL EEG STUDIES

The indication for video-iEEG monitoring is the absence of a unique focal hypothesis regarding the source of the patient's seizures (obtained with non-invasive investigation), or the need for cortical mapping of the epileptogenic cortex vs. eloquent cortex (7). Therefore, intracranial electrodes often sample from more than one lobe, although their spatial sampling remains limited and needs to be targeted using all available clinical and paraclinical information. Subdural grids allow dense sampling of the cortical convexity while intracerebral depth electrodes are able to reach deeper structures (e.g., medial temporal structures); combinations of both techniques are feasible. Therefore, iEEG studies represent a unique opportunity to investigate seizure networks in human beings with optimal temporal and excellent spatial resolution.

The concept of the seizure-onset zone as a single, circumscribed brain region implies that, assuming that intracranial electrodes sample this region, ictal iEEG activity should invariably start there. Careful observation of ictal iEEG recordings, however, reveals that this is not always the case. Rather, there are patients in whom clinically indistinguishable seizures seem to start at any of two or more distinct brain areas (100). Observations such as this were one of the major factors spurring the interest in considering seizure-generating brain regions as distributed networks. Therefore, the seizure-onset zone could be seen as the particular regions with the lowest seizure threshold while other regions could also give rise to independent seizure onsets, which explains the need to consider more than the sole seizure-onset zone for estimating the epileptogenic zone. In an attempt to quantitatively analyze seizure-onset patterns, Bartolomei and colleagues (185) developed the epileptogenicity index (EI), which takes into account the transition of iEEG activity toward higher frequencies (a general observation of ictal iEEG patterns) together with the delay in which the transition is observed compared to the ictal onset. This approach has revealed that in a significant portion of TLE patients, the medial and lateral temporal lobe display similar EI, implying that both structures could equally subtend seizure generation. Also of interest, some patients with what seemed like TLE before implantation actually displayed the highest values of EI in the fronto-orbital, opercular, or insular cortex rather than the temporal lobe, and these patients had poorer outcomes after resective surgery, suggesting that they harbored more distributed seizure-generating networks not easily amenable to full resection (186). The number of brain regions with a high EI increases with the duration of epilepsy, suggesting that epilepsy networks may extend over time as a result of plasticity triggered by pathological activity (185, 186).

The same authors analyzed the neurophysiological correlates of alterations of consciousness in TLE (187). They found that alteration of consciousness was associated with increased broadband synchronization in a network of structures, which were mainly extra-temporal, including the thalamus, cingulate cortex, and parieto-temporal association cortex. Consciousness was preserved as long as excessive synchrony was confined to the temporal lobe. Similarly, loss of consciousness in parietal seizures was associated with widespread parietal and frontal synchronization (188). The authors framed these observations into the context of the global workspace theory, in which the sustained synchronization of neuronal activity in widely distributed modules renders perceptions, memories, and intentions available to consciousness (189). This work rejoins observations made with single photon emission computed tomography that temporal lobe seizures causing altered consciousness were associated with widespread cortical and subcortical blood-flow alterations (190). That group later showed increases in the power of delta oscillations in the frontal and parietal association cortices during seizure-related loss of consciousness (191). Results from studies in a rat model of complex partial seizures suggest that these widespread changes are caused by transient alteration of activity in the subcortical septal nuclei (192), implying that the widespread effects of temporal lobe seizures on cortical networks could be mediated indirectly via the midline arousal structures (193).

Measures of directed connectivity in seizure networks are starting to reveal the internal organization of the individual nodes that make up the network. To date, most iEEG studies use mathematical approaches to determine the direction of connections. For instance, using focal cortical dysplasia as a model of a circumscribed seizure-onset zone and applying partial directed coherence analysis, Varotto et al. (12) found that the focal dysplasia indeed acted as the initial generator of ictal activity, as evidenced by its greater out-degree both interictally, pre-ictally, and during ictal onsets [the out-degree is a summary measure of the influence of one network node on all the others (194)]. Cortical-areas remote from the morphological lesion could also be involved in the onset or early propagation of ictal high-frequency activity and could thus represent secondary foci. Wilke et al. (195) used frequency-band-specific betweenness centrality, a graph theoretical measure of the "importance" of a node in network pathways, to demonstrate a significant overlap between the intracranial electrodes showing the highest betweenness centrality and the seizure-onset zone delineated visually by clinical neurophysiologists, as well as the resected cortical area. That correspondence was present both during ictal and interictal recordings and was highest for gamma-band frequencies. In addition, the analysis also revealed nodes with high betweenness centrality that had not been clinically identified as part of the seizure-onset zone. Van Mierlo et al. (196) showed that the single intracranial electrode with the highest out-degree during seizure onsets was included in the clinically defined seizure-onset zone as well as the resection area in all of eight patients. These first findings suggest that analyzing epileptic networks in the framework of graph theory, taking into account the direction of connections between nodes in the network, can help clinicians delineate the primary drivers from secondary nodes in seizure nodes [see also in Ref. (197) for a review]. In the near future, we expect that the tools of graph theory will be applied more generally to iEEG data to describe more fully the spatio-temporal dynamics of seizure networks. Another unique perspective could be offered by the analysis of simultaneous recordings of iEEG and fMRI (198, 199) to combine the spatial resolution of iEEG with the mapping of whole-brain BOLD changes related to epileptic activity. This could allow bridging the poorly understood gap between increased iEEG connectivity and reduced BOLD connectivity within epileptic networks (108).

Micro-electrode studies in human beings

Another potential breakthrough in the investigation of epileptic networks could stem, in a somewhat paradoxical fashion, from micro-electrode array recordings, which revealed new insights on the pathophysiology of epilepsy. Schevon et al. (200) inserted arrays comprising of 96 electrodes arranged in a 4-by-4-mm square pattern in the putative seizure-onset zone allowing to record single unit activity in cortical layers 4 and 5 as well as recording the local-field potentials. They showed that there is a sharp delineation (at a sub-millimetric scale) between cortical-areas involved in intense hypersynchronous firing (the hallmark of ictal activity, based on animal studies) and adjacent areas with only mildly increased firing rate and synchrony. Crucially, visual inspection of the iEEG alone did not allow distinguishing between what the authors termed the seizure core and its (presumably) inhibitory penumbra. The same investigators further proposed that ictal high-frequency oscillations phase-locked to the lower-frequency, high-amplitude ictal iEEG recorded by standard intracranial electrodes might represent a signature of increased firing in the seizure core (201). These new findings open the possibility of investigating neuronal firing in distributed seizure networks using conventional iEEG electrodes, without the need for micro-electrode arrays. Future work building on these exciting findings will likely increase our understanding of the ways in which seizures alter normal neuronal firing across the nodes of the involved networks.

Direct electrical stimulation studies

Direct electrical stimulation (DES) in epileptic patients consists of administering electrical currents to the brain tissue in order to transiently influence or perturb its function. A technique almost as old as epilepsy surgery, it has mostly been used to probe the function of the cortex directly underlying or surrounding the stimulation site (202–205). In that context, DES is generally delivered at high frequencies (e.g., 50–60 Hz) for a few seconds with the aim of inducing clinical changes in the patient (206). More recently, DES has also been used to investigate FC; in that case, single stimulation pulses are delivered at low frequencies (e.g., 1 Hz) and the readout consists of time-locked perturbations in the activity of points distant from the stimulation site (cortico-cortical evoked potentials, CCEPs) (207). An interesting aspect of DES-based FC assessments is that they are directed, i.e., the effect of stimulation at site A on site B is not necessarily symmetrical with the effect of stimulating B on A (**Figure 5**). There is an intuitive appeal to this "hands-on" interventional approach to reveal directional connectivity. Evoked effective connectivity was found to correlate with FC measured by resting-state fMRI (22) as well as with anatomical connectivity probed by diffusion tensor imaging (208). It has been pointed out, however, that DES can activate axons in the antidromic as well as the orthodromic direction, and could also stimulate *fibers de passage*, an important caveat to keep in mind when interpreting the directionality information provided by these data (209).

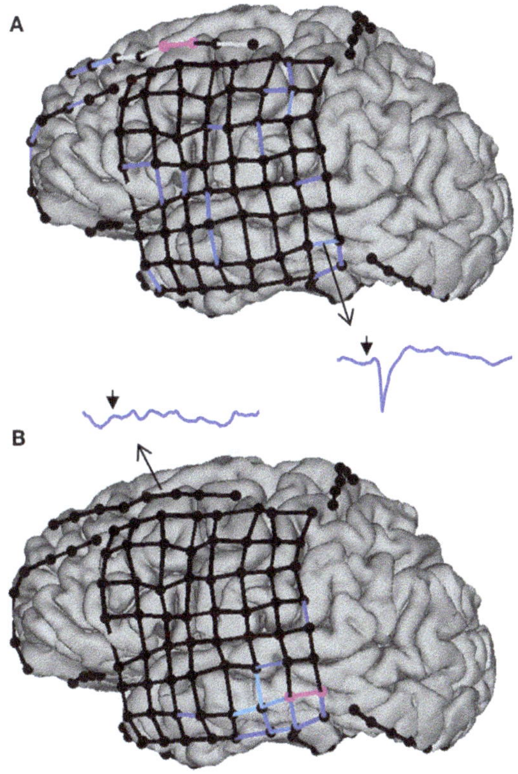

FIGURE 5 | Evoked effective connectivity reveals the directionality of neural connections in the human brain. In this example, subdural electrodes are represented by circles, and CCEP responses as lines linking bipolar electrode pairs. Missing (e.g., artifacted) data are indicated by light gray lines, sub-threshold (non-significant) responses by black lines, and significant responses by progressively lighter shades of blue.
(A) Stimulation of the middle frontal gyrus (electrode pair colored in pink) triggers widespread responses in the frontal and temporal lobes, including the middle temporal gyrus (inset: CCEP waveform from 50 ms before to 250 ms after stimulation; the arrow indicates the time of stimulation). By contrast, stimulation of the middle temporal gyrus **(B)** does not evoke any significant response in the frontal lobe, illustrating that effective connectivity between remote brain structures is not necessarily reciprocal.

This highlights the importance of aiming at obtaining multimodal functional and structural information to better understand brain connectivity and dynamics.

Evoked effective connectivity has revealed strong intralobar connectivity in the temporal and frontal lobes, as well as connections between the frontal and temporal lobes that are more prominent in the frontal-to-temporal than in the temporal-to-frontal direction (210, 211). An intriguing aspect of these studies is the observation that, whereas interhemispheric connections between the frontal lobes are relatively common, temporal-temporal connections appear sparse, being observed in <20% of patients (211). This begs the question of which neuronal pathways are responsible for bitemporal synchronized spiking as well as the propagation of seizures from one temporal lobe to the other one (212). Recently, David et al. (213) generalized this approach offering to develop an atlas of evoked effective connectivity that would eventually allow, through data sharing, sampling most of the human brain's volume.

Direct electrical stimulation has also been used to specifically evaluate epileptic networks, the general idea being that the responses of remote sites to stimulation of epileptogenic cortex (214) or the responses of epileptogenic cortex to stimulation of remote sites (215) differ from those involving only normal brain tissue. Interestingly, the network of brain areas that respond to DES of the seizure-onset zone overlaps partially but not completely with the areas of ictal propagation, suggesting both that seizures propagate sequentially through multiple nodes in the network and that some existing connections between the seizure-onset zone and distant brain areas "shut down" during seizures (216). Further research combining iEEG and DES, as well as integrating these techniques with fMRI and high-density non-invasive electromagnetic recordings, will improve our understanding of the physiology of seizure networks.

WHAT WE CAN LEARN FROM ANIMAL MODELS

Recording the activity of any node suspected to be determinant in the disease is not feasible in human beings, contrarily to animal research. Moreover, animal-related technologies offer the possibility to desiccate and manipulate cellular and molecular components of such networks, as well as scrutinizing the associated structural and functional alterations. A great perspective in pathological networks study is detecting features associated with the risk of recurrence after a first seizure as well as predicting the evolution toward pharmaco-resistance.

Animal models allow studying networks connectivity and recording the underlying brain activity with high spatial coverage and resolution (217), and addressing the process of epileptogenesis and ictogenesis, including their molecular and genetic mechanisms at cellular and subcellular levels (218–222). Imbalance between excitation and inhibition might not only occur at the local microscopic level (223, 224), but could also reflect dysregulation of excitatory and inhibitory neuronal interactions at a larger (network) scale. Recent evidence emphasizes the modifications of the network dynamic, or network configuration that characterizes, and sometimes precedes or even predicts a seizure. Network analysis could be a powerful tool to more precisely define the different epilepsies and develop new treatments that target networks, instead of focal activity (11, 100).

In animals and human beings, focal onsets have been identified in generalized epilepsy, and complex large-scale network involvement has been shown in focal epilepsies (8, 11, 14). Spontaneous epileptic disease occurs in animals, as in the case of the genetic absence epileptic rats of Strasbourg (GAERS) or in the WAG/Rij rats (225–227); other models studied are epileptic conditions induced by – mainly – chemical or electrical interventions (220). A major animal model of TLE is the kainate, or pilocarpine, model of hippocampal sclerosis (HS) (228–232). Kainate, a glutamatergic agonist, is injected either in the hippocampus or intraperitoneally. It is suspected that the kainate has a tropism for the hippocampus, which led several authors to consider that the kainate induces specifically a HS. Yet, the mechanisms by which kainate induces an epileptic activity is still debated; the immune system and leakage of the blood–brain barrier have been cited as critical for the expression of the disease (233, 234). Hence, it is not excluded that systemic kainate may have diffuse effects on the brain.

Models of focally induced epileptic disorders might avoid this limitation. One of them, electrical kindling, triggers focal epileptic activity using focal electrical stimulation in accordance with standard stimulation parameters, e.g., duration of the stimulation, frequency, and intensity of the stimulus (220, 235, 236). The emergence of a distant pathological activity can be related to remote effects of the focally induced epilepsy, and not to the direct diffuse effects of the electrical or chemical triggers. Electrical stimulation, in particular of the performant-path, has also been described as a model of induced status epilepticus (237, 238).

CONNECTIVITY STUDIES IN ANIMALS

Electrophysiology can assess connectivity and RS networks in animal models of epilepsy by recording several brain regions simultaneously. The great advantage is that the signal can be directly linked to neuronal activity. Using intrahippocampal recording in a rat model of induced TLE, Wang et al. (239) showed that neuronal pairs presented a decreased FC prior to the status epilepticus induced by an intraperitoneal injection of pilocarpine. Using Graph Theory measures in an *in vitro* Mg^{2+}-free model of hippocampal epilepsy, Gong et al. (240) reported the modifications in network configuration that appear in parallel to epileptiform discharges. More interestingly, they revealed that the changes in network configuration appeared before and lasted longer than the epileptiform discharges (240). These two observations suggest that the classical ictal activity, i.e., the presence of spikes in the EEG, could be the resultant of network reconfiguration, i.e., it could even be an epiphenomenon of a more profound alteration in brain connectivity, indicating that it could be possible to identify certain network alterations as a biomarker of epilepsy. Such studies aimed at identifying markers of an upcoming ictal activity and have mainly looked at the local activity changes (241). Knowledge on remote involvement is sparse. Recent works (224) showed structural alterations remote from the focus, but only a few evidence of distant, abnormal neuronal activity exists (242). Major advancement has been made to record as many neurons or neuronal populations as possible at the same time (145, 243–248); this shows the feasibility to investigate large-scale networks in animal models with high temporal and spatial resolution (**Figure 6**). Their combination with effective connectivity measures (25) will help to better understand the hierarchical organization of epileptic networks. Gong et al. (240) demonstrated the leading activity of pyramidal cells over granular cells in an *in vitro* model of TLE, illustrating the utility of effective connectivity in the field of epilepsy.

Research on animal models of epilepsy has been dominated by invasive electro-physiology technique. Recently, the combination of EEG and fMRI has emerged with interesting results, such as those reported by Englot et al. (192), where they describe how a partial limbic seizure lead to neocortical slow-wave activity; yet, technical issues makes difficult to obtain combined EEG-fMRI in awake animals. As in Englot et al. (192), fMRI could possibly be a powerful *in vivo* screening method for anatomical regions that could then be more deeply investigated with EEG.

Using fMRI, Mishra et al. (249) showed that rats submitted to traumatic brain injury through left parietal fluid percussion presented a decreased correlation coefficient between the left parietal cortex and other brain regions. Dysfunctional activity in the left parietal cortex, as highlighted by the decreased correlation coefficient could have been expected, yet the pattern of resting BOLD-fMRI connectivity showed that only certain regions were specifically affected, namely the left hippocampus and the contralateral parietal cortex. This illustrates that BOLD-fMRI can be used to identify secondary dysfunctional brain regions in rodents following a proepileptogenic injury (249). The same group investigated with fMRI the FC in WAG/Rij rats (250) and found an increased correlation between brain areas suspected to be involved in seizures when compared to non-epileptic rats; more importantly, this increase was observed outside of the ictal periods. Choi et al. (251) performed a FC study using the ^{18}fluorodeoxyglucose positron emission tomography (PET) signal in a rat model of TLE. They revealed the decreased correlation of several pairs of brain structures, most of them included left amygdala and left entorhinal cortex (251). Hence, despite the systemic injection of pilocarpine, the affected network appeared to be mainly restricted to the left hemisphere (251). It would have been very interesting to see if the electro-physiological counterpart of such functional deficit was also restricted to one hemisphere, yet no EEG recording was reported. Asymmetry in the central nervous system is well recognized, e.g., asymmetry of the temporal lobes, but the reason why the left hemisphere appears to be more functionally altered in this rat model of TLE is unclear, although electro-physiological experiments suggest that the left hemisphere is indeed more prone to develop epileptic discharges (252). The authors claimed that the PET images were acquired in the interictal period, but no EEG recording was used (251); yet, if true, this would suggest that epileptic animals can be identified as such on the basis of the FC

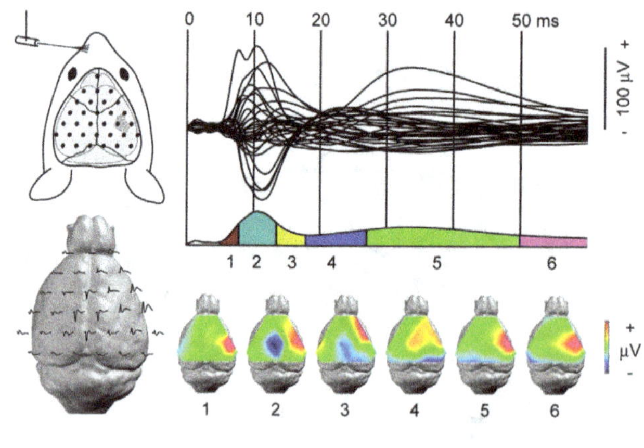

FIGURE 6 | Dynamic of somato-sensory network mapped with high-density EEG. Somato-sensory evoked potential (SEP) from left whisker stimulation. *Top left:* each black dot represents the position of one recording electrode; the most anterior one is ground. *Top right:* 31 electrode traces displaying the SEP with sub-milliseconds resolution. *Bottom left:* the same electrode traces represented over the mouse brain. In the lissencephalic mouse brain, dipoles are estimated to be generated below the recording electrodes. *Bottom right:* segmentation of the SEP in six stable configurations of potential maps. The technique's high spatial and temporal resolutions identify the first component, somato-sensory barrel field activity, followed by motor cortex and contra-lateral somato-sensory areas recruitment within a few milliseconds. Adapted from Megevand et al. (243) with permission.

of particular networks outside of any ictal activity. These studies (249–251) indicate that the pathological process in these rats is ongoing: the epileptic brain is not suffering from epilepsy only during seizures.

The anatomical basis of FC is largely unclear. Zhou et al. (253) nicely investigated the anatomical substrate and plasticity of such connections. They observed that after partial posterior callosotomy of wild-type rats, the FC of the auditory and visual cortices decreased at day 7 and returned to baseline at day 28, whereas this decrease was still present in rats submitted to complete callosotomy (253). The authors concluded that it could be possible to identify the anatomical basis of FC, and that these functional connections were also capable of plasticity. This is an important proof-of-concept: it is possible to identify morphological substrate of functional connections and manipulate them.

DIFFERENTIAL INVOLVEMENT OF SPECIFIC BRAIN REGIONS IN ANIMAL MODELS OF GENERALIZED EPILEPSY

Different rat models of generalized absence epilepsy have been studied and all share the presence of the characteristic SWDs (254, 255). Using combined EEG-fMRI in WAG/Rij rats, Mishra et al. (250) demonstrated that during SWDs, the associated fluctuations in the BOLD signal were specific to certain brain regions. Indeed, the somato-sensory barrel field showed an increase, whereas the striatum showed a decrease in the BOLD signal and cerebral blood-flow (225, 250). On the other hand, the local-field potential (LFP) and the multi-unit activity (MUA) were increased in both regions (225). Vascular steal or dopamine-regulated blood volume could account, at least in part, for this lack of matching between BOLD signal and CBF on the one hand and LFP and MUA on the other hand (225). An earlier study using surface and deep EEG recordings in the same rat-model showed that these rats shared a similar focus located in the ventrolateral part of the somato-sensory cortex (SC) (145). More importantly, the authors observed that the ictal activity of the cortical focus preceded the one in the thalamus, suggesting that the cortex was leading the thalamus (145). Nersesyan et al. (256) investigated the relation between SWDs and CBF in the same animal model. They showed that regions involved in SWDs, i.e., SC, presented a 1- to 2-s delayed increase in CBF during a SWD, whereas this increase did not appear in regions not involved in the SWDs, such as primary visual cortex (256). In a parallel work using the same animal model of absence epilepsy, they observed that the BOLD signal was not equally modified across brain regions during a SWD (257): the somato-sensory and motor cortices, as well as subcortical regions, i.e., thalamus, basal ganglia, and brainstem, showed an increased BOLD signal, whereas other regions such as the occipital cortex did not show such a modulation of the signal (257). Again, the increase in the BOLD signal appeared with a lag of a few seconds after the electro-physiological SWDs (257). This finding is in contrast with a work by Desalvo et al. (258), in which they used a rat model of generalized tonico-clonic seizures induced by injection of iv bicuculline, and observed that BOLD increased significantly in primary and secondary somato-sensory cortices, as well as in primary auditory cortex and thalamus *before* the onset of electro-physiological seizures. The role of the SC in initiating GSWDs was further investigated through inactivation of this cortical region in GAERS animals (259). The pharmacological inactivation of the SC with the sodium channel blocker tetrodotoxine prevented the spike-and-wave activity; yet unilateral application of the drug did not completely abolish the abnormal contra-lateral oscillations. On the whole, these studies highlight the importance of abnormal focal brain activity as a potential trigger of generalized seizures (258). The identification of interacting yet independent nodes within a network of suspected generalized epilepsy is a major advance in epilepsy research. Indeed, it will permit to refine the therapeutic intervention toward the manipulation of one particular and decisive node.

SHORT-RANGE AND LONG-RANGE NETWORK MODULATIONS IN ANIMAL MODELS OF FOCAL EPILEPSY

Different animal models of focal epilepsy exist (220), such as the kainate- or pilocarpine-models of MTLE (228, 229, 260), posttraumatic epilepsy (261, 262), or electrical kindling (227, 263). Despite an initially focal insult, recent evidence (e.g., 242) shows that remote brain areas become affected by the pathological activity of the epileptic focus.

The induction of a focal epileptic syndrome in a rat model of generalized epilepsy allows better understanding how these two entities interact. Carcak et al. (227) took advantage of the fact that absence epilepsy may increase the resistance to limbic seizures. They investigated the role of the cortico-thalamo-cortical circuitry, involved in SWDs, in the development of limbic seizures induced by unilateral electrical stimulation of the rat amygdala. Whereas control rats, i.e., those without absence epilepsy, presented all convulsive epileptic seizures following amygdala electrical stimulation, rats suffering from absence epilepsy did not (227). In order to understand how the circuit involved in absence epilepsy could affect the one of TLE, the authors investigated the spontaneous activity in the reticular thalamic nucleus (RTN), known to be involved in the slow-waves discharges that characterize absence epilepsy (227). Remarkably, the electrical stimulation of the amygdala had a different effect on the mean firing frequency of neurons of the RTN: in not-stimulated animals, there was no significant difference between epileptic and non-epileptic rats, whereas the increase after stimulation was higher in epileptic rats when compared to non-epileptic rats (227). This suggests first that the development of an epileptic focus alters the activity of neurons in the RTN and second that this alteration depends on the activity before the induction of the epilepsy. The use of Wistar rats as controls for GAERS rats in that study is commonly accepted, but could still be questioned; yet the conclusion would still remains the same: the effects of an epileptic focus seem to depend on the brain state in which it is being established. It would hence be interesting to investigate how an epileptic focus affects a given network, but also how a particular network configuration can modulate the effects of an epileptic focus. The involvement of the thalamus in propagation of temporal lobe seizures has already been the scope of several studies (156, 264). If the thalamus has a major role in the generation of SWDs (227), this could highlight the relevance of studying the interaction between hippocampus and thalamus, in the context of focal epilepsies.

Hippocampal sclerosis is a frequent lesion that has been deeply investigated, although, most of the works conducted local, intrahippocampal recordings. Yet, recent publications have shown the involvement of remote brain areas. Using 16 bipolar deep electrodes in the pilocarpine rat-model of HS, Toyoda et al. (247) showed that the initial focus varied from one seizure to another in each individual rat. The subiculum, the dorsal and ventral hippocampus, and the amygdala were the regions where seizure onsets were most often recorded. All regions could be considered as belonging to the same network; indeed, an interesting observation is that most seizures were convulsive, and this did not depend upon where the seizure started (247). This suggests that the involved network is more determining than the seizure-onset zone for the clinical expression of a seizure. Long-range modifications in the kainate mouse-model of TLE were also observed. It has been shown that non-injected hippocampus presented indeed morphological alterations, notably in the expression of the neuropeptide-Y, which is known to modulate neuronal activity (265, 266), and electro-physiological changes, such as significant decrease in the power of the theta frequency band (265). *In vitro*, Khalilov et al. (267) demonstrated that a mirror focus in the contra-lateral hippocampus appears after 10–15 successive applications of kainate in the ipsilateral hippocampus. These findings are in line with the hypothesis that an epileptic focus leads to permanent electrophysiological and morphological modifications in remote brain areas (268–270). Other works have also stressed the possibility that subcortical brain regions, such as the basal ganglia, could influence or even inhibit the progression of an ictal activity originating from the temporal lobe (271, 272).

Evidence of distant brain involvement arises also from electrically induced epilepsy. For instance, during hippocampal seizures induced by electrical stimulation in rats, the frontal neocortex presented a parallel modification in spontaneous activity, i.e., fast polyspike activity when the seizure was generalized and slow oscillations when it was partial (242). This example illustrates that distant brain areas are affected even after a few or only one focal epileptic seizure. It would be extremely interesting to study how this involvement evolves in a chronic disease.

On the whole, evidence exists that other brain areas are recruited in propagation or in inhibition of the seizure spread. Hence, the epileptic threshold does not seem to depend only on the imbalance between excitation and inhibition within the focus, but could also be determined by the intricate interactions between the components of a given network.

EXPERIMENTAL THERAPEUTIC INTERVENTIONS ON THE EPILEPTIC NETWORK

Conceiving epilepsy as a network disease has therapeutic consequences. The classical view is to modulate the activity of the so-called epileptic focus, or seizure-onset zone, in order to control the disease. Yet, any node of an epileptic network could possibly be a target. In this sense, open-loop or closed-loop devices, either through electrical or optogenetic stimulation, are promising tools for generalized (217) as well as for focal epilepsy (273, 274). Major work has shown that it is possible to identify critical nodes in a given epileptic network: the modification of their activation – mainly inhibition – could help to control, or even stop an ictal activity. Paz et al. (274) showed in a rat model of cortical epilepsy that the inactivation through optogenetics of the thalamic ventrobasal nucleus could stop an ongoing seizure. In the same line, Langlois et al. (264) showed in an *in vivo* model of TLE that DBS of the ipsilateral parafascicular nucleus of the thalamus (PF) stopped the ongoing hippocampal paroxysmal discharges (HPD), while higher current intensities were needed to stop the HPD if DBS was applied to neighboring areas (264), illustrating the specificity of PF in controlling HPDs. The anterior thalamic nucleus (ANT) appears also to be involved in control or spread of epileptic activity of mesial temporal onset (156). Ablation or electrical stimulation of ANT increases the epileptic threshold (263, 275–277); yet, opposite results have also been observed (278). On the whole, ANT is a recognized target for refractory epilepsy, although mechanisms by which manipulation of the ANT increases epileptic threshold are poorly understood. Use of animal research and the possibility to identify how the activity of ANT may modulate epileptic activity at remote sites, e.g., with the use of effective connectivity measures, is crucial to tailor therapeutic interventions. Such recent evidence shows that the manipulation of the primary epileptic focus does not seem to be the only possibility to achieve the control of an epileptic disease. The thalamus in particular, and other subcortical regions as well (272) have been identified as major targets for epileptic network modulation culminating in clinical applications in the form of DBS of ANT in focal epilepsies (279).

CONCLUSION

With increasingly complex methodological strategies and an ever-increasing wealth of possible approaches, the study of brain connectivity and its neuroscientific and clinical correlates are very promising. Nevertheless, the application of connectivity techniques for diagnostic or prognostic purposes requires further studies to be firmly grounded by invasive studies and sufficient follow-up investigations before it can be reliably applied to the clinical management of individual patients. Combining functional techniques can lead to the achievement of complementary information for improving each single technique.

Focal epilepsies, despite focal epileptogenic zone, are diseases affecting the whole brain: altered large-scale FC is reflected in neuropsychological features of individual specific syndrome. Hippocrates (400 years b.c.) considered epilepsy as a systemic disease, centered in the brain, due to an altered "defluxion of cold phlegm" through the body. In more recent times, the concept of epilepsy as "focus disease" has been largely developed (280–282), whereas in the last decade it has shifted to a "brain-network disease" (15). In parallel to the "brain-network" concept of epilepsy, psychiatric and neurological co-morbidities, such as strokes, dementia, and migraine are more and more defined. Interestingly, somatic co-morbidities have also come to light, since several medical conditions, such as cardiac, gastrointestinal, and respiratory disorders, are often associated with epilepsy (283). These findings may lead to re-consider epilepsy as a "systemic disease," this time with the diagnostic and therapeutic knowledge obtained recently by ground-breaking work on network analysis.

Concerning "generalized" epilepsy, neuro-imaging, and especially connectivity studies have allowed considering them as focal brain disorders with fast bilateral discharge propagation. This concept leads to the idea that focal and generalized epilepsies are the two extremes of a single spectrum and to a possible new way of studying mechanisms of AED: do they have an effect on particular nodes of a network where receptors are more expressed? Is it possible to detect an anatomical target to avoid generation/propagation of seizures, using disconnection or stimulation? For all these reasons, translational research in light of network analysis, based on fundamental science through animal experiments and clinical perspectives through human research, opens new opportunities to better understand the complexity of epilepsy and define new and more effective treatments for patients.

ACKNOWLEDGMENTS

Francesca Pittau is supported by the Swiss National Science Foundation (FNS SPUM grant 140332). Serge Vulliemoz is supported by grant FNS 141165 and the Gertrude von Meissner Foundation. Laurent Sheybani is supported by grant FNS 323530_158125). Frédéric Grouiller is supported by the Center for Biomedical Imaging of the Universities and Hospitals of Geneva and Lausanne, and EPFL. We thank Dr. Gaetano Cantalupo (Verona) for the thoughtful comments during the manuscript preparation.

REFERENCES

1. Hauser WA, Annegers JF, Kurland LT. Incidence of epilepsy and unprovoked seizures in Rochester, Minnesota: 1935-1984. *Epilepsia* (1993) **34**:453–68.
2. Sander JW. The epidemiology of epilepsy revisited. *Curr Opin Neurol* (2003) **16**:165–70. doi:10.1097/00019052-200304000-00008
3. Schuele SU, Luders HO. Intractable epilepsy: management and therapeutic alternatives. *Lancet Neurol* (2008) **7**:514–24. doi:10.1016/S1474-4422(08)70108-X
4. Bancaud J. Surgery of epilepsy based on stereotactic investigations – the plan of the SEEG investigation. *Acta Neurochir Suppl (Wien)* (1980) **30**:25–34. doi:10.1007/978-3-7091-8592-6_4
5. Spencer S, Huh L. Outcomes of epilepsy surgery in adults and children. *Lancet Neurol* (2008) **7**:525–37. doi:10.1016/S1474-4422(08)70109-1
6. De Tisi J, Bell GS, Peacock JL, McEvoy AW, Harkness WF, Sander JW, et al. The long-term outcome of adult epilepsy surgery, patterns of seizure remission, and relapse: a cohort study. *Lancet* (2011) **378**:1388–95. doi:10.1016/S0140-6736(11)60890-8
7. Rosenow F, Luders H. Presurgical evaluation of epilepsy. *Brain* (2001) **124**:1683–700. doi:10.1093/brain/124.9.1683
8. Laufs H, Hamandi K, Salek-Haddadi A, Kleinschmidt AK, Duncan JS, Lemieux L. Temporal lobe interictal epileptic discharges affect cerebral activity in "default mode" brain regions. *Hum Brain Mapp* (2007) **28**:1023–32. doi:10.1002/hbm.20323
9. Gotman J. Epileptic networks studied with EEG-fMRI. *Epilepsia* (2008) **49**(Suppl 3):42–51. doi:10.1111/j.1528-1167.2008.01509.x
10. Fahoum F, Lopes R, Pittau F, Dubeau F, Gotman J. Widespread epileptic networks in focal epilepsies-EEG-fMRI study. *Epilepsia* (2012) **53**:1618–27. doi:10.1111/j.1528-1167.2012.03533.x
11. Richardson MP. Large scale brain models of epilepsy: dynamics meets connectomics. *J Neurol Neurosurg Psychiatry* (2012) **83**:1238–48. doi:10.1136/jnnp-2011-301944
12. Varotto G, Tassi L, Franceschetti S, Spreafico R, Panzica F. Epileptogenic networks of type II focal cortical dysplasia: a stereo-EEG study. *Neuroimage* (2012) **61**:591–8. doi:10.1016/j.neuroimage.2012.03.090
13. Engel J Jr, Thompson PM, Stern JM, Staba RJ, Bragin A, Mody I. Connectomics and epilepsy. *Curr Opin Neurol* (2013) **26**:186–94. doi:10.1097/WCO.0b013e32835ee5b8
14. Stefan H, Lopes da Silva FH. Epileptic neuronal networks: methods of identification and clinical relevance. *Front Neurol* (2013) **4**:8. doi:10.3389/fneur.2013.00008
15. Berg AT, Berkovic SF, Brodie MJ, Buchhalter J, Cross JH, Van Emde Boas W, et al. Revised terminology and concepts for organization of seizures and epilepsies: report of the ILAE commission on classification and terminology, 2005-2009. *Epilepsia* (2010) **51**:676–85. doi:10.1111/j.1528-1167.2010.02522.x
16. Gotman J, Grova C, Bagshaw A, Kobayashi E, Aghakhani Y, Dubeau F. Generalized epileptic discharges show thalamocortical activation and suspension of the default state of the brain. *Proc Natl Acad Sci U S A* (2005) **102**:15236–40. doi:10.1073/pnas.0504935102
17. Smith SM, Fox PT, Miller KL, Glahn DC, Fox PM, MacKay CE, et al. Correspondence of the brain's functional architecture during activation and rest. *Proc Natl Acad Sci U S A* (2009) **106**:13040–5. doi:10.1073/pnas.0905267106
18. Biswal BB, Mennes M, Zuo XN, Gohel S, Kelly C, Smith SM, et al. Toward discovery science of human brain function. *Proc Natl Acad Sci U S A* (2010) **107**:4734–9. doi:10.1073/pnas.0911855107
19. Tomarken AJ, Waller NG. Structural equation modeling: strengths, limitations, and misconceptions. *Annu Rev Clin Psychol* (2005) **1**:31–65. doi:10.1146/annurev.clinpsy.1.102803.144239
20. Friston KJ, Harrison L, Penny W. Dynamic causal modelling. *Neuroimage* (2003) **19**:1273–302. doi:10.1016/S1053-8119(03)00202-7
21. Granger CWJ. Investigating causal relations by econometric models and cross-spectral methods. *Econometrica* (1969) **37**:424–38. doi:10.2307/1912791
22. Keller CJ, Bickel S, Entz L, Ulbert I, Milham MP, Kelly C, et al. Intrinsic functional architecture predicts electrically evoked responses in the human brain. *Proc Natl Acad Sci U S A* (2011) **108**:10308–13. doi:10.1073/pnas.1019750108
23. Astolfi L, Cincotti F, Mattia D, De Vico Fallani F, Lai M, Baccala L, et al. Comparison of different multivariate methods for the estimation of cortical connectivity: simulations and applications to EEG data. *Conf Proc IEEE Eng Med Biol Soc* (2005) **5**:4484–7. doi:10.1109/IEMBS.2005.1615463
24. Smith SM, Miller KL, Salimi-Khorshidi G, Webster M, Beckmann CF, Nichols TE, et al. Network modelling methods for FMRI. *Neuroimage* (2011) **54**:875–91. doi:10.1016/j.neuroimage.2010.08.063
25. Plomp G, Quairiaux C, Michel CM, Astolfi L. The physiological plausibility of time-varying Granger-causal modeling: normalization and weighting by spectral power. *Neuroimage* (2014) **97C**:206–16. doi:10.1016/j.neuroimage.2014.04.016
26. Bullmore E, Sporns O. Complex brain networks: graph theoretical analysis of structural and functional systems. *Nat Rev Neurosci* (2009) **10**:186–98. doi:10.1038/nrn2575
27. Ogawa S, Tank DW, Menon R, Ellermann JM, Kim SG, Merkle H, et al. Intrinsic signal changes accompanying sensory stimulation: functional brain mapping with magnetic resonance imaging. *Proc Natl Acad Sci U S A* (1992) **89**:5951–5. doi:10.1073/pnas.89.13.5951
28. Greicius MD, Krasnow B, Reiss AL, Menon V. Functional connectivity in the resting brain: a network analysis of the default mode hypothesis. *Proc Natl Acad Sci U S A* (2003) **100**:253–8. doi:10.1073/pnas.0135058100
29. Shmuel A, Leopold DA. Neuronal correlates of spontaneous fluctuations in fMRI signals in monkey visual cortex: implications for functional connectivity at rest. *Hum Brain Mapp* (2008) **29**:751–61. doi:10.1002/hbm.20580
30. Fahoum F, Zelmann R, Tyvaert L, Dubeau F, Gotman J. Epileptic discharges affect the default mode network – FMRI and intracerebral EEG evidence. *PLoS One* (2013) **8**:e68038. doi:10.1371/journal.pone.0068038
31. Raichle ME, MacLeod AM, Snyder AZ, Powers WJ, Gusnard DA, Shulman GL. A default mode of brain function. *Proc Natl Acad Sci U S A* (2001) **98**:676–82. doi:10.1073/pnas.98.2.676
32. Buckner RL, Andrews-Hanna JR, Schacter DL. The brain's default network: anatomy, function, and relevance to disease. *Ann N Y Acad Sci* (2008) **1124**:1–38. doi:10.1196/annals.1440.011
33. Cavanna AE, Trimble MR. The precuneus: a review of its functional anatomy and behavioural correlates. *Brain* (2006) **129**:564–83. doi:10.1093/brain/awl004

34. Biswal B, Yetkin FZ, Haughton VM, Hyde JS. Functional connectivity in the motor cortex of resting human brain using echo-planar MRI. *Magn Reson Med* (1995) **34**:537–41. doi:10.1002/mrm.1910340409
35. McKeown MJ, Makeig S, Brown GG, Jung TP, Kindermann SS, Bell AJ, et al. Analysis of fMRI data by blind separation into independent spatial components. *Hum Brain Mapp* (1998) **6**:160–88. doi:10.1002/(SICI)1097-0193(1998)6:5/6<368::AID-HBM7>3.3.CO;2-5
36. Bellec P, Rosa-Neto P, Lyttelton OC, Benali H, Evans AC. Multi-level bootstrap analysis of stable clusters in resting-state fMRI. *Neuroimage* (2010) **51**:1126–39. doi:10.1016/j.neuroimage.2010.02.082
37. Lemieux L, Daunizeau J, Walker MC. Concepts of connectivity and human epileptic activity. *Front Syst Neurosci* (2011) **5**:12. doi:10.3389/fnsys.2011.00012
38. Biswal BB. Resting state fMRI: a personal history. *Neuroimage* (2012) **62**:938–44. doi:10.1016/j.neuroimage.2012.01.090
39. De Vico Fallani F, Astolfi L, Cincotti F, Mattia D, Maglione AG, Vecchiato G, et al. Large-scale cortical networks estimated from scalp EEG signals during performance of goal-directed motor tasks. *Conf Proc IEEE Eng Med Biol Soc* (2010) **2010**:1738–41. doi:10.1109/IEMBS.2010.5626710
40. De Pasquale F, Della Penna S, Snyder AZ, Lewis C, Mantini D, Marzetti L, et al. Temporal dynamics of spontaneous MEG activity in brain networks. *Proc Natl Acad Sci U S A* (2010) **107**:6040–5. doi:10.1073/pnas.0913863107
41. Brookes MJ, Woolrich M, Luckhoo H, Price D, Hale JR, Stephenson MC, et al. Investigating the electrophysiological basis of resting state networks using magnetoencephalography. *Proc Natl Acad Sci U S A* (2011) **108**:16783–8. doi:10.1073/pnas.1112685108
42. Cabral J, Kringelbach ML, Deco G. Exploring the network dynamics underlying brain activity during rest. *Prog Neurobiol* (2014) **114**:102–31. doi:10.1016/j.pneurobio.2013.12.005
43. Lehmann D. Topography of spontaneous alpha EEG fields in humans. *Electroencephalogr Clin Neurophysiol* (1971) **30**:161–2.
44. Dierks T, Jelic V, Julin P, Maurer K, Wahlund LO, Almkvist O, et al. EEG-microstates in mild memory impairment and Alzheimer's disease: possible association with disturbed information processing. *J Neural Transm* (1997) **104**:483–95. doi:10.1007/BF01277666
45. Strelets V, Faber PL, Golikova J, Novototsky-Vlasov V, Koenig T, Gianotti LR, et al. Chronic schizophrenics with positive symptomatology have shortened EEG microstate durations. *Clin Neurophysiol* (2003) **114**:2043–51. doi:10.1016/S1388-2457(03)00211-6
46. Koenig T, Prichep L, Lehmann D, Sosa PV, Braeker E, Kleinlogel H, et al. Millisecond by millisecond, year by year: normative EEG microstates and developmental stages. *Neuroimage* (2002) **16**:41–8. doi:10.1006/nimg.2002.1070
47. Lehmann D, Strik WK, Henggeler B, Koenig T, Koukkou M. Brain electric microstates and momentary conscious mind states as building blocks of spontaneous thinking: I. Visual imagery and abstract thoughts. *Int J Psychophysiol* (1998) **29**:1–11.
48. Michel CM, Murray MM. Towards the utilization of EEG as a brain imaging tool. *Neuroimage* (2012) **61**:371–85. doi:10.1016/j.neuroimage.2011.12.039
49. Britz J, Van De Ville D, Michel CM. BOLD correlates of EEG topography reveal rapid resting-state network dynamics. *Neuroimage* (2010) **52**:1162–70. doi:10.1016/j.neuroimage.2010.02.052
50. Mantini D, Perrucci MG, Del Gratta C, Romani GL, Corbetta M. Electrophysiological signatures of resting state networks in the human brain. *Proc Natl Acad Sci U S A* (2007) **104**:13170–5. doi:10.1073/pnas.0700668104
51. Van De Ville D, Britz J, Michel CM. EEG microstate sequences in healthy humans at rest reveal scale-free dynamics. *Proc Natl Acad Sci U S A* (2010) **107**:18179–84. doi:10.1073/pnas.1007841107
52. Knowlton RC, Elgavish RA, Limdi N, Bartolucci A, Ojha B, Blount J, et al. Functional imaging: I. relative predictive value of intracranial electroencephalography. *Ann Neurol* (2008) **64**:25–34. doi:10.1002/ana.21389
53. Knowlton RC, Razdan SN, Limdi N, Elgavish RA, Killen J, Blount J, et al. Effect of epilepsy magnetic source imaging on intracranial electrode placement. *Ann Neurol* (2009) **65**:716–23. doi:10.1002/ana.21660
54. Brodbeck V, Spinelli L, Lascano AM, Wissmeier M, Vargas MI, Vulliemoz S, et al. Electroencephalographic source imaging: a prospective study of 152 operated epileptic patients. *Brain* (2011) **134**:2887–97. doi:10.1093/brain/awr243
55. Megevand P, Spinelli L, Genetti M, Brodbeck V, Momjian S, Schaller K, et al. Electric source imaging of interictal activity accurately localises the seizure onset zone. *J Neurol Neurosurg Psychiatry* (2014) **85**:38–43. doi:10.1136/jnnp-2013-305515
56. Schoffelen JM, Gross J. Source connectivity analysis with MEG and EEG. *Hum Brain Mapp* (2009) **30**:1857–65. doi:10.1002/hbm.20745
57. Plummer C, Harvey AS, Cook M. EEG source localization in focal epilepsy: where are we now? *Epilepsia* (2008) **49**:201–18. doi:10.1111/j.1528-1167.2007.01381.x
58. Kaiboriboon K, Luders HO, Hamaneh M, Turnbull J, Lhatoo SD. EEG source imaging in epilepsy – practicalities and pitfalls. *Nat Rev Neurol* (2012) **8**:498–507. doi:10.1038/nrneurol.2012.150
59. Birot G, Spinelli L, Vulliemoz S, Megevand P, Brunet D, Seeck M, et al. Head model and electrical source imaging: a study of 38 epileptic patients. *Neuroimage Clin* (2014) **5**:77–83. doi:10.1016/j.nicl.2014.06.005
60. Plummer C, Wagner M, Fuchs M, Harvey AS, Cook MJ. Dipole versus distributed EEG source localization for single versus averaged spikes in focal epilepsy. *J Clin Neurophysiol* (2010) **27**:141–62. doi:10.1097/WNP.0b013e3181dd5004
61. Dai Y, Zhang W, Dickens DL, He B. Source connectivity analysis from MEG and its application to epilepsy source localization. *Brain Topogr* (2012) **25**:157–66. doi:10.1007/s10548-011-0211-0
62. Jin SH, Jeong W, Chung CK. Information source in multiple MEG spike clusters can be identified by effective connectivity in focal cortical dysplasia. *Epilepsy Res* (2013) **105**:118–24. doi:10.1016/j.eplepsyres.2013.01.011
63. Tanaka N, Peters JM, Prohl AK, Takaya S, Madsen JR, Bourgeois BF, et al. Clinical value of magnetoencephalographic spike propagation represented by spatiotemporal source analysis: correlation with surgical outcome. *Epilepsy Res* (2014) **108**:280–8. doi:10.1016/j.eplepsyres.2013.11.006
64. Douw L, Van Dellen E, De Groot M, Heimans JJ, Klein M, Stam CJ, et al. Epilepsy is related to theta band brain connectivity and network topology in brain tumor patients. *BMC Neurosci* (2010) **11**:103. doi:10.1186/1471-2202-11-103
65. Van Dellen E, Douw L, Hillebrand A, De Witt Hamer PC, Baayen JC, Heimans JJ, et al. Epilepsy surgery outcome and functional network alterations in longitudinal MEG: a minimum spanning tree analysis. *Neuroimage* (2014) **86**:354–63. doi:10.1016/j.neuroimage.2013.10.010
66. Varotto G, Visani E, Canafoglia L, Franceschetti S, Avanzini G, Panzica F. Enhanced frontocentral EEG connectivity in photosensitive generalized epilepsies: a partial directed coherence study. *Epilepsia* (2012) **53**:359–67. doi:10.1111/j.1528-1167.2011.03352.x
67. Gupta D, Ossenblok P, Van Luijtelaar G. Space-time network connectivity and cortical activations preceding spike wave discharges in human absence epilepsy: a MEG study. *Med Biol Eng Comput* (2011) **49**:555–65. doi:10.1007/s11517-011-0778-3
68. Malinowska U, Badier JM, Gavaret M, Bartolomei F, Chauvel P, Benar CG. Interictal networks in magnetoencephalography. *Hum Brain Mapp* (2014) **35**:2789–805. doi:10.1002/hbm.22367
69. Kleen JK, Scott RC, Holmes GL, Roberts DW, Rundle MM, Testorf M, et al. Hippocampal interictal epileptiform activity disrupts cognition in humans. *Neurology* (2013) **81**:18–24. doi:10.1212/WNL.0b013e318297ee50
70. Ives JR, Warach S, Schmitt F, Edelman RR, Schomer DL. Monitoring the patient's EEG during echo planar MRI. *Electroencephalogr Clin Neurophysiol* (1993) **87**:417–20. doi:10.1016/0013-4694(93)90156-P
71. Gotman J, Kobayashi E, Bagshaw AP, Benar CG, Dubeau F. Combining EEG and fMRI: a multimodal tool for epilepsy research. *J Magn Reson Imaging* (2006) **23**:906–20. doi:10.1002/jmri.20577
72. Van Houdt PJ, De Munck JC, Leijten FS, Huiskamp GJ, Colon AJ, Boon PA, et al. EEG-fMRI correlation patterns in the presurgical evaluation of focal epilepsy: a comparison with electrocorticographic data and surgical outcome measures. *Neuroimage* (2013) **75**:238–48. doi:10.1016/j.neuroimage.2013.02.033
73. Pittau F, Grouiller F, Spinelli L, Seeck M, Michel CM, Vulliemoz S. The role of functional neuroimaging in pre-surgical epilepsy evaluation. *Front Neurol* (2014) **5**:31. doi:10.3389/fneur.2014.00031
74. Seeck M, Lazeyras F, Michel CM, Blanke O, Gericke CA, Ives J, et al. Non-invasive epileptic focus localization using EEG-triggered functional MRI and electromagnetic tomography. *Electroencephalogr Clin Neurophysiol* (1998) **106**:508–12. doi:10.1016/S0013-4694(98)00017-0

75. Benar CG, Gross DW, Wang Y, Petre V, Pike B, Dubeau F, et al. The BOLD response to interictal epileptiform discharges. *Neuroimage* (2002) **17**:1182–92. doi:10.1006/nimg.2002.1164
76. Thornton R, Vulliemoz S, Rodionov R, Carmichael DW, Chaudhary UJ, Diehl B, et al. Epileptic networks in focal cortical dysplasia revealed using electroencephalography-functional magnetic resonance imaging. *Ann Neurol* (2011) **70**:822–37. doi:10.1002/ana.22535
77. An D, Fahoum F, Hall J, Olivier A, Gotman J, Dubeau F. Electroencephalography/functional magnetic resonance imaging responses help predict surgical outcome in focal epilepsy. *Epilepsia* (2013) **54**:2184–94. doi:10.1111/epi.12434
78. Grouiller F, Thornton RC, Groening K, Spinelli L, Duncan JS, Schaller K, et al. With or without spikes: localization of focal epileptic activity by simultaneous electroencephalography and functional magnetic resonance imaging. *Brain* (2011) **134**:2867–86. doi:10.1093/brain/awr156
79. Glover GH. Deconvolution of impulse response in event-related BOLD fMRI. *Neuroimage* (1999) **9**:416–29. doi:10.1006/nimg.1998.0419
80. Bagshaw AP, Aghakhani Y, Benar CG, Kobayashi E, Hawco C, Dubeau F, et al. EEG-fMRI of focal epileptic spikes: analysis with multiple haemodynamic functions and comparison with gadolinium-enhanced MR angiograms. *Hum Brain Mapp* (2004) **22**:179–92. doi:10.1002/hbm.20024
81. Hawco CS, Bagshaw AP, Lu Y, Dubeau F, Gotman J. BOLD changes occur prior to epileptic spikes seen on scalp EEG. *Neuroimage* (2007) **35**:1450–8. doi:10.1016/j.neuroimage.2006.12.042
82. Grouiller F, Vercueil L, Krainik A, Segebarth C, Kahane P, David O. Characterization of the hemodynamic modes associated with interictal epileptic activity using a deformable model-based analysis of combined EEG and functional MRI recordings. *Hum Brain Mapp* (2010) **31**:1157–73. doi:10.1002/hbm.20925
83. Moeller F, Levan P, Muhle H, Stephani U, Dubeau F, Siniatchkin M, et al. Absence seizures: individual patterns revealed by EEG-fMRI. *Epilepsia* (2010) **51**:2000–10. doi:10.1111/j.1528-1167.2010.02698.x
84. Vaudano AE, Avanzini P, Tassi L, Ruggieri A, Cantalupo G, Benuzzi F, et al. Causality within the epileptic network: an EEG-fMRI study validated by intracranial EEG. *Front Neurol* (2013) **4**:185. doi:10.3389/fneur.2013.00185
85. Groening K, Brodbeck V, Moeller F, Wolff S, Van Baalen A, Michel CM, et al. Combination of EEG-fMRI and EEG source analysis improves interpretation of spike-associated activation networks in paediatric pharmacoresistant focal epilepsies. *Neuroimage* (2009) **46**:827–33. doi:10.1016/j.neuroimage.2009.02.026
86. Vulliemoz S, Thornton R, Rodionov R, Carmichael DW, Guye M, Lhatoo S, et al. The spatio-temporal mapping of epileptic networks: combination of EEG-fMRI and EEG source imaging. *Neuroimage* (2009) **46**:834–43. doi:10.1016/j.neuroimage.2009.01.070
87. Laufs H, Richardson MP, Salek-Haddadi A, Vollmar C, Duncan JS, Gale K, et al. Converging PET and fMRI evidence for a common area involved in human focal epilepsies. *Neurology* (2011) **77**:904–10. doi:10.1212/WNL.0b013e31822c90f2
88. Flanagan D, Badawy RA, Jackson GD. EEG-fMRI in focal epilepsy: local activation and regional networks. *Clin Neurophysiol* (2014) **125**:21–31. doi:10.1016/j.clinph.2013.06.182
89. Vaudano AE, Carmichael DW, Salek-Haddadi A, Rampp S, Stefan H, Lemieux L, et al. Networks involved in seizure initiation. A reading epilepsy case studied with EEG-fMRI and MEG. *Neurology* (2012) **79**:249–53. doi:10.1212/WNL.0b013e31825fdf3a
90. Piredda S, Gale K. A crucial epileptogenic site in the deep prepiriform cortex. *Nature* (1985) **317**:623–5. doi:10.1038/317623a0
91. Racine RJ, Mosher M, Kairiss EW. The role of the pyriform cortex in the generation of interictal spikes in the kindled preparation. *Brain Res* (1988) **454**:251–63. doi:10.1016/0006-8993(88)90825-6
92. Loscher W, Ebert U. The role of the piriform cortex in kindling. *Prog Neurobiol* (1996) **50**:427–81. doi:10.1016/S0301-0082(96)00036-6
93. Centeno M, Vollmar C, Stretton J, Symms MR, Thompson PJ, Richardson MP, et al. Structural changes in the temporal lobe and piriform cortex in frontal lobe epilepsy. *Epilepsy Res* (2014) **108**:978–81. doi:10.1016/j.eplepsyres.2014.03.001
94. Hamandi K, Powell HW, Laufs H, Symms MR, Barker GJ, Parker GJ, et al. Combined EEG-fMRI and tractography to visualise propagation of epileptic activity. *J Neurol Neurosurg Psychiatry* (2008) **79**:594–7. doi:10.1136/jnnp.2007.125401
95. Bhardwaj RD, Mahmoodabadi SZ, Otsubo H, Snead OC III, Rutka JT, Widjaja E. Diffusion tensor tractography detection of functional pathway for the spread of epileptiform activity between temporal lobe and Rolandic region. *Childs Nerv Syst* (2010) **26**:185–90. doi:10.1007/s00381-009-1017-1
96. Lascano AM, Lemkaddem A, Granziera C, Korff CM, Boex C, Jenny B, et al. Tracking the source of cerebellar epilepsy: hemifacial seizures associated with cerebellar cortical dysplasia. *Epilepsy Res* (2013) **105**:245–9. doi:10.1016/j.eplepsyres.2012.12.010
97. Kleen JK, Scott RC, Holmes GL, Lenck-Santini PP. Hippocampal interictal spikes disrupt cognition in rats. *Ann Neurol* (2010) **67**:250–7. doi:10.1002/ana.21896
98. Chaudhary UJ, Centeno M, Carmichael DW, Vollmar C, Rodionov R, Bonelli S, et al. Imaging the interaction: epileptic discharges, working memory, and behavior. *Hum Brain Mapp* (2013) **34**:2910–7. doi:10.1002/hbm.22115
99. Centeno M, Carmichael DW. Network connectivity in epilepsy: resting state fMRI and EEG-fMRI contributions. *Front Neurol* (2014) **5**:93. doi:10.3389/fneur.2014.00093
100. Spencer SS. Neural networks in human epilepsy: evidence of and implications for treatment. *Epilepsia* (2002) **43**:219–27. doi:10.1046/j.1528-1157.2002.26901.x
101. Voets NL, Adcock JE, Stacey R, Hart Y, Carpenter K, Matthews PM, et al. Functional and structural changes in the memory network associated with left temporal lobe epilepsy. *Hum Brain Mapp* (2009) **30**:4070–81. doi:10.1002/hbm.20830
102. Bettus G, Bartolomei F, Confort-Gouny S, Guedj E, Chauvel P, Cozzone PJ, et al. Role of resting state functional connectivity MRI in presurgical investigation of mesial temporal lobe epilepsy. *J Neurol Neurosurg Psychiatry* (2010) **81**:1147–54. doi:10.1136/jnnp.2009.191460
103. Pereira FR, Alessio A, Sercheli MS, Pedro T, Bilevicius E, Rondina JM, et al. Asymmetrical hippocampal connectivity in mesial temporal lobe epilepsy: evidence from resting state fMRI. *BMC Neurosci* (2010) **11**:66. doi:10.1186/1471-2202-11-66
104. Bettus G, Guedj E, Joyeux F, Confort-Gouny S, Soulier E, Laguitton V, et al. Decreased basal fMRI functional connectivity in epileptogenic networks and contralateral compensatory mechanisms. *Hum Brain Mapp* (2009) **30**:1580–91. doi:10.1002/hbm.20625
105. Addis DR, Moscovitch M, McAndrews MP. Consequences of hippocampal damage across the autobiographical memory network in left temporal lobe epilepsy. *Brain* (2007) **130**:2327–42. doi:10.1093/brain/awm166
106. Powell HW, Richardson MP, Symms MR, Boulby PA, Thompson PJ, Duncan JS, et al. Reorganization of verbal and nonverbal memory in temporal lobe epilepsy due to unilateral hippocampal sclerosis. *Epilepsia* (2007) **48**:1512–25. doi:10.1111/j.1528-1167.2007.01053.x
107. Morgan VL, Rogers BP, Sonmezturk HH, Gore JC, Abou-Khalil B. Cross hippocampal influence in mesial temporal lobe epilepsy measured with high temporal resolution functional magnetic resonance imaging. *Epilepsia* (2011) **52**:1741–9. doi:10.1111/j.1528-1167.2011.03196.x
108. Bettus G, Ranjeva JP, Wendling F, Benar CG, Confort-Gouny S, Regis J, et al. Interictal functional connectivity of human epileptic networks assessed by intracerebral EEG and BOLD signal fluctuations. *PLoS One* (2011) **6**:e20071. doi:10.1371/journal.pone.0020071
109. Pittau F, Grova C, Moeller F, Dubeau F, Gotman J. Patterns of altered functional connectivity in mesial temporal lobe epilepsy. *Epilepsia* (2012) **53**:1013–23. doi:10.1111/j.1528-1167.2012.03464.x
110. Waites AB, Briellmann RS, Saling MM, Abbott DF, Jackson GD. Functional connectivity networks are disrupted in left temporal lobe epilepsy. *Ann Neurol* (2006) **59**:335–43. doi:10.1002/ana.20733
111. Kobayashi E, Grova C, Tyvaert L, Dubeau F, Gotman J. Structures involved at the time of temporal lobe spikes revealed by interindividual group analysis of EEG/fMRI data. *Epilepsia* (2009) **50**:2549–56. doi:10.1111/j.1528-1167.2009.02180.x
112. Frings L, Schulze-Bonhage A, Spreer J, Wagner K. Remote effects of hippocampal damage on default network connectivity in the human brain. *J Neurol* (2009) **256**:2021–9. doi:10.1007/s00415-009-5233-0

113. Liao W, Zhang Z, Pan Z, Mantini D, Ding J, Duan X, et al. Altered functional connectivity and small-world in mesial temporal lobe epilepsy. *PLoS One* (2010) **5**:e8525. doi:10.1371/journal.pone.0008525
114. Liao W, Zhang Z, Pan Z, Mantini D, Ding J, Duan X, et al. Default mode network abnormalities in mesial temporal lobe epilepsy: a study combining fMRI and DTI. *Hum Brain Mapp* (2011) **32**:883–95. doi:10.1002/hbm.21076
115. Zhang Z, Lu G, Zhong Y, Tan Q, Liao W, Wang Z, et al. Altered spontaneous neuronal activity of the default-mode network in mesial temporal lobe epilepsy. *Brain Res* (2010) **1323**:152–60. doi:10.1016/j.brainres.2010.01.042
116. Haneef Z, Lenartowicz A, Yeh HJ, Engel J Jr, Stern JM. Effect of lateralized temporal lobe epilepsy on the default mode network. *Epilepsy Behav* (2012) **25**:350–7. doi:10.1016/j.yebeh.2012.07.019
117. Morgan VL, Sonmezturk HH, Gore JC, Abou-Khalil B. Lateralization of temporal lobe epilepsy using resting functional magnetic resonance imaging connectivity of hippocampal networks. *Epilepsia* (2012) **53**:1628–35. doi:10.1111/j.1528-1167.2012.03590.x
118. McCormick C, Quraan M, Cohn M, Valiante TA, McAndrews MP. Default mode network connectivity indicates episodic memory capacity in mesial temporal lobe epilepsy. *Epilepsia* (2013) **54**:809–18. doi:10.1111/epi.12098
119. Andrews-Hanna JR, Reidler JS, Sepulcre J, Poulin R, Buckner RL. Functional-anatomic fractionation of the brain's default network. *Neuron* (2010) **65**:550–62. doi:10.1016/j.neuron.2010.02.005
120. Damoiseaux JS, Rombouts SA, Barkhof F, Scheltens P, Stam CJ, Smith SM, et al. Consistent resting-state networks across healthy subjects. *Proc Natl Acad Sci U S A* (2006) **103**:13848–53. doi:10.1073/pnas.0601417103
121. Fransson P, Marrelec G. The precuneus/posterior cingulate cortex plays a pivotal role in the default mode network: evidence from a partial correlation network analysis. *Neuroimage* (2008) **42**:1178–84. doi:10.1016/j.neuroimage.2008.05.059
122. Yeo BT, Krienen FM, Chee MW, Buckner RL. Estimates of segregation and overlap of functional connectivity networks in the human cerebral cortex. *Neuroimage* (2013) **88C**:212–27. doi:10.1016/j.neuroimage.2013.10.046
123. Heimer L, Alheid GF, De Olmos JS, Groenewegen HJ, Haber SN, Harlan RE, et al. The accumbens: beyond the core-shell dichotomy. *J Neuropsychiatry Clin Neurosci* (1997) **9**:354–81.
124. Koob GF, Volkow ND. Neurocircuitry of addiction. *Neuropsychopharmacology* (2010) **35**:217–38. doi:10.1038/npp.2009.110
125. Bunzeck N, Doeller CF, Dolan RJ, Duzel E. Contextual interaction between novelty and reward processing within the mesolimbic system. *Hum Brain Mapp* (2012) **33**:1309–24. doi:10.1002/hbm.21288
126. Lieb JP, Dasheiff RM, Engel J Jr. Role of the frontal lobes in the propagation of mesial temporal lobe seizures. *Epilepsia* (1991) **32**:822–37. doi:10.1111/j.1528-1157.1991.tb05539.x
127. Yadid G, Friedman A. Dynamics of the dopaminergic system as a key component to the understanding of depression. *Prog Brain Res* (2008) **172**:265–86. doi:10.1016/S0079-6123(08)00913-8
128. Price JL, Drevets WC. Neurocircuitry of mood disorders. *Neuropsychopharmacology* (2010) **35**:192–216. doi:10.1038/npp.2009.104
129. Chen S, Wu X, Lui S, Wu Q, Yao Z, Li Q, et al. Resting-state fMRI study of treatment-naive temporal lobe epilepsy patients with depressive symptoms. *Neuroimage* (2012) **60**:299–304. doi:10.1016/j.neuroimage.2011.11.092
130. Butler T, Blackmon K, McDonald CR, Carlson C, Barr WB, Devinsky O, et al. Cortical thickness abnormalities associated with depressive symptoms in temporal lobe epilepsy. *Epilepsy Behav* (2012) **23**:64–7. doi:10.1016/j.yebeh.2011.10.001
131. Stretton J, Pope RA, Winston GP, Sidhu MK, Symms M, Duncan JS, et al. Temporal lobe epilepsy and affective disorders: the role of the subgenual anterior cingulate cortex. *J Neurol Neurosurg Psychiatry* (2014). doi:10.1136/jnnp-2013-306966
132. Meletti S, Benuzzi F, Rubboli G, Cantalupo G, Stanzani Maserati M, Nichelli P, et al. Impaired facial emotion recognition in early-onset right mesial temporal lobe epilepsy. *Neurology* (2003) **60**:426–31. doi:10.1212/WNL.60.3.426
133. Schacher M, Winkler R, Grunwald T, Kraemer G, Kurthen M, Reed V, et al. Mesial temporal lobe epilepsy impairs advanced social cognition. *Epilepsia* (2006) **47**:2141–6. doi:10.1111/j.1528-1167.2006.00857.x
134. Hlobil U, Rathore C, Alexander A, Sarma S, Radhakrishnan K. Impaired facial emotion recognition in patients with mesial temporal lobe epilepsy associated with hippocampal sclerosis (MTLE-HS): side and age at onset matters. *Epilepsy Res* (2008) **80**:150–7. doi:10.1016/j.eplepsyres.2008.03.018
135. Meletti S, Benuzzi F, Cantalupo G, Rubboli G, Tassinari CA, Nichelli P. Facial emotion recognition impairment in chronic temporal lobe epilepsy. *Epilepsia* (2009) **50**:1547–59. doi:10.1111/j.1528-1167.2008.01978.x
136. Broicher SD, Frings L, Huppertz HJ, Grunwald T, Kurthen M, Kramer G, et al. Alterations in functional connectivity of the amygdala in unilateral mesial temporal lobe epilepsy. *J Neurol* (2012) **259**:2546–54. doi:10.1007/s00415-012-6533-3
137. Bonelli SB, Powell R, Yogarajah M, Thompson PJ, Symms MR, Koepp MJ, et al. Preoperative amygdala fMRI in temporal lobe epilepsy. *Epilepsia* (2009) **50**:217–27. doi:10.1111/j.1528-1167.2008.01739.x
138. Cataldi M, Avoli M, De Villers-Sidani E. Resting state networks in temporal lobe epilepsy. *Epilepsia* (2013) **54**:2048–59. doi:10.1111/epi.12400
139. Negishi M, Martuzzi R, Novotny EJ, Spencer DD, Constable RT. Functional MRI connectivity as a predictor of the surgical outcome of epilepsy. *Epilepsia* (2011) **52**:1733–40. doi:10.1111/j.1528-1167.2011.03191.x
140. Luo C, An D, Yao D, Gotman J. Patient-specific connectivity pattern of epileptic network in frontal lobe epilepsy. *Neuroimage Clin* (2014) **4**:668–75. doi:10.1016/j.nicl.2014.04.006
141. Centeno M, Vollmar C, O'Muircheartaigh J, Stretton J, Bonelli SB, Symms MR, et al. Memory in frontal lobe epilepsy: an fMRI study. *Epilepsia* (2012) **53**:1756–64. doi:10.1111/j.1528-1167.2012.03570.x
142. Meeren H, Van Luijtelaar G, Da Silva F, Coenen A. Evolving concepts on the pathophysiology of absence seizures: the cortical focus theory. *Arch Neurol* (2005) **62**:371–6. doi:10.1001/archneur.62.3.371
143. Blumenfeld H. Cellular and network mechanisms of spike-wave seizures. *Epilepsia* (2005) **46**(Suppl 9):21–33. doi:10.1111/j.1528-1167.2005.00311.x
144. Gloor P. Generalized cortico-reticular epilepsies. Some considerations on the pathophysiology of generalized bilaterally synchronous spike and wave discharge. *Epilepsia* (1968) **9**:249–63. doi:10.1111/j.1528-1157.1968.tb04624.x
145. Meeren HK, Pijn JP, Van Luijtelaar EL, Coenen AM, Da Silva FH. Cortical focus drives widespread corticothalamic networks during spontaneous absence seizures in rats. *J Neurosci* (2002) **22**:1480–95.
146. Manning JP, Richards DA, Leresche N, Crunelli V, Bowery NG. Cortical-area specific block of genetically determined absence seizures by ethosuximide. *Neuroscience* (2004) **123**:5–9. doi:10.1016/j.neuroscience.2003.09.026
147. Polack PO, Guillemain I, Hu E, Deransart C, Depaulis A, Charpier S. Deep layer somatosensory cortical neurons initiate spike-and-wave discharges in a genetic model of absence seizures. *J Neurosci* (2007) **27**:6590–9. doi:10.1523/JNEUROSCI.0753-07.2007
148. Archer JS, Abbott DF, Waites AB, Jackson GD. fMRI "deactivation" of the posterior cingulate during generalized spike and wave. *Neuroimage* (2003) **20**:1915–22. doi:10.1016/S1053-8119(03)00294-5
149. Aghakhani Y, Bagshaw AP, Benar CG, Hawco C, Andermann F, Dubeau F, et al. fMRI activation during spike and wave discharges in idiopathic generalized epilepsy. *Brain* (2004) **127**:1127–44. doi:10.1093/brain/awh136
150. Masterton RA, Carney PW, Abbott DF, Jackson GD. Absence epilepsy subnetworks revealed by event-related independent components analysis of functional magnetic resonance imaging. *Epilepsia* (2013) **54**:801–8. doi:10.1111/epi.12163
151. Salek-Haddadi A, Lemieux L, Merschhemke M, Friston KJ, Duncan JS, Fish DR. Functional magnetic resonance imaging of human absence seizures. *Ann Neurol* (2003) **53**:663–7. doi:10.1002/ana.10586
152. Labate A, Briellmann RS, Abbott DF, Waites AB, Jackson GD. Typical childhood absence seizures are associated with thalamic activation. *Epileptic Disord* (2005) **7**:373–7.
153. Laufs H, Lengler U, Hamandi K, Kleinschmidt A, Krakow K. Linking generalized spike-and-wave discharges and resting state brain activity by using EEG/fMRI in a patient with absence seizures. *Epilepsia* (2006) **47**:444–8. doi:10.1111/j.1528-1167.2006.00443.x
154. Moeller F, Siebner HR, Wolff S, Muhle H, Granert O, Jansen O, et al. Simultaneous EEG-fMRI in drug-naive children with newly diagnosed absence epilepsy. *Epilepsia* (2008) **49**:1510–9. doi:10.1111/j.1528-1167.2008.01626.x

155. Hamandi K, Salek-Haddadi A, Laufs H, Liston A, Friston K, Fish DR, et al. EEG-fMRI of idiopathic and secondarily generalized epilepsies. *Neuroimage* (2006) **31**:1700–10. doi:10.1016/j.neuroimage.2006.02.016
156. Child ND, Benarroch EE. Anterior nucleus of the thalamus: functional organization and clinical implications. *Neurology* (2013) **81**:1869–76. doi:10.1212/01.wnl.0000436078.95856.56
157. Carney PW, Masterton RA, Harvey AS, Scheffer IE, Berkovic SF, Jackson GD. The core network in absence epilepsy. Differences in cortical and thalamic BOLD response. *Neurology* (2010) **75**:904–11. doi:10.1212/WNL.0b013e3181f11c06
158. Westmijse I, Ossenblok P, Gunning B, Van Luijtelaar G. Onset and propagation of spike and slow wave discharges in human absence epilepsy: a MEG study. *Epilepsia* (2009) **50**:2538–48. doi:10.1111/j.1528-1167.2009.02162.x
159. Roche-Labarbe N, Zaaimi B, Berquin P, Nehlig A, Grebe R, Wallois F. NIRS-measured oxy- and deoxyhemoglobin changes associated with EEG spike-and-wave discharges in children. *Epilepsia* (2008) **49**:1871–80. doi:10.1111/j.1528-1167.2008.01711.x
160. Seneviratne U, Cook M, D'Souza W. Focal abnormalities in idiopathic generalized epilepsy: a critical review of the literature. *Epilepsia* (2014) **55**:1157–69. doi:10.1111/epi.12688
161. Tyvaert L, Chassagnon S, Sadikot A, Levan P, Dubeau F, Gotman J. Thalamic nuclei activity in idiopathic generalized epilepsy: an EEG-fMRI study. *Neurology* (2009) **73**:2018–22. doi:10.1212/WNL.0b013e3181c55d02
162. Wang Z, Lu G, Zhang Z, Zhong Y, Jiao Q, Tan Q, et al. Altered resting state networks in epileptic patients with generalized tonic-clonic seizures. *Brain Res* (2011) **1374**:134–41. doi:10.1016/j.brainres.2010.12.034
163. McGill ML, Devinsky O, Kelly C, Milham M, Castellanos FX, Quinn BT, et al. Default mode network abnormalities in idiopathic generalized epilepsy. *Epilepsy Behav* (2012) **23**:353–9. doi:10.1016/j.yebeh.2012.01.013
164. Zhang Z, Liao W, Chen H, Mantini D, Ding JR, Xu Q, et al. Altered functional-structural coupling of large-scale brain networks in idiopathic generalized epilepsy. *Brain* (2011) **134**:2912–28. doi:10.1093/brain/awr223
165. Maneshi M, Moeller F, Fahoum F, Gotman J, Grova C. Resting-state connectivity of the sustained attention network correlates with disease duration in idiopathic generalized epilepsy. *PLoS One* (2012) **7**:e50359. doi:10.1371/journal.pone.0050359
166. Kay BP, Difrancesco MW, Privitera MD, Gotman J, Holland SK, Szaflarski JP. Reduced default mode network connectivity in treatment-resistant idiopathic generalized epilepsy. *Epilepsia* (2013) **54**:461–70. doi:10.1111/epi.12057
167. Kim JB, Suh SI, Seo WK, Oh K, Koh SB, Kim JH. Altered thalamocortical functional connectivity in idiopathic generalized epilepsy. *Epilepsia* (2014) **55**:592–600. doi:10.1111/epi.12580
168. Vollmar C, O'Muircheartaigh J, Barker GJ, Symms MR, Thompson P, Kumari V, et al. Motor system hyperconnectivity in juvenile myoclonic epilepsy: a cognitive functional magnetic resonance imaging study. *Brain* (2011) **134**:1710–9. doi:10.1093/brain/awr098
169. Vulliemoz S, Vollmar C, Koepp MJ, Yogarajah M, O'Muircheartaigh J, Carmichael DW, et al. Connectivity of the supplementary motor area in juvenile myoclonic epilepsy and frontal lobe epilepsy. *Epilepsia* (2011) **52**:507–14. doi:10.1111/j.1528-1167.2010.02770.x
170. Vollmar C, O'Muircheartaigh J, Symms MR, Barker GJ, Thompson P, Kumari V, et al. Altered microstructural connectivity in juvenile myoclonic epilepsy: the missing link. *Neurology* (2012) **78**:1555–9. doi:10.1212/WNL.0b013e3182563b44
171. Wandschneider B, Centeno M, Vollmar C, Stretton J, O'Muircheartaigh J, Thompson PJ, et al. Risk-taking behavior in juvenile myoclonic epilepsy. *Epilepsia* (2013) **54**:2158–65. doi:10.1111/epi.12413
172. Moeller F, Stephani U, Siniatchkin M. Simultaneous EEG and fMRI recordings (EEG-fMRI) in children with epilepsy. *Epilepsia* (2013) **54**:971–82. doi:10.1111/epi.12197
173. Siniatchkin M, Coropceanu D, Moeller F, Boor R, Stephani U. EEG-fMRI reveals activation of brainstem and thalamus in patients with Lennox-Gastaut syndrome. *Epilepsia* (2011) **52**:766–74. doi:10.1111/j.1528-1167.2010.02948.x
174. Pillay N, Archer JS, Badawy RA, Flanagan DF, Berkovic SF, Jackson G. Networks underlying paroxysmal fast activity and slow spike and wave in Lennox-Gastaut syndrome. *Neurology* (2013) **81**:665–73. doi:10.1212/WNL.0b013e3182a08f6a
175. Archer JS, Warren AE, Stagnitti MR, Masterton RA, Abbott DF, Jackson GD. Lennox-Gastaut syndrome and phenotype: secondary network epilepsies. *Epilepsia* (2014) **55**:1245–54. doi:10.1111/epi.12682
176. Moeller F, Groening K, Moehring J, Muhle H, Wolff S, Jansen O, et al. EEG-fMRI in myoclonic astatic epilepsy (Doose syndrome). *Neurology* (2014) **82**:1508–13. doi:10.1212/WNL.0000000000000359
177. Archer JS, Briellman RS, Abbott DF, Syngeniotis A, Wellard RM, Jackson GD. Benign epilepsy with centro-temporal spikes: spike triggered fMRI shows somato-sensory cortex activity. *Epilepsia* (2003) **44**:200–4. doi:10.1046/j.1528-1157.2003.02502.x
178. Boor S, Vucurevic G, Pfleiderer C, Stoeter P, Kutschke G, Boor R. EEG-related functional MRI in benign childhood epilepsy with centrotemporal spikes. *Epilepsia* (2003) **44**:688–92. doi:10.1046/j.1528-1157.2003.27802.x
179. Lengler U, Kafadar I, Neubauer BA, Krakow K. fMRI correlates of interictal epileptic activity in patients with idiopathic benign focal epilepsy of childhood. A simultaneous EEG-functional MRI study. *Epilepsy Res* (2007) **75**:29–38. doi:10.1016/j.eplepsyres.2007.03.016
180. Masterton RA, Harvey AS, Archer JS, Lillywhite LM, Abbott DF, Scheffer IE, et al. Focal epileptiform spikes do not show a canonical BOLD response in patients with benign rolandic epilepsy (BECTS). *Neuroimage* (2010) **51**:252–60. doi:10.1016/j.neuroimage.2010.01.109
181. Siniatchkin M, Groening K, Moehring J, Moeller F, Boor R, Brodbeck V, et al. Neuronal networks in children with continuous spikes and waves during slow sleep. *Brain* (2010) **133**:2798–813. doi:10.1093/brain/awq183
182. Mirandola L, Cantalupo G, Vaudano AE, Avanzini P, Ruggieri A, Pisani F, et al. Centrotemporal spikes during NREM sleep: the promoting action of thalamus revealed by simultaneous EEG and fMRI coregistration. *Epilepsy Behav Case Rep* (2013) **1**:106–9. doi:10.1016/j.ebcr.2013.06.005
183. Moeller F, Moehring J, Ick I, Steinmann E, Wolff S, Jansen O, et al. EEG-fMRI in atypical benign partial epilepsy. *Epilepsia* (2013) **54**:e103–8. doi:10.1111/epi.12243
184. Vaudano AE, Ruggieri A, Vignoli A, Avanzini P, Benuzzi F, Gessaroli G, et al. Epilepsy-related brain networks in ring chromosome 20 syndrome: an EEG-fMRI study. *Epilepsia* (2014) **55**:403–13. doi:10.1111/epi.12539
185. Bartolomei F, Chauvel P, Wendling F. Epileptogenicity of brain structures in human temporal lobe epilepsy: a quantified study from intracerebral EEG. *Brain* (2008) **131**:1818–30. doi:10.1093/brain/awn111
186. Bartolomei F, Cosandier-Rimele D, McGonigal A, Aubert S, Regis J, Gavaret M, et al. From mesial temporal lobe to temporoperisylvian seizures: a quantified study of temporal lobe seizure networks. *Epilepsia* (2010) **51**:2147–58. doi:10.1111/j.1528-1167.2010.02690.x
187. Arthuis M, Valton L, Regis J, Chauvel P, Wendling F, Naccache L, et al. Impaired consciousness during temporal lobe seizures is related to increased long-distance cortical-subcortical synchronization. *Brain* (2009) **132**:2091–101. doi:10.1093/brain/awp086
188. Lambert I, Arthuis M, McGonigal A, Wendling F, Bartolomei F. Alteration of global workspace during loss of consciousness: a study of parietal seizures. *Epilepsia* (2012) **53**:2104–10. doi:10.1111/j.1528-1167.2012.03690.x
189. Bartolomei F, McGonigal A, Naccache L. Alteration of consciousness in focal epilepsy: the global workspace alteration theory. *Epilepsy Behav* (2014) **30**:17–23. doi:10.1016/j.yebeh.2013.09.012
190. Blumenfeld H, McNally KA, Vanderhill SD, Paige AL, Chung R, Davis K, et al. Positive and negative network correlations in temporal lobe epilepsy. *Cereb Cortex* (2004) **14**:892–902. doi:10.1093/cercor/bhh048
191. Englot DJ, Yang L, Hamid H, Danielson N, Bai X, Marfeo A, et al. Impaired consciousness in temporal lobe seizures: role of cortical slow activity. *Brain* (2010) **133**:3764–77. doi:10.1093/brain/awq316
192. Englot DJ, Modi B, Mishra AM, Desalvo M, Hyder F, Blumenfeld H. Cortical deactivation induced by subcortical network dysfunction in limbic seizures. *J Neurosci* (2009) **29**:13006–18. doi:10.1523/JNEUROSCI.3846-09.2009
193. Blumenfeld H. Impaired consciousness in epilepsy. *Lancet Neurol* (2012) **11**:814–26. doi:10.1016/S1474-4422(12)70188-6
194. Rubinov M, Sporns O. Complex network measures of brain connectivity: uses and interpretations. *Neuroimage* (2010) **52**:1059–69. doi:10.1016/j.neuroimage.2009.10.003
195. Wilke C, Worrell G, He B. Graph analysis of epileptogenic networks in human partial epilepsy. *Epilepsia* (2011) **52**:84–93. doi:10.1111/j.1528-1167.2010.02785.x

196. Van Mierlo P, Carrette E, Hallez H, Raedt R, Meurs A, Vandenberghe S, et al. Ictal-onset localization through connectivity analysis of intracranial EEG signals in patients with refractory epilepsy. *Epilepsia* (2013) **54**:1409–18. doi:10.1111/epi.12206
197. Panzica F, Varotto G, Rotondi F, Spreafico R, Franceschetti S. Identification of the epileptogenic zone from stereo-EEG signals: a connectivity-graph theory approach. *Front Neurol* (2013) **4**:175. doi:10.3389/fneur.2013.00175
198. Vulliemoz S, Carmichael DW, Rosenkranz K, Diehl B, Rodionov R, Walker MC, et al. Simultaneous intracranial EEG and fMRI of interictal epileptic discharges in humans. *Neuroimage* (2011) **54**:182–90. doi:10.1016/j.neuroimage.2010.08.004
199. Carmichael DW, Vulliemoz S, Rodionov R, Thornton JS, McEvoy AW, Lemieux L. Simultaneous intracranial EEG-fMRI in humans: protocol considerations and data quality. *Neuroimage* (2012) **63**:301–9. doi:10.1016/j.neuroimage.2012.05.056
200. Schevon CA, Weiss SA, McKhann G Jr, Goodman RR, Yuste R, Emerson RG, et al. Evidence of an inhibitory restraint of seizure activity in humans. *Nat Commun* (2012) **3**:1060. doi:10.1038/ncomms2056
201. Weiss SA, Banks GP, McKhann GM Jr, Goodman RR, Emerson RG, Trevelyan AJ, et al. Ictal high frequency oscillations distinguish two types of seizure territories in humans. *Brain* (2013) **136**:3796–808. doi:10.1093/brain/awt276
202. Penfield W, Boldrey E. Somatic motor and sensory representation in the cerebral cortex of man as studied by electrical stimulation. *Brain* (1937) **60**:389–443. doi:10.1093/brain/60.4.389
203. Hamberger MJ. Cortical language mapping in epilepsy: a critical review. *Neuropsychol Rev* (2007) **17**:477–89. doi:10.1007/s11065-007-9046-6
204. Selimbeyoglu A, Parvizi J. Electrical stimulation of the human brain: perceptual and behavioral phenomena reported in the old and new literature. *Front Hum Neurosci* (2010) **4**:46. doi:10.3389/fnhum.2010.00046
205. Megevand P, Groppe DM, Goldfinger MS, Hwang ST, Kingsley PB, Davidesco I, et al. Seeing scenes: topographic visual hallucinations evoked by direct electrical stimulation of the parahippocampal place area. *J Neurosci* (2014) **34**:5399–405. doi:10.1523/JNEUROSCI.5202-13.2014
206. Parvizi J, Rangarajan V, Shirer WR, Desai N, Greicius MD. The will to persevere induced by electrical stimulation of the human cingulate gyrus. *Neuron* (2013) **80**:1359–67. doi:10.1016/j.neuron.2013.10.057
207. Matsumoto R, Nair DR, Lapresto E, Najm I, Bingaman W, Shibasaki H, et al. Functional connectivity in the human language system: a cortico-cortical evoked potential study. *Brain* (2004) **127**:2316–30. doi:10.1093/brain/awh246
208. Conner CR, Ellmore TM, Disano MA, Pieters TA, Potter AW, Tandon N. Anatomic and electro-physiologic connectivity of the language system: a combined DTI-CCEP study. *Comput Biol Med* (2011) **41**:1100–9. doi:10.1016/j.compbiomed.2011.07.008
209. David O, Bastin J, Chabardes S, Minotti L, Kahane P. Studying network mechanisms using intracranial stimulation in epileptic patients. *Front Syst Neurosci* (2010) **4**:148. doi:10.3389/fnsys.2010.00148
210. Wilson CL, Isokawa M, Babb TL, Crandall PH. Functional connections in the human temporal lobe. I. analysis of limbic system pathways using neuronal responses evoked by electrical stimulation. *Exp Brain Res* (1990) **82**:279–92.
211. Lacruz ME, Garcia Seoane JJ, Valentin A, Selway R, Alarcon G. Frontal and temporal functional connections of the living human brain. *Eur J Neurosci* (2007) **26**:1357–70. doi:10.1111/j.1460-9568.2007.05730.x
212. Gloor P, Salanova V, Olivier A, Quesney LF. The human dorsal hippocampal commissure. An anatomically identifiable and functional pathway. *Brain* (1993) **116**(Pt 5):1249–73. doi:10.1093/brain/116.5.1249
213. David O, Job AS, De Palma L, Hoffmann D, Minotti L, Kahane P. Probabilistic functional tractography of the human cortex. *Neuroimage* (2013) **80**:307–17. doi:10.1016/j.neuroimage.2013.05.075
214. Iwasaki M, Enatsu R, Matsumoto R, Novak E, Thankappen B, Piao Z, et al. Accentuated cortico-cortical evoked potentials in neocortical epilepsy in areas of ictal onset. *Epileptic Disord* (2010) **12**:292–302. doi:10.1684/epd.2010.0334
215. Valentin A, Anderson M, Alarcon G, Seoane JJ, Selway R, Binnie CD, et al. Responses to single pulse electrical stimulation identify epileptogenesis in the human brain in vivo. *Brain* (2002) **125**:1709–18. doi:10.1093/brain/awf187
216. Enatsu R, Jin K, Elwan S, Kubota Y, Piao Z, O'Connor T, et al. Correlations between ictal propagation and response to electrical cortical stimulation: a cortico-cortical evoked potential study. *Epilepsy Res* (2012) **101**:76–87. doi:10.1016/j.eplepsyres.2012.03.004
217. Berenyi A, Belluscio M, Mao D, Buzsaki G. Closed-loop control of epilepsy by transcranial electrical stimulation. *Science* (2012) **337**:735–7. doi:10.1126/science.1223154
218. Buckmaster PS. Laboratory animal models of temporal lobe epilepsy. *Comp Med* (2004) **54**:473–85.
219. Mishra AM, Bai H, Gribizis A, Blumenfeld H. Neuroimaging biomarkers of epileptogenesis. *Neurosci Lett* (2011) **497**:194–204. doi:10.1016/j.neulet.2011.01.076
220. Coppola A, Moshe SL. Animal models. *Handb Clin Neurol* (2012) **107**:63–98. doi:10.1016/B978-0-444-52898-8.00004-5
221. Guillemain I, Kahane P, Depaulis A. Animal models to study aetiopathology of epilepsy: what are the features to model? *Epileptic Disord* (2012) **14**:217–25. doi:10.1684/epd.2012.0528
222. Galanopoulou AS. Basic mechanisms of catastrophic epilepsy – overview from animal models. *Brain Dev* (2013) **35**:748–56. doi:10.1016/j.braindev.2012.12.005
223. Cossart R, Dinocourt C, Hirsch JC, Merchan-Perez A, De Felipe J, Ben-Ari Y, et al. Dendritic but not somatic GABAergic inhibition is decreased in experimental epilepsy. *Nat Neurosci* (2001) **4**:52–62. doi:10.1038/82900
224. Soussi R, Boulland JL, Bassot E, Bras H, Coulon P, Chaudhry FA, et al. Reorganization of supramammillary-hippocampal pathways in the rat pilocarpine model of temporal lobe epilepsy: evidence for axon terminal sprouting. *Brain Struct Funct* (2014). doi:10.1007/s00429-014-0800-2
225. Mishra AM, Ellens DJ, Schridde U, Motelow JE, Purcaro MJ, Desalvo MN, et al. Where fMRI and electrophysiology agree to disagree: corticothalamic and striatal activity patterns in the WAG/Rij rat. *J Neurosci* (2011) **31**:15053–64. doi:10.1523/JNEUROSCI.0101-11.2011
226. Elms J, Powell KL, Van Raay L, Dedeurwaerdere S, O'Brien TJ, Morris MJ. Long-term valproate treatment increases brain neuropeptide Y expression and decreases seizure expression in a genetic rat model of absence epilepsy. *PLoS One* (2013) **8**:e73505. doi:10.1371/journal.pone.0073505
227. Carcak N, Zheng T, Ali I, Abdullah A, French C, Powell KL, et al. The effect of amygdala kindling on neuronal firing patterns in the lateral thalamus in the GAERS model of absence epilepsy. *Epilepsia* (2014) **55**:654–65. doi:10.1111/epi.12592
228. Bouilleret V, Ridoux V, Depaulis A, Marescaux C, Nehlig A, La Salle G. Recurrent seizures and hippocampal sclerosis following intrahippocampal kainate injection in adult mice: electroencephalography, histopathology and synaptic reorganization similar to mesial temporal lobe epilepsy. *Neuroscience* (1999) **89**:717–29. doi:10.1016/S0306-4522(98)00401-1
229. Leite JP, Garcia-Cairasco N, Cavalheiro EA. New insights from the use of pilocarpine and kainate models. *Epilepsy Res* (2002) **50**:93–103. doi:10.1016/S0920-1211(02)00072-4
230. Riban V, Bouilleret V, Pham-Le BT, Fritschy JM, Marescaux C, Depaulis A. Evolution of hippocampal epileptic activity during the development of hippocampal sclerosis in a mouse model of temporal lobe epilepsy. *Neuroscience* (2002) **112**:101–11. doi:10.1016/S0306-4522(02)00064-7
231. Marchi N, Oby E, Batra A, Uva L, De Curtis M, Hernandez N, et al. In vivo and in vitro effects of pilocarpine: relevance to ictogenesis. *Epilepsia* (2007) **48**:1934–46. doi:10.1111/j.1528-1167.2007.01185.x
232. Curia G, Longo D, Biagini G, Jones RS, Avoli M. The pilocarpine model of temporal lobe epilepsy. *J Neurosci Methods* (2008) **172**:143–57. doi:10.1016/j.jneumeth.2008.04.019
233. Deprez F, Zattoni M, Mura ML, Frei K, Fritschy JM. Adoptive transfer of T lymphocytes in immunodeficient mice influences epileptogenesis and neurodegeneration in a model of temporal lobe epilepsy. *Neurobiol Dis* (2011) **44**:174–84. doi:10.1016/j.nbd.2011.06.011
234. Zattoni M, Mura ML, Deprez F, Schwendener RA, Engelhardt B, Frei K, et al. Brain infiltration of leukocytes contributes to the pathophysiology of temporal lobe epilepsy. *J Neurosci* (2011) **31**:4037–50. doi:10.1523/JNEUROSCI.6210-10.2011
235. Lothman EW, Hatlelid JM, Zorumski CF, Conry JA, Moon PF, Perlin JB. Kindling with rapidly recurring hippocampal seizures. *Brain Res* (1985) **360**:83–91. doi:10.1016/0006-8993(85)91223-5

236. Morales JC, Alvarez-Ferradas C, Roncagliolo M, Fuenzalida M, Wellmann M, Nualart FJ, et al. A new rapid kindling variant for induction of cortical epileptogenesis in freely moving rats. *Front Cell Neurosci* (2014) **8**:200. doi:10.3389/fncel.2014.00200
237. Kowski AB, Kanaan H, Schmitt FC, Holtkamp M. Deep hypothermia terminates status epilepticus – an experimental study. *Brain Res* (2012) **1446**:119–26. doi:10.1016/j.brainres.2012.01.022
238. Reddy DS, Kuruba R. Experimental models of status epilepticus and neuronal injury for evaluation of therapeutic interventions. *Int J Mol Sci* (2013) **14**:18284–318. doi:10.3390/ijms140918284
239. Wang CH, Hung CP, Chen MT, Shih YH, Lin YY. Hippocampal desynchronization of functional connectivity prior to the onset of status epilepticus in pilocarpine-treated rats. *PLoS One* (2012) **7**:e39763. doi:10.1371/journal.pone.0039763
240. Gong XW, Li JB, Lu QC, Liang PJ, Zhang PM. Effective connectivity of hippocampal neural network and its alteration in Mg2+-free epilepsy model. *PLoS One* (2014) **9**:e92961. doi:10.1371/journal.pone.0092961
241. Cymerblit-Sabba A, Schiller Y. Network dynamics during development of pharmacologically induced epileptic seizures in rats in vivo. *J Neurosci* (2010) **30**:1619–30. doi:10.1523/JNEUROSCI.5078-09.2010
242. Englot DJ, Mishra AM, Mansuripur PK, Herman P, Hyder F, Blumenfeld H. Remote effects of focal hippocampal seizures on the rat neocortex. *J Neurosci* (2008) **28**:9066–81. doi:10.1523/JNEUROSCI.2014-08.2008
243. Megevand P, Quairiaux C, Lascano AM, Kiss JZ, Michel CM. A mouse model for studying large-scale neuronal networks using EEG mapping techniques. *Neuroimage* (2008) **42**:591–602. doi:10.1016/j.neuroimage.2008.05.016
244. Megevand P, Troncoso E, Quairiaux C, Muller D, Michel CM, Kiss JZ. Long-term plasticity in mouse sensorimotor circuits after rhythmic whisker stimulation. *J Neurosci* (2009) **29**:5326–35. doi:10.1523/JNEUROSCI.5965-08.2009
245. Quairiaux C, Sizonenko SV, Megevand P, Michel CM, Kiss JZ. Functional deficit and recovery of developing sensorimotor networks following neonatal hypoxic-ischemic injury in the rat. *Cereb Cortex* (2010) **20**:2080–91. doi:10.1093/cercor/bhp281
246. Quairiaux C, Megevand P, Kiss JZ, Michel CM. Functional development of large-scale sensorimotor cortical networks in the brain. *J Neurosci* (2011) **31**:9574–84. doi:10.1523/JNEUROSCI.5995-10.2011
247. Toyoda I, Bower MR, Leyva F, Buckmaster PS. Early activation of ventral hippocampus and subiculum during spontaneous seizures in a rat model of temporal lobe epilepsy. *J Neurosci* (2013) **33**:11100–15. doi:10.1523/JNEUROSCI.0472-13.2013
248. Berenyi A, Somogyvari Z, Nagy AJ, Roux L, Long JD, Fujisawa S, et al. Large-scale, high-density (up to 512 channels) recording of local circuits in behaving animals. *J Neurophysiol* (2014) **111**:1132–49. doi:10.1152/jn.00785.2013
249. Mishra AM, Bai X, Sanganahalli BG, Waxman SG, Shatillo O, Grohn O, et al. Decreased resting functional connectivity after traumatic brain injury in the rat. *PLoS One* (2014) **9**:e95280. doi:10.1371/journal.pone.0095280
250. Mishra AM, Bai X, Motelow JE, Desalvo MN, Danielson N, Sanganahalli BG, et al. Increased resting functional connectivity in spike-wave epilepsy in WAG/Rij rats. *Epilepsia* (2013) **54**:1214–22. doi:10.1111/epi.12227
251. Choi H, Kim YK, Kang H, Lee H, Im HJ, Hwang DW, et al. Abnormal metabolic connectivity in the pilocarpine-induced epilepsy rat model: a multiscale network analysis based on persistent homology. *Neuroimage* (2014) **99C**:226–36. doi:10.1016/j.neuroimage.2014.05.039
252. Xia Y, Lai Y, Lei L, Liu Y, Yao D. Left hemisphere predominance of pilocarpine-induced rat epileptiform discharges. *J Neuroeng Rehabil* (2009) **6**:42. doi:10.1186/1743-0003-6-42
253. Zhou IY, Liang YX, Chan RW, Gao PP, Cheng JS, Hu Y, et al. Brain resting-state functional MRI connectivity: morphological foundation and plasticity. *Neuroimage* (2014) **84**:1–10. doi:10.1016/j.neuroimage.2013.08.037
254. Tenney JR, Duong TQ, King JA, Ludwig R, Ferris CF. Corticothalamic modulation during absence seizures in rats: a functional MRI assessment. *Epilepsia* (2003) **44**:1133–40. doi:10.1046/j.1528-1157.2003.61002.x
255. Chahboune H, Mishra AM, Desalvo MN, Staib LH, Purcaro M, Scheinost D, et al. DTI abnormalities in anterior corpus callosum of rats with spike-wave epilepsy. *Neuroimage* (2009) **47**:459–66. doi:10.1016/j.neuroimage.2009.04.060
256. Nersesyan H, Herman P, Erdogan E, Hyder F, Blumenfeld H. Relative changes in cerebral blood flow and neuronal activity in local microdomains during generalized seizures. *J Cereb Blood Flow Metab* (2004) **24**:1057–68. doi:10.1097/01.WCB.0000131669.02027.3E
257. Nersesyan H, Hyder F, Rothman DL, Blumenfeld H. Dynamic fMRI and EEG recordings during spike-wave seizures and generalized tonic-clonic seizures in WAG/Rij rats. *J Cereb Blood Flow Metab* (2004) **24**:589–99. doi:10.1097/01.WCB.0000117688.98763.23
258. Desalvo MN, Schridde U, Mishra AM, Motelow JE, Purcaro MJ, Danielson N, et al. Focal BOLD fMRI changes in bicuculline-induced tonic-clonic seizures in the rat. *Neuroimage* (2010) **50**:902–9. doi:10.1016/j.neuroimage.2010.01.006
259. Polack PO, Mahon S, Chavez M, Charpier S. Inactivation of the somatosensory cortex prevents paroxysmal oscillations in cortical and related thalamic neurons in a genetic model of absence epilepsy. *Cereb Cortex* (2009) **19**:2078–91. doi:10.1093/cercor/bhn237
260. Straessle A, Loup F, Arabadzisz D, Ohning GV, Fritschy JM. Rapid and long-term alterations of hippocampal GABAB receptors in a mouse model of temporal lobe epilepsy. *Eur J Neurosci* (2003) **18**:2213–26. doi:10.1046/j.1460-9568.2003.02964.x
261. Timofeev I, Bazhenov M, Avramescu S, Nita DA. Posttraumatic epilepsy: the roles of synaptic plasticity. *Neuroscientist* (2010) **16**:19–27. doi:10.1177/1073858409333545
262. Pitkanen A, Kemppainen S, Ndode-Ekane XE, Huusko N, Huttunen JK, Grohn O, et al. Posttraumatic epilepsy – disease or comorbidity? *Epilepsy Behav* (2014). doi:10.1016/j.yebeh.2014.01.013
263. Zhang Q, Wu ZC, Yu JT, Zhong XL, Xing YY, Tian Y, et al. Anticonvulsant effect of unilateral anterior thalamic high frequency electrical stimulation on amygdala-kindled seizures in rat. *Brain Res Bull* (2012) **87**:221–6. doi:10.1016/j.brainresbull.2011.11.023
264. Langlois M, Polack PO, Bernard H, David O, Charpier S, Depaulis A, et al. Involvement of the thalamic parafascicular nucleus in mesial temporal lobe epilepsy. *J Neurosci* (2010) **30**:16523–35. doi:10.1523/JNEUROSCI.1109-10.2010
265. Arabadzisz D, Antal K, Parpan F, Emri Z, Fritschy JM. Epileptogenesis and chronic seizures in a mouse model of temporal lobe epilepsy are associated with distinct EEG patterns and selective neurochemical alterations in the contralateral hippocampus. *Exp Neurol* (2005) **194**:76–90. doi:10.1016/j.expneurol.2005.01.029
266. Marx M, Haas CA, Haussler U. Differential vulnerability of interneurons in the epileptic hippocampus. *Front Cell Neurosci* (2013) **7**:167. doi:10.3389/fncel.2013.00167
267. Khalilov I, Holmes GL, Ben-Ari Y. In vitro formation of a secondary epileptogenic mirror focus by interhippocampal propagation of seizures. *Nat Neurosci* (2003) **6**:1079–85. doi:10.1038/nn1125
268. Morrell F. Experimental focal epilepsy in animals. *Arch Neurol* (1959) **1**:141–7. doi:10.1001/archneur.1959.03840020015003
269. Ben-Ari Y, Lagowska J, Tremblay E, La Salle G. A new model of focal status epilepticus: intra-amygdaloid application of kainic acid elicits repetitive secondarily generalized convulsive seizures. *Brain Res* (1979) **163**:176–9. doi:10.1016/0006-8993(79)90163-X
270. Sobayo T, Mogul DJ. Rapid onset of a kainate-induced mirror focus in rat hippocampus is mediated by contralateral AMPA receptors. *Epilepsy Res* (2013) **106**:35–46. doi:10.1016/j.eplepsyres.2013.03.010
271. Sabatino M, Gravante G, Ferraro G, Vella N, La Grutta G, La Grutta V. Striatonigral suppression of focal hippocampal epilepsy. *Neurosci Lett* (1989) **98**:285–90. doi:10.1016/0304-3940(89)90415-1
272. Rektor I, Kuba R, Brazdil M, Chrastina J. Do the basal ganglia inhibit seizure activity in temporal lobe epilepsy? *Epilepsy Behav* (2012) **25**:56–9. doi:10.1016/j.yebeh.2012.04.125
273. Krook-Magnuson E, Armstrong C, Oijala M, Soltesz I. On-demand optogenetic control of spontaneous seizures in temporal lobe epilepsy. *Nat Commun* (2013) **4**:1376. doi:10.1038/ncomms2376
274. Paz JT, Davidson TJ, Frechette ES, Delord B, Parada I, Peng K, et al. Closed-loop optogenetic control of thalamus as a tool for interrupting seizures after cortical injury. *Nat Neurosci* (2013) **16**:64–70. doi:10.1038/nn.3269
275. Mirski MA, Rossell LA, Terry JB, Fisher RS. Anticonvulsant effect of anterior thalamic high frequency electrical stimulation in the rat. *Epilepsy Res* (1997) **28**:89–100. doi:10.1016/S0920-1211(97)00034-X

276. Hamani C, Ewerton FI, Bonilha SM, Ballester G, Mello LE, Lozano AM. Bilateral anterior thalamic nucleus lesions and high-frequency stimulation are protective against pilocarpine-induced seizures and status epilepticus. *Neurosurgery* (2004) **54**:191–5. doi:10.1227/01.NEU.0000097552.31763.AE
277. Takebayashi S, Hashizume K, Tanaka T, Hodozuka A. The effect of electrical stimulation and lesioning of the anterior thalamic nucleus on kainic acid-induced focal cortical seizure status in rats. *Epilepsia* (2007) **48**:348–58. doi:10.1111/j.1528-1167.2006.00948.x
278. Lado FA. Chronic bilateral stimulation of the anterior thalamus of kainate-treated rats increases seizure frequency. *Epilepsia* (2006) **47**:27–32. doi:10.1111/j.1528-1167.2006.00366.x
279. Fisher R, Salanova V, Witt T, Worth R, Henry T, Gross R, et al. Electrical stimulation of the anterior nucleus of thalamus for treatment of refractory epilepsy. *Epilepsia* (2010) **51**:899–908. doi:10.1111/j.1528-1167.2010.02536.x
280. Jackson JH. Lectures on the diagnosis of epilepsy. *Br Med J* (1879) **1**:33–6. doi:10.1136/bmj.1.941.33
281. Jackson JH. Lectures on the diagnosis of epilepsy. *Br Med J* (1879) **1**:141–3. doi:10.1136/bmj.1.944.141
282. Jackson JH. Lectures on the diagnosis of epilepsy. *Br Med J* (1879) **1**:109–12. doi:10.1136/bmj.1.943.109
283. Sander JW. Comorbidity and premature mortality in epilepsy. *Lancet* (2013) **382**:1618–9. doi:10.1016/S0140-6736(13)61136-8

5

Metabolic changes in occipital lobe epilepsy with automatisms

Chong H. Wong*[1,2]*, Armin Mohamed*[1,3]*, Lingfeng Wen*[3,4]*, Stefan Eberl*[3,4]*, Ernest Somerville*[2,5]*, Michael Fulham*[1,3] *and Andrew F. Bleasel*[1,2]*

[1] *Sydney Medical School, University of Sydney, Sydney, NSW, Australia*
[2] *Department of Neurology, Westmead Hospital, Westmead, NSW, Australia*
[3] *Department of PET and Nuclear Medicine, Royal Prince Alfred Hospital, Camperdown, NSW, Australia*
[4] *School of Information Technologies, University of Sydney, Sydney, NSW, Australia*
[5] *Institute of Neurological Sciences, Prince of Wales Hospital, Randwick, NSW, Australia*

***Correspondence:**
Andrew F. Bleasel, Department of Neurology, Westmead Hospital, Darcy Road, Westmead, NSW 2145, Australia
e-mail: andrew.bleasel@sydney.edu.au

Purpose: Some studies suggest that the pattern of glucose hypometabolism relates not only to the ictal-onset zone but also reflects seizure propagation. We investigated metabolic changes in patients with occipital lobe epilepsy (OLE) that may reflect propagation of ictal discharge during seizures with automatisms.

Methods: Fifteen patients who had undergone epilepsy surgery for intractable OLE and had undergone interictal Fluorine-18-fluorodeoxyglucose positron-emission tomography (^{18}F-FDG-PET) between 1994 and 2004 were divided into two groups (with and without automatisms during seizure). Significant regions of hypometabolism were identified by comparing ^{18}F-FDG-PET results from each group with 16 healthy controls by using statistical parametric mapping.

Key Findings: Significant hypometabolism was confined largely to the epileptogenic occipital lobe in the patient group without automatisms. In patients with automatisms, glucose hypometabolism extended from the epileptogenic occipital lobe into the ipsilateral temporal lobe.

Significance: We identified a distinctive hypometabolic pattern that was specific for OLE patients with automatisms during a seizure. This finding supports the postulate that seizure propagation is a cause of glucose hypometabolism beyond the region of seizure onset.

Keywords: epilepsies, focal, epilepsy, occipital lobe, positron-emission tomography, fluorodeoxyglucose, automatisms, automotor seizure

INTRODUCTION

Fluorine-18-fluorodeoxyglucose positron-emission tomography (^{18}F-FDG-PET) is often used for localization of the epileptogenic region during an epilepsy presurgical evaluation. However, the interictal ^{18}F-FDG-PET hypometabolism often extends beyond the epileptogenic region into the adjacent and remote cortical and subcortical structures (1). Several studies investigating this phenomenon demonstrated the patterns of interictal glucose hypometabolism may reflect metabolic disturbances from propagation of seizures to functionally connected remote brain areas or networks (2–6).

In occipital lobe epilepsy (OLE), oral and manual automatisms are common and are often attributed to seizure propagation from the occipital to the temporal lobe (7, 8). This study examines ^{18}F-FDG-PET of patients with OLE to identify specific pattern of functional disturbances in brain areas that may reflect an ictal pathway during seizures with automatisms.

MATERIALS AND METHODS

We included all 15 patients with medically intractable epilepsy, who had undergone occipital lobe resections and interictal ^{18}F-FDG-PET between 1994 and 2004 at the Westmead and Royal Prince Alfred Hospitals, Australia. The study was approved by the ethics committees in Central Sydney (Protocol no. X03-0161) and Western Sydney Area Health Services [HREC reference no: HS/TG HREC 2003/6/4.13 (1670)]. Patients with resection of the parieto-occipital cortex were not included. The occipital lobe boundaries were established as defined by the Tzourio-Mazoyer atlas (9).

Seizure semiology was determined from the review of the in-patient video-EEG recording and was classified according to the seizure semiologic classification developed at the Cleveland Clinic Foundation in the 1990s (10). Based on the presence or absence of seizures with automatisms during in-patient video-EEG recording, patients were assigned into a seizure with automatisms group or a seizure without automatisms group. Seizures with automatisms were defined as seizures with oro-alimentary and manual automatisms, usually, but not always, with impairment of consciousness (10, 11).

Methods for FDG-PET acquisition and for statistical parametric mapping (SPM2; Wellcome Department of Cognitive Neurology, UK) and spatial pre-processing of FDG-PET images of patients and 16 healthy controls have been described in detail elsewhere (6, 12, 13). In brief, ^{18}F-FDG-PET images were realigned, spatially normalized, and smoothed by convolution with a 10-mm FWHM Gaussian kernel. The ^{18}F-FDG-PET images of patients with left occipital ictal onset were transposed horizontally so that all ictal-onset foci were lateralized to the right side. Both patients and controls had regional metabolic rates of glucose hypometabolism estimated using a population-based input function calibrated by using two arterialized-venous blood sampling procedures (14). For statistical analysis, ^{18}F-FDG-PET images of each patient group were compared with images of the 16 healthy controls (8 males, median age 31.5 years, interquartile range 25–75%; 25–42 years) at the voxel-by-voxel level using two-sample t-tests to identify all clusters of voxels exhibiting significant hypometabolism. SPM analysis identifies regions with

Table 1 | Summary of clinical features, investigation results, and surgical outcome.

Patient (age/gender)	Age of onset	MRI findings	Lobe of ictal onset[a]	Typical semiology[b]	Seizure outcome	Pathology
PATIENTS WITHOUT AUTOMATISM DURING SEIZURES						
1. 25 yr/M	12yr	Lt mesial occipital lesion	Lt OLE	Cephalic aura > tonic seizure (Rt arm)	Engel 2	Type 1 cortical dysplasia
2. 20 yr/F	7 yr	Rt inf-mesial occipital lobe lesion	Rt OLE	Visual aura > Lt versive seizure > dialeptic seizure	Engel 1	Type 2 cortical dysplasia
3. 15 yr/M	12 yr	Normal MRI	Rt OLE	Visual aura > Lt versive seizure > SGTCS	Engel 1	Type 2 cortical dysplasia
4. 32 yr/M	18 yr	Rt inf-mesial occipital lobe lesion	Rt OLE	Visual aura > SGTCS	Engel 2	Gliosis
5. 30 yr/F	20 yr	Normal MRI	Lt OLE	Visual aura > SGTCS	Engel 1	Type 1 cortical dysplasia
6. 25 yr/F	17 yr	Lt dorsolateral occipital lobe lesion	Lt OLE	SGTCS	Engel 1	Ganglioglioma
PATIENTS WITH AUTOMATISMS DURING SEIZURES						
7. 15 yr/F	4 yr	Normal MRI	Rt OLE	Visual aura > automotor seizure	Engel 1	Type 2 cortical dysplasia
8. 10 yr/F	6 yr	Rt inf-mesial occipital lobe atrophy	Rt OLE	Visual aura > automotor seizure	Engel 1	Gliosis
9. 15 yr/F	3 yr	Rt inf-mesial occipital lobe lesion	Rt OLE	Visual aura > automotor seizure	Engel 1	Ganglioglioma
10. 18 yr/M	6 yr	Normal MRI	Lt OLE	Visual aura > automotor seizure	Engel 1	Type 2 cortical dysplasia
11. 26 yr/M	7 yr	Lt inf-mesial occipital lobe lesion	Lt OLE	Visual aura > automotor seizure > tonic seizure (Rt arm)	Engel 1	Dysembryoplastic neuroepithelial tumor
12. 26 yr/F	11 yr	Normal MRI	Lt OLE	Cephalic aura > automotor seizures > SGTCS	Engel 1	Type 1 cortical dysplasia
13. 13 yr/F	2 yr	Lt dorsolateral occipital lobe lesion	Rt OLE	Visual aura > automotor seizure	Engel 1	Dysembryoplastic neuroepithelial tumor
14. 30 yr/M	17 yr	Rt inf-mesial occipital lobe lesion	Rt OLE	Visual aura > automotor seizure	Engel 3	Ganglioglioma
15. 27 yr/M	14 yr	Normal MRI	Rt OLE	Visual aura > automotor seizure	Engel 2	Type 1 cortical dysplasia

[a] *Origin of seizures was based on clinical history, scalp, and intracranial video-EEG monitoring, MRI, ^{18}F-FDG-PET, ^{99m}Tc-hexamethyl-propylene-amine-oxime single photon emission computed tomography and neuropsychological studies.*

[b] *Seizure semiology determined on video review of in-patient video-electroencephalography and classified according to the seizure semiologic classification (10). Automotor seizures refer to seizures with oro-alimentary and manual automatisms.*

Cephalic aura refers a sensation in the head (15).

M, male; F, female; Lt, left; Rt, right; yr, years; inf, inferior; OLE, occipital lobe epilepsy; SGTCS, secondarily generalized tonic clonic seizures.

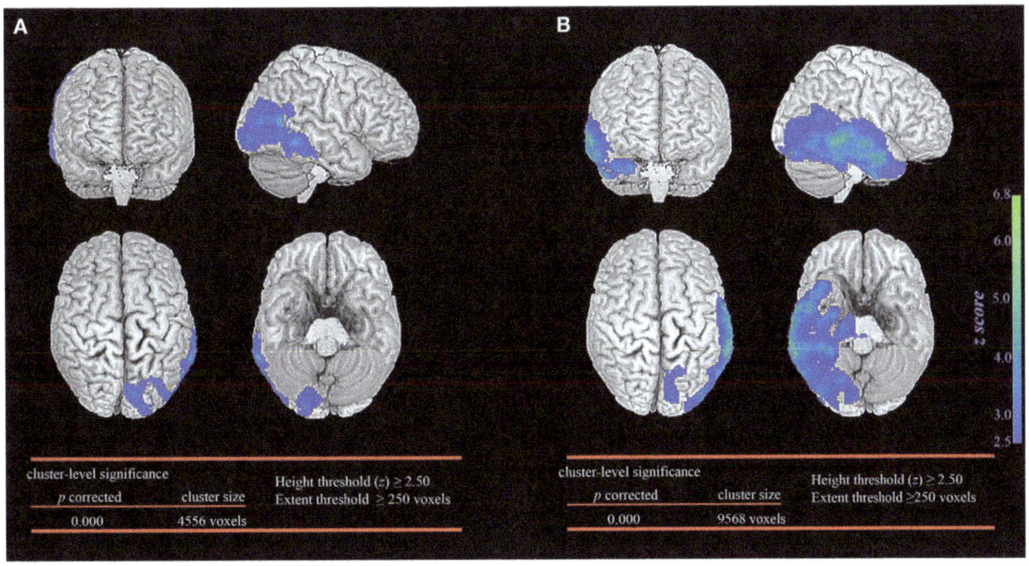

FIGURE 1 | Statistical parametric mapping comparison between patient groups and healthy controls. Significant glucose hypometabolism was observed in the ipsilateral occipital lobe in the group of occipital lobe epilepsy patients without automatisms during seizures **(A)**. In the group of occipital lobe epilepsy patients with automatisms during seizures, significant decrease in glucose hypometabolism extends to involve the ispsilateral temporal lobe **(B)**.

cluster size (extent threshold) larger than 250 contiguous voxels and with voxel-level significance (height threshold) of $p \geq 0.01$. Only regions with clusters of voxels that exceeds this extent and height threshold and achieved corrected cluster-level significance of $p < 0.05$ were considered significant. Group analysis was performed to eliminate interindividual metabolic variability. The analysis allowed the identification and comparison of hypometabolic patterns for the seizures with automatisms and the seizures without automatisms groups when compared to normal healthy controls.

RESULTS

Fifteen patients (eight females and seven males) with age of seizure onset between 2 and 20 years (median age 11 years; IQR 25–75%, 6–17 years) were studied. The median age of the study population was 25 years old (IQR 25–75%, 15–27 years). Ten patients were admitted to hospital for in-patient prolonged video EEG on at least two occasions (range 1–4 video-EEG monitoring). The median number of seizures recorded was 16 seizures (IQR 25–75%, 11–35 seizures; range 10–50 seizures). Among the patients, 13 had intracranial video-EEG studies and showed an ictal-onset zone within the occipital lobe. Two patients (patient 6 and 13) did not undergo invasive monitoring but showed a MRI abnormality with concordant scalp video-EEG findings; both became seizure free after surgery. The median follow-up duration following surgery was 10.1 years (IQR 25–75%, 8–15.8 years). Twelve patients achieved Engel class 1 outcome, 2 had significant seizure improvement (Engel 2) and 1 had worthwhile improvement (Engel 3). The histopathology was summarized in **Table 1**.

Nine patients had seizures with automatisms occurring as a component of their habitual seizures. The other six patients, who never had automatisms as a feature of their habitual seizures, were assigned to the group without automatisms for SPM group analysis. **Table 1** summarizes the seizure semiology of all patients studied.

In the seizure without automatisms group, SPM analysis revealed significant glucose hypometabolism involving primarily the epileptogenic occipital lobe and extending marginally into the posterior temporal region (**Figure 1A**). In contrast, the patient group with automatisms not only demonstrated prominent glucose hypometabolism in the epileptogenic occipital lobe but also a significant decrease in glucose metabolism in the basal temporal, lateral temporal, and anteromesial temporal structures (**Figure 1B**).

The extent of temporal lobe involvement was significantly associated with the presence of automatisms during seizures ($p < 0.001$, median 1223 voxels; IQR 928–4207 voxels) when compared to patients without automatisms during seizures (median 101 voxels; IQR 0–300 voxels). No significant association was found between the extent of temporal lobe involvement, duration of epilepsy before FDG-PET, age when FDG-PET was performed and seizure outcome.

DISCUSSION

In this study, we determined the interictal metabolic patterns of glucose in patients with OLE with and without automatisms. The major difference in OLE patients with automatisms was the presence of significant glucose hypometabolism in the temporal lobe. We suggest that this interictal metabolic change reflects evidence for the propagation pathway of seizures in patients with automatisms.

Significant hypometabolism was present in the occipital lobe in both groups of patients with OLE. ^{18}F-FDG-PET has been used to localize ictal focus by showing regional glucose hypometabolism in the epileptogenic occipital lobe in OLE (16, 17). Our finding was not unexpected given that ^{18}F-FDG-PET revealed focal areas of relative hypometabolism that was associated with the epileptogenic zone.

The occipital lobe is connected to the mesial and lateral temporal structures by abundant multisynaptic projections (18, 19). Several studies have shown seizures originating from the occipital lobe readily propagate to the temporal lobe (7, 8, 20, 21), and the occipital to temporal seizure spread coincides with the appearance of oral and manual automatisms (7, 8, 22). Our patient group with seizures and automatisms demonstrated significant glucose hypometabolism extending from the epileptogenic occipital lobe into the temporal lobe. We postulate this hypometabolism reflects neuronal dysfunction from the spread of electrical activity into the ipsilateral temporal lobe during the evolution of seizures with automatisms.

Several studies support the hypothesis that the topography of glucose hypometabolism relates, at least in part, to brain regions involved in the ictal onset and to pathways of seizure propagation generating the clinical manifestations (3, 4, 23). Schlaug et al. examined the relationship between seizure semiology and interictal abnormalities in cerebral glucose metabolism in 48 patients with neocortical focal epilepsy. The investigators found patients with focal clonic seizures had prominent glucose hypometabolism in the contralateral primary motor area and unilateral tonic seizures were associated with markedly decreased metabolism in the supplementary motor area (2). Others reported ictal dystonic posturing to be correlated with contralateral basal ganglia hypometabolism (3, 5). Several brain regions have been reported to produce automatisms by direct cortical electrical stimulation. These include the amygdala, hippocampus, peri-insular temporal cortex, anterior cingulate gyrus, and mesial frontal cortex (24–26). In our cohort of OLE patients with oral and manual automatisms, our analysis found extension of interictal glucose hypometabolism outside of the epileptogenic occipital lobe into basal, lateral, and anteromesial temporal cortices. These structures overlap with regions described in the literature as regions producing automatisms with electrical stimulation. These findings provide confirmatory evidence of occipital lobe seizures often spread to the temporal lobe, and oral and manual automatisms can be a marker of the spread. These same patients overall had a good outcome following surgery on the occipital lobe, leaving the temporal lobe *in situ*. This suggests involvement of the temporal lobe reflects spread of ictal activity, rather than the temporal lobe being a key part of the epileptogenic network.

ACKNOWLEDGMENTS

This work was supported in part by University of Sydney Postgraduate Award and Millennium Institute Stipend to Dr. Chong H. Wong.

REFERENCES

1. Sperling MR, Gur RC, Alavi A, Gur RE, Resnick S, O'Connor MJ, et al. Subcortical metabolic alterations in partial epilepsy. *Epilepsia* (1990) **31**:145–55. doi:10.1111/j.1528-1167.1990.tb06299.x
2. Schlaug G, Antke C, Holthausen H, Arnold S, Ebner A, Tuxhorn I, et al. Ictal motor signs and interictal regional cerebral hypometabolism. *Neurology* (1997) **49**:341–50. doi:10.1212/WNL.49.2.341
3. Dupont S, Semah F, Baulac M, Samson Y. The underlying pathophysiology of ictal dystonia in temporal lobe epilepsy: an FDG-PET study. *Neurology* (1998) **51**:1289–92. doi:10.1212/WNL.51.5.1289
4. Chassoux F, Semah F, Bouilleret V, Landre E, Devaux B, Turak B, et al. Metabolic changes and electro-clinical patterns in mesio-temporal lobe epilepsy: a correlative study. *Brain* (2004) **127**:164–74. doi:10.1093/brain/awh014
5. Rusu V, Chassoux F, Landre E, Bouilleret V, Nataf F, Devaux BC, et al. Dystonic posturing in seizures of mesial temporal origin: electroclinical and metabolic patterns. *Neurology* (2005) **65**:1612–9. doi:10.1212/01.wnl.0000184510.44808.50
6. Wong CH, Bleasel A, Wen L, Eberl S, Byth K, Fulham M, et al. The topography and significance of extratemporal hypometabolism in refractory mesial temporal lobe epilepsy examined by FDG-PET. *Epilepsia* (2010) **51**:1365–73. doi:10.1111/j.1528-1167.2010.02552.x
7. Salanova V, Andermann F, Olivier A, Rasmussen T, Quesney LF. Occipital lobe epilepsy: electroclinical manifestations, electrocorticography, cortical stimulation and outcome in 42 patients treated between 1930 and 1991. Surgery of occipital lobe epilepsy. *Brain* (1992) **115**(Pt 6):1655–80. doi:10.1093/brain/115.6.1655
8. Williamson PD, Thadani VM, Darcey TM, Spencer DD, Spencer SS, Mattson RH. Occipital lobe epilepsy: clinical characteristics, seizure spread patterns, and results of surgery. *Ann Neurol* (1992) **31**:3–13. doi:10.1002/ana.410310103
9. Tzourio-Mazoyer N, Landeau B, Papathanassiou D, Crivello F, Etard O, Delcroix N, et al. Automated anatomical labeling of activations in SPM using a macroscopic anatomical parcellation of the MNI MRI single-subject brain. *Neuroimage* (2002) **15**:273–89. doi:10.1006/nimg.2001.0978
10. Luders H, Acharya J, Baumgartner C, Benbadis S, Bleasel A, Burgess R, et al. Semiological seizure classification. *Epilepsia* (1998) **39**:1006–13. doi:10.1111/j.1528-1157.1998.tb01452.x
11. Kotagal P. Automotor seizures. In: Lüders HO, Noachtar S, editors. *Epileptic Seizures: Pathophysiology and Clinical Semiology*. Philadelphia, PA: Churchill Livingstone (2000). p. 449–57.
12. Mohamed A, Eberl S, Fulham MJ, Kassiou M, Zaman A, Henderson D, et al. Sequential 123I-iododexetimide scans in temporal lobe epilepsy: comparison with neuroimaging scans (MR imaging and 18F-FDG PET imaging). *Eur J Nucl Med Mol Imaging* (2005) **32**:180–5. doi:10.1007/s00259-004-1654-2
13. Wong CH, Bleasel A, Wen L, Eberl S, Byth K, Fulham M, et al. Relationship between preoperative hypometabolism and surgical outcome in neocortical epilepsy surgery. *Epilepsia* (2012) **53**:1333–40. doi:10.1111/j.1528-1167.2012.03547.x
14. Eberl S, Anayat AR, Fulton RR, Hooper PK, Fulham MJ. Evaluation of two population-based input functions for quantitative neurological FDG PET studies. *Eur J Nucl Med* (1997) **24**:299–304. doi:10.1007/BF01728767
15. Blume WT, Luders HO, Mizrahi E, Tassinari C, Van Emde Boas W, Engel J Jr. Glossary of descriptive terminology for ictal semiology: report of the ILAE task force on classification and terminology. *Epilepsia* (2001) **42**:1212–8. doi:10.1046/j.1528-1157.2001.22001.x
16. Sturm JW, Newton MR, Chinvarun Y, Berlangieri SU, Berkovic SF. Ictal SPECT and interictal PET in the localization of occipital lobe epilepsy. *Epilepsia* (2000) **41**:463–6. doi:10.1111/j.1528-1157.2000.tb00190.x
17. Kim SK, Lee DS, Lee SK, Kim YK, Kang KW, Chung CK, et al. Diagnostic performance of [18F]FDG-PET and ictal [99mTc]-HMPAO SPECT in occipital lobe epilepsy. *Epilepsia* (2001) **42**:1531–40. doi:10.1046/j.1528-1157.2001.21901.x
18. Turner BH, Mishkin M, Knapp M. Organization of the amygdalopetal projections from modality-specific cortical association areas in the monkey. *JComp Neurol* (1980) **191**:515–43. doi:10.1002/cne.901910402
19. Catani M, Jones DK, Donato R, Ffytche DH. Occipito-temporal connections in the human brain. *Brain* (2003) **126**:2093–107. doi:10.1093/brain/awg203
20. Collins RC, Caston TV. Functional anatomy of occipital lobe seizures: an experimental study in rats. *Neurology* (1979) **29**:705–16. doi:10.1212/WNL.29.5.705
21. Usui N, Mihara T, Baba K, Matsuda K, Tottori T, Umeoka S, et al. Early seizure propagation from the occipital lobe to medial temporal structures and its surgical implication. *Epileptic Disord* (2008) **10**:260–5. doi:10.1684/epd.2008.0223

22. Babb TL, Halgren E, Wilson C, Engel J, Crandall P. Neuronal firing patterns during the spread of an occipital lobe seizure to the temporal lobes in man. *Electroencephalogr Clin Neurophysiol* (1981) **51**:104–7. doi:10.1016/0013-4694(81)91513-3
23. Savic I, Altshuler L, Baxter L, Engel J Jr. Pattern of interictal hypometabolism in PET scans with fludeoxyglucose F 18 reflects prior seizure types in patients with mesial temporal lobe seizures. *Arch Neurol* (1997) **54**:129–36. doi:10.1001/archneur.1997.00550140011006
24. Jasper HH. Some physiological mechanisms involved in epileptic automatisms. *Epilepsia* (1964) **5**:1–20. doi:10.1111/j.1528-1157.1964.tb04341.x
25. Talairach J, Bancaud J, Geier S, Bordas-Ferrer M, Bonis A, Szikla G, et al. The cingulate gyrus and human behaviour. *Electroencephalogr Clin Neurophysiol* (1973) **34**:45–52. doi:10.1016/0013-4694(73)90149-1
26. Fish DR, Gloor P, Quesney FL, Oliver A. Clinical responses to electrical brain stimulation of the temporal and frontal lobes in patients with epilepsy. *Brain* (1993) **116**:397–414. doi:10.1093/brain/116.2.397

6

The dynamics of the epileptic brain reveal long-memory processes

Mark J. Cook[1]*, Andrea Varsavsky[2], David Himes[3], Kent Leyde[3], Samuel Frank Berkovic[4], Terence O'Brien[5] and Iven Mareels[2]

[1] Department of Medicine, St. Vincent's Hospital, University of Melbourne, Fitzroy, VIC, Australia
[2] Department of Electrical and Electronic Engineering, University of Melbourne, Fitzroy, VIC, Australia
[3] Neurovista Corporation, Seattle, WA, USA
[4] Department of Medicine, Austin and Repatriation Medical Centre, University of Melbourne, Fitzroy, VIC, Australia
[5] Department of Medicine, Royal Melbourne Hospital, University of Melbourne, Fitzroy, VIC, Australia

***Correspondence:**
Mark J. Cook, Department of Medicine, St. Vincent's Hospital, Fitzroy Victoria 3065, VIC, Australia
e-mail: markcook@unimelb.edu.au

The pattern of epileptic seizures is often considered unpredictable and the interval between events without correlation. A number of studies have examined the possibility that seizure activity respects a power-law relationship, both in terms of event magnitude and inter-event intervals. Such relationships are found in a variety of natural and man-made systems, such as earthquakes or Internet traffic, and describe the relationship between the magnitude of an event and the number of events. We postulated that human inter-seizure intervals would follow a power-law relationship, and furthermore that evidence for the existence of a long-memory process could be established in this relationship. We performed a *post hoc* analysis, studying eight patients who had long-term (up to 2 years) ambulatory intracranial EEG data recorded as part of the assessment of a novel seizure prediction device. We demonstrated that a power-law relationship could be established in these patients ($\beta = -1.5$). In five out of the six subjects whose data were sufficiently stationary for analysis, we found evidence of long memory between epileptic events. This memory spans time scales from 30 min to 40 days. The estimated Hurst exponents range from 0.51 to 0.77 ± 0.01. This finding may provide evidence of phase-transitions underlying the dynamics of epilepsy.

Keywords: epilepsy, long-range memory, power-law phenomena, neural dynamics in cortical networks, seizure clustering

INTRODUCTION

Epilepsy is a common and serious neurological disorder characterized by recurrent seizures. Though cycles of seizure activity associated with biological rhythms (circadian and menstrual) have long been recognized, Poisson processes have been felt to describe the pattern of seizure occurrence, with departures perhaps explained by external factors (1). Many authors have noted more variability in seizure frequency than would be expected if their distribution followed a simple Poisson model, with overdispersion in series of seizure counts (2–6).

Identification of a *power law* in epileptic inter-event times has received considerable interest (7). Power laws describe a relationship between quantities, where the frequency of an event varies as a power of another feature of the event, such as size. In such a relationship, small events occur very more frequently than large events, although the probability of the large events is non-trivial. The existence of power-law relationships is necessary for certain types of system behavior, such as critical dynamics, to exist. By itself, the presence of a power law is not a sufficient condition to prove critical system behavior, but its absence is strong evidence against such dynamics.

A *long-memory process* (or *long-range-dependent* process) is another type of dynamic behavior that can be identified by the existence of a power law in the higher order statistics of a system. This describes a situation where the decay of dependence of system dynamics on past events is slower than exponential, and correlation of events extends far beyond immediate values. This contrasts with short memory processes in which the system dynamics can be described using a short and finite memory. A parameter typically used to characterize the length of this dependence is the *Hurst exponent* (H). A value of $H = 0.5$ defines a system that is random (i.e., no dependence), and $0.5 < H < 1$ defines a positive correlation, or clustering of extremes, so that long intervals are likely to be followed by long intervals, and short intervals by short intervals. Values of $0 < H < 0.5$ imply anti-correlation, and $H > 1$ implies non-stationarity in the data. We have previously demonstrated the existence of long-memory processes in epileptic seizures in animal and limited human datasets (8).

Recognizing and understanding any long-term dynamic processes underlying epilepsy would have significant implications for its management; however, the data required for the estimation of this have not previously been available. Human scalp EEG data are easily obtainable, but has poor localization properties that obscure seizure initiation dynamics (8–10), and are typically only very short term (~1 day duration). Intracranial EEG (iEEG) improves localization, but such limited duration

(~1 week) records are obtained during pre-resection assessment of hospitalized patients, under artificial circumstances of sleep and medication withdrawal, and show different seizure dynamics to those observed in ambulatory recordings.

We present here a study of the dynamics of epileptic seizure generation using intracranial, ambulatory, human EEG data with continuous records up to 2 years duration. This unique dataset was acquired for the purpose of epileptic seizure anticipation (11). To our knowledge, this is the first time data of this nature has been available for the study of epilepsy. The volume and uniqueness of the data make the possibilities for analysis immense, but we restrict our work here to the study of the distribution and correlation of seizure event times.

SUBJECTS

Data acquired for a clinical feasibility study of a seizure prediction device involving long-term implantation of iEEG recording electrodes were used. More details of the study can be found in Cook et al. (11). Subjects were selected primarily on the basis of medically refractory nature, with 2–12 reported seizures/month, as confirmed through patient diaries. Approval for the study was obtained though the Human Research Ethics Committees of the participating clinical centers. All subjects gave written informed consent to participate prior to any study procedures being performed.

Seventeen subjects were enrolled from the three tertiary referral epilepsy centers comprising the Melbourne University Epilepsy Group. Two of these elected to pursue other treatment options prior to implantation, and so are not included in any further results. These adult subjects were selected chiefly on the basis of suitable seizure frequency (2–12 seizures/month) and all had a level of independence sufficient to make the device useful in the management of daily activities. Nine males and six females with a mean age of 44.5 years (range 20–62 years) were implanted. Six subjects had undergone previous epilepsy resective surgery and one had used vagus nerve stimulation (VNS), which was explanted at the time of predictive system implant.

Subjects meeting inclusion/exclusion criteria were implanted with the SAS and initially entered a Data Collection Phase, where the hand-held device remained passive (where no advisories were given to the subject) and iEEG data was collected. When sufficient data was obtained, a subject-specific algorithm was created. The algorithm was then evaluated against minimum performance criteria and if satisfactory, the subject entered the Advisory Phase. In the Advisory Phase, the algorithm was enabled to provide visual and audible advisories to the subject. Throughout the study, ambulatory iEEG data were analyzed for seizure statistics and other relevant electroencephalographic events. Subjects served as their own controls for the purpose of evaluating study outcomes.

PROCEDURES

The major components of the implanted seizure prediction system are: (1) the implantable lead assemblies, (2) the implantable telemetry unit, (3) the external hand-held personal advisory device, and (4) the external charging accessory. In addition to these components, a cluster-computing system and associated software was used to configure algorithms for each individual subject.

A total of 15 subjects were implanted with the device, 9 males and 6 females with a mean age of 44.5 years (range 20–62). Two silicone implantable lead assemblies, each with eight platinum iridium contacts distributed across two electrode arrays (16 electrodes in total), were used to collect iEEG on the cortical surface. Leads were placed regionally, unilaterally over the quadrant believed to contain the epileptogenic zone, as determined by prior EEG studies, imaging studies, and/or seizure etiology, via a small craniotomy or through prior craniotomy sites if surgery had been performed in the past. A typical implantation scheme is shown in **Figure 1**. For those subjects diagnosed with bilateral temporal lobe onset seizures, leads were placed over the hemisphere that generated the most frequent, stereotypical seizures. System operation and integrity was verified prior to wound closure. The leads were tunneled down the neck and terminated at a subclavicularly placed, titanium encased, hermetically sealed, implantable telemetry unit, which sampled 16 channels of iEEG acquired at 400 Hz and wirelessly transmitted it to an external, hand-held personal advisory device. The external, hand-held personal advisory device received the telemetered iEEG and stored iEEG on standard flash memory cards for subsequent analysis. An important component was that it also supported audio recordings, both manually triggered by the subject for diary purposes, and also automatically activated when a seizure was detected by the system to aid in establishing a clinical correlate with iEEG activity. The duration of implantation varied between ~0.5 and ~1.8 years.

The clinical study algorithm utilized a layered structure consisting of a filtering layer, a feature extraction layer, and a classification

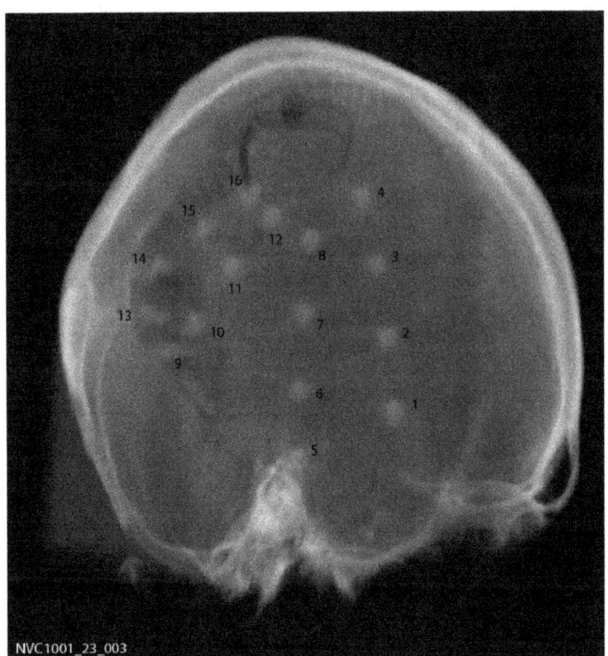

FIGURE 1 | Plain skull radiograph of subject post implantation, showing typical implantation scheme.

layer. Each layer could be configured using a number of subject-specific parameters that were created as part of an algorithm training process.

The filtering and feature extraction layers were used to implement a form of spectral analysis. Input signals were filtered by a collection of octave-wide digital filters covering the range from 2 to 128 Hz. A wide band filter complemented these filters and optional notch filters designed to eliminate interference from AC-mains sources. Filter outputs could be analyzed for average energy or line-length over a 5 s analysis window. These outputs could be normalized using previously derived parameters or by other signals. The combination of 16 available iEEG input channels and many different filtering options created a list of several 100-candidate features. During algorithm training, the list of candidates was analyzed to find the best 16 features. This 16-dimension feature vector was then passed to the classification layer.

The classifier design was intended to create a computationally efficient implementation that was functionally similar to a k-nearest neighbor (kNN) classifier. This was accomplished through use of a partitioning approach that reduced the need to search through long lists of training data points. The classifier output was filtered, thresholded, and then passed to the user interface state machine used to control the three likelihood indicators. The main function of the state machine was to latch a condition in the case where the classifier output was repeatedly alternating across a decision threshold, preventing rapidly changing advisories and possible subject confusion.

To support the study, a revised cluster-computing environment was developed. The main function of this new cluster computer was to train subject-specific algorithms to generate the required algorithm configuration parameters. The system could also apply hold-out or cross validation quasi-prospective methods to provide an estimate of algorithm performance needed to inform the decision to proceed into the Advisory Phase of the study. The system could also be used to calculate algorithm performance using prospective data collected during the Advisory Phase.

Post processing was applied to the iEEG data to determine the time and the length of both clinical and sub-clinical seizures (defined as electroencephalographic events with no clinically relevant manifestation). Study investigators annotated the iEEG acquired and events were detected by a validated seizure detection algorithm based on an unsupervised learning approach that identifies statistically significant outliers in iEEG features associated with seizures (12). Accumulated iEEG was annotated by clinical staff and verified by study investigators utilizing subject diaries, hand-held audio recordings, and a seizure detection algorithm (12). Events were categorized as clinically reported, and found in EEG (type 1), events not clinically reported, but found in EEG, and having a similar envelope to type 1 events (type 2), and those not clinically reported, but found in EEG, without evidence of clinical manifestations (type 3). Events clinically reported but without EEG changes were excluded. A large number of events were necessary for accurate analysis, and so the 8 subjects who had more than 400 recorded events were studied. The inter-event intervals, defined as the time between the onset of one seizure and the onset of the next were used for analysis. To estimate the Hurst exponent, point processes were generated by quantizing the timescale to 1-min resolution, and the presence or absence of seizure onset at a particular time was represented with the value of 1 or 0, respectively. A summary of all data included for analysis can be found in **Table 1**.

MATERIALS AND METHODS

ESTIMATING POWER LAWS

Mathematically, a quantity x follows a power law if it is drawn from a probability distribution $f(x) \propto x^{\beta}$. The scaling exponent β is a constant that can be estimated as the (linear) gradient of the log–log plot $\log[f(x)] = \beta \log(x) + c$. This estimate is highly susceptible to errors when the dataset is not ideal, such as brevity, non-stationarity, or inaccurate records.

ESTIMATING THE HURST EXPONENT

To estimate the Hurst exponent (H) of a long-memory process, a power law must be identified in the second order statistics (such as the variance) of the dataset. The relationship between β and H depends on the method used to derive the power law (13–15).

Recent research has shown that a reliable and robust estimate of H is possible with the use of wavelets (15–17), designed to isolate activity at different frequencies and timescales (14, 15). Recursively applying a wavelet transform with dyadic sampling to a dataset yields wavelet coefficients $d_m(n)$ at each time scale m. The larger the m, the lower the frequency that $d_m(n)$ describe, with the highest frequency occurring at $m = 0$, that is, at the sampling frequency. H is estimated by

Table 1 | Summary of data.

	P1	P2	P3	P4	P5	P6	P7	P8
Age	22	52	48	51	50	53	43	50
Sex	F	M	M	F	F	F	M	M
Epileptogenic zone	PT	FT	FT	OP	FT	FT	T	T
AED's	CBZ, LTG, PHT	CBZ, CLZ, LEV	CBZ, LEV	CBZ	LEV, OXC, ZNS	LCM, PHT, PRP	LTG, LCM, PHT, RTG	CBZ, CLZ, LEV, LCM
Record length (days)	523	182	504	305	313	646	650	618
Total seizures	1569	574	446	750	1088	479	4561	985
Median ISI	3 min	41 min	11.5 h	3 h	21 min	13 h	5 min	1 h

AED's: CBZ, carbamazepine; CLZ, clonazepam; LCM, lacosamide; LEV, levetiracetam; LTG , lamotrigine; OXC, oxcarbazepine; PHT, phenytoin; PRP, perampanel; RTG, retigabine; ZNS, zonisamide; epileptogenic zones: FT, frontotemporal; OP, occipitoparietal; PT, parietal-temporal; T, temporal.

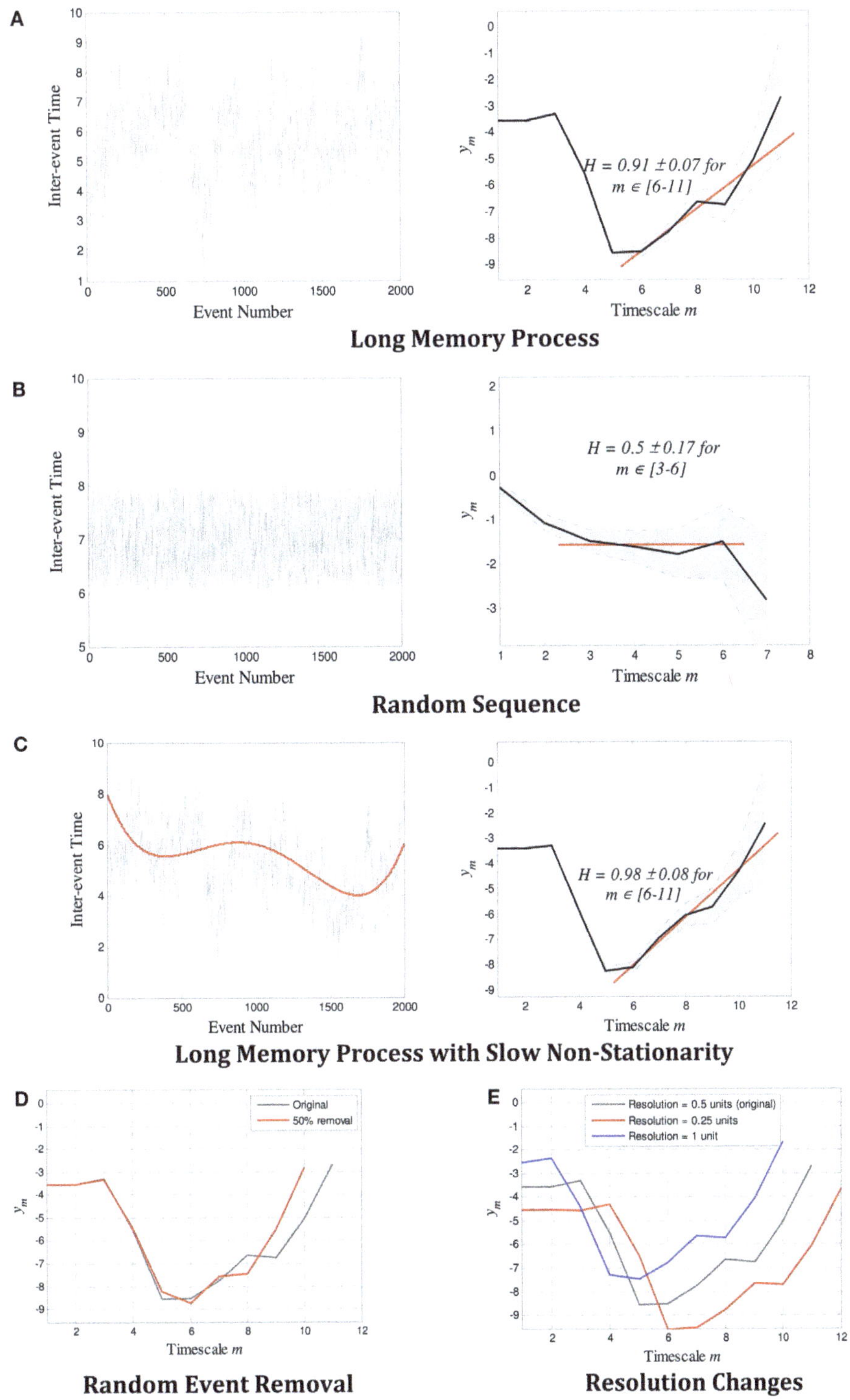

FIGURE 2 | Example estimates of the Hurst exponent H for (A) a long-memory process with $H = 0.9$, and (B) a random process with $H = 0.5$. In each case, the *scalogram* (a log–log plot of m versus y_m) shows a region of alignment of at least four scales that correctly identifies a power law with gradient β and $H = 0.5(\beta + 1)$. **(C–E)** show the robustness properties of wavelet estimation tools. The gradient β (and therefore H) is not affected by **(C)** slow non-stationarity, **(D)** a large number of missing events, or **(E)** the resolution of the point process. In **(A–C)**, the 95% confidence limits as defined by the variance σ_m^2 at each scale is denoted by the gray shaded region between dotted lines, and the red line shows the gradient β identified over the region of alignment. The error bounds and the linear fit are not shown in **(D–E)** for easier visualization, though they are similar in magnitude and quality as those in **(A–C)**.

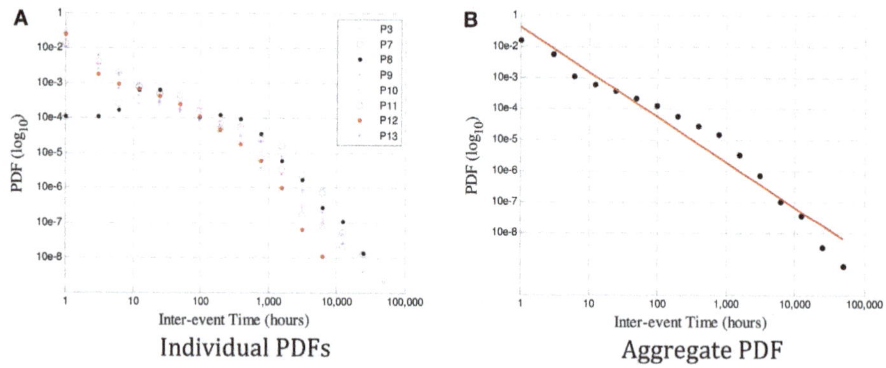

FIGURE 3 | In (A) are the PDF distributions (in a log-log plot) for each of P1–8. A power law is evident, but the gradient for each subject varies, and estimates of the scaling exponent β may be influenced by insufficient data in some subjects. The aggregate PDF in **(B)** shows an estimated power law with gradient β = − 1.5. The deviation from linearity that occurs at ~1000 h is also observed at a different time in ~10% of the subjects in Ref. (18), and could be caused by insufficient data at large time scales (leading to an under-estimate of β) or by a genuine excursion from a true power law in the data.

identifying the power-law exponent β that occurs in the *scalogram*, that is, the plot of m versus the variance of wavelet coefficients,

$$y_m = \frac{1}{N_m}\sum_{n=1}^{N_m} |d_m(n)|^2 - \hat{g}_m.$$

The parameter $\hat{g}_m \approx -\frac{1}{N_m \ln 2}$ is a correction factor used to so that the estimate of H is unbiased. When this method is used, the Hurst exponent H is computed as $H = 0.5(\beta + 1)$. The variance at each m is given by $\sigma_m^2 \approx -\frac{2}{N_m \ln^2 2}$ and can be used to infer the confidence of the estimate. For stationary processes, the estimated values of H range between 0.5 and 1. When $H = 0.5$ is found, the underlying process cannot be determined: it may infer a true system with $H = 0.5$, that is, with no memory between events, but may also result from systems with long memory but unpredictable variance. Our methods fail to identify the type of memory involved. When $0.5 < H < 1$, there is evidence of memory in the system, and thus there is a correlation between past and present events. The higher the H, the longer this memory is (15, 16).

Example estimates of H for both random and long-memory processes are shown in **Figures 2A,B. Figures 2C–E** show that wavelet estimation tools are robust in the presence of smooth non-stationarity, accurate even when a large number of events are removed, and not affected by the resolution of the records. More detailed description of the methods can be found in the on-line methods section.

RESULTS

THE EXISTENCE OF POWER LAW

In **Figure 3A**, it is the probability density function (PDF, or normalized histogram) of the inter-seizure times of each of the eight viable datasets. It is evident that a power law likely exists in all datasets, although the variability in the number of events used to derive individual PDFs would make an estimate of each slope error-prone. So as to obtain a better estimate, the events of all eight subjects were grouped together to derive a combined PDF, shown in **Figure 3B**.

THE EXISTENCE OF LONG-MEMORY PROCESSES

The existence of long-memory processes was evaluated for the eight subjects, and the resulting scalograms shown in **Figure 4**.

The Daubechies wavelet was used for all calculations of H. The order of this wavelet transform dictates the level of non-stationarity tolerated in the data. To select an appropriate number, the wavelet order was systematically increased until the resulting scalograms were approximately constant. In all cases, wavelet order 4 was sufficient. To test for more abrupt non-stationarity that is not tolerated by this method, data were divided into segments of approximately 250–500 events (depending on the total length of the record), and the scalograms for each segment were recomputed. The range of scales where the gradients coincide across all segments was identified as the stationary scales for each subject. These are shown as the shaded background of **Figure 4**. Two subjects (P2 and P4) were completely non-stationary and were not included in further analysis.

To compute the Hurst exponent, regions of alignment were defined as any four or more scales within the stationary regions over which a straight line could be drawn (15). A Hurst exponent consistent with the existence of long memory was found in five out of the six subjects with sufficiently stationary data, with H ranging between 0.66 and 0.77. Conservative estimates of the time scales where dependence was evident ranged between 30 min and 40 days (**Table 2**).

DISCUSSION

We have confirmed previous findings of a power-law relationship in inter-seizure intervals, on a large and unique human dataset. A scaling exponent of β = − 1.5 was shown to exist in the averaged PDF of all eight subjects (**Figure 3B**), consistent with earlier finding (18). Wavelet-based tools were used to compute a *patient-specific* estimate of the Hurst exponent H. In five subjects, H was consistent with the existence of a long-memory process, while in one subject the correlation between seizures

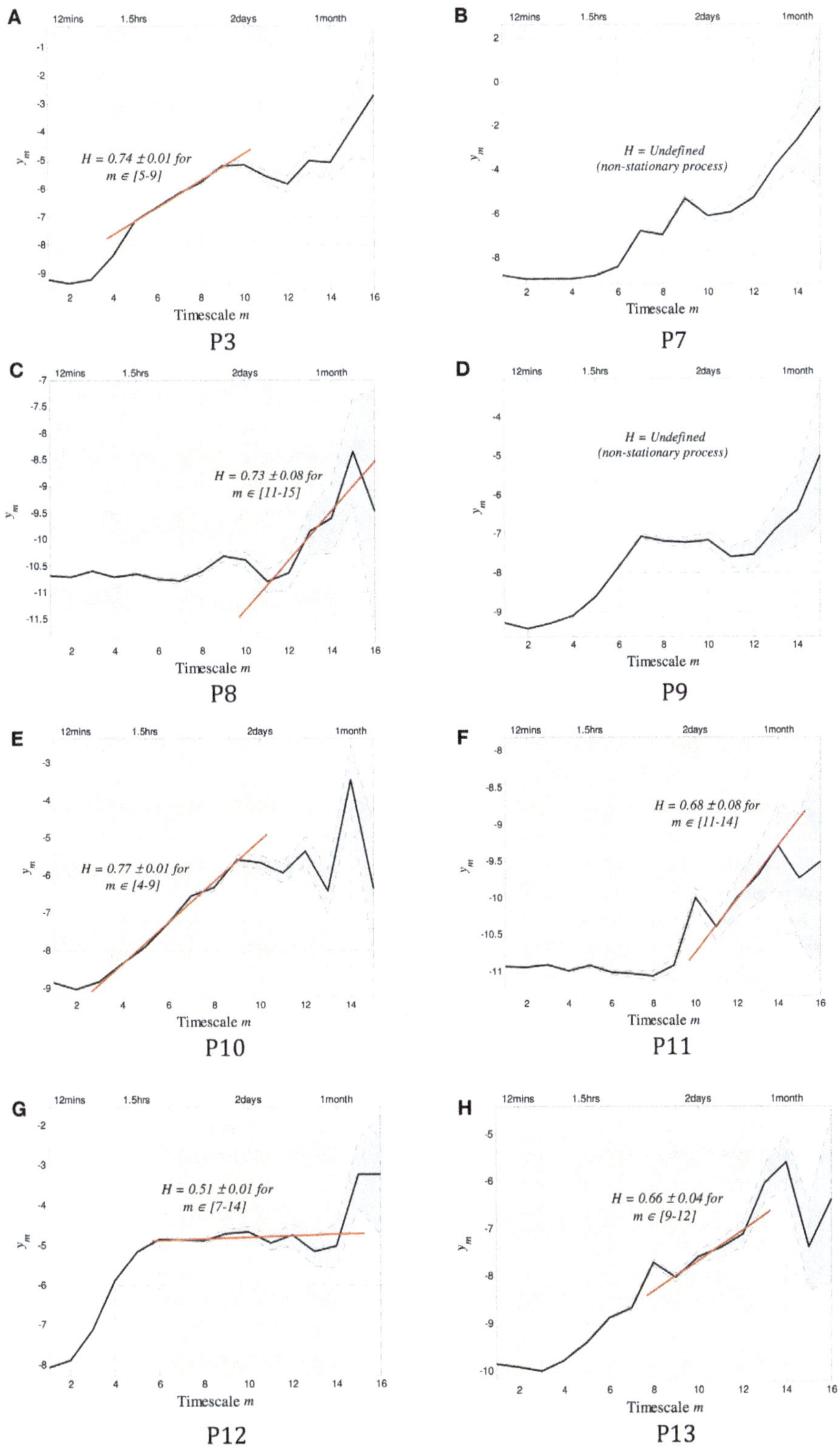

FIGURE 4 | The scalograms for P1–8 are shown. In addition to the conventions used in **Figure 1**, the orange shaded background denotes scales over which the data were stationary and that can be used to estimate *H*. Of the eight subjects, all but two (P2 and P4) showed stationary scales from which a Hurst exponent *H* could be computed. Of the remaining six subjects, five were found to have regions of alignment with scaling exponents consistent with the existence of long memory, with *H* ranging from 0.66 to 0.77. The last subject (P7) showed potentially random correlations between time scales ($H = 0.51 \pm 0.01$). Note that to infer stationarity for P7, the data were divided into three segments containing ~1500 events each. At the small time scales, two of the segments agreed with the results, and one did not. This may imply a sharp dynamic change occurring sometimes during the 1.8 years of recording. A summary of all results can be found in **Table 2**.

Table 2 | Summary of results.

	P1	P2	P3	P4	P5	P6	P7	P8
Stationary	YES	NO	YES	NO	YES	YES	YES	YES
Long Memory found	YES	–	YES	–	YES	YES	NO	YES
Hurst exponent *H*	0.74 ± 0.01	–	0.73 ± 0.08	–	0.77 ± 0.01	0.68 ± 0.08	0.51 ± 0.01	0.66 ± 0.04
Region of Alignment (scales *m*)	5–9	–	11–15	–	4–9	11–14	7–14	9–12
Length of Dependence (time)	1 h–1.5 days	–	3–40 days	–	30 min–1.5 days	3–20 days	4 h–20 days	17 h–6 days

was indeterminable and potentially negligible. This estimate was shown to be robust even when the length of the data is relatively short and when the likelihood of inaccurate records (in the form of missing events) is high. To our knowledge, this is the first time that long-range memory has been identified in human seizure frequency, and similarly the first time a Hurst exponent has been estimated.

The advantage of using wavelet tools to identify the existence of a power law (and, in this case, the existence of long memory) is that the scaling exponent β can be computed on a patient-specific basis. Traditional methods of estimating β require very high quality data over a very long period of time for a robust fit (19). Data must often be aggregated over many subjects, leading to conclusions that are only relevant on average and losing any patient-specific information (e.g., related to differing pathology or site of origin). This is demonstrated in **Figure 3**, where the variability in exponent between subjects in (a), as well as the deviation from a true power law in some cases (e.g., P3) are lost when the aggregate $\beta = -1.5$ estimated in (b).

A range of time scales that are involved in these long-memory processes can be identified using this method of estimating *H*. For example, in P3 dependence exists from ~3 to 40 days, implying that the dynamics that led to the generation of a seizure are affected by events that took place in the range up to 40 days prior.

In one subject (P7), no dependence could be identified in the stationary region of the scalogram ($H = 0.5$). It is possible that some dependence exists at smaller time scales, but the process was not sufficiently stationary to make for a robust estimate at those scales.

There are a number of potential limitations to this study. The patient group suffering refractory seizures may not be typical, and the medication used in treatment, as well as routine changes in doses made during the study, may have effects on the timing and occurrence of events not considered in our analysis. Data dropouts through brief telemetry failure may also have influenced our findings, but these were not felt to be significant, and modeling indicates that random loss of data, even at high rates, does not affect our estimates (see **Figure 2D**).

There was a marked discrepancy between seizure frequencies as estimated from patient diaries and those captured by the implanted system. While this was to some degree accounted for by a high number of sub-clinical (type 3) events, both the clinically reported (type 1 events) and clinically confirmed but unreported (type 2 events, as ascertained through analysis of event-triggered audio recordings) were still often orders of magnitude greater than expected, confirming the poor reliability of subjects ability to recognize events.

Existence of long memory is useful in the analysis and interpretation of signals such as the EEG. In the study of epileptic seizure prediction, over 20 years of research has yielded a few success stories (20–22), but none have been readily generalized to wider datasets. The existence (or otherwise) of long memory could explain the differences in performance between different people – if long memory is present then the underlying dynamics are relatively less complex than one where memory cannot be established. In effect, the system becomes more predictable. As an example, we can look at the prediction algorithm proposed in Cook et al. (11), which uses the same data as in this study. Of the 8 subjects included here, the seizures of P2, P4 and P7 were unpredictable. Interestingly, we have shown that the dynamics of P2 and P4 are non-stationary, and that only random (or alternatively, highly complex) correlations exist between events in P7. A long-memory process was identified for all other subjects, and between 54 and 100% of seizures were correctly predicted for these subjects. Although the dataset is limited, it appears that the existence of memory between events is necessary for successful prediction.

The results presented here can be applied in algorithm design directly – it is now known, in a patient-specific way, the dependence of epileptic seizures on past events, and data that reflects this should be included (or accounted for) in any predictive analysis. When analyzing the dynamics of epilepsy, we have shown that an appropriate mathematical model should incorporate mechanisms that allow for interactions stretching far into the past, and that the length of dependence should be tunable.

These findings also have implications for the clinical management of epilepsy. Many authors have remarked on the inadequacy of current methods of assessing the efficacy of anticonvulsants, exclusively based currently on patient diaries (7, 23). More sophisticated methods of analysis based on better understanding of the non-random occurrence of events may permit recognition of treatment effects at a much earlier time point (4). Determination of the optimum time for medication withdrawal after a suitable seizure-free interval may also be more accurately estimated (24). The findings here do not, however, confirm Gower's dictum that "seizures beget seizures" (25), with progressive escalation in the frequency of events, but rather that there is a deep structure to the timing and occurrence of seizures, with a complex inter-relationship between past and future events.

ACKNOWLEDGMENTS

The basis of the code used to estimate *H* in this work is freely available for non-commercial purposes from http://www.cubinlab.ee.unimelb.edu.au/~darryl/secondorder_code.html. The authors, Patrice Abry and Darryl Veitch, retain copyright of this code.

REFERENCES

1. Milton JG, Gotman J, Remillard GM, Andermann F. Timing of seizure recurrence in adult epileptic patients: a statistical analysis. *Epilepsia* (1987) **28**:471–8. doi:10.1111/j.1528-1157.1987.tb03675.x
2. Balish M, Albert PS, Theodore WH. Seizure frequency in intractable partial epilepsy: a statistical analysis. *Epilepsia* (1991) **32**:642–9. doi:10.1111/j.1528-1157.1991.tb04703.x
3. Greenwood M, Yule GU. An inquiry into the nature of frequency distributions representative of multiple happenings with particular reference to the occurrence of multiple attacks of disease or of repeated accidents. *J R Stat Soc* (1920) **83**:255–79. doi:10.2307/2341080
4. Hopkins A, Davies P, Dobson C. Mathematical models of patterns of seizures: their use in the evaluation of drugs. *Arch Neurol* (1985) **42**:463–7. doi:10.1001/archneur.1985.04060050061009
5. Iasemidis LD, Olson LD, Savit RS, Sackellares JC. Time dependencies in the occurrences of epileptic seizures. *Epilepsy Res* (1994) **17**:81–94. doi:10.1016/0920-1211(94)90081-7
6. Tauboll E, Lundervold A, Gjerstad L. Temporal distribution of seizures in epilepsy. *Epilepsy Res* (1991) **8**:153–65. doi:10.1016/0920-1211(91)90084-S
7. Osorio I, Frei MG, Sornette D, Milton J, Lai Y-C. Epileptic seizures: quakes of the brain? *Phys Rev E* (2010) **82**:021919. doi:10.1103/PhysRevE.82.021919
8. Varsavsky A, Mareels I, Cook M. *Epileptic Seizures and the EEG: Measurement, Models, Detection and Prediction.* CRC Press (2010).
9. Malmivuo J, Plonsey R. *Bioelectromagnetism: Principles and Applications of Bioelectric and Biomagnetic Fields.* New York: Oxford University Press (1995).
10. Nunez P, Srinivasan R. *Electric Fields of the Brain: The Neurophysics of the EEG.* 2nd ed. New York: Oxford University Press (2006).
11. Cook MJ, O'Brien TJ, Berkovic SF, Murphy M, Morokoff A, Fabinyi G, et al. Prediction of seizure likelihood with a long-term, implanted seizure advisory system in patients with drug-resistant epilepsy: a first-in-man study. *Lancet Neurol* (2013) **12**:563–71. doi:10.1016/S1474-4422(13)70075-9
12. Gardner AB, Krieger AM, Vachtsevanos G, Litt B. One-class novelty detection for seizure analysis from intracranial EEG. *J Mach Learn Res* (2006) **7**: 1025–44.
13. Beran J. *Statistics for Long-Memory Processes: Monographs on Statistics and Applied Probability.* New York: Chapman & Hail (1994).
14. Doukhan P, Khezour A, Lang G. *Theory and Applications of Long-Range Dependence.* Boston: Birkhauser (2003).
15. Park K, Willinger W. Self-similar network traffic and performance evaluation. In: Park K, Willinger W, editors. *Wavelets for the Analysis, Estimation, and Synthesis of Scaling Data.* New York, USA: John Wiley & Sons, Inc (2000). p. 1–38.
16. Abry P, Flandrin P, Taqqu MS, Veitch D. Wavelets for the analysis, estimation, and synthesis of scaling data. In: Park K, Willinger W, editors. *Self-Similar Network Traffic and Performance Evaluation.* New York, USA: John Wiley & Sons, Inc (2000). p. 39–88.
17. Aldroubi A, Unser M. *Wavelets in Medicine and Biology.* CRC Press (1996).
18. Osorio I, Frei MG, Sornette D, Milton J. Pharmaco-resistant seizures: self-triggering capacity, scale-free properties and predictability? *Eur J Neurosci* (2009) **30**:1554–8. doi:10.1111/j.1460-9568.2009.06923.x
19. Clauset A, Shalizi CR, Newman MEJ. Power-law distributions in empirical data. *SIAM Rev* (2009) **51**:661–703. doi:10.1137/070710111
20. Iasemidis LD. Epileptic seizure prediction and control. *IEEE Trans Biomed Eng* (2003) **50**:549–58. doi:10.1109/TBME.2003.810689
21. Lehnertz K, Mormann F, Osterhage H, Müller A, Prusseit J, Chernihovskyi A, et al. State-of-the-art of seizure prediction. *J Clin Neurophysiol* (2007) **24**:147–53. doi:10.1097/WNP.0b013e3180336f16
22. Mormann F, Andrzejak RG, Elger CE, Lehnertz K. Seizure prediction: the long and winding road. *Brain* (2007) **130**:314–33. doi:10.1093/brain/awl241
23. Hoppe C, Poepel A, Elger CE. Epilepsy: accuracy of patient seizure counts. *Arch Neurol* (2007) **64**:1595–9. doi:10.1001/archneur.64.11.1595
24. Beghi E. AED discontinuation may not be dangerous in seizure-free patients. *J Neural Transm* (2010) **118**:187–91. doi:10.1007/s00702-010-0528-y
25. Gowers WR. *Epilepsy and Other Chronic Convulsive Disorders: Their Causes, Symptoms and Treatment.* London: J&A Churchill (1881).

7

The piriform cortex and human focal epilepsy

David N. Vaughan[1,2]* and Graeme D. Jackson[1,2,3]

[1] Florey Institute of Neuroscience and Mental Health, Heidelberg, VIC, Australia
[2] Department of Neurology, Austin Health, Heidelberg, VIC, Australia
[3] Department of Medicine, University of Melbourne, Melbourne, VIC, Australia

Correspondence:
David N. Vaughan, Melbourne Brain Centre, Florey Institute of Neuroscience and Mental Health, 245 Burgundy Street, Heidelberg, VIC 3084, Australia
e-mail: d.vaughan@brain.org.au

It is surprising that the piriform cortex, when compared to the hippocampus, has been given relatively little significance in human epilepsy. Like the hippocampus, it has a phylogenetically preserved three-layered cortex that is vulnerable to excitotoxic injury, has broad connections to both limbic and cortical areas, and is highly epileptogenic – being critical to the kindling process. The well-known phenomenon of early olfactory auras in temporal lobe epilepsy highlights its clinical relevance in human beings. Perhaps because it is anatomically indistinct and difficult to approach surgically, as it clasps the middle cerebral artery, it has, until now, been understandably neglected. In this review, we emphasize how its unique anatomical and functional properties, as primary olfactory cortex, predispose it to involvement in focal epilepsy. From recent convergent findings in human neuroimaging, clinical epileptology, and experimental animal models, we make the case that the piriform cortex is likely to play a facilitating and amplifying role in human focal epileptogenesis, and may influence progression to epileptic intractability.

Keywords: pyriform, area tempestas, claustrum, olfaction, olfactory aura, EEG-fMRI, temporal lobe epilepsy, intracranial electrodes

INTRODUCTION

One of the important human senses and one of life's great pleasures is olfaction. From the aroma of a floral bouquet, to the flavor of a meal, and even to the familiar scent of a family member, odors provide us with rich information about our environment that influences our decisions, emotions, and memories.

The piriform cortex is a unique brain region that underlies the mechanisms that produce these olfactory experiences. It forms the major part of the primary olfactory cortex and has extensive connections with other parts of the olfactory network. It is a phylogenetically old structure that can also be found in amphibians, reptiles, and other mammals, and as such has a number of special properties. Unlike other primary cortical regions, it receives input directly from the olfactory bulb without this information being relayed through the thalamus. Additionally, it has a three-layered allocortical structure, which in human beings is otherwise only found in the hippocampus – one of the regions most implicated in focal epilepsy.

Historically, the role that the piriform cortex may play in epilepsy has not been widely recognized. In the study of human focal epilepsy, attention has mostly been given to mesial temporal structures, especially the hippocampus, and to regions of abnormal brain structure. The earliest indications that seizures may involve olfactory cortex were descriptions in the late nineteenth century of "uncinate seizures," which begin with an olfactory hallucination, and were generally thought to herald a progressive tumor of the temporal lobe. Separately, the clinical observation that some people with epilepsy have impaired olfactory function also hinted at seizure involvement of olfactory cortex. It was not until the 1980s that the particular epileptogenicity of the piriform cortex in animal models was discovered, although this finding did not have an immediate impact on human clinical epileptology.

Over the last two decades, the application of functional neuroimaging to human brain function has led to many new insights into the role of the piriform cortex in olfactory perception. In the field of epilepsy, similar techniques have emphasized a network view of seizures. Most recently, several studies using data from electroencephalography, functional MRI and nuclear medicine imaging, have suggested that the human piriform cortex may be a common node in focal epilepsy arising from different brain regions.

Therefore, it is now timely to revisit the piriform cortex and to re-examine its relevance to focal epilepsy. Beginning with a description of the anatomy and function of the piriform cortex, we go on to review the literature regarding seizures that arise within olfactory cortex in animal models and human beings, the involvement of piriform cortex in distant inter-ictal discharges, and the impact of epilepsy on olfaction. Finally, we discuss the potential for the piriform cortex to become a therapeutic target in treatment of epilepsy, and describe a case of possible piriform epilepsy where resection of the piriform cortex was performed. From consideration of these convergent lines of evidence, we argue that the piriform cortex is critically placed between limbic and cortical networks, to distribute epileptic activity, facilitate epileptogenesis, and potentially contribute toward the development of intractable human epilepsy.

THE ANATOMY AND FUNCTION OF THE PIRIFORM CORTEX HAS PROPERTIES THAT PREDISPOSE IT TO EPILEPTIC SEIZURES

Synonymously referred to as "piriform," "pyriform," and sometimes "prepyriform" (indicating the anterior piriform), the piriform cortex is the largest component of primary olfactory cortex (1–3).

Odors are first detected in the nasal epithelium by olfactory sensory neurons. These cells project to the olfactory bulb, where inputs from similar receptor types are collected together in glomeruli. Here, they synapse onto mitral and tufted cells, which project to cortical regions via the olfactory tract (4).

Primary olfactory cortex is defined as regions that receive direct input from the lateral olfactory tract. In addition to piriform cortex this includes the anterior olfactory nucleus, olfactory tubercle, periamygdaloid cortex, and the anterior part of the entorhinal cortex (5). Beyond these regions, the olfactory network includes orbitofrontal cortex, thalamus, and insula cortex (6) and interactions with other cortical networks.

ANATOMICAL LOCATION OF THE PIRIFORM CORTEX

The human piriform cortex is located at the junction of the temporal and frontal lobes, medial to the temporal stem (7), and lines the superior and inferior banks of the endorhinal sulcus (**Figures 1** and **2**). The name piriform comes from its "pear-shaped" appearance in some mammals such as cats (3), although in human beings, it is a relatively smaller structure and does not have this shape (8).

In human beings, it can be subdivided anatomically into frontal or temporal lobe parts. In the temporal lobe it begins anteriorly at the level of the limen insulae, and extends posteriorly to overlie the amygdaloid nuclei (10), becoming contiguous with the cortical amygdala. Medially, the piriform cortex transitions into the perirhinal or entorhinal cortex, with this border marked more posteriorly by a small depression, the sulcus semiannularis. In the frontal lobe, the piriform cortex extends from the fundus of the endorhinal sulcus, forming a triangular region that is bounded medially by the olfactory tubercle and lateral olfactory tract (11, 12). Laterally, it merges into the insular neocortex (7).

In rats, the piriform cortex is comparatively much larger, and does not have the curvature around a deep sulcus that is seen in human beings. It lies along a rostrocaudal axis, and can be divided into an anterior and posterior part on the basis of the thickness of cell layer III, and the presence of the overlying lateral olfactory tract (3).

Histological studies in the macaque (5) indicate that the primate frontal and temporal piriform cortex correspond to the rodent anterior and posterior piriform, respectively. Despite this, some human MRI studies have divided the piriform cortex into anterior and posterior parts, using at a given y-axis value in the MNI coordinate system (13), or at the most anterior coronal slice where frontal and temporal lobes meet (14). Therefore, the specific criteria used in each study to subdivide the piriform should be carefully noted when comparing results.

HISTOLOGY OF THE PIRIFORM CORTEX

The defining histological feature of piriform cortex is its allocortical three-layered structure (11).

The main excitatory neuron types are superficial pyramidal cells, deep pyramidal cells, and semilunar cells. The pyramidal cells are found densely packed in layer IIb and more sparsely in layer III, with dendrites projecting up to layer I to receive inputs from the olfactory bulb (15, 16). Semilunar cells are a distinct population found in layer IIa, which also receive olfactory bulb inputs, and are similar to pyramidal cells but do not have basal dendrites and show a distinct firing pattern (15, 17).

The interneurons of the piriform cortex are mostly inhibitory GABAergic cells. They are found across all layers and multiple classes can be identified on the basis of unique electrophysiological and morphological properties (18, 19). They variously provide both feed-forward and feedback inhibition onto the pyramidal cells (20–23), which allows the pyramidal cells to produce temporally sparse but accurate responses to trains of olfactory bulb input.

The endopiriform nucleus is a separate population of neurons that lies deep to the piriform cortex (24), being found along its full rostrocaudal extent. These multipolar cells project widely to piriform cortex, orbitofrontal, and thalamic regions (25). In rats, the endopiriform nucleus provides a layer of integration between olfactory and gustatory processing (26). The endopiriform nucleus is also found in primates (5). In human beings, it corresponds to the parts of the ventral claustrum that lie adjacent to the piriform cortex and amygdala (27), which have been labeled "prepiriform claustrum" and "periamygdalar claustrum," respectively (7). These areas should not be confused with the dorsal (or insular) part of the claustrum (28), which has a different embryological origin and different patterns of connectivity (29).

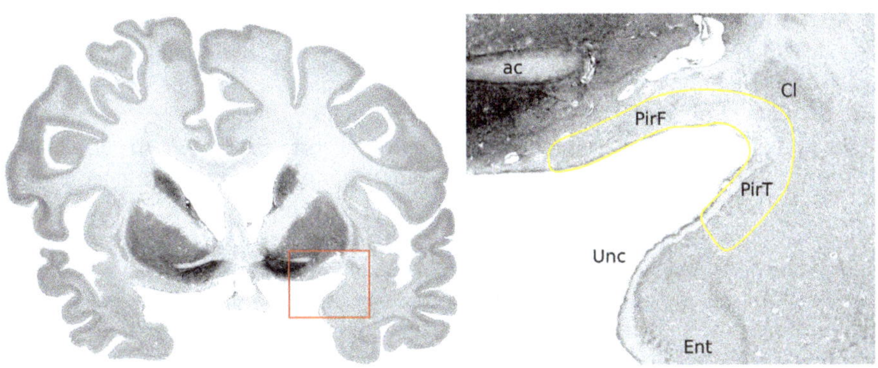

FIGURE 1 | Anatomical location of the piriform cortex. Nissl stained coronal brain slice at the level of the anterior commissure of a 65-year-old woman, from the BigBrain dataset (9). Labels were placed with reference to Mai et al. (7): ac, anterior commissure; PirF, frontal piriform cortex; PirT, temporal piriform cortex; Cl, claustrum; Unc, uncus; Ent, entorhinal cortex.

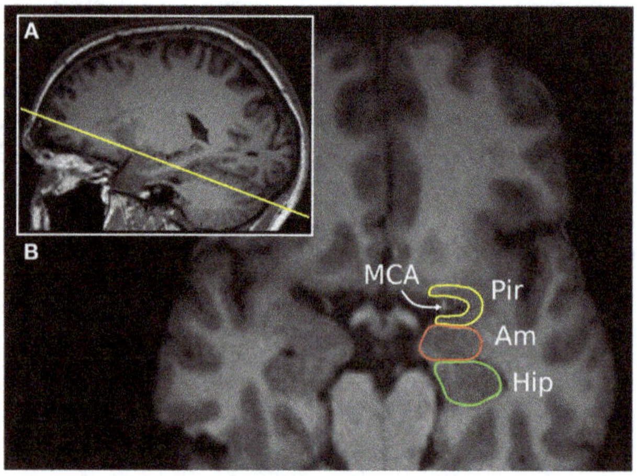

FIGURE 2 | The "piriform axis". T1-weighted MPRAGE image of a 37-year-old man, displayed in a **(A)** para-sagittal and **(B)** oblique-axial orientation, approximately +20° relative to the anterior commissure-posterior commissure axis. This orientation allows the relationship between the piriform cortex (Pir), amygdala (Am), and hippocampus (Hip) to be seen. The arrow indicates the position of the middle cerebral artery within the endorhinal sulcus.

There are several striking similarities between the structure of piriform cortex and that of the hippocampus (8). As paleocortex, both have a phylogenetically conserved structure with three layers, pyramidal neurons with similar morphology, a predominantly horizontal arrangement of fiber projections, and the presence of GABAergic interneurons. Analogous microcircuits in both piriform cortex and hippocampus provide excitation, feedforward inhibition, and feedback inhibition (30). Their main structural difference is that the piriform does not have a distinct zone that corresponds to the dentate gyrus, although the distributed semilunar cells do have morphology that is similar to granule cells.

STRUCTURAL CONNECTIVITY OF THE PIRIFORM CORTEX

The main input to the piriform cortex is from mitral cells, and to a lesser extent tufted cells, of the olfactory bulb (15). Each glomerulus in the olfactory bulb, which represents a specific olfactory chemoreceptor type, projects to a broad region of the piriform cortex to synapse with many pyramidal cells (31, 32). Each pyramidal cell receives input from a random selection of glomeruli, allowing cells to respond to complex features of odor mixtures (33).

Additional inputs to the piriform are from the anterior olfactory nucleus and association fibers from all other olfactory cortical regions, as well as lighter commissural projections from the contralateral piriform cortex (34). Neuromodulatory inputs include cholinergic modulation from the horizontal limb of the diagonal band, serotonergic modulation from the raphe nuclei (activating inhibitory GABAergic interneurons), noradrenergic input from the locus coeruleus (35), and dopaminergic modulation from the ventral tegmental area (3, 6).

Within the piriform cortex, pyramidal cells are strongly interconnected, by recurrent projections onto many other pyramidal cells (1). A single pyramidal cell has an arbor that extends over much of the piriform cortex, and in the rat, synapses with more than 1000 other cells (36). This forms a large excitatory network that requires strong local feedback inhibition to prevent runaway activation (20). However, the benefit of this arrangement of diffusely projecting inputs, combined with extensive intra-piriform connectivity, is the ability to perform pattern matching in an architecture described as "content-addressable memory" (37). This allows partially degraded patterns of input to produce consistent reproducible responses that are spatially distributed across the piriform cortex (38).

The outputs from piriform cortex pyramidal cells are widespread to cortical and subcortical regions (15, 39). There are strong limbic connections, especially to the entorhinal cortex and to the amygdala (36, 40, 41), frontal lobe connections to multiple parts of the orbitofrontal cortex, and projections to agranular insular cortex (5). Important subcortical connections are to the mediodorsal nucleus of the thalamus (42, 43), and to the hypothalamus (44). There are also return projections from the piriform to the ipsilateral olfactory bulb, which has been likened to the cortico-thalamic circuit in other sensory modalities by some authors (45).

Based on these connections, several local recurrent circuits may provide a substrate for seizure activity (3). Firstly, the projections from piriform pyramidal cells to amygdala nuclei are returned by projections from the basolateral amygdala to the endopiriform nucleus. Secondly, projections to the subiculum link the piriform with the hippocampus, a loop that is returned to the piriform via the entorhinal cortex. Finally, piriform feedback to the olfactory bulb could also form a reentrant circuit (46).

FUNCTIONAL ROLE OF THE PIRIFORM CORTEX WITHIN OLFACTORY NETWORKS

The perception of odors involves activation of distributed cortical and subcortical networks, with regional nodes that are variably recruited depending on the nature and complexity of the olfactory task (47). Activation of the piriform cortex is seen commonly across all olfactory tasks, and it appears to be the key region for representation of the "olfactory object" (48). However, the piriform also has an important role in discrimination of odors (49), in olfactory working memory (50), and acts as an information distributing node to other brain regions (51).

Within piriform cortex, odors are represented as spatially distributed ensembles (52, 53). This activity is not static over time, and shows variability with the phase of the respiratory cycle (54), and especially with sniffing (55). The anterior piriform cortex encodes for molecular features of the odorant, whereas the posterior piriform encodes for the quality of the odor (14). There is rapid habituation of the piriform response to a sustained odor within seconds (56), which is a property that may be the basis for figure-ground segmentation, that is, to allow a novel odor to stand out in a complex olfactory environment (48). Piriform activation can also occur in the absence of an odorant, for example, by imagining a smell (57), or on viewing a picture or word that has a strong olfactory association (58, 59), which is consistent with the behavior of primary cortical regions for other sensory modalities.

Larger scale network interactions of the piriform cortex can be conceptualized as including an orbitofrontal-thalamic circuit, a limbic stream, and a fronto-temporal cortical stream. Additional cortical regions including the anterior insula are important for integration of olfaction into taste and flavor (60).

The orbitofrontal cortex is the principal higher-order target for piriform cortex, both directly and indirectly via the thalamus. The olfactory functions of orbitofrontal cortex include involvement in encoding for odor identity and valence, predicting anticipated olfactory stimuli (61), multisensory integration of olfactory information, assessment of reward and value signals, and a role in emotion (62). The mediodorsal nucleus of the thalamus provides an indirect pathway between piriform cortex and the orbitofrontal cortex, and is therefore well placed to provide assessment of prediction error (63), or to control olfactory attention (64). Furthermore, the connectivity between these three regions is modulated during olfactory learning (65), and by olfactory attention (66).

Limbic processing of olfactory stimuli plays an important role in memory, emotion and social behavior. Indeed the spontaneous recall of a vivid memory or emotion on smelling a particular odor is a common human experience (67). Entorhinal cortex and hippocampal activation occurs during odor identification and memory tasks, reflecting the involvement of autobiographical memory systems (68). Exposure to odors of varying degrees of pleasantness produces amygdala activation that reflects the valence (69) and also the intensity and overall emotional value of an odor (70).

The semantic network, which involves the dominant inferior frontal gyrus and its downstream influence on the fusiform gyrus and posterior temporal regions, is important for naming odors and for olfactory working memory when odors are nameable (50, 71). The temporal pole may be the critical area for interaction between olfactory and semantic networks based on an apparent disconnection syndrome in people with atrophy of this region (72).

PIRIFORM CORTEX IS THE MOST SUSCEPTIBLE REGION TO EPILEPTOGENIC STIMULATION

PIRIFORM CORTEX SENSITIVITY TO CHEMICAL STIMULATION

A unique property of the piriform cortex is its sensitivity for inducing epileptic seizures in experimental animals. In 1985, Piredda and Gale identified a site in the forebrain of the rat, which is exquisitely responsive to pro-convulsant chemical stimulation (73), naming it the "area tempestas" (74). Injections into this region produced bilateral clonic seizures, at much lower concentrations than are required when applied to other brain regions. Picomolar amounts of bicuculline (a GABA antagonist), carbachol (a cholinergic agonist), kainic acid (an excitatory amino acid), and micromolar concentrations of glutamate all demonstrated this effect. Preventing glutamatergic excitation via either AMPA or NMDA receptors in the area tempestas can prevent seizures, indicating that both receptor types are needed for this regions to become epileptogenic (75, 76).

The location of the area tempestas is deep to the anterior piriform cortex, overlapping cellular layer III and the adjacent endopiriform nucleus (25, 73). Some studies have shown wider sensitivity to bicuculline across both anterior and posterior piriform cortex, however, and some variability in the expression of seizures between different rat strains (77).

The area tempestas cannot be ethically demonstrated in human beings, as it is defined by an epileptic response to chemical stimulation, and is not a circumscribed anatomical structure. This study has been performed in non-human primates, however (78), using bicuculline injections into the frontal piriform cortex. A highly focal 2 mm region of chemosensitivity was identified. The resulting seizures consisted of automatisms and myoclonus of the mouth and face, contralateral arm clonus, salivation, behavioral arrest, and unresponsiveness, with retained postural control (79), consistent with the features of focal dycognitive and focal motor seizures in human beings.

The brain regions most affected by seizure activity triggered from area tempestas, are the posterior piriform cortex and ipsilateral entorhinal cortex (80), the olfactory bulbs, perirhinal cortex, amygdala, and the mediodorsal thalamus (81). This has been demonstrated by ictal uptake of radiolabeled glucose, and also by the ictal expression of *c-fos* and other immediate-early genes *in vivo* (82–84). Examination of *in vitro* slice preparations shows that discharge propagation from the endopiriform nucleus up to the superficial layers of piriform cortex is via longitudinally orientated rostrocaudal association fibers (85).

The posterior piriform cortex, perirhinal cortex, and mediodorsal thalamus are important regions for seizure propagation from the area tempestas. Blockade of glutamatergic transmission at these locations prevents such seizures occurring (76, 80, 81). This is mediated primarily by the action of AMPA receptors, as selective blockade of NMDA receptors did not prevent seizures occurring.

PIRIFORM SUSCEPTIBILITY TO ELECTRICAL KINDLING

Seizures may also be produced from the piriform cortex by repeated electrical stimulation (3, 86). Comparison to other nearby structures shows that perirhinal cortex and dorsal claustrum also kindle as rapidly, or even faster (87). The amygdala, entorhinal cortex, and hippocampus are less sensitive (88).

The location within piriform cortex for the most rapid kindling in rodents has been reported as the central part (layer III of the rostral part of the posterior piriform cortex) (89) or in the endopiriform nucleus (90). Deep layers of the posterior piriform cortex also show the lowest afterdischarge thresholds. In human beings, these areas correspond to the frontal piriform close to the temporal stem, or to the prepiriform claustrum. Several authors have emphasized that the region corresponding to area tempestas (in the deep anterior piriform cortex) does not respond to electrical kindling as quickly (91, 92).

Seizures produced during the course of piriform kindling follow the same progression of motor features as kindling in other limbic regions (93). During piriform-kindled status epilepticus (type 2), where the animals show intermittent freezing and exploratory behaviors, the affected regions are the olfactory cortex and amygdala. When facial and limb clonus was also present (type 3), the hippocampus, prefrontal cortex, and insular cortex were also seen to be involved (94). Piriform kindling produces chronic network-wide changes, for example, altered potentiation at the entorhinal cortex (95), which may relate to emergence of spontaneous seizure after kindling is completed.

Therefore, the piriform cortex is highly susceptible to the induction of seizures by both chemical and electrical means, although the exact positioning of the intervention within the piriform appears to be less important, than whether an extended olfactory-limbic network can be recruited.

HUMAN SEIZURES WITH OLFACTORY AURAS TELL US ABOUT EPILEPTIC INVOLVEMENT OF THE OLFACTORY NETWORK

Focal seizures that begin with an olfactory sensation as their earliest feature can be inferred to arise within the olfactory network. In human beings, this is a relatively uncommon type of seizure, but examining these events in detail can tells us about the patterns seizure spread from the piriform cortex. The most common olfactory ictal phenomenon is a hallucination, where the perception of an odor is unrelated to any environmental stimulus. There can also be olfactory illusions, where odors in the environment are misperceived (96, 97), or vaguer episodes with the quality of a reminiscence (98).

The earliest influential descriptions of seizures with an olfactory aura were by Hughlings Jackson in 1889. He described a woman who developed stereotyped episodes of a horrible smell of "dirty burning stuff" associated with a complicated visual hallucination and a feeling of suffocation. A sarcoma of the "temporo-sphenoidal lobe" was found at postmortem. Review of their diagrams shows invasion of the piriform cortex, temporal pole, amygdala, adjacent white matter, and compression of the lenticular nucleus (99). Subsequently the name "uncinate group of fits" was given to seizures beginning with a crude sensation of smell or taste, and variably associated with oral automatisms and the "dreamy state" (100, 101). Importantly, this label was intended to convey that these seizures involved a broad region of which the uncus is a part, and should not be interpreted as a precise anatomical localization.

CLINICAL CHARACTERISTICS OF SEIZURES WITH AN OLFACTORY AURA

Estimates of the prevalence of olfactory epileptic auras are quite variable due to patient selection criteria and how auras were ascertained. Considering all people with focal epilepsy, rates between 0.9 and 8.1% are reported (102–107). If restricted to epilepsy arising from the temporal lobe, with or without selection for epilepsy surgery, olfactory auras are present in 0.6–16% (108–113). Out of people who experience an epileptic aura of any kind, between 19 and 30% have an olfactory aura (114–116).

The character of olfactory hallucinations is usually unpleasant, and may be described as rotten, fetid, sulfurous, or burned (110, 117). This may correspond to epileptic activity causing particularly intense activation of the piriform cortex and amygdala, as occurs with non-pathological smelling of unpleasant odors in the environment (57). Less commonly the olfactory hallucination is neutral and only rarely pleasant (102, 106). Some descriptions have emphasized the "crude" nature of the experience, without having the full experiential quality of smelling an actual odor (100). Indeed many patients find the hallucination "indescribable," or refer to it as "like" the aroma of something else (98), suggesting that the engagement of the olfactory network is not the full physiological pattern of olfactory perception. The olfactory hallucination is usually pervasive, but in rare cases is experienced as coming from one nostril (98), or from one side of the body (118), which may be due to lateralized involvement of primary olfactory cortex or activation of the superior temporal gyrus (12).

A particular "rhinostomal" sensation of tickling or pressure in the nose or pharynx often accompanies olfactory hallucinations (98). This may be analogous to the trigeminal nerve stimulation that is physiologically produced by many odorants. A similar sensation of unilateral itching inside the nose has also been triggered by electrical stimulation near the olfactory bulb (119).

Olfactory auras may be accompanied by other aura symptoms, pointing to epileptic activation of multiple sensory or cognitive networks. The association of olfactory auras with ictal emotion (120) suggests epileptic co-involvement of olfactory and limbic networks. Olfactory auras are often accompanied by gustatory or psychic auras when the underlying epileptogenic lesion is a tumor (102, 105, 106). However, patients with mesial temporal sclerosis tended to have epigastic sensations and autonomic phenomena accompanying the olfactory aura (110), indicating different spread patterns depending on etiology.

When there are multiple aura types during the same seizure, the order of progression indicates the direction of epileptic spread. In a small case series, one patient with a neocortical temporal lesion had an olfactory aura followed by a sensory aura. Another similar patient had a concurrent olfactory and psychic aura (116). These examples may represent epileptic spread from the olfactory network into cortical networks and limbic networks respectively. Two further patients with mesial temporal sclerosis were described in this cohort. The first had a concurrent olfactory-abdominal aura, and the second had a progression of autonomic, sensory, and psychic symptoms before the olfactory aura emerged. This latter case is an example where the seizure likely began outside the olfactory network, but it became engaged as the seizure progressed. In patients with mesial temporal sclerosis, imaging data has shown that patients with an olfactory aura are more likely to have an accompanying abnormality of the amygdala (121). This suggests that the amygdala may be a possible gateway for seizure spread from mesial temporal into olfactory networks.

The etiology of seizures with an olfactory aura is commonly found to be a tumor (102, 108, 113) or mesial temporal sclerosis (109, 110, 114), with debate over which of these is more common. Other cases have been caused by intracerebral hemorrhage (122), middle cerebral artery aneurysm (118), arteriovenous malformation, head injury (103, 123), and previous encephalitis (124). In rare cases, there is no obvious cause and no structural abnormality is found on MRI (110). It is the anatomical location of these lesions, rather than the nature of the pathology, that is most relevant to the occurrence of olfactory auras, although the close relationship of the middle cerebral artery to the piriform cortex at the endorhinal sulcus should be noted.

THE POST-ICTAL NOSE-WIPE COULD BE EXPLAINED BY AN ICTAL RHINOSTOMAL SENSATION

A movement of the hand to wipe or rub the nose is often observed in the immediate post-ictal phase following focal seizures. It is most common in seizures from the mesial temporal lobe, occurring in more than half of mesial temporal lobe epilepsy patients having video-EEG prior to surgery (125, 126), but it may also be seen in frontal lobe epilepsy. It may be accompanied by post-ictal coughing (127), and does not occur if the seizure evolves to a bilateral convulsion (119). Typically, the hand ipsilateral to the seizure focus is used, because of contralateral neglect or weakness (125).

We hypothesize that the ictal nose-wipe is a voluntary action performed in response to the ictal rhinostomal sensation, as a result of epileptic activation of olfactory regions. Geyer et al. (119) have previously suggested that olfactory hallucinations and post-ictal nose-rubbing are linked by epileptic involvement arising from the uncus. However, many patients with post-ictal nose-wiping do not have awareness of any olfactory aura (128). Hirsch et al. (125) proposed that the nose-wipe is caused by increased nasal secretions from ictal activation of autonomic pathways, particularly the amygdala (129). Intracranial EEG recordings from the amygdala can show early ictal involvement in seizures, which include nose-wiping, but this is neither sufficient nor necessary for nose-wiping to occur (130).

LESION "LOCALIZATION" IN SEIZURES WITH AN OLFACTORY HALLUCINATION

The anatomical location of epileptogenic lesions indicates how seizure discharges gain access to the olfactory network. It should not be assumed however that the lesion equates to the location where the aura is produced, as emergence of an olfactory percept likely requires coordinated activation of multiple olfactory brain regions (131, 132).

Olfactory auras are not lateralizing, and are associated with similar rates of left and right-sided lesions (107, 110, 111). The most common location is in the anteromesial temporal lobe, with some tumors extending into the frontal lobe (102, 108). Other series have found only temporal lobe lesions, both with and without involvement of mesial temporal structures (107, 114). In a few cases, lesions have been isolated to the amygdala (102, 110, 123).

The case most strongly indicating primary involvement of the piriform cortex is provided by Mizobuchi et al. (118). The cause of seizures was a 1 cm aneurysm of the middle cerebral artery, "between the tip of the right temporal lobe and the orbitofrontal gyrus." MRI clearly shows compression of both frontal and temporal piriform cortex, although the authors do not label it as such. The olfactory aura was followed by a phase of retained awareness and speech, but impaired memory, suggesting limited seizure spread to either autobiographical (limbic) or perhaps semantic (cortical) memory networks.

Whether purely frontal lobe lesions can cause seizures with an olfactory hallucination is less clear, even though this is often said to be the case (106, 133). In some series of patients with frontal lobe epilepsy, confirmed by curative frontal lobe resection, there have been no instances of olfactory auras (134). Possible cases include one out of a series of 28 patients with extra-temporal focal epilepsy studied by intracranial stereo-EEG, although this patient was cured by temporal lobe resection (135). Another study described two patients under the heading of an olfactory-gustatory-fear aura, who had frontal lobe lesions at the supplementary motor area and lateral premotor cortex, respectively (105).

The only unequivocal report of a frontal lobe lesion causing an epileptic olfactory aura was due to an abscess at the frontal pole (136). Several pathways to involvement of the olfactory network are possible here; seizure activity could have spread from the lesion into adjacent orbitofrontal cortex, activity could have propagated via the uncinate fasciculus into the temporal lobe, or there may have been local inflammatory or epileptic irritation of the olfactory tract. Of these sites, an olfactory hallucination has been produced most consistently by electrical stimulation of the olfactory tract (137).

ICTAL EEG IN SEIZURES WITH OLFACTORY AURAS

Scalp EEG during seizures with an olfactory aura has shown epileptiform discharges at the ipsilateral sphenoidal electrode, consistent with seizure involvement of mesial temporal structures (102, 120, 138). This confirms that these olfactory hallucinations are epileptic in origin, and are not due to mere inter-ictal dysfunction of the olfactory network.

Intracranial EEG recording has much greater sensitivity for detecting focal epileptic activity, but sparse spatial sampling often limits the precision of localization. Electrodes have typically been placed into mesial temporal structures, over the lateral and inferior temporal lobes, and into frontal regions, with the piriform cortex seldom being an explicit target for recording.

The following five reports demonstrate intracranial recordings of epileptic activity in the temporal and/or frontal lobe associated with an olfactory aura, although it must be noted that no cases had an electrode directly in piriform cortex. (i) Epileptic activity at the amygdala and hippocampus was seen in a patient who had a temporo-basal cyst and habitually experienced an epigastric-olfactory-gustatory aura (139). (ii) Discharges from the hippocampus were seen in two patients who had mesial temporal sclerosis, during an olfactory aura (140). (iii) A patient with a more elaborate aura, consisting of initial déjà vu then an olfactory hallucination, detachment, fear, and auditory illusions, had ictal rhythms that were widespread across the right hippocampus, amygdala, anterior cingulate, middle, and superior temporal gyri (141). (iv) A patient who experienced seizures with a sense of foreboding, dissociation, and a "sickening" smell, showed initial activity in superior temporal electrodes, with consistent spread of the discharge into orbital areas (135). (v) A further three patients had simultaneous epileptic activity in the temporal and orbitofrontal regions during the olfactory aura, however, no aura occurred in seizures when only the frontal lobe was involved, or when temporal lobe involvement was late (142).

Therefore, the seizures that produce olfactory hallucinations typically involve relatively widespread activity in the orbitofrontal and anterior temporal lobe. Although recordings directly from piriform cortex were not obtained in these cases, we infer its involvement from its location at the center of the regions that were sampled, and its core role in olfactory perception.

INTRACRANIAL STIMULATION DEMONSTRATES SITES THAT MAY PRODUCE AN OLFACTORY HALLUCINATION

Direct electrical stimulation of the human brain, either during surgery or via long-term implanted electrodes, has identified locations that may trigger an olfactory sensation similar to the epileptic aura. Findings are somewhat variable, and several large studies of temporal lobe stimulations have induced no olfactory sensations at all (143).

The earliest reports are of a crude sense of smell produced by stimulation of the uncus, or of the olfactory bulb (144). Only a few authors have applied stimulation near the piriform (145). Overall, stimulation of the amygdala is the location that most often produces an olfactory percept, although reproducibility in individual patients is not consistent (145–148).

In one patient with epilepsy, amygdala stimulation produced an afterdischarge that propagated to the hippocampus, at the same time accompanied by a "foul rotten odor" typical of their usual seizures. Transection adjacent to the amygdala prevented propagation to the hippocampus, but the olfactory aura on amygdala stimulation still occurred. The patient became seizure free after resection of the amygdala and overlying anterior cortex, including temporal piriform cortex (123). This suggests that either amygdala activity itself or spread into the adjacent piriform cortex is the relevant pathway, and that amygdala-to-hippocampus spread is less important.

Stimulation over the orbitofrontal cortex does not elicit an olfactory hallucination, unless the electrodes are in a position to stimulate the olfactory bulb or tract (137). The induced odor is always unpleasant. This could be because a large number of fibers are stimulated through the use of macro-electrodes, and the subsequent activation of olfactory cortex, which is relatively intense.

SEIZURES MAY INVOLVE THE PIRIFORM CORTEX WITHOUT AN OLFACTORY HALLUCINATION

An intriguing possibility is that some human seizures may arise from the piriform cortex, without being accompanied by an olfactory aura. This has been demonstrated in a single case of reading epilepsy, that was intensively investigated using combined imaging techniques and advanced statistical modeling (149). Clinically, covert reading induced peri-oral myoclonus, however, no accompanying olfactory hallucination was described. Both magnetoencephalography and EEG-fMRI demonstrated seizure-related activity at the dominant left premotor cortex, with fMRI showing a more extensive network of activation involving left piriform cortex, left thalamus, and right inferior frontal gyrus, consistent with findings from a larger group of people with reading epilepsy (150). Modeling of fMRI timecourses showed the earliest BOLD response was in the left piriform cortex. An effective connectivity analysis identified a model where piriform cortex activity drives activation of the premotor cortex and then onto other regions. While this case report suggests a possible role of piriform cortex in driving seizures into premotor regions, whether this is generally the case in patients with reading epilepsy remains to be confirmed.

PIRIFORM CORTEX IS A NODE FOR SECONDARY SPREAD OF INTER-ICTAL DISCHARGES IN HUMAN BEINGS

Beyond its role in olfactory auras, the piriform cortex may be one of the common pathways for propagation of epileptic discharges in focal epilepsy. The first study to suggest this used combined encephalography and functional MRI (EEG-fMRI) (151). They studied a diverse group of 19 patients, who had focal epilepsy arising from all lobes. After aligning the epileptic side between patients, a second-level random effects analysis was performed, and showed significant clusters with peak BOLD response overlying the ipsilateral piriform cortex (**Figure 3A**). Regions of

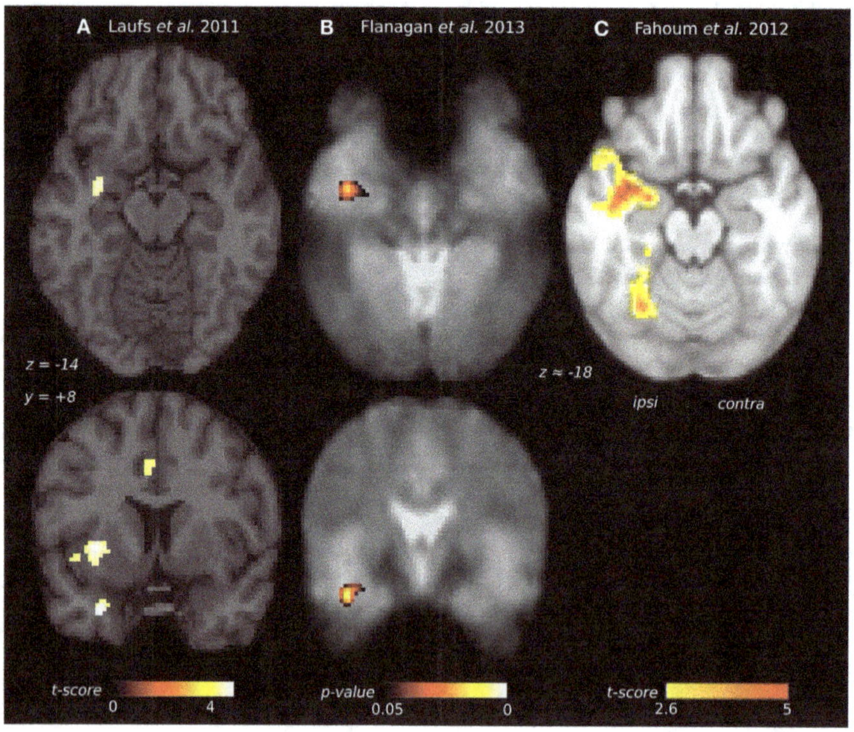

FIGURE 3 | Comparison of piriform cortex activation in EEG-fMRI studies of focal epilepsy. (A) Group EEG-fMRI analysis for a mixed cohort of focal epilepsy at threshold $p < 0.001$ ($n = 19$). **(B)** Group EEG-fMRI random effects analysis for a mixed epilepsy cohort ($n = 27$) showing *p*-values <0.05 FWE corrected. Reproduced from Flanagan et al. (153) with permission from Elsevier. **(C)** Group EEG-fMRI analysis of a purely TLE cohort ($n = 32$), with hemodynamic response function peaking at 5 s ($p < 0.05$ cluster corrected). Reproduced from Fahoum et al. (154) with permission from Wiley Periodicals, Inc. ©2012 International League against Epilepsy.

activation also extended over the ipsilateral dorsal claustrum and anterior cingulate. The interpretation is that these areas are activated by inter-ictal discharges in many individuals, regardless of the site where the discharge begins. A recent paper has commented that the peak coordinates in this study favor activation of the dorsal claustrum (152), although the shape of the activation clusters do not entirely follow this structure, and activation specifically within the thin sheet of the claustrum would be difficult to resolve at this fMRI resolution.

Replication of this analysis using functional MRI acquired at 3 T, in an independent cohort of 27 patients with heterogeneous epileptic foci, again identified a common area of temporal lobe activation, in the region of the ipsilateral piriform cortex (**Figure 3B**) (153).

A further EEG-fMRI study analyzed subjects with focal epilepsy, this time grouped by lobe (154, 155). In total, 32 patients had temporal lobe epilepsy, 14 frontal lobe epilepsy, and 20 posterior quadrant epilepsy. The activations detected by this approach were more extensive than in previous studies, suggesting greater homogeneity of epileptic networks within these selected groups. The temporal lobe epilepsy cohort showed an ipsilateral network of activation over the insula, claustrum, temporal piriform cortex, and amygdala (**Figure 3C**), as well as anterior hippocampus, mid-cingulate and cerebellum. The frontal lobe epilepsy group did not have significant activation of piriform cortex, although other sites of activation were seen in the mid-cingulate, ipsilateral frontal operculum, thalamus, and cerebellum. The posterior quadrant epilepsy group had no significant regions of common activation (154).

Taken together, these results indicate that inter-ictal discharges arising from the temporal lobe, and perhaps those from the frontal lobe, can produce common activation within the piriform cortex, along with other ipsilateral brain regions. This occurs in the absence of positive olfactory symptoms. Whether discharges from parietal and occipital lobe foci also engage the piriform cortex in this way requires further clarification.

PIRIFORM CORTEX IS SUSCEPTIBLE TO SEIZURE-INDUCED INJURY AND FACILITATES PROGRESSION OF FOCAL EPILEPTOGENESIS

STATUS EPILEPTICUS INJURES THE HUMAN PIRIFORM CORTEX

A characteristic property of the piriform cortex is its tendency to sustain neuronal injury as a consequence of repeated seizures. This is demonstrated by three unusual human cases of status epilepticus, in people who had no prior history of epilepsy (156). The causes were neuroleptic malignant syndrome, carcinomatous meningitis, and unknown, respectively. The duration of status epilepticus on EEG was between 9 h and 3 days. The three individuals died between 11 and 27 days after status epilepticus. At postmortem, neuronal loss was most prominent in the piriform cortex, hippocampal subfields, and amygdala, although with some asymmetry and variability between individuals. Milder widespread changes were seen in the deep layers of the neocortex, the Purkinje cell layer of the cerebellum, and the dorsomedial nucleus of the thalamus. Glutamate-mediated excitotoxicity has been suggested as the mechanism of neuronal necrosis, by analogy to animal studies of status epilepticus.

Domoic acid, a glutamate analog, has also been seen to cause neuronal toxicity in the human piriform cortex following status epilepticus. The most prominent injury is to the hippocampus, which is likely related to kainate receptor excitotoxicity (157), but more widespread injury also occurs, affecting the piriform cortex, olfactory tubercle, amygdala, mediodorsal thalamus, and nucleus accumbens (158). The same pattern is seen with domoic acid in experimental animals (159), although one study in rats has suggested that the most significant early changes are in the olfactory bulb and endopiriform nucleus (160). The mechanism of piriform cortex injury in these cases may be either the direct effect of the toxin, or the kindling effect of repeated seizures.

INDUCED STATUS EPILEPTICUS INJURES THE PIRIFORM CORTEX IN EXPERIMENTAL ANIMALS

Status epilepticus induced by pilocarpine or kainic acid also produces early injury to the piriform cortex, even though greater attention is often given to the hippocampus in these studies.

Rodents treated with pilocarpine, a potent muscarinic agonist, are often presented as a model of human chronic temporal lobe epilepsy (161, 162). Following systemic administration of pilocarpine, there is an initial phase of limbic status epilepticus, then a latent period of several weeks, before spontaneous recurrent seizures develop. Here, we discuss the initial phase only. Although many brain regions are affected, serial MRI shows the earliest changes in the piriform and entorhinal cortex, as early as 6 h after the status epilepticus (163, 164), reflecting cellular edema, and neuronal loss in these regions (165). Cellular hyperactivity, imaged by *c-fos* expression, is first seen (at 30 min) at the piriform cortex, olfactory tubercle, thalamus, caudate, and lateral habenula, with later changes (at 60–90 min) in hippocampus, amygdala, and basal ganglia (166). Early neuronal loss and gliosis occur in the piriform cortex, hippocampus, amydala, thalamus, and substantia nigra (167). More specifically within the piriform cortex and endopiriform nucleus, it is the posterior two-thirds that are affected, which reflects the pattern of arborization of efferents from the endopiriform nucleus (168). It is primarily the pyramidal cells that are lost, but immunocytochemistry also shows loss of distinct populations of piriform GABAergic interneurons, some of which have analogous labeling to hippocampal basket cells (169). Involvement of the piriform cortex may be explained by cholinergic innervation from the diagnonal band of Broca (170), or the tendency of piriform cortex to produce burst firing with muscarinic antagonism (171). Subsequent neuronal loss may be caused by excitotoxic glutamate release and neuronal calcium influx during seizures (172) or by concurrent ischemic mechanisms (173).

Kainic acid is an analog of glutamate, which like pilocarpine, produces limbic status epilepticus after systemic administration. This results in damage to the hippocampus, amygdala, piriform cortex, entorhinal cortex, thalamus, and septal regions, although with some differences in timing relative to the pilocarpine model (174). The regions showing greatest oxidative stress are the piriform cortex, hippocampus, and cerebellum (175), and the greatest subsequent volume loss is again in the posterior olfactory cortex and amygdala, with loss of approximately one-third loss of neurons in these areas (176). GABAergic neurons of the piriform cortex also show a unique property in this situation, of increasing mRNA expression for glutamate decarboxylase (GAD), perhaps in an attempt to control excitotoxic injury in the face of ongoing neuronal loss (177). The mechanisms of piriform cortex injury here are either the direct excitotoxic effect of the kainic acid, or via release of glutamate during the seizure, and although disentangling these possibilities is difficult, the ability of specific blockade of glutamatergic NMDA receptors to prevent neuronal loss in this model favors the latter (178).

Lesion studies of the piriform cortex further indicate that piriform cortex involvement may be a critical for the development of chemically induced seizures. In the administration of soman, a powerful inhibitor of acetylcholinesterase that causes seizures via stimulation of muscarinic and nicotinic receptors, pre-lesioning of posterior piriform cortex or perirhinal cortex significantly increased the latency to seizure onset. This prevention did not occur with ablation of the amygdala, entorhinal cortex, or hippocampus (179).

AMYGDALA KINDLING CAUSES CHANGES WITHIN PIRIFORM CORTEX

Neuronal injury at the piriform cortex, and subsequent change in its function, is seen following electrical kindling at sites such as the amygdala or hippocampus (3). During amygdala kindling, afterdischarges are induced from the piriform from the very first stimulation, indicating the high connectivity from the amygdala and propensity of piriform cortex to sustain epileptic discharges (180). During this process, neuronal loss not only occurs at the primary kindling site, but is also at the central piriform cortex, particularly with loss of GABAergic interneurons (181, 182). Once amygdala kindling is completed, there is increased background firing of neurons in the upper layers of the central piriform. These are most likely inhibitory interneurons, which have pathologically reduced sensitivity to glutamate, and are compensating for loss of feed-forward inhibition (183, 184). There is also increased excitability at the piriform cortex, which is demonstrated by a significant drop in its afterdischarge threshold (185).

Many other changes occur in the piriform cortex following amygdala kindling, which may underlie this increased excitability. These include expression of markers of synaptogenesis on excitatory neurons (186, 187), altered regulation of glutamate transporters (188), abnormal transcription of AMPA and GABA receptor subunits (189, 190), altered expression of voltage gated potassium channels on multipolar inhibitory interneurons (191), alteration of chloride transport that further exacerbates the failure of GABAergic inhibition (192) and proliferation of astrocytes (193). The most recent observation has been the breakdown of perineuronal nets around specific interneurons, leading to increased sites of GABA release, and the pathological rewiring of local microcircuits (194).

PIRIFORM CORTEX FACILITATES EPILEPTOGENESIS IN THE AMYGDALA KINDLING MODEL

As the epileptic state develops, the piriform cortex plays a key role in the facilitation and distribution of kindled afterdischarges. Early in the process, uptake of radiolabeled deoxyglucose during seizures shows involvement only of the amygdala and the regions it is directly connected to, including the piriform. After kindling is completed, much more widespread activation is seen during seizures, affecting substantia nigra, thalamic nuclei, basal ganglia, and bilateral neocortex (3, 195). Similarly using *c-fos* expression as a marker of cellular activity, a limited expression of seizures is seen in the early phases, confined to either a unilateral amygdala-insula-temporal network, or a bilateral amygdala-hippocampal network. Following kindling, this becomes much more extensive involving extensive amygdala, olfactory, hippocampal, and neocortical regions bilaterally (196). Furthermore, during amygdala kindling, spontaneous discharges arise most frequently from the piriform cortex (197). Together this suggests that the piriform is involved in converting the kindled seizure discharge from one that is confined to the stimulation site and immediate projections, into an event having more widespread distribution (3).

The role of the piriform cortex in facilitating epileptogenesis can be further explored by blocking it prior to the kindling process. This approach has given variable results depending on the site and method of piriform inhibition. Permanent lesions that alter the progression of amygdala or hippocampal kindling have included the destruction of the central piriform cortex with ibotenate (198, 199), electrical ablation of the ipsilateral piriform, and knife-cut disconnection of the anterior piriform (200). These increased the number of stimulations to achieve kindling, prolonging either during the early or later phases, and increased the post-kindling seizure threshold. Other approaches such as injecting the anterior piriform, or bilateral radio-ablation of the area tempestas did not alter kindling (91), re-enforcing that it is the posterior piriform, which is the critical site for discharge propagation.

Chemical modulation of the piriform cortex also can alter the course of amygdala kindling. Microinjection of a $GABA_A$ receptor agonist, or an NMDA receptor antagonist reduces the duration of kindled afterdischarges (92, 201). Microinjection of vigabatrin, an antiepileptic medication, which elevates local GABA levels, inhibited seizures in previously kindled animals, showing greatest effect when applied to the central piriform cortex (201, 202). Finally, local application of adenosine to the piriform cortex (an endogenous neurotransmitter that may have an antiepileptic effect by decreasing glutamate release), inhibited kindling from both the amygdala and the hippocampus (203, 204). Kindling of the amygdala can also be blocked by lesions at the dorsal claustrum (205), demonstrating that the piriform cortex is not the only critical structure in limbic epileptogenesis.

In summary, the available evidence shows that either chemical or repeated electrical stimulation applied to limbic sites can produce complex changes in the piriform cortex, which ultimately results in increased piriform cortex excitability. Therefore, the piriform cortex can provide a pathway for focal epileptogenesis, via the facilitation and widespread distribution of epileptic discharges.

As a corollary, we should consider whether the piriform cortex has any influence on the progression to intractable epilepsy. Defined in clinical populations as ongoing seizures despite adequate trials of two appropriate and tolerated medications (206), medication resistance in epilepsy is likely to be a multifactorial process (207), and is often related to the intrinsic severity of the epilepsy syndrome (208). The epilepsy most strongly associated with piriform cortex involvement is temporal lobe epilepsy (as discussed in Sections "Human Seizures with Olfactory Auras Tell us About Epileptic Involvement of the Olfactory Network" and

"The Impact of Epilepsy on Olfaction and its Imaging Correlates in Human Beings"), which has high rates of medical intractability that may either be present from the onset, or develop over time (209). Hippocampal atrophy is a particular marker for progression to intractability in this group, and an association between hippocampal atrophy and piriform atrophy has been noted (10). High initial seizure frequency and the occurrence of status epilepticus are known to cause piriform cortex injury and are also risk factors for intractability (210). A further mechanism of pharmacoresistance is the expression of the multi-drug transporter P-glycoprotein, which can cause efflux of medications from epileptogenic sites (211). Marked P-glycoprotein expression has been seen at both hippocampus and piriform cortex in phenobarbitone-resistant rat models (212). However, there may be significant interspecies variation for this mechanism, and recent *in vivo* human imaging of P-glycoprotein did not detect significant changes at the piriform cortex (213). Lastly, alterations in neural networks due to axonal sprouting and synaptic reorganization may contribute to pharmacoresistance (214). Therefore, the piriform cortex has anatomical and functional characteristics that position it to contribute to the phenomena associated with intractability.

THE IMPACT OF EPILEPSY ON OLFACTION AND ITS IMAGING CORRELATES IN HUMAN BEINGS

OLFACTORY FUNCTION IS IMPAIRED BY FOCAL EPILEPSY

A common theme in focal epilepsy is that overlap of epileptic regions with sensory networks produces dysfunction of that modality (215). In patients with temporal lobe epilepsy, many aspects of olfactory function are abnormal (115), which is most likely caused by epileptic involvement of the olfactory network.

The threshold for detection of odors is normal for people with temporal lobe epilepsy, on standard testing with n-butanol or phenyl ethyl alcohol (124, 216–220). However, some studies have found reduced sensitivity for odors by using broader panels of odorants (115, 221). The occurrence of seizures may transiently alter odor detection thresholds, with heightened olfactory sensitivity during the seizure prodrome, and reduced sensitivity lasting for hours or days in the post-ictal phase (115).

In contrast, odor discrimination, memory, and identification/naming are all commonly impaired in temporal lobe epilepsy. Odor discrimination relies on the piriform cortex, orbitofrontal regions, and the hippocampus (222), and failure on this task reflects dysfunction of these networks (219, 220, 223, 224), although this deficit has not been confirmed on all studies (217). Single-nostril presentation of odorants lateralizes the deficit to the same side as the epileptic focus (220).

Memory recall of odors activates an extensive network including olfactory cortex, semantic networks, and attention systems (13). Impaired odor memory has been demonstrated with a variety of protocols (216, 220). Some studies have detected abnormality only in left sided (225), or in right-sided temporal lobe epilepsy (226), probably related to the relative involvement of the autobiographical memory network versus semantic networks on a given task (227). Single-nostril presentation again shows an ipsilateral deficit, being more pronounced in left sided epilepsy (223).

Identification of odors, for example by selecting from a list of names, is also impaired (124, 217, 219). This deficit occurs equally with left and right-sided temporal lobe epilepsy (216, 225) or can have a right temporal lobe predominance (218). Correct odor identification activates olfactory, limbic and semantic networks, plus other primary cortical areas (68), but may have more pronounced involvement of the non-dominant hemisphere when non-verbal identification is used (228, 229).

Olfactory function in patients with generalized or extra-temporal focal epilepsy has rarely been tested. Impaired odor identification was found in a mixed group mostly with generalized epilepsy (225). Another group with extra-temporal epilepsies had normal odor detection, discrimination, and memory (220). This may be surprising in light of the EEG-fMRI findings indicating common involvement of the piriform cortex in some extra-temporal focal epilepsies, although more behavioral data is clearly needed to address this discordance.

NEUROIMAGING OF PIRIFORM CORTEX SHOWS OLFACTORY DYSFUNCTION IN FOCAL EPILEPSY

Multiple neuroimaging modalities have shown changes to piriform cortex in focal epilepsy, which parallel the dysfunction of olfactory processing we have described above.

Volumetric MRI shows piriform cortex atrophy in temporal lobe epilepsy. This was examined by manual tracing of the temporal and periamygdaloid cortex, identifying reduced volume on the same side as the epileptic focus (10). This effect is greater with right-sided epilepsy. Piriform cortex atrophy is bilateral in a subgroup of patients with left temporal lobe epilepsy. There is a significant correlation between atrophy of piriform cortex and atrophy of the hippocampus, amygdala, and entorhinal cortex, indicating that the piriform changes are not isolated, but are part of a distributed network effect. The olfactory bulb volume is also reduced in temporal lobe epilepsy (230), which may be a "top-down" effect driven by pathology within primary olfactory cortex.

In frontal lobe epilepsy, voxel-based morphometry has surprisingly shown increased volumes of the piriform cortex and amygdala bilaterally compared to controls, and no regions of atrophy were found (231). The meaning of increased gray matter volume in this context is uncertain.

Chemosensory evoked potentials (CSERPs) can tell us about the relative timing of olfactory processing. In temporal lobe epilepsy, evoked potentials are delayed when an odor is presented to the side of the epileptic focus (232). This effect was most pronounced in right temporal lobe epilepsy, reflecting the relative importance of the right hemisphere in olfaction.

The functional activity of olfactory brain regions in epilepsy has been investigated with positron emission tomography (PET) using an $[^{15}O]$-H_2O tracer (233). People with temporal lobe epilepsy failed to activate the ipsilateral piriform cortex, amygdala, and anterior insula when smelling various odors. Furthermore, when smelling familiar (nameable) odors patients with left mesial temporal lobe epilepsy failed to activate left inferior frontal cortex, which the authors suggest may be due to impairment of connections between olfactory and semantic networks.

PET using a $[^{11}C]$-flumazenil tracer has been used to probe $GABA_A$ receptor expression. In a group of patients with focal epilepsy from all lobes, flumazenil binding was inversely correlated with seizure frequency in the frontal piriform cortex (151). The finding that people with more seizures have the weaker expression of $GABA_A$ receptors, suggests that altered GABAergic inhibition in the piriform cortex may be a consequence of increased seizure frequency, and potentially even a cause for frequent seizures.

CAN STIMULATION OF THE PIRIFORM CORTEX BE USED THERAPEUTICALLY?

ABORTING SEIZURES WITH AN OLFACTORY STIMULUS

As early as 1881, Gowers suggested that the application of a strong aroma, such as ammonia or amyl nitrite, may in some cases arrest the course of a seizure (234). Other historical accounts have described the use of other unpleasant odors such as "shoe-smell" (235). Setting aside any direct pharmacological effect of these odors, a plausible hypothesis is that strong physiological activation of olfactory cortex can temporarily prevent or disrupt the progression of epileptic discharges. An alternative interpretation would be that the smell produces a change in cognitive state, for example alertness, which is less permissive for seizures to evolve.

In a detailed clinical account of this technique, Efron describes a woman with "uncinate" seizures, who had an exceptionally long olfactory prodrome that would reliably evolve into an olfactory hallucination and eventually a generalized convulsion (236, 237). Medial temporal epileptic discharges during her attacks were confirmed using sphenoidal electrodes. Smelling an unpleasant odor in the early phase of her attacks (such as hydrogen sulfide, dimercaprol or jasmine) would reliably prevent the seizure progressing, and she was able to use this approach for seizure control.

Experimental evidence from the amygdala-kindling model supports olfactory stimulation as a plausible treatment. After rats had been fully kindled, olfactory presentation of toluene was effective at preventing seizures (238). Smelling either toluene or ammonia increased the amygdala stimulation threshold for inducing events, and with ammonia the seizure duration was also decreased.

Conversely, there are rare reports of seizures being triggered by an olfactory stimulus. During depth-electrode recording from the amygdala in an awake patient (239), smelling various odors induced an amygdala discharge accompanied by similar symptoms to her usual focal seizures.

The therapeutic use of an odor to abort seizures is unfortunately only applicable to a very small number of patients. It requires that the patient have a long aura phase with preserved awareness where they can take this action, and the even then, the probability of this intervention being successful is unknown. Nonetheless, it does demonstrate an important mechanism of relevance to more invasive treatment approaches.

DEEP BRAIN STIMULATION OF PIRIFORM CORTEX

If physiological stimulation of piriform cortex can interrupt or prevent seizures, then perhaps direct electrical stimulation at this site could have the same effect. Deep brain stimulation (DBS) for focal epilepsy in human beings has shown promising results, particularly with stimulation of the anterior nucleus of the thalamus (240, 241). However, piriform DBS has not been performed in human beings, and only a few studies have been done in experimental animals.

In rats, low-frequency electrical stimulation of the piriform cortex at 1Hz has been used. With an amygdala-kindling model, piriform stimulation inhibits the kindling process (242), and also decreases the incidence of generalized seizures in fully kindled animals. More specifically, this was achieved by stimulation of the ipsilateral central piriform cortex, with contralateral stimulation being less effective (243, 244). On the other hand, when the kindling was initially directed at the piriform cortex, inhibitory piriform stimulation was not effective (245). Therefore, piriform stimulation may be most useful when it is a secondary relay for discharges, rather than the primary epileptogenic site, with the aim being to preventing piriform-mediated amplification and distribution of widespread discharges.

Therefore, whether piriform cortex or endopiriform nucleus DBS may be of any benefit in human focal epilepsy is currently unknown. At a minimum, further studies of DBS to these targets in animal models of epilepsy will be needed to approach this question.

CASE REPORT: SURGICAL TREATMENT OF POSSIBLE PIRIFORM EPILEPSY

Surgical intervention involving the piriform cortex may be beneficial for carefully selected patients, but poses a particular diagnostic and anatomical challenge. Here, we report a 37-year-old woman who had seizures from the second year of life, which consisted of an aura of feeling scared, followed by screaming and wild flailing of all limbs or cycling leg movements. She did not have an olfactory aura. Events were brief, lasting less than 1 min. Ictal scalp EEG showed bitemporal rhythmic delta. High-resolution MRI did not identify any lesion. FDG-PET was non-localizing. One ictal-interictal SPECT suggested right orbitofrontal hyperperfusion.

Video-EEG monitoring was performed with multiple frontal and temporal intracranial electrodes, including a depth-electrode targeting the frontal piriform cortex, placed via the lateral frontal lobe (**Figures 4A,B**). Inter-ictal recordings showed bursts of epileptiform gamma over the orbitofrontal cortex, and spiking at the hippocampus and temporal pole. Sub-clinical electrographic seizures (**Figure 4D**) were recorded from the piriform cortex electrode, showing 1–2 min runs of rhythmic sharp waves. Her stereotyped clinical seizures (**Figure 4E**) showed attenuation and gamma frequencies at the piriform and orbitofrontal electrodes, then an evolving ictal rhythm at these locations and over the right temporal lobe.

A right temporal lobectomy was performed, and was extended into the frontal lobe to remove frontal piriform cortex, along with posterior parts of the inferior frontal gyrus and lateral orbital gyrus. Resection was also extended to remove temporal piriform cortex, the antero-inferior amygdala, and the hippocampus (**Figure 4C**). Histology of the orbitofrontal tissue showed some disorganized architecture and prominent single white matter neurons, interpreted by the neuropathologist as possible focal cortical dysplasia (MCD 1) although no balloon cells or dysmorphic neurons were seen. No tissue abnormality was found in temporal lobe structures.

Following surgery, she had a marked reduction of seizure frequency, from several events per day to occasional and mainly nocturnal events. There was immediate improvement in her

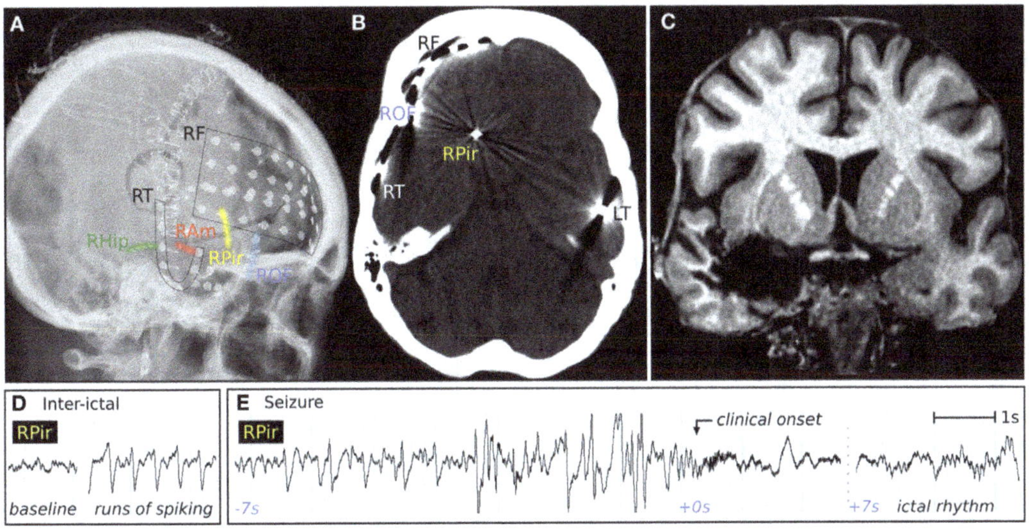

FIGURE 4 | Clinical imaging of a patient with possible piriform epilepsy. **(A)** Lateral skull X-ray showing positions of intracranial electrodes. RF, right frontal subdural electrodes; RT, right temporal subdural electrode strip; RHip, right hippocampal depth electrode; RAm, right amygdala depth electrodes; RPir, right piriform electrodes; ROF, right orbitofrontal subdural electrodes; LT, left temporal subdural electrode strip. **(B)** CT performed in the piriform axis showing the position of the most inferomesial RPir electrode contact, in orbitofrontal cortex adjacent to frontal piriform cortex. **(C)** Coronal T1-weighted MRI, showing posterior extent of surgical resection, with removal of right frontal piriform cortex. **(D)** EEG recorded from most inferomesial RPir electrode, showing trains of inter-ictal spiking, and **(E)** a seizure from sleep, with progressively building discharges, then gamma activity and attenuation, followed 7 s later by an evolving ictal rhythm. At the "clinical onset," there was explosive onset of screaming and flailing movements of the limbs.

responsiveness and speed of processing compared to her preoperative psychomotor slowness. Although the semiology in this case simultaneously suggested frontal lobe (ictal hypermotor activity) and amygdala activity (prolonged episodes of fear), the implantation identified orbitofrontal cortex or frontal piriform cortex as the most likely regions of onset. Resection of these structures was by necessity incomplete, in part because of the dangerous proximity of the middle cerebral artery and other vessels traversing the anterior perforated substance.

DISCUSSION

In this review, we have examined several lines of evidence that associate the piriform cortex with focal epilepsy. The central question is therefore, what role does the piriform cortex play?

It is clearly the generator of seizures in animal models where chemical or electrical stimulation is applied directly to the piriform cortex. The human piriform cortex is very likely to share this exquisite sensitivity to pro-convulsive stimulation. However, only very rare cases of human epilepsy arising directly from piriform cortex have been described, such as that of Mizobuchi et al. (118), and arguably the case report described above.

Conversely, the piriform cortex will be an unrelated bystander in some forms of epilepsy, with no role in seizure onset or spread. Focal seizures from the occipital or parietal lobes may be examples in this category, although only limited data about the piriform cortex has been reported for these patients so far (154, 220, 225).

Of greater clinical relevance, the piriform cortex is a common target of discharge spread, particularly in frontal lobe and temporal lobe epilepsy. This is indicated by the site of lesions that can produce an olfactory epileptic aura (102), the impact of fronto-temporal epilepsy on olfactory function (115), and the detection of piriform cortex activity on EEG-fMRI in these cases (151).

A role for the piriform cortex during human epileptogenesis is probable, but remains to be confirmed. Its tendency to suffer preferential neuronal loss following seizures, as observed in both human status epilepticus (156), and in animal models of induced epilepsy (181), may lead to electrophysiological and local microcircuit changes (185), which result in piriform hyper-excitability. We hypothesize that when the piriform cortex is a target of discharge spread, it can be readily recruited as a secondary hyper-excitable node in the epileptic network by this mechanism. However, inhibition of the piriform cortex only partially blocks the development of epilepsy (86), meaning that it is still possible for epileptogenesis to occur via other less sensitive pathways.

Subsequently the piriform cortex can act as a distributor of epileptic discharges, by facilitating seizures with a limbic origin to spread into olfactory and cortical networks, and vice versa. The evidence for this comes from the amygdala-kindling model of focal epilepsy (3), and clinical descriptions of aura progression (116).

This predisposition of piriform cortex to become involved in focal epilepsy may be understood from the perspective of the architecture that has developed to achieve its normal function. The high inter-connectivity of excitatory neurons provides the basis for a spatially distributed representation of odors, with an intrinsic method for template completion and pattern matching (37). However, this same architecture makes it prone to forming hyper-excitable local networks if local inhibitory circuits are altered or lost. Furthermore, strong reciprocal connectivity to nearby structures such as the olfactory bulb, amygdala, and hippocampus-entorhinal cortex are essential for top-down modulation of olfactory inputs, olfactory memory, and the processing of emotional salience. However, these loops pose the risk of becoming reentrant circuits that sustain seizure activity (3).

Therefore the piriform cortex is highly relevant to the understanding of human focal epilepsy arising from the temporal or frontal lobes. It is a common node of discharge spread, can be injured and kindled by seizure activity, and may be involved in the facilitation and distribution of epileptic discharges throughout limbic and cortical networks. It is a potential target for invasive therapies, including EEG recording and surgical resection, and its unique properties and anatomical relationships must be taken into account.

ACKNOWLEDGMENTS

We thank Prof Matthias Koepp for providing the imaging data for **Figure 3A**. We acknowledge the work of Dr John Archer, Prof Gavin Fabinyi, and Prof Renate Kalnins in providing the electrophysiology, neurosurgery and histopathological data presented in the case report. This study was supported by the National Health and Medical Research Council of Australia (NHMRC Project Grant 628952, Practitioner Fellowship 1060312 and Postgraduate Scholarship 1055877), and by the Operational Infrastructure Support Program of the State Government of Victoria.

REFERENCES

1. Haberly LB. Neuronal circuitry in olfactory cortex: anatomy and functional implications. *Chem Senses* (1985) **10**:219–38. doi:10.1093/chemse/10.2.219
2. Haberly LB, Price JL. Association and commissural fiber systems of the olfactory cortex of the rat. I. Systems originating in the piriform cortex and adjacent areas. *J Comp Neurol* (1978) **178**:711–40. doi:10.1002/cne.901780408
3. Löscher W, Ebert U. The role of the piriform cortex in kindling. *Prog Neurobiol* (1996) **50**:427–81. doi:10.1016/S0301-0082(96)00036-6
4. Giessel AJ, Datta SR. Olfactory maps, circuits and computations. *Curr Opin Neurobiol* (2014) **24**:120–32. doi:10.1016/j.conb.2013.09.010
5. Carmichael ST, Clugnet M-C, Price JL. Central olfactory connections in the macaque monkey. *J Comp Neurol* (1994) **346**:403–34. doi:10.1002/cne.903460306
6. Shipley M, Reyes P. Anatomy of the human olfactory bulb and central olfactory pathways. In: Laing DG, Doty RL, Breipohl W, editors. *The Human Sense of Smell*. Berlin: Springer (1991). p. 29–60.
7. Mai JK, Paxinos G, Voss T. *Atlas of the Human Brain*. Amsterdam: Elsevier (2008).
8. Haberly LB. Comparative aspects of olfactory cortex. In: Jones EG, Peters A, editors. *Cerebral Cortex*. New York, NY: Plenum Press (1990). p. 137–66.
9. Amunts K, Lepage C, Borgeat L, Mohlberg H, Dickscheid T, Rousseau M-É, et al. BigBrain: an ultrahigh-resolution 3d human brain model. *Science* (2013) **340**:1472–5. doi:10.1126/science.1235381
10. Gonçalves Pereira PM, Insausti R, Artacho-Pérula E, Salmenperä T, Kälviäinen R, Pitkänen A. MR volumetric analysis of the piriform cortex and cortical amygdala in drug-refractory temporal lobe epilepsy. *AJNR Am J Neuroradiol* (2005) **26**:319–32. Available from: http://www.ajnr.org/content/26/2/319.long
11. Allison AC. The secondary olfactory areas in the human brain. *J Anat* (1954) **88**:481.
12. Porter J, Anand T, Johnson B, Khan RM, Sobel N. Brain mechanisms for extracting spatial information from smell. *Neuron* (2005) **47**:581–92. doi:10.1016/j.neuron.2005.06.028
13. Royet J-P, Morin-Audebrand L, Cerf-Ducastel B, Haase L, Issanchou S, Murphy C, et al. True and false recognition memories of odors induce distinct neural signatures. *Front Hum Neurosci* (2011) **5**:65. doi:10.3389/fnhum.2011.00065
14. Gottfried JA, Winston JS, Dolan RJ. Dissociable codes of odor quality and odorant structure in human piriform cortex. *Neuron* (2006) **49**:467–79. doi:10.1016/j.neuron.2006.01.007
15. Neville KR, Haberly LB. Olfactory cortex. In: Shepherd GM, editor. *The Synaptic Organization of the Brain*. Oxford: Oxford University Press (2004). p. 415–71.
16. Price JL. An autoradiographic study of complementary laminar patterns of termination of afferent fibers to the olfactory cortex. *J Comp Neurol* (1973) **150**:87–108. doi:10.1002/cne.901500105
17. Suzuki N, Bekkers JM. Neural coding by two classes of principal cells in the mouse piriform cortex. *J Neurosci* (2006) **26**:11938–47. doi:10.1523/jneurosci.3473-06.2006
18. Suzuki N, Bekkers JM. Inhibitory neurons in the anterior piriform cortex of the mouse: classification using molecular markers. *J Comp Neurol* (2010) **518**:1670–87. doi:10.1002/cne.22295
19. Young A, Sun Q-Q. GABAergic inhibitory interneurons in the posterior piriform cortex of the GAD67-GFP mouse. *Cereb Cortex* (2009) **19**:3011–29. doi:10.1093/cercor/bhp072
20. Franks KM, Russo MJ, Sosulski DL, Mulligan AA, Siegelbaum SA, Axel R. Recurrent circuitry dynamically shapes the activation of piriform cortex. *Neuron* (2011) **72**:49–56. doi:10.1016/j.neuron.2011.08.020
21. Luna VM, Schoppa NE. GABAergic circuits control input-spike coupling in the piriform cortex. *J Neurosci* (2008) **28**:8851–9. doi:10.1523/jneurosci.2385-08.2008
22. Stokes CCA, Isaacson JS. From dendrite to soma: dynamic routing of inhibition by complementary interneuron microcircuits in olfactory cortex. *Neuron* (2010) **67**:452–65. doi:10.1016/j.neuron.2010.06.029
23. Suzuki N, Bekkers JM. Microcircuits mediating feedforward and feedback synaptic inhibition in the piriform cortex. *J Neurosci* (2012) **32**:919–31. doi:10.1523/jneurosci.4112-11.2012
24. Behan M, Haberly LB. Intrinsic and efferent connections of the endopiriform nucleus in rat. *J Comp Neurol* (1999) **408**:532–48. doi:10.1002/(SICI)1096-9861(19990614)408:4<532::AID-CNE7>3.3.CO;2-J
25. Ekstrand JJ, Domroese ME, Johnson DM, Feig SL, Knodel SM, Behan M, et al. A new subdivision of anterior piriform cortex and associated deep nucleus with novel features of interest for olfaction and epilepsy. *J Comp Neurol* (2001) **434**:289–307. doi:10.1002/cne.1178
26. Sugai T, Yamamoto R, Yoshimura H, Kato N. Multimodal cross-talk of olfactory and gustatory information in the endopiriform nucleus in rats. *Chem Senses* (2012) **37**:681–8. doi:10.1093/chemse/bjs046
27. Kowianski P, Dziewiatkowski J, Kowianska J, Morys J. Comparative anatomy of the claustrum in selected species: a morphometric analysis. *Brain Behav Evol* (1999) **53**:44–54. doi:10.1159/000006581
28. Crick FC, Koch C. What is the function of the claustrum? *Philos Trans R Soc Lond B Biol Sci* (2005) **360**:1271–9. doi:10.1098/rstb.2005.1661
29. Zhang X, Hannesson D, Saucier D, Wallace A, Howland J, Corcoran M. Susceptibility to kindling and neuronal connections of the anterior claustrum. *J Neurosci* (2001) **21**:3674–87. Available from: http://www.jneurosci.org/content/21/10/3674.long
30. Shepherd GM. The microcircuit concept applied to cortical evolution: from three-layer to six-layer cortex. *Front Neuroanat* (2011) **5**:30. doi:10.3389/fnana.2011.00030
31. Ghosh S, Larson SD, Hefzi H, Marnoy Z, Cutforth T, Dokka K, et al. Sensory maps in the olfactory cortex defined by long-range viral tracing of single neurons. *Nature* (2011) **472**:217–20. doi:10.1038/nature09945
32. Ojima H, Mori K, Kishi K. The trajectory of mitral cell axons in the rabbit olfactory cortex revealed by intracellular HRP injection. *J Comp Neurol* (1984) **230**:77–87. doi:10.1002/cne.902300107
33. Davison IG, Ehlers MD. Neural circuit mechanisms for pattern detection and feature combination in olfactory cortex. *Neuron* (2011) **70**:82–94. doi:10.1016/j.neuron.2011.02.047
34. Wilson DA. Binaral interactions in the rat piriform cortex. *J Neurophysiol* (1997) **78**:160–9.
35. Bouret S, Sara SJ. Locus coeruleus activation modulates firing rate and temporal organization of odour-induced single-cell responses in rat piriform cortex. *Eur J Neurosci* (2002) **16**:2371–82. doi:10.1046/j.1460-9568.2002.02413.x
36. Johnson DM, Illig KR, Behan M, Haberly LB. New features of connectivity in piriform cortex visualized by intracellular injection of pyramidal cells suggest that "primary" olfactory cortex functions like "association" cortex in other sensory systems. *J Neurosci* (2000) **20**:6974–82. Available from: http://www.jneurosci.org/content/20/18/6974.long

37. Ambros-Ingerson J, Granger R, Lynch G. Simulation of paleocortex performs hierarchical clustering. *Science* (1990) **247**:1344–8. doi:10.1126/science.2315702
38. Barnes DC, Hofacer RD, Zaman AR, Rennaker RL, Wilson DA. Olfactory perceptual stability and discrimination. *Nat Neurosci* (2008) **11**:1378–80. doi:10.1038/nn.2217
39. Shipley MT, Ennis M. Functional organization of olfactory system. *J Neurobiol* (1996) **30**:123–76. doi:10.1002/(SICI)1097-4695(199605)30:1<123::AID-NEU11>3.3.CO;2-S
40. Kajiwara R, Tominaga T, Takashima I. Olfactory information converges in the amygdaloid cortex via the piriform and entorhinal cortices: observations in the guinea pig isolated whole-brain preparation. *Eur J Neurosci* (2007) **25**:3648–58. doi:10.1111/j.1460-9568.2007.05610.x
41. Krettek JE, Price JL. Projections from the amygdaloid complex and adjacent olfactory structures to the entorhinal cortex and to the subiculum in the rat and cat. *J Comp Neurol* (1977) **172**:723–52. doi:10.1002/cne.901720409
42. Kuroda M, Murakami K, Kishi K, Price JL. Distribution of the piriform corticalterminals to cells in the central segment of the mediodorsal thalamic nucleus of the rat. *Brain Res* (1992) **595**:159–63. doi:10.1016/0006-8993(92)91468-T
43. Russchen FT, Amaral DG, Price JL. The afferent input to the magnocellular division of the mediodorsal thalamic nucleus in the monkey, *Macaca fascicularis*. *J Comp Neurol* (1987) **256**:175–210. doi:10.1002/cne.902560202
44. Price JL, Slotnick BM, Revial MF. Olfactory projections to the hypothalamus. *J Comp Neurol* (1991) **306**:447–61. doi:10.1002/cne.903060309
45. Kay LM, Sherman SM. An argument for an olfactory thalamus. *Trends Neurosci* (2007) **30**:47–53. doi:10.1016/j.tins.2006.11.007
46. Ramsdell JS, Gulland FM. Domoic acid epileptic disease. *Mar Drugs* (2014) **12**:1185–207. doi:10.3390/md12031185
47. Savic I, Gulyas B, Larsson M, Roland P. Olfactory functions are mediated by parallel and hierarchical processing. *Neuron* (2000) **26**:735–45. doi:10.1016/S0896-6273(00)81209-X
48. Gottfried JA. Central mechanisms of odour object perception. *Nat Rev Neurosci* (2010) **11**:628–41. doi:10.1038/nrn2883
49. Howard JD, Plailly J, Grueschow M, Haynes J-D, Gottfried JA. Odor quality coding and categorization in human posterior piriform cortex. *Nat Neurosci* (2009) **12**:932–8. doi:10.1038/nn.2324
50. Zelano C, Montag J, Khan R, Sobel N. A specialized odor memory buffer in primary olfactory cortex. *PLoS One* (2009) **4**:e4969. doi:10.1371/journal.pone.0004965
51. Nigri A, Ferraro S, D'Incerti L, Critchley HD, Bruzzone MG, Minati L. Connectivity of the amygdala, piriform, and orbitofrontal cortex during olfactory stimulation: a functional MRI study. *Neuroreport* (2013) **24**:171–5. doi:10.1097/WNR.0b013e32835d5d2b
52. Illig KR, Haberly LB. Odor-evoked activity is spatially distributed in piriform cortex. *J Comp Neurol* (2003) **457**:361–73. doi:10.1002/cne.10557
53. Stettler DD, Axel R. Representations of odor in the piriform cortex. *Neuron* (2009) **63**:854–64. doi:10.1016/j.neuron.2009.09.005
54. Litaudon P, Amat C, Bertrand B, Vigouroux M, Buonviso N. Piriform cortex functional heterogeneity revealed by cellular responses to odours. *Eur J Neurosci* (2003) **17**:2457–61. doi:10.1046/j.1460-9568.2003.02654.x
55. Mainland J. The sniff is part of the olfactory percept. *Chem Senses* (2005) **31**:181–96. doi:10.1093/chemse/bjj012
56. Rennaker RL, Chen C-FF, Ruyle AM, Sloan AM, Wilson DA. Spatial and temporal distribution of odorant-evoked activity in the piriform cortex. *J Neurosci* (2007) **27**:1534–42. doi:10.1523/jneurosci.4072-06.2007
57. Bensafi M, Sobel N, Khan RM. Hedonic-specific activity in piriform cortex during odor imagery mimics that during odor perception. *J Neurophysiol* (2007) **98**:3254–62. doi:10.1152/jn.00349.2007
58. González J, Barros-Loscertales A, Pulvermüller F, Meseguer V, Sanjuán A, Belloch V, et al. Reading cinnamon activates olfactory brain regions. *Neuroimage* (2006) **32**:906–12. doi:10.1016/j.neuroimage.2006.03.037
59. Gottfried JA, Smith APR, Rugg MD, Dolan RJ. Remembrance of odors past: human olfactory cortex in cross-modal recognition memory. *Neuron* (2004) **42**:687–95. doi:10.1016/S0896-6273(04)00270-3
60. Veldhuizen MG, Small DM. Modality-specific neural effects of selective attention to taste and odor. *Chem Senses* (2011) **36**:747–60. doi:10.1093/chemse/bjr043
61. Gottfried JA, Zelano C. The value of identity: olfactory notes on orbitofrontal cortex function: olfactory perspectives on OFC function. *Ann N Y Acad Sci* (2011) **1239**:138–48. doi:10.1111/j.1749-6632.2011.06268.x
62. Kringelbach ML, Rolls ET. The functional neuroanatomy of the human orbitofrontal cortex: evidence from neuroimaging and neuropsychology. *Prog Neurobiol* (2004) **72**:341–72. doi:10.1016/j.pneurobio.2004.03.006
63. Zelano C, Mohanty A, Gottfried JA. Olfactory predictive codes and stimulus templates in piriform cortex. *Neuron* (2011) **72**:178–87. doi:10.1016/j.neuron.2011.08.010
64. Tham WWP, Stevenson RJ, Miller LA. The role of the mediodorsal thalamic nucleus in human olfaction. *Neurocase* (2011) **17**:148–59. doi:10.1080/13554794.2010.504728
65. Cohen Y, Wilson DA, Barkai E. Differential modifications of synaptic weights during odor rule learning: dynamics of interaction between the piriform cortex with lower and higher brain areas. *Cereb Cortex* (2013). doi:10.1093/cercor/bht215
66. Plailly J, Howard JD, Gitelman DR, Gottfried JA. Attention to odor modulates thalamocortical connectivity in the human brain. *J Neurosci* (2008) **28**:5257–67. doi:10.1523/JNEUROSCI.5607-07.2008
67. Chu S, Downes JJ. Odour-evoked autobiographical memories: psychological investigations of proustian phenomena. *Chem Senses* (2000) **25**:111–6. doi:10.1093/chemse/25.1.111
68. Kjelvik G, Evensmoen HR, Brezova V, Håberg AK. The human brain representation of odor identification. *J Neurophysiol* (2012) **108**:645–57. doi:10.1152/jn.01036.2010
69. Royet J-P, Plailly J, Delon-Martin C, Kareken DA, Segebarth C. fMRI of emotional responses to odors. *Neuroimage* (2003) **20**:713–28. doi:10.1016/S1053-8119(03)00388-4
70. Winston JS. Integrated neural representations of odor intensity and affective valence in human amygdala. *J Neurosci* (2005) **25**:8903–7. doi:10.1523/jneurosci.1569-05.2005
71. Savic I, Berglund H. Passive perception of odors and semantic circuits. *Hum Brain Mapp* (2004) **21**:271–8. doi:10.1002/hbm.20009
72. Olofsson JK, Rogalski E, Harrison T, Mesulam M-M, Gottfried JA. A cortical pathway to olfactory naming: evidence from primary progressive aphasia. *Brain* (2013) **136**:1245–59. doi:10.1093/brain/awt019
73. Piredda S, Gale K. A crucial epileptogenic site in the deep prepiriform cortex. *Nature* (1985) **317**:623–5. doi:10.1038/317623a0
74. Gale K. Progression and generalization of seizure discharge: anatomical and neurochemical substrates. *Epilepsia* (1988) **29**:S15–34. doi:10.1111/j.1528-1157.1988.tb05795.x
75. Piredda S, Gale K. Role of excitatory amino acid transmission in the genesis of seizures elicited from the deep prepiriform cortex. *Brain Res* (1986) **377**:205–10. doi:10.1016/0006-8993(86)90859-0
76. Tortorella A, Halonen T, Sahibzada N, Gale K. A crucial role of the α-amino-3-hydroxy-5-methylisoxazole-4-propionic acid subtype of glutamate receptors in piriform and perirhinal cortex for the initiation and propagation of limbic motor seizures. *J Pharmacol Exp Ther* (1997) **280**:1401–5.
77. Ebert U, Wlaź P, Löscher W. High susceptibility of the anterior and posterior piriform cortex to induction of convulsions by bicuculline. *Eur J Neurosci* (2000) **12**:4195–205. doi:10.1111/j.1460-9568.2000.01315.x
78. Gale K. Chemoconvulsant seizures: advantages of focally-evoked seizure models. *Ital J Neurol Sci* (1995) **16**:17–25. doi:10.1007/BF02229070
79. Gale K, Dubach M. Localization of area tempestas in the piriform cortex of the monkey. In: AES proceedings. Annual meeting of the American Epilepsy Society, Miami, Florida. *Epilepsia* (1993) **34**(Suppl 6):21.
80. Halonen T, Tortorella A, Zrebeet H, Gale K. Posterior piriform and perirhinal cortex relay seizures evoked from the area tempestas: role of excitatory and inhibitory amino acid receptors. *Brain Res* (1994) **652**:145–8. doi:10.1016/0006-8993(94)90328-X
81. Cassidy RM, Gale K. Mediodorsal thalamus plays a critical role in the development of limbic motor seizures. *J Neurosci* (1998) **18**:9002–9.
82. Eells JB, Clough RW, Browning RA, Jobe PC. Comparative fos immunoreactivity in the brain after forebrain, brainstem, or combined seizures induced by electroshock, pentylenetetrazol, focally induced and audiogenic seizures in rats. *Neuroscience* (2004) **123**:279–92. doi:10.1016/j.neuroscience.2003.08.015

83. Lanaud P, Maggio R, Gale K, Grayson DR. Temporal and spatial patterns of expression of c-fos, zif/268, c-Jun and Jun-B mRNAs in rat brain following seizures evoked focally from the deep prepiriform cortex. *Exp Neurol* (1993) **119**:20–31. doi:10.1006/exnr.1993.1003
84. Maggio R, Lanaud P, Grayson DR, Gale K. Expression of c-fos mRNA following seizures evoked from an epileptogenic site in the deep prepiriform cortex: regional distribution in brain as shown by in situ hybridization. *Exp Neurol* (1993) **119**:11–9. doi:10.1006/exnr.1993.1002
85. Demir R, Haberly LB, Jackson MB. Epileptiform discharges with in-vivo-like features in slices of rat piriform cortex with longitudinal association fibers. *J Neurophysiol* (2001) **86**:2445–60. Available from: http://jn.physiology.org/content/86/5/2445.long
86. Morimoto K, Fahnestock M, Racine RJ. Kindling and status epilepticus models of epilepsy: rewiring the brain. *Prog Neurobiol* (2004) **73**:1–60. doi:10.1016/j.pneurobio.2004.03.009
87. Mohapel P, Zhang X, Gillespie G, Chlan-Fourney J, Hannesson D, Corley S, et al. Kindling of the claustrum and insular cortex: comparison to perirhinal cortex in the rat. *Eur J Neurosci* (2001) **13**:1501–19. doi:10.1046/j.0953-816x.2001.01532.x
88. McIntyre DC, Gilby KL. Mapping seizure pathways in the temporal lobe. *Epilepsia* (2008) **49**(Suppl 3):23–30. doi:10.1111/j.1528-1167.2008.01507.x
89. Honack D, Wahnschaffe U, Loscher W. Kindling from stimulation of a highly sensitive locus in the posterior part of the piriform cortex. Comparison with amygdala kindling and effects of antiepileptic drugs. *Brain Res* (1991) **538**:196–202. doi:10.1016/0006-8993(91)90430-4
90. Löscher W, Ebert U, Wahnschaffe U, Rundfeldt C. Susceptibility of different cell layers of the anterior and posterior part of the piriform cortex to electrical stimulation and kindling: comparison with the basolateral amygdala and "area tempestas". *Neuroscience* (1995) **66**:265–76. doi:10.1016/0306-4522(94)00614-B
91. Cain DP, Corcoran ME, Desborough KA, McKitrick DJ. Kindling in the deep prepyriform cortex of the rat. *Exp Neurol* (1988) **100**:203–9. doi:10.1016/0014-4886(88)90212-9
92. Morimoto K, Dragunow M, Goddard GV. Deep prepyriform cortex kindling and its relation to amygdala kindling in the rat. *Exp Neurol* (1986) **94**:637–48. doi:10.1016/0014-4886(86)90243-8
93. Inoue K, Morimoto K, Sato K, Yamada N, Otsuki S. Mechanisms in the development of limbic status epilepticus and hippocampal neuron loss: an experimental study in a model of status epilepticus induced by kindling-like electrical stimulation of the deep prepyriform cortex in rats. *Acta Med Okayama* (1992) **46**:129–39.
94. White LE, Price JL. The functional anatomy of limbic status epilepticus in the rat. I. Patterns of 14C-2-deoxyglucose uptake and Fos immunocytochemistry. *J Neurosci* (1993) **13**:4787–809.
95. Chapman A, Racine RJ. Piriform cortex efferents to the entorhinal cortex in vivo: kindling-induced potentiation and the enhancement of long-term potentiation by low-frequency piriform cortex or medial septal stimulation. *Hippocampus* (1997) **7**:257–70. doi:10.1002/(SICI)1098-1063(1997)7:3<257:AID-HIPO2>3.0.CO;2-I
96. Elliott B, Joyce E, Shorvon S. Delusions, illusions and hallucinations in epilepsy: 1. Elementary phenomena. *Epilepsy Res* (2009) **85**:162–71. doi:10.1016/j.eplepsyres.2009.03.018
97. Jacek S, Stevenson RJ, Miller LA. Olfactory dysfunction in temporal lobe epilepsy: a case of ictus-related parosmia. *Epilepsy Behav* (2007) **11**:466–70. doi:10.1016/j.yebeh.2007.05.016
98. Daly D. Uncinate fits. *Neurology* (1958) **8**:250–250. doi:10.1212/WNL.8.4.250
99. Jackson JH, Beevor CE. Case of tumour of the right temporosphenoidal lobe bearing on the localisation of the sense of smell and on the interpretation of a particular variety of epilepsy. *Brain* (1889) **12**:346–9. doi:10.1093/brain/12.3.346
100. Jackson JH, Stewart P. Epileptic attacks with a warning of a crude sensation of smell and with the intellectual aura (dreamy state) in a patient who had symptoms pointing to gross organic disease of the right temporo-sphenoidal lobe. *Brain* (1899) **22**:534–49. doi:10.1093/brain/22.4.534
101. Mills CK. The cerebral centers for taste and smell and the uncinate group of fits, based on the study of a case of tumor of the temporal lobe with necropsy. *J Am Med Assoc* (1908) **LI**:879–85. doi:10.1001/jama.1908.25410110001001
102. Acharya V, Acharya J, Lüders H. Olfactory epileptic auras. *Neurology* (1998) **51**:56–61. doi:10.1212/WNL.51.1.56
103. Howe JG, Gibson JD. Uncinate seizures and tumors, a myth reexamined. *Ann Neurol* (1982) **12**:227–227. doi:10.1002/ana.410120238
104. Lennox WG, Cobb S. Epilepsy: XIII. Aura in epilepsy; a statistical review of 1,359 cases. *Arch Neurol Psychiatry* (1933) **30**:374–87. doi:10.1001/archneurpsyc.1933.02240140138007
105. Manford M, Fish DR, Shorvon SD. An analysis of clinical seizure patterns and their localizing value in frontal and temporal lobe epilepsies. *Brain* (1996) **119**:17–40. doi:10.1093/brain/119.1.17
106. Mauguière F. Scope and presumed mechanisms of hallucinations in partial epileptic seizures. *Epileptic Disord* (1999) **1**:81–91.
107. Ye BS, Cho Y-J, Jang SH, Lee MK, Lee BI, Heo K. The localizing and lateralizing value of auras in lesional partial epilepsy patients. *Yonsei Med J* (2012) **53**:477–85. doi:10.3349/ymj.2012.53.3.477
108. Arseni C, Petrovici IN. Epilepsy in temporal lobe tumours. *Eur Neurol* (1971) **5**:201–14. doi:10.1159/000114072
109. Binder DK, Garcia PA, Elangovan GK, Barbaro NM. Characteristics of auras in patients undergoing temporal lobectomy: clinical article. *J Neurosurg* (2009) **111**:1283–9. doi:10.3171/2009.3.JNS081366
110. Chen C, Shih Y-H, Yen D-J, Lirng J-F, Guo Y-C, Yu H-Y, et al. Olfactory auras in patients with temporal lobe epilepsy. *Epilepsia* (2003) **44**:257–60. doi:10.1046/j.1528-1157.2003.25902.x
111. Gupta AK, Jeavons PM, Hughes RC, Covanis A. Aura in temporal lobe epilepsy: clinical and electroencephalographic correlation. *J Neurol Neurosurg Psychiatry* (1983) **46**:1079–83. doi:10.1136/jnnp.46.12.1079
112. Mulder DW, Daly D. Psychiatric symptoms associated with lesions of temporal lobe. *J Am Med Assoc* (1952) **150**:173–6. doi:10.1001/jama.1952.03680030005003
113. Penfield W, Perot P. The brain's record of auditory and visual experience. A final summary and discussion. *Brain* (1963) **86**:595–696. doi:10.1093/brain/86.4.595
114. Fried I, Spencer DD, Spencer SS. The anatomy of epileptic auras: focal pathology and surgical outcome. *J Neurosurg* (1995) **83**:60–6. doi:10.3171/jns.1995.83.1.0060
115. West SE, Doty RL. Influence of epilepsy and temporal lobe resection on olfactory function. *Epilepsia* (1995) **36**:531–42. doi:10.1111/j.1528-1157.1995.tb02565.x
116. Widdess-Walsh P, Kotagal P, Jeha L, Wu G, Burgess R. Multiple auras: clinical significance and pathophysiology. *Neurology* (2007) **69**:755–61. doi:10.1212/01.wnl.0000267650.50269.5d
117. Kasper BS, Kasper EM, Pauli E, Stefan H. Phenomenology of hallucinations, illusions, and delusions as part of seizure semiology. *Epilepsy Behav* (2010) **18**:13–23. doi:10.1016/j.yebeh.2010.03.006
118. Mizobuchi M, Ito N, Tanaka C, Sako K, Sumi Y, Sasaki T. Unidirectional olfactory hallucination associated with ipsilateral unruptured intracranial aneurysm. *Epilepsia* (1999) **40**:516–9. doi:10.1111/j.1528-1157.1999.tb00751.x
119. Geyer JD, Payne TA, Faught E, Drury I. Postictal nose-rubbing in the diagnosis, lateralization, and localization of seizures. *Neurology* (1999) **52**:743–743. doi:10.1212/WNL.52.4.743
120. Weil AA. Depressive reactions associated with temporal lobe-uncinate seizures. *J Nerv Ment Dis* (1955) **121**:505–10. doi:10.1097/00005053-195506000-00002
121. Van Paesschen W, King MD, Duncan JS, Connelly A. The amygdala and temporal lobe simple partial seizures: a prospective and quantitative MRI study. *Epilepsia* (2001) **42**:857–62. doi:10.1046/j.1528-1157.2001.042007857.x
122. Nye E, Arendts G. Intracerebral haemorrhage presenting as olfactory hallucinations. *Emerg Med* (2002) **14**:447–9. doi:10.1046/j.1442-2026.2002.00385.x
123. Andy OJ, Jurko MF, Hughes JR. The amygdala in relation to olfaction. *Confin Neurol* (1975) **37**:215–22. doi:10.1159/000102743
124. Lehrner J, Baumgartner C, Serles W, Olbrich A, Pataraia E, Bacher J, et al. Olfactory prodromal symptoms and unilateral olfactory dysfunction are associated in patients with right mesial temporal lobe epilepsy. *Epilepsia* (1997) **38**:1042–4. doi:10.1111/j.1528-1157.1997.tb01490.x
125. Hirsch LJ, Lain AH, Walczak TS. Postictal nosewiping lateralizes and localizes to the ipsilateral temporal lobe. *Epilepsia* (1998) **39**:991–7. doi:10.1111/j.1528-1157.1998.tb01449.x
126. Leutmezer F, Serles W, Lehrner J, Pataraia E, Zeiler K, Baumgartner C. Postictal nose wiping: a lateralizing sign in temporal lobe complex partial seizures. *Neurology* (1998) **51**:1175–7. doi:10.1212/WNL.51.4.1175

127. Wennberg R. Postictal coughing and noserubbing coexist in temporal lobe epilepsy. *Neurology* (2001) **56**:133–4. doi:10.1212/WNL.56.1.133-a
128. Meletti S, Cantalupo G, Stanzani-Maserati M, Rubboli G, Alberto Tassinari C. The expression of interictal, preictal, and postictal facial-wiping behavior in temporal lobe epilepsy: a neuro-ethological analysis and interpretation. *Epilepsy Behav* (2003) **4**:635–43. doi:10.1016/j.yebeh.2003.09.004
129. Wennberg R. Electroclinical analysis of postictal noserubbing. *Can J Neurol Sci* (2000) **27**:131–6. Available from: http://cjns.metapress.com/content/yjr532r895nw1ayy/fulltext.pdf
130. Catenoix H, Guenot M, Isnard J, Fischer C, Mauguiere F, Ryvlin P. Intracranial EEG study of seizure-associated nose wiping. *Neurology* (2004) **63**:1127–9. doi:10.1212/01.WNL.0000138573.62251.59
131. Baars BJ. Multiple sources of conscious odor integration and propagation in olfactory cortex. *Front Psychol* (2013) **4**:930. doi:10.3389/fpsyg.2013.00930
132. Keller A. Attention and olfactory consciousness. *Front Psychol* (2011) **2**:380. doi:10.3389/fpsyg.2011.00380
133. Bancaud J, Talairach J. Clinical semiology of frontal lobe seizures. *Adv Neurol* (1992) **57**:3–58.
134. Kotagal P, Arunkumar G, Hammel J, Mascha E. Complex partial seizures of frontal lobe onset statistical analysis of ictal semiology. *Seizure* (2003) **12**:268–81. doi:10.1016/S1059-1311(02)00276-5
135. Ludwig BI, Marsan CA, Van Buren J. Depth and direct cortical recording in seizure disorders of extratemporal origin. *Neurology* (1976) **26**:1085–1085. doi:10.1212/WNL.26.11.1085
136. Schneider RC, Crosby EC, Bagchi BK, Calhoun HD. Temporal or occipital lobe hallucinations triggered from frontal lobe lesions. *Neurology* (1961) **11**:172–172. doi:10.1212/WNL.11.2.172
137. Kumar G, Juhász C, Sood S, Asano E. Olfactory hallucinations elicited by electrical stimulation via subdural electrodes: effects of direct stimulation of olfactory bulb and tract. *Epilepsy Behav* (2012) **24**:264–8. doi:10.1016/j.yebeh.2012.03.027
138. King DW, Marsan CA. Clinical features and ictal patterns in epileptic patients with EEG temporal lobe foci. *Ann Neurol* (1977) **2**:138–47. doi:10.1002/ana.410020209
139. Wieser HG. Depth recorded limbic seizures and psychopathology. *Neurosci Biobehav Rev* (1983) **7**:427–40. doi:10.1016/0149-7634(83)90050-7
140. Gil-Nagel A, Risinger MW. Ictal semiology in hippocampal versus extrahippocampal temporal lobe epilepsy. *Brain* (1997) **120**:183–92. doi:10.1093/brain/120.1.183
141. Bancaud J, Brunet-Bourgin F, Chauvel P, Halgren E. Anatomical origin of déjà vu and vivid "memories" in human temporal lobe epilepsy. *Brain* (1994) **117**:71–90. doi:10.1093/brain/117.1.71
142. Munari C, Bancaud J. Electroclinical symptomatology of partial seizures of orbital frontal origin. *Adv Neurol* (1992) **57**:257–65.
143. Greenberg MS. Olfactory hallucinations. In: Serby MH, Chobor KL, editors. *Science of Olfaction*. New York, NY: Springer-Verlag (1992). p. 467–99.
144. Penfield W, Jasper HH. *Epilepsy and The Functional Anatomy of The Human Brain*. Boston: Little, Brown & Co (1954).
145. Van Buren JM. Sensory, motor and autonomic effects of mesial temporal stimulation in man. *J Neurosurg* (1961) **18**:273–88. doi:10.3171/jns.1961.18.3.0273
146. Bartolomei F, Barbeau E, Gavaret M, Guye M, McGonigal A, Régis J, et al. Cortical stimulation study of the role of rhinal cortex in déjà vu and reminiscence of memories. *Neurology* (2004) **63**:858–64. doi:10.1212/01.WNL.0000137037.56916.3F
147. Fish DR, Gloor P, Quesney FL, Oliver A. Clinical responses to electrical brain stimulation of the temporal and frontal lobes in patients with epilepsy Pathophysiological implications. *Brain* (1993) **116**:397–414. doi:10.1093/brain/116.2.397
148. Gloor P, Olivier A, Quesney LF, Andermann F, Horowitz S. The role of the limbic system in experiential phenomena of temporal lobe epilepsy. *Ann Neurol* (1982) **12**:129–44. doi:10.1002/ana.410120203
149. Vaudano AE, Carmichael DW, Salek-Haddadi A, Rampp S, Stefan H, Lemieux L, et al. Networks involved in seizure initiation. A reading epilepsy case studied with EEG-fMRI and MEG. *Neurology* (2012) **79**:249–53. doi:10.1212/WNL.0b013e31825fdf3a
150. Salek-Haddadi A, Mayer T, Hamandi K, Symms M, Josephs O, Fluegel D, et al. Imaging seizure activity: a combined EEG/EMG-fMRI study in reading epilepsy. *Epilepsia* (2009) **50**:256–64. doi:10.1111/j.1528-1167.2008.01737.x
151. Laufs H, Richardson MP, Salek-Haddadi A, Vollmar C, Duncan JS, Gale K, et al. Converging PET and fMRI evidence for a common area involved in human focal epilepsies. *Neurology* (2011) **77**:904–10. doi:10.1212/WNL.0b013e31822c90f2
152. Koubeissi M, Bartolomei F, Abdelrahman B, Picard F. Electrical stimulation of a small brain area reversibly disrupts consciousness. *Epilepsy Behav* (2014) **37**:32–5. doi:10.1016/j.yebeh.2014.05.027
153. Flanagan D, Badawy RAB, Jackson GD. EEG–fMRI in focal epilepsy: local activation and regional networks. *Clin Neurophysiol* (2014) **125**:21–31. doi:10.1016/j.clinph.2013.06.182
154. Fahoum F, Lopes R, Pittau F, Dubeau F, Gotman J. Widespread epileptic networks in focal epilepsies: EEG-fMRI study. *Epilepsia* (2012) **53**:1618–27. doi:10.1111/j.1528-1167.2012.03533.x
155. Kobayashi E, Grova C, Tyvaert L, Dubeau F, Gotman J. Structures involved at the time of temporal lobe spikes revealed by interindividual group analysis of EEG/fMRI data. *Epilepsia* (2009) **50**:2549–56. doi:10.1111/j.1528-1167.2009.02180.x
156. Fujikawa DG, Itabashi HH, Wu A, Shinmei SS. Status epilepticus-induced neuronal loss in humans without systemic complications or epilepsy. *Epilepsia* (2000) **41**:981–91. doi:10.1111/j.1528-1157.2000.tb00283.x
157. Cendes F, Andermann F, Carpenter S, Zatorre RJ, Cashman NR. Temporal lobe epilepsy caused by domoic acid intoxication: evidence for glutamate receptor–mediated excitotoxicity in humans. *Ann Neurol* (1995) **37**:123–6. doi:10.1002/ana.410370125
158. Teitelbaum JS, Zatorre RJ, Carpenter S, Gendron D, Evans AC, Gjedde A, et al. Neurologic sequelae of domoic acid intoxication due to the ingestion of contaminated mussels. *N Engl J Med* (1990) **322**:1781–7. doi:10.1056/NEJM199006213222505
159. Pulido OM. Domoic acid toxicologic pathology: a review. *Mar Drugs* (2008) **6**:180–219. doi:10.3390/md20080010
160. Tiedeken JA, Muha N, Ramsdell JS. A Cupric silver histochemical analysis of domoic acid damage to olfactory pathways following status epilepticus in a rat model for chronic recurrent spontaneous seizures and aggressive behavior. *Toxicol Pathol* (2013) **41**:454–69. doi:10.1177/0192623312453521
161. Curia G, Longo D, Biagini G, Jones RSG, Avoli M. The pilocarpine model of temporal lobe epilepsy. *J Neurosci Methods* (2008) **172**:143–57. doi:10.1016/j.jneumeth.2008.04.019
162. Scorza FA, Arida RM, Naffah-Mazzacoratti Mda G, Scerni DA, Calderazzo L, Cavalheiro EA. The pilocarpine model of epilepsy: what have we learned? *An Acad Bras Cienc* (2009) **81**:345–65. doi:10.1590/S0001-37652009000300003
163. André V, Dubé C, François J, Leroy C, Rigoulot M-A, Roch C, et al. Pathogenesis and pharmacology of epilepsy in the lithium-pilocarpine model. *Epilepsia* (2007) **48**:41–7. doi:10.1111/j.1528-1167.2007.01288.x
164. Wall CJ, Kendall EJ, Obenaus A. Rapid alterations in diffusion-weighted images with anatomic correlates in a rodent model of status epilepticus. *AJNR Am J Neuroradiol* (2000) **21**:1841–52. Available from: http://www.ajnr.org/content/21/10/1841.long
165. Roch C, Leroy C, Nehlig A, Namer IJ. Magnetic resonance imaging in the study of the lithium–pilocarpine model of temporal lobe epilepsy in adult rats. *Epilepsia* (2002) **43**:325–35. doi:10.1046/j.1528-1157.2002.11301.x
166. Sinel'nikova VV, Shubina LV, Gol'tyaev MV, Loseva EV, Kichigina VF. Detection of c-fos expression in the brains of animals with a pilocarpine model of temporal lobe epilepsy. *Neurosci Behav Physiol* (2013) **43**:1084–91. doi:10.1007/s11055-013-9853-6
167. Peredery O, Persinger MA, Parker G, Mastrosov L. Temporal changes in neuronal dropout following inductions of lithium/pilocarpine seizures in the rat. *Brain Res* (2000) **881**:9–17. doi:10.1016/S0006-8993(00)02730-X
168. Druga R, Kubova H, Suchomelova L, Haugvicova R. Lithium/pilocarpine status epilepticus-induced neuropathology of piriform cortex and adjoining structures in rats is age-dependent. *Physiol Res* (2003) **52**:251–64. Available from: http://www.biomed.cas.cz/physiolres/pdf/52/52_251.pdf
169. Chen S, Kobayashi M, Honda Y, Kakuta S, Sato F, Kishi K. Preferential neuron loss in the rat piriform cortex following pilocarpine-induced status epilepticus. *Epilepsy Res* (2007) **74**:1–18. doi:10.1016/j.eplepsyres.2006.11.008
170. de Almeida L, Idiart M, Linster C. A model of cholinergic modulation in olfactory bulb and piriform cortex. *J Neurophysiol* (2013) **109**:1360–77. doi:10.1152/jn.00577.2012
171. Whalley BJ, Postlethwaite M, Constanti A. Further characterization of muscarinic agonist-induced epileptiform bursting activity in immature rat piriform

cortex, in vitro. *Neuroscience* (2005) **134**:549–66. doi:10.1016/j.neuroscience.2005.04.018

172. McDonough JH, Shih T-M. Neuropharmacological mechanisms of nerve agent-induced seizure and neuropathology. *Neurosci Biobehav Rev* (1997) **21**:559–79. doi:10.1016/S0149-7634(96)00050-4
173. Fabene PF, Merigo F, Galiè M, Benati D, Bernardi P, Farace P, et al. Pilocarpine-induced status epilepticus in rats involves ischemic and excitotoxic mechanisms. *PLoS One* (2007) **2**:e1105. doi:10.1371/journal.pone.0001105
174. Covolan L, Mello LEAM. Temporal profile of neuronal injury following pilocarpine or kainic acid-induced status epilepticus. *Epilepsy Res* (2000) **39**:133–52. doi:10.1016/S0920-1211(99)00119-9
175. Candelario-Jalil E, Al-Dalain SM, Castillo R, Martínez G, León Fernández OS. Selective vulnerability to kainate-induced oxidative damage in different rat brain regions. *J Appl Toxicol* (2001) **21**:403–7. doi:10.1002/jat.768
176. Chen S, Buckmaster PS. Stereological analysis of forebrain regions in kainate-treated epileptic rats. *Brain Res* (2005) **1057**:141–52. doi:10.1016/j.brainres.2005.07.058
177. Freichel C, Potschka H, Ebert U, Brandt C, Löscher W. Acute changes in the neuronal expression of GABA and glutamate decarboxylase isoforms in the rat piriform cortex following status epilepticus. *Neuroscience* (2006) **141**:2177–94. doi:10.1016/j.neuroscience.2006.05.040
178. Brandt C, Potschka H, Löscher W, Ebert U. N-methyl-D-aspartate receptor blockade after status epilepticus protects against limbic brain damage but not against epilepsy in the kainate model of temporal lobe epilepsy. *Neuroscience* (2003) **118**:727–40. doi:10.1016/S0306-4522(03)00027-7
179. Myhrer T, Enger S, Aas P. Anticonvulsant impact of lesions in the ventrolateral forebrain of rats challenged with soman. *Brain Res* (2008) **1226**:241–7. doi:10.1016/j.brainres.2008.06.014
180. Ebert U, Rundfeldt C, Löscher W. Development and pharmacological suppression of secondary afterdischarges in the hippocampus of amygdala-kindled rats. *Eur J Neurosci* (1995) **7**:732–41. doi:10.1111/j.1460-9568.1995.tb00677.x
181. Bolkvadze T, Dzhaparidze ND, Zhvaniya MG, Kotariya NT, Tsitsishvili AS. Cellular composition of the piriform cortex of the rat brain in experimental epilepsy. *Neurosci Behav Physiol* (2006) **36**:271–4. doi:10.1007/s11055-006-0010-3
182. Lehmann H, Ebert U, Löscher W. Amygdala-kindling induces a lasting reduction of GABA-immunoreactive neurons in a discrete area of the ipsilateral piriform cortex. *Synapse* (1998) **29**:299–309. doi:10.1002/(SICI)1098-2396(199808)29:4<299::AID-SYN2>3.0.CO;2-0
183. Gernert M, Bloms-Funke P, Ebert U, Löscher W. Kindling causes persistent in vivo changes in firing rates and glutamate sensitivity of central piriform cortex neurons in rats. *Neuroscience* (2000) **99**:217–27. doi:10.1016/S0306-4522(00)00195-0
184. Teskey GC, Racine RJ. Increased spontaneous unit discharge rates following electrical kindling in the rat. *Brain Res* (1993) **624**:11–8. doi:10.1016/0006-8993(93)90054-Q
185. Scott BW, Park H, Han H, Wahidie A, Burnham WM. Extrafocal threshold reductions in amygdala-kindled rats. *Epilepsia* (2010) **51**:1729–35. doi:10.1111/j.1528-1167.2010.02524.x
186. Foster JA, Puchowicz MJ, McIntyre DC, Herkenham M. Activin mRNA induced during amygdala kindling shows a spatiotemporal progression that tracks the spread of seizures. *J Comp Neurol* (2004) **476**:91–102. doi:10.1002/cne.20197
187. Li S, Reinprecht I, Fahnestock M, Racine RJ. Activity-dependent changes in synaptophysin immunoreactivity in hippocampus, piriform cortex, and entorhinal cortex of the rat. *Neuroscience* (2002) **115**:1221–9. doi:10.1016/S0306-4522(02)00485-2
188. Miller HP, Levey AI, Rothstein JD, Tzingounis AV, Conn PJ. Alterations in glutamate transporter protein levels in kindling-induced epilepsy. *J Neurochem* (1997) **68**:1564–70. doi:10.1046/j.1471-4159.1997.68041564.x
189. Henderson AK, Galic MA, Teskey GC. Cortical kindling induces elevated levels of AMPA and GABA receptor subunit mRNA within the amygdala/piriform region and is associated with behavioral changes in the rat. *Epilepsy Behav* (2009) **16**:404–10. doi:10.1016/j.yebeh.2009.08.015
190. Prince HC, Tzingounis AV, Levey AI, Conn PJ. Functional downregulation of GluR2 in piriform cortex of kindled animals. *Synapse* (2000) **38**:489–98. doi:10.1002/1098-2396(20001215)38:4<489:AID-SYN15>3.0.CO;2-N
191. Gavrilovici C, Pollock E, Everest M, Poulter MO. The loss of interneuron functional diversity in the piriform cortex after induction of experimental epilepsy. *Neurobiol Dis* (2012) **48**:317–28. doi:10.1016/j.nbd.2012.07.002
192. Okabe A, Ohno K, Toyoda H, Yokokura M, Sato K, Fukuda A. Amygdala kindling induces upregulation of mRNA for NKCC1, a Na+, K+–2Cl-cotransporter, in the rat piriform cortex. *Neurosci Res* (2002) **44**:225–9. doi:10.1016/S0168-0102(02)00093-7
193. Vessal M, Dugani CB, Solomon DA, McIntyre Burnham W, Ivy GO. Might astrocytes play a role in maintaining the seizure-prone state? *Brain Res* (2005) **1044**:190–6. doi:10.1016/j.brainres.2005.02.058
194. Pollock E, Everest M, Brown A, Poulter MO. Metalloproteinase inhibition prevents inhibitory synapse reorganization and seizure genesis. *Neurobiol Dis* (2014) **70**:21–31. doi:10.1016/j.nbd.2014.06.003
195. Engel J, Wolfson L, Brown L. Anatomical correlates of electrical and behavioral events related to amygdaloid kindling. *Ann Neurol* (1978) **3**:538–44. doi:10.1002/ana.410030615
196. Clark M, Post RM, Weiss SR, Cain CJ, Nakajima T. Regional expression of c-fos mRNA in rat brain during the evolution of amygdala kindled seizures. *Brain Res Mol Brain Res* (1991) **11**:55–64. doi:10.1016/0169-328X(91)90021-O
197. Racine RJ, Mosher M, Kairiss EW. The role of the pyriform cortex in the generation of interictal spikes in the kindled preparation. *Brain Res* (1988) **454**:251–63. doi:10.1016/0006-8993(88)90825-6
198. Schwabe K, Ebert U, Löscher W. Bilateral lesions of the central but not anterior or posterior parts of the piriform cortex retard amygdala kindling in rats. *Neuroscience* (2000) **101**:513–21. doi:10.1016/S0306-4522(00)00407-3
199. Wahnschaffe U, Ebert U, Löscher W. The effects of lesions of the posterior piriform cortex on amygdala kindling in the rat. *Brain Res* (1993) **615**:295–303. doi:10.1016/0006-8993(93)90041-K
200. Racine RJ, Paxinos G, Mosher JM, Kairiss EW. The effects of various lesions and knife-cuts on septal and amygdala kindling in the rat. *Brain Res* (1988) **454**:264–74. doi:10.1016/0006-8993(88)90826-8
201. Stevens JR, Phillips I, de Beaurepaire R. γ-Vinyl GABA in endopiriform area suppresses kindled amygdala seizures. *Epilepsia* (1988) **29**:404–11. doi:10.1111/j.1528-1157.1988.tb03739.x
202. Schwabe K, Ebert U, Löscher W. The central piriform cortex: anatomical connections and anticonvulsant effect of GABA elevation in the kindling model. *Neuroscience* (2004) **126**:727–41. doi:10.1016/j.neuroscience.2004.04.022
203. Namvar S, Mirnajafi-Zadeh J, Fathollahi Y, Zeraati M. The role of piriform cortex adenosine A1 receptors on hippocampal kindling. *Can J Neurol Sci* (2008) **35**:226–31. Available from: http://cjns.metapress.com/content/34R82677JQ3H2404
204. Rezvani ME, Mirnajafi-Zadeh J, Fathollahi Y, Palizvan MR. Anticonvulsant effect of A1 but not A2A adenosine receptors of piriform cortex in amygdala-kindled rats. *Can J Physiol Pharmacol* (2007) **85**:606–12. doi:10.1139/y07-046
205. Wada J, Tsuchimochi H. Role of the claustrum in convulsive evolution of visual afferent and partial nonconvulsive seizures in primates. *Epilepsia* (1997) **38**:897–906. doi:10.1111/j.1528-1157.1997.tb01255.x
206. Kwan P, Arzimanoglou A, Berg AT, Brodie MJ, Allen Hauser W, Mathern G, et al. Definition of drug resistant epilepsy: consensus proposal by the ad hoc Task Force of the ILAE Commission on Therapeutic Strategies. *Epilepsia* (2010) **51**:1069–77. doi:10.1111/j.1528-1167.2009.02397.x
207. Schmidt D, Löscher W. Drug resistance in epilepsy: putative neurobiologic and clinical mechanisms. *Epilepsia* (2005) **46**:858–77. doi:10.1111/j.1528-1167.2005.54904.x
208. Rogawski MA, Johnson MR. Intrinsic severity as a determinant of antiepileptic drug refractoriness. *Epilepsy Curr* (2008) **8**:127–30. doi:10.1111/j.1535-7511.2008.00272.x
209. Berg AT, Langfitt J, Shinnar S, Vickrey BG, Sperling MR, Walczak T, et al. How long does it take for partial epilepsy to become intractable? *Neurology* (2003) **60**:186–90. doi:10.1212/01.WNL.0000031792.89992.EC
210. Kwong KL, Sung WY, Wong SN, So KT. Early predictors of medical intractability in childhood epilepsy. *Pediatr Neurol* (2003) **29**:46–52. doi:10.1016/S0887-8994(03)00028-6
211. Sisodiya SM, Lin W-R, Harding BN, Squier MV, Thom M. Drug resistance in epilepsy: expression of drug resistance proteins in common causes of refractory epilepsy. *Brain* (2002) **125**:22–31. doi:10.1093/brain/awf002
212. Volk HA, Löscher W. Multidrug resistance in epilepsy: rats with drug-resistant seizures exhibit enhanced brain expression of P-glycoprotein compared with rats with drug-responsive seizures. *Brain* (2005) **128**:1358–68. doi:10.1093/brain/awh437
213. Feldmann M, Asselin M-C, Liu J, Wang S, McMahon A, Anton-Rodriguez J, et al. P-glycoprotein expression and function in patients with temporal lobe

epilepsy: a case-control study. *Lancet Neurol* (2013) **12**:777–85. doi:10.1016/S1474-4422(13)70109-1
214. Fang M, Xi Z-Q, Wu Y, Wang X-F. A new hypothesis of drug refractory epilepsy: neural network hypothesis. *Med Hypotheses* (2011) **76**:871–6. doi:10.1016/j.mehy.2011.02.039
215. Grant AC. Interictal perceptual function in epilepsy. *Epilepsy Behav* (2005) **6**:511–9. doi:10.1016/j.yebeh.2005.03.016
216. Eskenazi B, Cain WS, Novelly RA, Mattson R. Odor perception in temporal lobe epilepsy patients with and without temporal lobectomy. *Neuropsychologia* (1986) **24**:553–62. doi:10.1016/0028-3932(86)90099-0
217. Haehner A, Henkel S, Hopp P, Hallmeyer-Elgner S, Reuner U, Reichmann H, et al. Olfactory function in patients with and without temporal lobe resection. *Epilepsy Behav* (2012) **25**:477–80. doi:10.1016/j.yebeh.2012.09.011
218. Kohler CG, Moberg PJ, Gur RE, O'Connor MJ, Sperling MR, Doty RL. Olfactory dysfunction in schizophrenia and temporal lobe epilepsy. *Neuropsychiatry Neuropsychol Behav Neurol* (2001) **14**:83–8.
219. Martinez BA, Cain WS, de Wijk RA, Spencer DD, Novelly RA, Sass KJ. Olfactory functioning before and after temporal lobe resection for intractable seizures. *Neuropsychology* (1993) **7**:351–63. doi:10.1037/0894-4105.7.3.351
220. Savic I, Bookheimer SY, Fried I, Engel J Jr. Olfactory bedside test. A simple approach to identify temporo-orbitofrontal dysfunction. *Arch Neurol* (1997) **54**:162–8. doi:10.1001/archneur.1997.00550140038010
221. Dimov D. [Olfactory function in epilepsy]. *Vestn Otorinolaringol* (1973) **35**:22–3.
222. Kareken DA, Mosnik DM, Doty RL, Dzemidzic M, Hutchins GD. Functional anatomy of human odor sensation, discrimination, and identification in health and aging. *Neuropsychology* (2003) **17**:482–95. doi:10.1037/0894-4105.17.3.482
223. Hudry J. Olfactory short-term memory and related amygdala recordings in patients with temporal lobe epilepsy. *Brain* (2003) **126**:1851–63. doi:10.1093/brain/awg192
224. West SE, Doty RL, O'Connor MJ, Sperling MR. Pre- and post-operative studies of olfactory function in patients with anterior temporal lobectomy. In: Proceedings of the Fifteenth Annual Meeting of the Association for Chemoreception Sciences, Sarasota, Florida. *Chem Senses* (1993) **21**:649.
225. Carroll B, Richardson JT, Thompson P. Olfactory information processing and temporal lobe epilepsy. *Brain Cogn* (1993) **22**:230–43. doi:10.1006/brcg.1993.1036
226. Abraham A, Mathai KV. The effect of right temporal lobe lesions on matching of smells. *Neuropsychologia* (1983) **21**:277–81. doi:10.1016/0028-3932(83)90045-3
227. Rausch R, Serafetinides EA, Crandall PH. Olfactory memory in patients with anterior temporal lobectomy. *Cortex* (1977) **13**:445–52. doi:10.1016/S0010-9452(77)80024-5
228. Gordon HW, Sperry RW. Lateralization of olfactory perception in the surgically separated hemispheres of man. *Neuropsychologia* (1969) **7**:111–20. doi:10.1016/0028-3932(69)90009-8
229. Savage R, Combs DR, Pinkston JB, Advokat C, Gouvier WD. The role of temporal lobe and orbitofrontal cortices in olfactory memory function. *Arch Clin Neuropsychol* (2002) **17**:305–18. doi:10.1016/S0887-6177(01)00114-7
230. Hummel T, Henkel S, Negoias S, Galván JRB, Bogdanov V, Hopp P, et al. Olfactory bulb volume in patients with temporal lobe epilepsy. *J Neurol* (2013) **260**:1004–8. doi:10.1007/s00415-012-6741-x
231. Centeno M, Vollmar C, Stretton J, Symms MR, Thompson PJ, Richardson MP, et al. Structural changes in the temporal lobe and piriform cortex in frontal lobe epilepsy. *Epilepsy Res* (2014) **108**:978–81. doi:10.1016/j.eplepsyres.2014.03.001
232. Hummel T, Pauli E, Schüler P, Kettenmann B, Stefan H, Kobal G. Chemosensory event-related potentials in patients with temporal lobe epilepsy. *Epilepsia* (1995) **36**:79–85. doi:10.1111/j.1528-1157.1995.tb01670.x
233. Ciumas C, Lindström P, Aoun B, Savic I. Imaging of odor perception delineates functional disintegration of the limbic circuits in mesial temporal-lobe epilepsy. *Neuroimage* (2008) **39**:578–92. doi:10.1016/j.neuroimage.2007.09.004
234. Gowers W. *Epilepsy and Other Chronic Convulsive Disorders: Their Causes, Symptoms and Treatment.* London: J & A Churchill (1881).
235. Jaseja H. Scientific basis behind traditional practice of application of "shoe-smell" in controlling epileptic seizures in the eastern countries. *Clin Neurol Neurosurg* (2008) **110**:535–8. doi:10.1016/j.clineuro.2008.02.006
236. Efron R. The effect of olfactory stimuli in arresting uncinate fits. *Brain* (1956) **79**:267–81. doi:10.1093/brain/79.2.267
237. Efron R. The conditioned inhibition of uncinate fits. *Brain* (1957) **80**:251–62. doi:10.1093/brain/80.2.251
238. Ebert U, Löscher W. Strong olfactory stimulation reduces seizure susceptibility in amygdala-kindled rats. *Neurosci Lett* (2000) **287**:199–202. doi:10.1016/S0304-3940(00)01161-7
239. Hughes JR, Andy OJ. The human amygdala. I. Electrophysiological responses to odorants. *Electroencephalogr Clin Neurophysiol* (1979) **46**:428–43. doi:10.1016/0013-4694(79)90144-5
240. Pereira EAC, Green AL, Stacey RJ, Aziz TZ. Refractory epilepsy and deep brain stimulation. *J Clin Neurosci* (2012) **19**:27–33. doi:10.1016/j.jocn.2011.03.043
241. Wyckhuys T, Geerts PJ, Raedt R, Vonck K, Wadman W, Boon P. Deep brain stimulation for epilepsy: knowledge gained from experimental animal models. *Acta Neurol Belg* (2009) **109**:63–80. Available from: http://www.actaneurologica.be/acta/download/2009-2/01-wyckhuys%20et%20al.pdf
242. Esmaeilpour K, Masoumi-Ardakani Y, Sheibani V, Shojaei A, Harandi S, Mirnajafi-Zadeh J. Comparing the anticonvulsant effects of low frequency stimulation of different brain sites on the amygdala kindling acquisition in rats. *Basic Clin Neurosci* (2013) **4**:68–74. Available from: http://bcn.iums.ac.ir/browse.php?a_code=A-10-1-170&slc_lang=en&sid=1
243. Yang L-X, Jin C-L, Zhu-Ge Z-B, Wang S, Wei E-Q, Bruce IC, et al. Unilateral low-frequency stimulation of central piriform cortex delays seizure development induced by amygdaloid kindling in rats. *Neuroscience* (2006) **138**:1089–96. doi:10.1016/j.neuroscience.2005.12.006
244. Zhu-Ge Z-B, Zhu Y-Y, Wu D-C, Wang S, Liu L-Y, Hu W-W, et al. Unilateral low-frequency stimulation of central piriform cortex inhibits amygdaloid-kindled seizures in Sprague–Dawley rats. *Neuroscience* (2007) **146**:901–6. doi:10.1016/j.neuroscience.2007.02.014
245. Ghorbani P, Mohammad-Zadeh M, Mirnajafi-Zadeh J, Fathollahi Y. Effect of different patterns of low-frequency stimulation on piriform cortex kindled seizures. *Neurosci Lett* (2007) **425**:162–6. doi:10.1016/j.neulet.2007.08.023

8

Temporal lobe epilepsy and surgery selectively alter the dorsal, not the ventral, default-mode network

Gaelle Eve Doucet*[1,2]*, Christopher Skidmore*[1]*, James Evans*[2]*, Ashwini Sharan*[2]*, Michael R. Sperling*[1]*, Dorian Pustina*[1]* and Joseph I. Tracy*[1]**

[1] Department of Neurology, Thomas Jefferson University, Philadelphia, PA, USA
[2] Department of Neurosurgery, Thomas Jefferson University, Philadelphia, PA, USA

***Correspondence:**
Joseph I. Tracy, Cognitive Neuroscience and Brain Imaging Laboratory, Department of Neurology, Jefferson Medical College, Thomas Jefferson University, 901 Walnut Street, Suite 447, Philadelphia, PA 19107, USA
e-mail: joseph.tracy@jefferson.edu

The default-mode network (DMN) is a major resting-state network. It can be divided in two distinct networks: one is composed of dorsal and anterior regions [referred to as the dorsal DMN (dDMN)], while the other involves the more posterior regions [referred to as the ventral DMN (vDMN)]. To date, no studies have investigated the potentially distinct impact of temporal lobe epilepsy (TLE) on these networks. In this context, we explored the effect of TLE and anterior temporal lobectomy (ATL) on the dDMN and vDMN. We utilized two resting-state fMRI sessions from left, right TLE patients (pre-/post-surgery) and normal controls (sessions 1/2). Using independent component analysis, we identified the two networks. We then evaluated for differences in spatial extent for each network between the groups, and across the scanning sessions. The results revealed that, pre-surgery, the dDMN showed larger differences between the three groups than the vDMN, and more particularly between right and left TLE than between the TLE patients and controls. In terms of change post-surgery, in both TLE groups, the dDMN also demonstrated larger changes than the vDMN. For the vDMN, the only changes involved the resected temporal lobe for each ATL group. For the dDMN, the left ATL group showed post-surgical increases in several regions outside the ictal temporal lobe. In contrast, the right ATL group displayed a large reduction in the frontal cortex. The results highlight that the two DMNs are not impacted by TLE and ATL in an equivalent fashion. Importantly, the dDMN was the more affected, with right ATL having a more deleterious effects than left ATL. We are the first to highlight that the dDMN more strongly bears the negative impact of TLE than the vDMN, suggesting there is an interaction between the side of pathology and DM sub-network activity. Our findings have implications for understanding the impact TLE and subsequent ATL on the functions implemented by the distinct DMNs.

Keywords: default-mode network, dorsal and ventral subdivisions, temporal lobe epilepsy, anterior temporal lobectomy, resting-state, fMRI

INTRODUCTION

The default-mode network (DMN) has been identified as one of the most robust and consistent resting-state network [see review of Ref. (1, 2)]. While much about its function remains unclear, research has suggested it is engaged in the maintenance of "tonic" or baseline cognitive processing related to self-awareness, episodic memory, or the modulation of internal (mental) versus external tasks. Others have linked it to anticipatory cognitive processes, the strength of cognitive reserve, or consciousness [see review of Ref. (1)]. Most recently, there has been new evidence that this network is also modulated by the nature of the spontaneous thoughts during a conscious resting-state (3, 4). It primarily consists of posterior cingulate cortex (PCC)/precuneus, ventral anterior cingulate cortex (ACC)/mesial prefrontal cortex, angular gyri, lateral temporal cortex, and mesial temporal lobes. However, a growing number of studies consider this network to be comprised of at least two functionally distinct subdivisions (5, 6): one is composed of dorsal and anterior regions [referred to as the dorsal DMN (dDMN)], and appears active when people engage in self-relevant decisions or affectively laden cognitive processes. The second division involves posterior and mesial temporal regions [referred to as the ventral DMN (vDMN)], and engages during decision-making related to constructing a mental scene, particularly a scene called up from episodic or semantic memory.

Investigated as a functional marker for neurological pathologies, several studies have reported that DMN activity is, indeed, altered by neurologic pathologies such as Alzheimer's disease (7) or schizophrenia (8). Given the role of the DMN in temporal lobe functions such as memory processing and conscious awareness, increasing our understanding of temporal lobe epilepsy (TLE) will require sophisticated analysis of this disorder's impact on the DMN. With regard to epilepsy, this network has been described as perturbed during both ictal (and subsequently, transitory loss of consciousness) (9) and interictal (10–13) states. To our knowledge, however, only a few studies have specifically investigated the DMN in unilateral TLE patients at rest through fMRI (10–12). Existing studies demonstrate abnormal reduced activity in this network compared to healthy controls, with distinct effects depending on the hemisphere with epileptic pathology. The effects of the standard surgery for intractable epilepsy [e.g., anterior temporal lobectomy (ATL)] on the DMN are still largely unknown. Indeed, to date, only one study has investigated this network and its changes prior to and after epilepsy surgery (10). In this study, McCormick et al. described connectivity changes involving the precuneus post-surgery relative to pre-surgery. These authors, however, did not explore the two specific sub-networks (dDMN and vDMN). Therefore, questions remain as to how the DMN subdivisions may be differentially affected by the resection of the temporal lobe, the laterality of the pathology, and the potential neuroplastic or compensatory responses generated post-surgery. In this sense, ATL provides a valuable model for testing the impact of structural changes in the DMN, as this procedure includes resection of several parts of the network, most notably the lateral and the mesial temporal regions.

In this context, we sought to expand our knowledge about the effect of both TLE and ATL on the DMN's subdivisions (dDMN and vDMN). We utilize resting-state fMRI data from 29 unilateral TLE patients (13 left, 16 right), who underwent standard en bloc resection of their epileptogenic temporal lobe (standard ATL), and 14 healthy matched controls. Using group independent component analysis (ICA), we identified the ventral and dDMNs. We hypothesized that the spatial extent of each DMN subdivision will differ between left and right TLE patients. More specifically, we expected that the left TLE patients will show more abnormalities than the right TLE, as it has been suggested that left TLE patients generally have more functional impairments at rest than right-sided patients (14, 15). We also hypothesized that ATL surgery will not affect the two networks in the same manner, as it will remove distinct regions in the temporal lobe within each network. We expected the vDMN to show more changes that the dDMN as it is this sub-network that includes the epileptogenic mesial temporal lobe, potentially fostering distinct neuroplasticity mechanisms and compensatory responses. It will increase our understanding of the neuroplasticity responses that one can expect to emerge for each DMN network post-surgery.

MATERIALS AND METHODS

PARTICIPANTS

A total of 14 healthy age-matched controls and 29 patients with refractory unilateral TLE (13 left and 16 right) were recruited from the Thomas Jefferson University Comprehensive Epilepsy Center. All the patients underwent a standard en bloc ATL to remove their epileptogenic temporal lobe. In detail, this surgery included a unilateral ATL and amygdalohippocampectomy [approximately 4–6 cm from the temporal pole with the size smaller for the left (language dominant) temporal lobe patients]. Note that all of our participants, controls and patients, were left hemisphere (LH) dominant as verified by task-fMRI (e.g., verb generation procedure). Details of the Thomas Jefferson Comprehensive Epilepsy Center algorithm for surgical decision-making are described by Sperling et al. (16). A combination of video/surface EEG (at least 96 h), MRI, PET, and neuropsychological testing was used to lateralize the side of seizure focus. All patient participants met the following inclusion criteria: unilateral temporal lobe seizure focus, concordant MRI, and/or PET findings of temporal lobe abnormality with no non-concordant data. TLE patients were excluded from the study for any of the following reasons: previous brain surgery; extra-temporal lesions; medical illness with central nervous system impact other than epilepsy; extra-temporal or multi-focal epilepsy; contraindications to MRI; psychiatric diagnosis other than an axis-I depression or anxiety disorder; or hospitalization for any axis-I disorder listed in the Diagnostic and Statistical Manual of Mental Disorders, IV. Patients provided written informed consent. **Table 1** outlines the patients' demographic and clinical characteristics.

Healthy normal controls (NCs) were recruited from the Thomas Jefferson University community, in order to match the patient participants in age and gender. All controls were free of psychiatric or neurological (central nervous system) disorders based on a health screening measure. This study was approved by the Institutional Review Board for Research with Human Subjects at Thomas Jefferson University and all participants provided a written informed consent.

MRI DATA ACQUISITION

All participants underwent magnetic resonance imaging on a 3-T X-series Philips Achieva clinical MRI scanner (Amsterdam, the Netherlands) using an 8-channel head coil. Both the NCs and the TLE patients underwent two identical fMRI scanning sessions. In detail, each patient underwent one pre-surgical (mean = 217 days prior to surgery) and one post-surgical ($m = 530$ days after surgery, minimum of 6 months) scan, while the NCs participated in two fMRI sessions, with parameters identical to the TLE patients at a time interval of at least 6 months. A total of 5 min of a resting-state condition was collected from all participants. Anatomical and functional acquisitions were similar for all patients. A single shot echoplanar gradient echo imaging sequence acquiring T2* signal was used with the following parameters: 120 volumes, 34 axial slices acquired parallel to the AC–PC line, TR = 2.5 s, TE = 35 ms, FOV = 256 mm, 128 × 128 data matrix isotropic voxels, flip angle = 90°, bandwidth = 1.802 (±241.1 kHz). The in-plane resolution was 2 mm × 2 mm and the slice thickness was 4 mm. Prior to collection of the T2* images, T1-weighted images (180 slices) were collected using an MPRage sequence (256 × 256 isotropic voxels; TR = 640 ms, TE = 3.2 ms, FOV = 256 mm, flip angle = 8°) in positions identical to the functional scans to provide an anatomical reference. The in-plane resolution for each T1 slice was 1 mm × 1 mm × 1 mm (axial oblique; angle following the anterior, posterior commissure line). Survey and field reference inhomogeneity images were collected prior to the start of the study. Each EPI imaging series started with three discarded scans to allow for T1 signal stabilization. Subjects lay in a foam pad to comfortably stabilize the head, were instructed to remain still throughout the scan, not fall asleep, and keep their eyes closed during the entirety of the scan.

IMAGE PROCESSING

Data from the patients (pre- and post-surgery scans) and NCs (sessions 1 and 2) were preprocessed identically using SPM8[1]. Slice timing correction was used to adjust for variable acquisition time

[1] http://www.fil.ion.ucl.ac.uk/spm/software/spm8

Table 1 | Clinical information and characteristics of the patients.

Pathology	Participants	Gender	Age at the pre-surgery scan date (years)	Age at seizure onset	Seizure type	Temporal pathology[a]	Duration of first scan-surgery (days)	Duration of second scan-surgery (days)	Seizure outcome class
Left TLE	1	M	56.4	16	SPS; rare CPS	Cavernoma	38	915	1
Left TLE	2	F	43.9	3	CPS; rare GTCS	HS	311	251	1
Left TLE	3	F	60.2	53	CPS/SPS	Mild subpial gliosis, no HS	90	1062	1
Left TLE	4	M	35.9	20	CPS	Gliosis and HS	61	1055	1
Left TLE	5	F	41.2	5	CPS/SPS	Gliosis and HS	586	181	5
Left TLE	6	F	42.3	38	CPS	Gliosis and HS	19	244	1
Left TLE	7	F	60.5	13	CPS	Gliosis and HS	34	364	1
Left TLE	8	M	60.0	50	CPS	Gliosis and HS	23	237	1
Left TLE	9	F	25.4	18	CPS with sec GTCS	Low grade glioma	200	238	1
Left TLE	10	F	31.3	14	CPS	Mild gliosis and HS	14	1705	1
Left TLE	11	F	34.7	19	CPS/SPS	Mild subpial gliosis, no HS	42	890	1
Left TLE	12	F	52.2	42	CPS	Gliosis and cavernous angioma	25	1360	1
Left TLE	13	M	34.1	31	CPS/GTCS	Gliosis, no HS	68	208	1
Right TLE	1	F	48.2	16	CPS/SPS	Gliosis and HS	172	787	1
Right TLE	2	F	33.1	2	CPS/rare GTCS	Gliosis and HS	76	641	1
Right TLE	3	F	30.0	10	CPS	Gliosis, no HS	271	530	1
Right TLE	4	F	26.0	21	CPS	Gliosis, cortical dysplasia	36	398	1
Right TLE	5	F	52.4	11	CPS/sec GTCS	Gliosis	64	227	2
Right TLE	6	M	55.3	5	CPS; rare sec GTCS	Gliosis and HS	38	159	1
Right TLE	7	M	57.5	27	CPS	Gliosis, no HS	628	282	2
Right TLE	8	M	28.1	16	CPS	Gliosis	35	255	1
Right TLE	9	M	25.6	19	CPS/SPS	Gliosis	23	245	3
Right TLE	10	M	65.3	20	CPS	Gliosis and HS	36	243	1
Right TLE	11	F	29.7	27	CPS/SPS	Mild gliosis	472	146	4
Right TLE	12	M	39.6	35	CPS	Mild gliosis	101	169	4
Right TLE	13	F	34.5	32	CPS	Gliosis	886	548	1
Right TLE	14	F	47.5	34	CPS	Mild gliosis	109	329	1
Right TLE	15	F	23.4	17	CPS	Gliosis	1451	1391	1
Right TLE	16	M	60.0	51	CPS/GTCS	Gliosis	394	297	2

F, female; M, male; HS, hippocampal sclerosis; CPS, complex partial seizures; SPS, simple partial seizures; sec GTCS, secondarily generalized tonic/clonic seizures. The seizure outcome classification, from class 1 to 4 is based on the Engel classification (25), class 5 reflects the presence of post-operative pseudo-seizures.
[a]Temporal pathology resulted from the surgical pathology report regarding the resected tissue after the ATL.

over slices in a volume, with the middle slice in every volume used as reference. Next, a six-parameter variance cost-function rigid body affine registration was used to realign all images within a session to the first volume. Motion regressors were computed and later used as regressors of no interest. To maximize mutual information, co-registration between functional scans and the MNI305 (Montreal Neurological Institute) template was carried out using six iterations and re-sampled with a seventh-degree B-spline interpolation. Functional images were then normalized and warped into standard space (MNI305) to allow for signal averaging across subjects. We utilized the standard normalization method in SPM8, which minimizes the sum-of-squared differences between the subject's image and the template (MNI305), while maximizing the prior probability of the transformation. This spatial normalization provided a reliable matching to the MNI template without causing aberrant distortions in the images, both in patients with no brain lesions and those having brain resections and abnormal signal (17). This enabled us to compare brain structures and define the same seed region (see next step) between pre- and post-surgical data. Segmentation of the data in the gray matter, white matter

(WM), and cerebro-spinal fluid (CSF) classes was also carried out. All normalized images were smoothed by convolution with a Gaussian kernel, with a full width at half maximum of 8 mm in all directions. For each individual, the time-courses of both WM and CSF were estimated in the relevant brain tissue classes defined at the segmentation step. Sources of spurious variance were then removed from the data through linear regression: six parameters obtained by rigid body correction of head motion and the CSF and WM signals. Finally, fMRI data were temporally filtered using the REST Toolbox (low cutoff frequency = 0.008 Hz – high cutoff frequency = 0.1 Hz) (18, 19). As head motion has been reported to potentially influence resting-state results (20), we utilized t-tests to check for differences either across scanning sessions or between our experimental groups. For each individual, we computed the maximum difference (i.e., minimum to maximum) within each of the six realignment parameters computed during preprocessing. No significant differences were observed either across the scanning sessions (pre- to post-) or between the experimental groups (Bonferroni corrected for the six parameters, for an effective alpha of $p = 0.05$).

STATISTICAL ANALYSES

Independent component analysis

Spatial probabilistic ICA (temporal concatenation method) was used to identify resting-state networks. Briefly, preprocessed images from each scan (a total of 86 inputs) were entered into the FMRIB software library (FSL) 4.0.8 Melodic ICA software[2] (21). This technique performs a spatio-temporal decomposition of the signal without any *a priori* seed, by simultaneously analyzing data from all the subjects (22). We used the Laplace approximation to estimate the number of components. The output resulted in 16 independent components (ICs) common for the entire group of participants. Each IC was associated with a Z-map and a time-series. Also, for each component, an effect size value is available for each participant, indicative of the strength of the component in each subject's data. Each map was thresholded at a posterior probability threshold of $p = 0.5$, using an alternative hypothesis-testing approach based on the fit of a Gaussian/Gamma mixture model (22). In a second step, based on these group ICs, we then applied a dual regression approach to characterize each IC in each subject, through a Z-map and an individual time-series (23).

[2]http://fsl.fmrib.ox.ac.uk/fsl/fslwiki/

Selection of the dorsal and ventral default-mode networks

Based on this group decomposition, we identified the two best-fit components for the dDMN and vDMN (**Figure 1**). For this, we computed the goodness-of-fit (GOF) for each IC, using the dDMN and vDMN templates provided by Shirer et al. (24). In detail, applying Greicius et al.'s method, a linear template-matching procedure was used, which takes the average z-score of voxels falling within the template minus the average z-score of voxels outside the template (7). These best-fit components reflect the degree to which their best-fit component network matched the default-mode networks template.

The IC selected as the best-fit for the dDMN (**Figure 1A**) includes a major cluster in the medial prefrontal cortex/ACC, the bilateral caudate nuclei. To a lesser degree, the PCC was also included as well as the right angular gyrus, the left superior temporal cortex, and right calcarine. The IC selected as the best-fit for the vDMN (**Figure 1B**) includes a large cluster in the medial parietal cortex, including the precuneus, PCC, and retrosplenial cortex. Bilateral angular gyri, the anterior ventral area of the medial prefrontal cortex as well as bilateral parahippocampal gyri (more extensive on the left), bilateral inferior temporal cortices, and bilateral superior/middle frontal cortices were also part of the vDMN.

Computation of goodness-of-fit or each individual network

After identifying the two best-fit networks, we computed the GOF for each network and each individual. These GOFs were used to indicate the fit or degree to which each individual's network was normative, with a higher GOF indicating a more normative network. These procedures yielded four GOF values for each individual (two pre-surgery and two post-surgery, one for each network). A repeated-measure ANOVA was run to test the effects

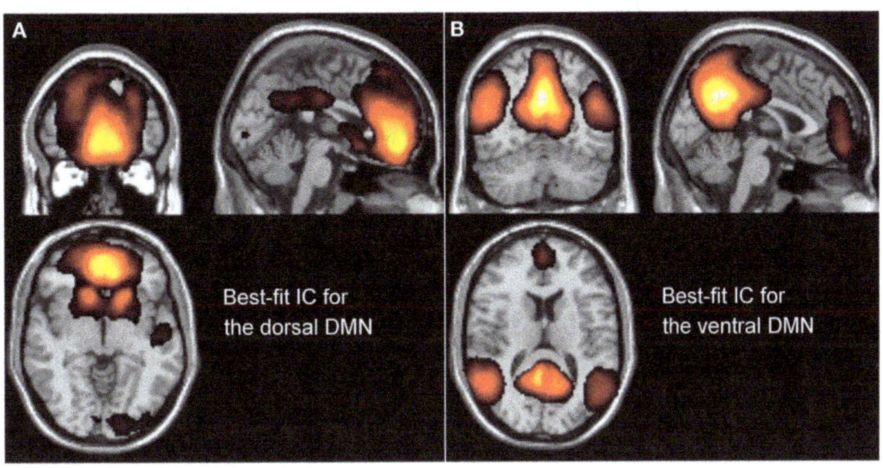

FIGURE 1 | Description of the best-fit independent components (ICs) for the dorsal DMN (A) and ventral DMN (B), resulted from the group ICA.

of sessions (pre-/post-surgery for patients, or session one and two for the NCs) and experimental group (RTLE, LTLE, NCs) on the GOF, run separately for each network.

Regional differences

At the group level, statistical analyses were computed in order to determine spatial extent differences for each network between the groups and the sessions. For this, individual Z-maps were entered into a second-level random-effects analyses, for each network separately. The first analysis was done on the pre-surgery data only. In other words, we tested the differences between the three experimental groups, pre-surgery, for each DMN subdivision independently. Second, to analyze within-subject pre- to post-surgery changes, a difference image was created for each participant. This image was obtained by subtracting pre- to post-surgery Z-maps, for each subject and each network. This allowed us to test both for decreases (pre > post-surgery) and increases (post > pre-surgery) in spatial extent across the scanning sessions. As the number of days between the two scans was significantly different between the groups (see Results), we added this as a continuous variable, a covariate of no-interest, in the model. Each comparison was restricted to changes involving positive voxels losing or gaining their engagement in the network of interest. In other words, we did not report the clusters of voxels remaining below the threshold defining during the ICA (posterior probability threshold of $p = 0.5$; corresponding to a $Z = 1.9$ and 2.2 for the dorsal and vDMN, respectively) at both sessions despite a possible significant change between the two sessions, as any such pattern would indicate the regions were not part of the network of interest at either session.

In order to avoid any confounding effect between normal and true post-surgery changes, we utilized two independent additional analyses. First, at the whole-brain level, we recomputed the relevant patient contrast (i.e., post- versus pre-surgery), and applied an exclusive mask involving the regions associated with significant changes between the two sessions for the control group ($p < 0.001$, uncorrected). Second, for each cluster showing a significant change in either patient group, we computed the averaged Z-values in the control group and computed a paired t-test between the two sessions. Any clusters significant in the control group were excluded, as these would represent normative, not patient related, changes, and, therefore, are not presented in the Section "Results."

Lastly, the height threshold of the statistical analyses was fixed at $p < 0.001$ (uncorrected, $T > 3.31$) and the spatial extent threshold at 50 voxels minimum for a cluster (e.g., corresponding to a corrected alpha level of $p < 0.045$).

Correlation with clinical characteristics

Lastly, we computed Pearson correlations to test the relation between the age of seizure onset and the GOFs, within each patient group. Also, regarding the analysis of regional differences, age of seizure onset was added as a covariate in the second-level analyses in order to test potential effects on pre-surgery DMN activity.

RESULTS

BEHAVIORAL DATA

The three experimental groups did not differ by age ($p = 0.7$), nor gender ($p = 0.09$). With regard to the patient groups, the RTLE and LTLE groups did not differ by age of seizure onset, illness duration, number of anti-epileptic drugs (pre- or post-surgery), presence/absence of unilateral mesial temporal sclerosis (MTS) (pre-surgery), nor the time interval between the fMRI scans and surgery (**Table 1**). With regards to the specialization of the LH for language, the left TLE patients had a smaller resection than the right TLE patients. However, this difference was not significantly different between the patient groups. Regarding the seizure outcome of the patients, we used a classification based on the Engel classes [class I–IV; (25)], with an additional class V reflecting the report of post-operative pseudo-seizures. Overall, all of the LTLE patients were seizure free (Engel class I, at least 1 year after surgery), except one who was in class V at 1 year (e.g., reporting pseudo-seizures with no epileptic seizures). For the RTLE group, 14 of 16 patients also had a good seizure outcome [classes I ($N = 10$), II ($N = 3$), or III ($N = 1$)], with two patients in class IV with no change in seizure frequency (see **Table 1**).

The only difference that emerged between the groups involved the number of days between the two scans ($p = 0.02$). In detail, the time interval between scans was shorter for the control group ($m = 380$ days), than for the LTLE ($m = 786$ days; $p = 0.02$), but not for the RTLE group ($m = 609$ days, $p = 0.3$). Note that the TLE groups did not differ ($p = 0.6$). To correct for this difference, the time interval between scans variable was added as a covariate of no interest in the second-level analysis involving pre- versus post-surgery comparisons.

GOODNESS-OF-FIT ANALYSES

A repeated-measure ANOVA applied on the GOF revealed no significant differences for the vDMN between the experimental groups ($p = 0.4$) or sessions ($p = 0.3$) (**Figure 2**). In contrast, for the dDMN, the RTLE showed higher GOF values than the LTLE, pre-surgery ($p = 0.013$). This difference between left and right TLE disappeared post-surgery, as we observed a significant reduction of the RTLE's post-surgery GOF ($p = 0.013$), reaching a level almost identical to that of the LTLE group. This effect was mostly driven by the high pre-surgery GOF of the RTLE, as it did not remain significant when accounting for this parameter in the model (by adding the pre-surgery GOF values as a baseline covariate). Of note, neither of the TLE patient groups' GOF significantly differed from the controls', for either network, pre- or post-surgery.

Within the patient groups, a negative correlation was revealed between the age of seizure onset and the GOF for the pre-surgery dDMN ($r = -0.42$; $p = 0.02$), indicating that more normative dDMN was associated with earlier age of seizure onset. Both TLE groups had similar effects (LTLE: $r = -0.45$, RTLE: $r = -0.47$). No other significant correlations were observed between age of seizure onset and the GOF values for either sub-network at either the pre- or post-surgery testing point.

REGIONAL ANALYSES

Pre-surgery

Consistent with the GOF analysis, the dDMN showed more regional differences between the three experimental groups than the vDMN (**Table 2**). In detail, both networks showed significant differences between the experimental groups, or more specifically

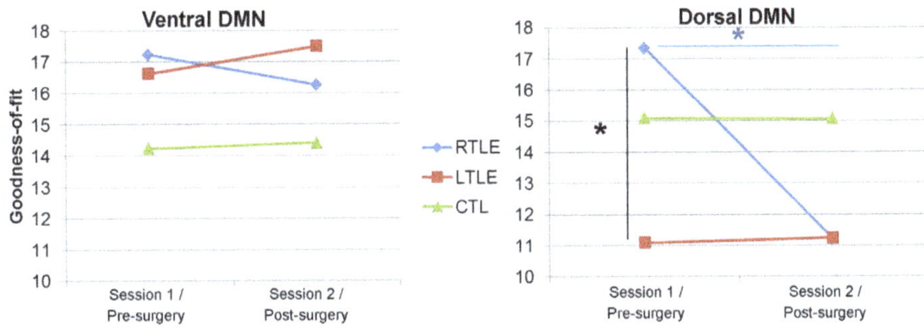

FIGURE 2 | Goodness-of-fit (GOF) for each default-mode network. Left panel: dorsal DMN (dDMN), right panel: ventral DMN (vDMN). *Significant difference at $p < 0.05$.

larger differences between the right and left TLE, than between the patient groups (RTLE and LTLE separately) and NCs.

Regarding the dDMN, the largest differences in pre-surgery emerged between the TLE groups. Indeed, the RTLE patients showed increased engagement of three large clusters located in the right superior frontal cortex and one cluster in the left PCC (**Figure 3**). In contrast, the LTLE did not display regions with significantly increased engagement in the dDMN, relative to the RTLE group. Compared to the NCs, the RTLE group showed reduced engagement of the right superior temporal cortex, while the LTLE group had an increased engagement of the left cerebellum (Crus I) in this DM subnetwork.

Regarding the vDMN, the RTLE group also showed increased engagement of large clusters, compared to the LTLE patients (**Table 2**). They were located in the left paracentral lobe, extending to the precuneus (**Figure 3**), and in the right middle temporal cortex. In contrast, the LTLE group showed increased involvement in the VIIB lobule of the left cerebellum, relative to the RTLE group. But the LTLE also displayed reduced involvement in the lobule V of the left-sided cerebellum, relative to the control group. Finally, we revealed that the RTLE group demonstrated increased engagement in the right calcarine and the left precuneus but no significant reduction compared to controls.

No association was revealed between the age of seizure onset and either pre-surgery DMN within each patient group.

Change from pre- to post-surgery

Overall, comparisons between the pre- and post-surgery sessions demonstrated larger changes in the dDMN than in the vDMN for both patient groups (**Table 3**). For the dDMN, the LTLE demonstrated increased involvement in several regions outside the ictal temporal lobe, post-surgery in comparison to pre-surgery. In detail, the right precuneus, right inferior parietal, and left middle temporal (posterior to the resection area) clusters showed positive involvement in the dDMN, post-surgery relative to pre-surgery (**Figure 4**). In contrast, as expected, the LTLE group lost the engagement of the left parahippocampal gyrus, located in the resected area, but also a cluster in the right middle temporal gyrus, post-surgery. The RTLE patients did not show any significant increased involvement of other regions in the dDMN, post-surgery. On the contrary, there was greatly reduced involvement of ipsilateral regions in their dDMN. Most notably, a particularly large focal cluster located in the right frontal lobe showed lower participation in the dDMN activity (**Figure 4**). To a lesser degree, the right caudate nucleus and insula also lost their functional involvement in this network post-surgery. Importantly, none of these changes were significant in the control group. NCs only showed a small reduction of engagement of the right thalamus in the dDMN during the session 2, relative to the session 1. We did not observe any significant increase at session 2 for the controls.

Regarding the vDMN, the only changes evident post-surgery were in the ictal/resected temporal lobe for each patient group, with reduced engagement, as expected (see **Table 3**). Also, the NCs showed reduced activity in two clusters located in the left precuneus and left middle temporal lobe for the session 2, relative to the session 1.

DISCUSSION

The present study investigated differences in the spatial extent of the two major subdivisions of the well-known DMN at rest in TLE patients. We tested for differences before and after ATL, with close examination of side of pathology (i.e., ictal focus) as a mediating factor. Prior work has described aberrant activity in the overall DMN in TLE patients' pre-surgery (11). We go further by clearly showing the unique effects of left versus right TLE, with further demonstration of the effects of ATL on the two main subdivisions of the DMN. Indeed, in contrast to our initial hypothesis, we found more evidence of TLE group differences in the dorsal rather than the vDMN, including distinct patterns of change for dDMN post-surgery. Thus, we show that ATL does not affect the DM networks in an equivalent fashion, and the nature of its impact varies depending on the pathologic hemisphere involved. Our results, therefore, imply that ATL has distinct effects on the cognitive functions associated with the DMN subdivisions, and that these effects will vary as a function of right and left TLE.

Importantly, our data show little evidence that the ventral subdivision of the DMN was affected by either TLE pre-surgery or ATL. Indeed, at the whole-brain level, using GOF measures, our analyses failed to produce significant differences, while we did observe substantive differences in the dDMN between the groups and the sessions. This seems counter-intuitive as the vDMN

Table 2 | Description of the significant differences within each DMN subdivision, between the experimental groups, pre-surgery.

Contrast	Region	Cluster voxel	*Z*-value	*x*	*y*	*z*	*Z* (RTLE)[a]	*Z* (LTLE)[a]
DORSAL DMN								
RTLE–LTLE	R Sup Ft	167	5.03	20	52	10	17	4
	R Sup Ft		3.71	20	56	22		
	R Sup Ft	139	4.25	14	26	−16	27	12
	R Rectus		4.22	8	44	−14		
	R Sup Ft	194	4.18	12	44	48	22	4
	R Sup Ft		3.84	12	28	44		
	R Sup Ft		3.81	24	38	48		
	L PCC	59	4.05	−4	−38	30	10	−1
	L PCC		3.45	−10	−44	26		
LTLE–RTLE	Null							
							Z (TLE)[a]	*Z* (NC)[a]
NC–LTLE	Null							
NC–RTLE	R Sup Tp	58	4.27	58	6	4	−4	9
LTLE–NC	L Cereb	63	4.11	−48	−76	−30	3	−11
	L Cereb		3.39	−42	−88	−32		
RTLE–NC	Null							
VENTRAL DMN								
RTLE–LTLE	L PCL	125	5	−10	−30	68	6	−2
	L Precu		3.47	−8	−44	68		
	R Mid Tp	124	4.02	52	−40	4	14	1
	R Mid Tp		3.28	60	−52	0		
LTLE–RTLE	L Cereb	92	3.99	−12	−72	−34	−3	7
	Cereb		3.42	0	−72	−38		
							Z (TLE)[a]	*Z* (NC)[a]
NC–LTLE	L Cereb	68	4.19	−16	−50	−18	−9	5
NC–RTLE	Null							
LTLE–NC	Null							
RTLE–NC	R Calcar	51	4.12	28	−66	12	3	−4
	L Precu	63	3.87	−6	−42	68	26	9
	L Precu		3.69	−2	−50	64		

NC, normal controls; LTLE, left temporal lobe epilepsy; RTLE, right temporal lobe epilepsy; Cereb, cerebellum; Calcar, calcarine; Precu, precuneus; Tp, temporal cortex; Mid, middle; L, left; R, right; PCL, paracentral lobule; Sup, superior; Ft, frontal cortex; PCC, posterior cingulate cortex.

[a]The last two columns indicate the averaged Z-values within each cluster for each group of interest, for each contrast, indicating the degree of difference between the two groups.

includes the epileptogenic mesial temporal lobe in TLE. However, within the vDMN, the mesial temporal lobe has a much less pivotal role than the precuneus, a region considered to be a major hub in the DMN (26). Therefore, the relative integrity of this network may suggest that the precuneus plays a compensatory role, reducing the negative impact of mesial temporal disease over the rest of the network, and otherwise helping to maintain network integrity. As a matter of fact, our regional analyses revealed little differences between the patient and control groups, supporting this interpretation. Further emphasizing a compensatory role for the precuneus in our data is that the RTLE group showed more engagement of the precuneus in the vDMN, than either the LTLE or controls. This finding is consistent with Zhang et al.'s study (11), which suggested that the PCC may play a compensatory role for the altered DMN in right but not left TLE. Our findings in LTLE for the vDMN stand in stark contrast to this, compelling consideration of an alternative interpretation. For example, rather than proposing that the RTLE is displaying a compensatory response involving the precuneus/PCC area (suggesting that the LTLE is associated with a normal activity in this region), instead the LTLE

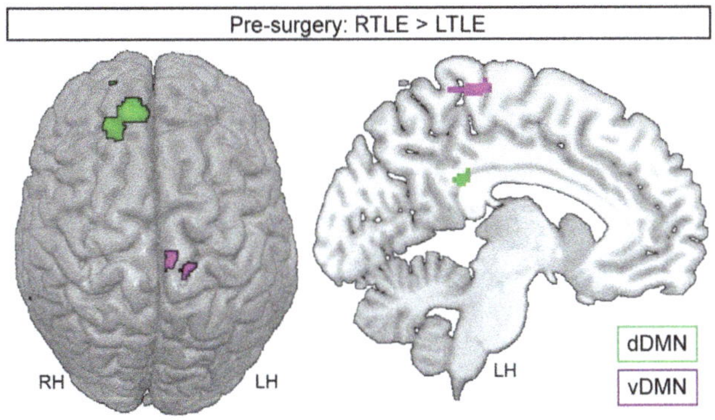

FIGURE 3 | Regions showing increased engagement in RTLE, relative to LTLE group, for the dorsal DMN (green) or the ventral DMN (purple). The images are shown in radiological orientation [e.g., the right side is the left hemisphere (LH)]. LH, left hemisphere; RH, right hemisphere.

patients can be seen as showing a pathologic loss of engagement of this region in the vDMN.

It is also worth noting that the LTLE group showed distinctly different engagement of the left-sided cerebellum with the rest of the vDMN, relative to the two other experimental groups. The exact reason for this cortical-cerebellar alteration is unclear, pre-surgery. It is interesting to note that in our previous study we observed a specific modulation of the functional connectivity between the left hippocampus and the left-sided cerebellum during a working memory task in the LTLE but not the RTLE (27). Thus, in combination, these separate results for LTLE patients may represent accruing evidence for altered functional connectivity between the cortex and the left-sided cerebellum. Overall, the absence of large alterations within the vDMN indicates that the abnormalities of unilateral temporal lobe seizures do not cause major perturbation of the whole vDMN. As was the case with the right TLE group, we again suggest that the precuneus/PCC has a protective role within this mostly posterior network, preventing major changes that might otherwise be caused by TLE pathology. This role is supported by previous studies describing the precuneus/PCC as a principal hub in the DMN (26, 28), perhaps generating activity or signals that limit seizure spread or epileptogenesis in TLE patients (29).

In contrast, our data show that TLE and ATL do have a significant effect on the regional extent of the dDMN, a sub-network whose major hub is prefrontal cortex, with precuneus involvement present, but to a much smaller degree. Indeed, large discrepancies were evident as a function of the side of the pathology. Pre-surgery, based on the GOF, the RTLE showed a more normative network than the LTLE (i.e., higher GOF as a sign of a better matching to the template). Also, the present data demonstrate that, pre-surgery, the LTLE group showed reduced involvement of the major regions in this network such as frontal cortex and PCC, relative to the RTLE group. Differences between the impact of right and left TLE have been described previously, associated with the (dominant) function of the LH in language-related processes (14, 15). It is important to note that the majority of our participants were right-handed, suggesting LH dominance for language was prominent in our sample. Thus, our data support the notion that the functions of the dDMN may be more strongly implemented by the LH, and is consistent with previous finding suggesting that the DMN is left-lateralized, heavily involved, for instance, in functions such as inner, covert speech (30). Given this lateralized bias in function, it makes sense that left-sided seizures are more harmful to this network than right-sided seizures. Conversely, our data suggest that the vDMN is less engaged in language processing, and will be less sensitive to left-lateralized pathology such as LTLE.

Another striking result is the negative correlation revealed between the age of seizure onset and the dDMN's GOF in patients, pre-surgery, regardless of the side of the pathology. In other words, this indicates that earlier age of seizure onset is associated with a more normative network. Indeed, higher GOF is indicative of a better match between the patients' network and the "normative" dDMN obtained by Shirer et al. (24) on healthy participants. We failed to find evidence of an association with onset at the regional level, suggesting that age of seizure onset has more of a global influence on the whole network, rather than selectively impacting a specific network region. This negative correlation is consistent with literature addressing the influence of early versus late seizure onset on brain plasticity. Indeed, previous studies describe how a mature brain is less plastic, allowing late onset seizures to cause irreversible impairment in the setting of fully acquired and developed cognitive functions (31). Our result suggests that this developmental feature is at work with the dDMN, implying that when a young brain is confronted with seizures it is more capable than an older brain of generating functional adaptation and plasticity in the dDMN. We observed no such developmental relationship in the vDMN.

Our study is the first to investigate the effect of ATL on DMN subdivisions, and, in addition, reporting different effects according to the side of the ATL. It is important to remember that the majority of our patients were confirmed to have good seizure outcome (seizure free or significant reduction of their seizures) at least 1 year after their surgery, confirming that the ATL surgery likely resected the primary seizure onset zone. Our data show that right ATL causes more damage in the dDMN than left ATL. More specifically, right ATL, but not left ATL, was associated with a large reduction in engagement of ipsilateral regions, especially the right frontal cortex in the dDMN. The reason for such loss of activity is still not clear, and we are the first to report this finding. This loss of frontal activity in the RTLE patients implies that right frontal cognitive deficits are likely to be more prominent in these patients following ATL, though neuropsychological studies, involving measures of executive function, do not support this (32). One possibility for this discrepancy is that diminished right frontal dDMN activity may impact other types of cognitive processing not measured by standard neuropsychological testing such as spontaneous cognition (e.g., mind wandering). Indeed, DMN activity has been associated with spontaneous mental processes in healthy subjects (3, 4), but no study has explored nature and integrity of spontaneous thoughts in TLE patients with concurrent measures of DMN subdivision activity.

With regard to the unique effects of the side of the ATL, left but not right ATL patients showed recruitment of additional posterior regions into the dDMN post-surgery. This finding speaks to the

Table 3 | Description of the changes between the two sessions, within each experimental group, for each DMN subdivision.

Contrast	Region	Cluster voxel	*Z*-value	*x*	*y*	*z*	*Z* (pre)[a]	*Z* (post)[a]
DORSAL DMN								
LTLE: post > pre	R Precu	138	4.68	16	−54	66	−9	3
	R Inf Pt	50	4.43	66	−30	52	0	7
	L Mid Tp	65	4.09	−52	−34	−4	−2	7
LTLE: pre > post	L Parahip – resected area	123	4.27	−28	−22	−22	2	N/A
	R Mid Tp	98	3.89	60	−60	4	4	−6
RTLE: post > pre	Null							
RTLE: pre > post	R Sup Ft	690	4.49	12	46	50	19	4
	R Sup Ft		4.34	22	36	48		
	R Sup Ft		4.18	26	26	50		
	R Caudate	69	3.59	14	16	16	9	−1
	R Insula	119	3.82	40	16	−14	22	3
NC: ses 2 > ses 1	Null							
NC: ses 1 > ses 2	R Thalamus	61	3.9	2	−6	10	6	−2
VENTRAL DMN								
LTLE: post > pre	Null							
LTLE: pre > post	L Inf Tp – resected area	61	4.31	−56	−2	−32	13	N/A
RTLE: post > pre	Null							
RTLE: pre > post	R inf Tp – resected area	294	5.05	66	−34	−16	9	N/A
	R inf Tp – resected area		4.23	60	−30	−26		
NC: ses 2 > ses 1	Null							
NC: ses 1 > ses 2	L Precu	143	4.66	−14	−54	26	24	19
	L Mid Tp	66	3.89	70	−34	−4	7	1

NC, normal controls; LTLE, left temporal lobe epilepsy; RTLE, right temporal lobe epilepsy; Cereb, cerebellum; Precu, precuneus; Tp, temporal cortex; Mid, middle; L, left; R, right; Inf, inferior; Sup, superior; Ft, frontal cortex; Parahip, parahippocampal gyrus; Pt, parietal cortex.

[a]The last two columns indicate the averaged Z-values within each cluster for each session (pre- and post-surgery for the patients, sessions 1 and 2 for the controls), indicating the degree of change between the sessions within the experimental group.

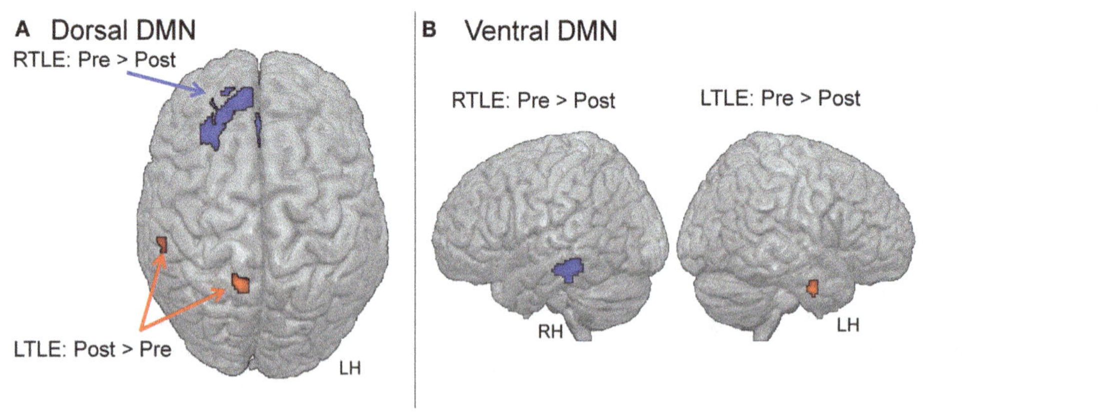

FIGURE 4 | Major changes between pre- and post-surgery for the dorsal DMN (A) or the ventral DMN (B), within each patient group. The images are shown in radiological orientation (e.g., the right side is the left hemisphere). LH, left hemisphere; RH, right hemisphere.

differential effect of temporal lobe seizures on the dominant versus non-dominant hemisphere. It has been previously demonstrated that LTLE patients are more prone to brain activity abnormalities than RTLE, pre-surgery (14, 15). Yet, we observed an increased engagement of the precuneus in this network for the LTLE patients post-surgery relative to pre-surgery. This is consistent with our previous interpretation regarding the positive and possible compensatory effect of this region on the network as a whole. Recalling that our left TLE patients had good seizure outcomes, we suggest that, released from seizure burden, the left dominant hemisphere is able to function more normally, with this normalization supported through the compensatory benefits conferred by adding new regions to bolster dDMN activity. This idea is also convergent with the findings of McCormick et al. (10), who described that post-surgical enhancement of functional connectivity involving the PCC correlated with better post-surgical episodic memory performance.

Overall, our data indicate that right TLE is associated with greater disruption of the dDMN post-surgery. In terms of lateralized effects, our data differs from the most common reports in the neuropsychological literature, which generally indicate that left (i.e., dominant hemisphere) TLE patients fare worse than right TLE patients after ATL surgery (33, 34), particularly in areas such as episodic memory. While our data may imply left, not right, sided ATL engender adaptive mechanisms and compensatory network responses after surgery, we cannot presume that the post-surgical changes observed in our right TLE are either associated with cognitive outcome or could explain any observed neurocognitive findings. Further investigations are needed to fill the gap between our knowledge of functional reorganization and its consequences for cognitive change following ATL and other surgical interventions.

With regard to the vDMN and surgery, our data suggest that ATL had very limited effects. Indeed, we only found expected changes within the resected temporal lobe for each of the patient groups. This lack of change is consistent with our interpretation of the pre-surgical finding. That is, the engagement of the precuneus/PCC area may have worked to limit or constrain some of the disruptions in the network caused by resection of the epileptogenic temporal lobe. More generally, these findings for the vDMN imply that TLE and ATL surgery, regardless of side, has less of an impact on vDMN functionality (e.g., decision-making related to constructing/recalling a mental scene) than might be expected.

Some limitations in our study should be noted. We cannot exclude the possibility that some changes revealed between pre- and post-surgery in the patient groups were partially caused by normal aging or the normal effects of time. Related to this, we were not able to match exactly the NC and the LTLE participants on the time interval between the scans. As described, we checked that the brain regions displaying change between the two sessions for the TLE patients were not areas of change in the NC group. Furthermore, we did not find any regions with increased engagement in the control group, suggesting that such DMN alterations are quite specific to the effects of ATL surgery and are not likely related to normal, time-related change in the healthy participants. Thus, we believe that we have highlighted the reliable effects of the ATL procedure on DMN activity at rest in TLE patients.

Another limitation is that the patients were not all seizure free. The right TLE group had slightly fewer seizure-free patients than the left TLE group, post-surgery (11/16 versus 12/13), although this difference was not significant. Unfortunately, the low sample size of the non-seizure free group precluded statistical analyses of the potential effect of different seizure outcomes on our findings. We acknowledge that patterns of seizure recurrence versus control may influence the status of the DMN. Indeed, it could be playing a role in our finding that the right, but not the left, TLE patients suffer from a large reduction of frontal activity in the dDMN as a result of factors such as seizure spread or secondary epileptogenesis [see Ref. (35)]. Further investigation is needed to explain such phenomenon, using a more balance sample size of TLE patients with poor versus good seizure outcome.

Regarding other clinical factors, AEDs could potentially effect network connectivity and changes post-surgery. However, AED status did not vary or change after surgery in our sample. We considered analyzing collected clinical data on seizure frequency. However, the experience at our epilepsy center is that age of onset is a more reliable measure than other historical measures such as seizure frequency or age at first risk (e.g., first signs of pathology). The former because awareness and recall of seizure occurrence is so poor; the latter because of the potential delay between the start and the discovery of pathology. We chose to focus on age of seizure onset as this may best capture developmental differences in response to neuroplasticity. For instance, younger compared to older age brains appear more disposed to plasticity and cognitive reorganization (36), factors that likely play a role in DMN strength and organization. With these issues of neuroplasticity in mind, variables such as – the age at which seizures fail to respond to medications – would not be as accurate, nor as meaningful. Moreover, our algorithm for ATL candidacy requires that all patients fail at least three seizure medications, with a large number having many more such failed trials. Therefore, it would be very difficult to accurately determine the age at which seizures failed to respond to medication. Lastly, illness duration is highly correlated with age at seizure onset, and thus constitutes a redundant variable.

Regarding pathology, it should be noted that all our patients did not have the same temporal pathology, especially with regard to the presence or absence of MTS. While we are aware that this variable is an important and relevant factor in TLE (37), our sample size was too low for any meaningful statistical comparison between patients with and without MTS. It should be noted that our major purpose was to explore the extra-temporal effects of TLE on network connectivity, and these extra-temporal regions were not "lesioned" in any of our patients.

CONCLUSION

We demonstrate that the subdivisions of the well-known default-mode resting-state network are effected differently by both the original TLE pathology, and subsequent ATL procedure. Overall, and somewhat unexpectedly, the dDMN appears more impacted by these factors. Prior to surgery, major whole-brain differences were observed in the dDMN, with right TLE displaying a more normative pattern based on the GOF measures. In terms of regional dDMN effects, the TLE group differences observed in frontal and precuneal regions, imply that left-sided, dominant hemisphere, pathology is more damaging to the network. In contrast, the status of the vDMN prior to surgery showed no differences among our groups at a whole-brain level, suggesting that neither left nor right pathology has a detrimental effect. Regionally for the vDMN, the RTLE group demonstrated increases, particularly in the precuneus, increases we believe reflect an adaptive, neuroprotective response, compensating for the right mesial pathology. Regarding the impact of ATL and post-surgical change in the DMN subdivisions, the vDMN, which includes most of the mesial temporal lobe, did not demonstrate any significant loss of activity outside the resected epileptogenic cortex, a finding that again suggests that the vDMN is less affected by epileptogenic pathology. For the dDMN post-surgery, contrasting effects were obtained for the TLE groups. LTLE patients demonstrated increased engagement of new posterior regions such as the precuneus, while the RTLE patients showed lost engagement of a large right anterior cluster. Here, we again see an adaptive or compensatory role for the precuneus, though in this case in the setting of left TLE.

Overall our data demonstrate that right ATL has a more deleterious effect on the dDMN, and that left, not right, sided ATL appears more likely to engender adaptive mechanisms and compensatory network responses after surgery. This latter suggests a possible inconsistency with the neuropsychological data, which tend to associate dominant hemisphere ATL with greater functional problems post-surgery in domains such as episodic memory. In this sense, our data raise questions about the nature and extent of the correspondence between resting-state networks associated with memory (i.e., the DMN) and neuropsychological measures of functionality. Further investigations are needed to fill the gap between knowledge about functional reorganization, as reported here, and its impact on cognitive status post-surgery.

To our knowledge, we are the first to highlight the differential impact of right and left TLE and subsequent ATL on the major subdivisions of the DMN, at rest. Our data show that the dDMN is more closely associated with the impact of TLE pathology and resective surgery than the vDMN, suggesting that studying the cognitive and behavioral correlates of this DMN subdivision and its changes with surgery may be fruitful, particularly as resting-state becomes better integrated into pre-surgical algorithms for predicting neurocognitive, neurobehavioral, and seizure outcomes.

AUTHOR CONTRIBUTIONS

Gaëlle E. Doucet conducted, performed, analyzed imaging experiments, and wrote the manuscript. Dorian Pustina performed imaging experiments. Christopher Skidmore and Michael R. Sperling designed and supervised the project. James Evans and Ashwini Sharan performed ATL surgeries. Joseph I. Tracy designed, supervised the project, and wrote the manuscript.

ACKNOWLEDGMENTS

The authors thank Dr. Karol Osipowicz for his participation in data acquisition. This work was supported, in part, by the National Institute for Neurological Disorders and Stroke (NINDS) (grant number R21 NS056071-01A1) to Dr. Joseph I. Tracy.

REFERENCES

1. Buckner RL, Andrews-Hanna JR, Schacter DL. The brain's default network: anatomy, function, and relevance to disease. *Ann N Y Acad Sci* (2008) **1124**:1–38. doi:10.1196/annals.1440.011
2. Raichle ME, MacLeod AM, Snyder AZ, Powers WJ, Gusnard DA, Shulman GL. A default mode of brain function. *Proc Natl Acad Sci USA* (2001) **98**(2):676–82. doi:10.1073/pnas.98.2.676
3. Andrews-Hanna JR, Reidler JS, Huang C, Buckner RL. Evidence for the default network's role in spontaneous cognition. *J Neurophysiol* (2010) **104**(1):322–35. doi:10.1152/jn.00830.2009
4. Doucet G, Naveau M, Petit L, Zago L, Crivello F, Jobard G, et al. Patterns of hemodynamic low-frequency oscillations in the brain are modulated by the nature of free thought during rest. *Neuroimage* (2012) **59**(4):3194–200. doi:10.1016/j.neuroimage.2011.11.059
5. Andrews-Hanna JR, Reidler JS, Sepulcre J, Poulin R, Buckner RL. Functional-anatomic fractionation of the brain's default network. *Neuron* (2010) **65**(4):550–62. doi:10.1016/j.neuron.2010.02.005
6. Doucet G, Naveau M, Petit L, Delcroix N, Zago L, Crivello F, et al. Brain activity at rest: a multiscale hierarchical functional organization. *J Neurophysiol* (2011) **105**:2753–63. doi:10.1152/jn.00895.2010
7. Greicius MD, Srivastava G, Reiss AL, Menon V. Default-mode network activity distinguishes Alzheimer's disease from healthy aging: evidence from functional MRI. *Proc Natl Acad Sci USA* (2004) **101**(13):4637–42. doi:10.1073/pnas.0308627101
8. Garrity AG, Pearlson GD, McKiernan K, Lloyd D, Kiehl KA, Calhoun VD. Aberrant "default mode" functional connectivity in schizophrenia. *Am J Psychiatry* (2007) **164**(3):450–7. doi:10.1176/appi.ajp.164.3.450
9. Dupont P, Zaknun JJ, Maes A, Tepmongkol S, Vasquez S, Bal CS, et al. Dynamic perfusion patterns in temporal lobe epilepsy. *Eur J Nucl Med Mol Imaging* (2009) **36**(5):823–30. doi:10.1007/s00259-008-1040-6
10. McCormick C, Quraan M, Cohn M, Valiante TA, McAndrews MP. Default mode network connectivity indicates episodic memory capacity in mesial temporal lobe epilepsy. *Epilepsia* (2013) **54**(5):809–18. doi:10.1111/epi.12098
11. Zhang Z, Lu G, Zhong Y, Tan Q, Liao W, Wang Z, et al. Altered spontaneous neuronal activity of the default-mode network in mesial temporal lobe epilepsy. *Brain Res* (2010) **1323**:152–60. doi:10.1016/j.brainres.2010.01.042
12. Haneef Z, Lenartowicz A, Yeh HJ, Engel J Jr, Stern JM. Effect of lateralized temporal lobe epilepsy on the default mode network. *Epilepsy Behav* (2012) **25**(3):350–7. doi:10.1016/j.yebeh.2012.07.019
13. Laufs H, Hamandi K, Salek-Haddadi A, Kleinschmidt AK, Duncan JS, Lemieux L. Temporal lobe interictal epileptic discharges affect cerebral activity in "default mode" brain regions. *Hum Brain Mapp* (2007) **28**(10):1023–32. doi:10.1002/hbm.20323
14. Doucet G, Osipowicz K, Sharan A, Sperling MR, Tracy JI. Extratemporal functional connectivity impairments at rest are related to memory performance in mesial temporal epilepsy. *Hum Brain Mapp* (2013) **34**(9):2202–16. doi:10.1002/hbm.22059
15. Pereira FR, Alessio A, Sercheli MS, Pedro T, Bilevicius E, Rondina JM, et al. Asymmetrical hippocampal connectivity in mesial temporal lobe epilepsy: evidence from resting state fMRI. *BMC Neurosci* (2010) **11**:66. doi:10.1186/1471-2202-11-66
16. Sperling MR, O'Connor MJ, Saykin AJ, Phillips CA, Morrell MJ, Bridgman PA, et al. A noninvasive protocol for anterior temporal lobectomy. *Neurology* (1992) **42**(2):416–22. doi:10.1212/WNL.42.2.416
17. Crinion J, Ashburner J, Leff A, Brett M, Price C, Friston K. Spatial normalization of lesioned brains: performance evaluation and impact on fMRI analyses. *Neuroimage* (2007) **37**(3):866–75. doi:10.1016/j.neuroimage.2007.04.065
18. Song XW, Dong ZY, Long XY, Li SF, Zuo XN, Zhu CZ, et al. REST: A toolkit for resting-state functional magnetic resonance imaging data processing. *PLoS One* (2011) **6**(9):e25031. doi:10.1371/journal.pone.0025031
19. Cordes D, Haughton VM, Arfanakis K, Carew JD, Turski PA, Moritz CH, et al. Frequencies contributing to functional connectivity in the cerebral cortex in "resting-state" data. *AJNR Am J Neuroradiol* (2001) **22**(7):1326–33.
20. Van Dijk KR, Sabuncu MR, Buckner RL. The influence of head motion on intrinsic functional connectivity MRI. *Neuroimage* (2012) **59**(1):431–8. doi:10.1016/j.neuroimage.2011.07.044
21. Smith SM, Jenkinson M, Woolrich MW, Beckmann CF, Behrens TE, Johansen-Berg H, et al. Advances in functional and structural MR image analysis and

implementation as FSL. *Neuroimage* (2004) **23**(Suppl 1):S208–19. doi:10.1016/j.neuroimage.2004.07.051

22. Beckmann CF, Smith SM. Probabilistic independent component analysis for functional magnetic resonance imaging. *IEEE Trans Med Imaging* (2004) **23**(2):137–52. doi:10.1109/TMI.2003.822821
23. Beckmann CF, Mackay CE, Filippini N, Smith SM. Group comparison of resting-state FMRI data using multi-subject ICA and dual regression. *15th Annual Meeting of Organization for Human Brain Mapping.* San Francisco, CA (2009).
24. Shirer WR, Ryali S, Rykhlevskaia E, Menon V, Greicius MD. Decoding subject-driven cognitive states with whole-brain connectivity patterns. *Cereb Cortex* (2012) **22**(1):158–165. doi:10.1093/cercor/bhr099
25. Engel JJ, Van Ness PC, Rasmussen TB, Ojemann LM. Outcome with respect to epileptic seizures. In: Engel J Jr, editor. *Surgical Treatment of the Epilepsies.* New York: Raven Press (1993). p. 609–21.
26. Fransson P, Marrelec G. The precuneus/posterior cingulate cortex plays a pivotal role in the default mode network: evidence from a partial correlation network analysis. *Neuroimage* (2008) **42**(3):1178–84. doi:10.1016/j.neuroimage.2008.05.059
27. Doucet G, Osipowicz K, Sharan A, Sperling M, Tracy JI. Hippocampal functional connectivity patterns during spatial working memory differ in right versus left temporal lobe epilepsy. *Brain Connect* (2013) **3**(4):398–406. doi:10.1089/brain.2013.0158
28. Achard S, Salvador R, Whitcher B, Suckling J, Bullmore E. A resilient, low-frequency, small-world human brain functional network with highly connected association cortical hubs. *J Neurosci* (2006) **26**(1):63–72. doi:10.1523/JNEUROSCI.3874-05.2006
29. Tracy JI, Osipowicz K, Spechler P, Sharan A, Skidmore C, Doucet G, et al. Functional connectivity evidence of cortico-cortico inhibition in temporal lobe epilepsy. *Hum Brain Mapp* (2014) **35**(1):353–66. doi:10.1002/hbm.22181
30. Mazoyer B, Zago L, Mellet E, Bricogne S, Etard O, Houde O, et al. Cortical networks for working memory and executive functions sustain the conscious resting state in man. *Brain Res Bull* (2001) **54**(3):287–98. doi:10.1016/S0361-9230(00)00437-8
31. Helmstaedter C, Witt JA. Neuropsychology in epilepsy. *Fortschr Neurol Psychiatr* (2009) **77**(11):639–45. doi:10.1055/s-0028-1109796
32. Stretton J, Thompson PJ. Frontal lobe function in temporal lobe epilepsy. *Epilepsy Res* (2012) **98**(1):1–13. doi:10.1016/j.eplepsyres.2011.10.009
33. Chelune GJ. Hippocampal adequacy versus functional reserve: predicting memory functions following temporal lobectomy. *Arch Clin Neuropsychol* (1995) **10**(5):413–32. doi:10.1093/arclin/10.5.413
34. Helmstaedter C, Roeske S, Kaaden S, Elger CE, Schramm J. Hippocampal resection length and memory outcome in selective epilepsy surgery. *J Neurol Neurosurg Psychiatry* (2011) **82**(12):1375–81. doi:10.1136/jnnp.2010.240176
35. Lieb JP, Dasheiff RM, Engel J Jr. Role of the frontal lobes in the propagation of mesial temporal lobe seizures. *Epilepsia* (1991) **32**(6):822–37. doi:10.1111/j.1528-1157.1991.tb05539.x
36. Helmstaedter C, Kurthen M, Lux S, Reuber M, Elger CE. Chronic epilepsy and cognition: a longitudinal study in temporal lobe epilepsy. *Ann Neurol* (2003) **54**(4):425–32. doi:10.1002/ana.10692
37. Mueller SG, Laxer KD, Barakos J, Cheong I, Garcia P, Weiner MW. Widespread neocortical abnormalities in temporal lobe epilepsy with and without mesial sclerosis. *Neuroimage* (2009) **46**(2):353–9. doi:10.1016/j.neuroimage.2009.02.020

9

Low consistency of four brain connectivity measures derived from intracranial electrode measurements

Stephen E. Jones[1]*, Erik B. Beall[1], Imad Najm[1], Ken E. Sakaie[1], Michael D. Phillips[1], Myron Zhang[2] and Jorge A. Gonzalez-Martinez[1]

[1] *Cleveland Clinic, Cleveland, OH, USA*
[2] *Ohio State University College of Medicine, Columbus, OH, USA*

****Correspondence:***
Stephen E. Jones, U15, 9500 Euclid Avenue, Cleveland, OH 44195, USA
e-mail: joness19@ccf.org

Measures of brain connectivity are currently subject to intense scientific and clinical interest. Multiple measures are available, each with advantages and disadvantages. Here, we study epilepsy patients with intracranial electrodes, and compare four different measures of connectivity. Perhaps the most direct measure derives from intracranial electrodes; however, this is invasive and spatial coverage is incomplete. These electrodes can be actively stimulated to trigger electrophysical responses to provide the first measure of connectivity. A second measure is the recent development of simultaneous BOLD fMRI and intracranial electrode stimulation. The resulting BOLD maps form a measure of effective connectivity. A third measure uses low frequency BOLD fluctuations measured by MRI, with functional connectivity defined as the temporal correlation coefficient between their BOLD waveforms. A fourth measure is structural, derived from diffusion MRI, with connectivity defined as an integrated diffusivity measure along a connecting pathway. This method addresses the difficult requirement to measure connectivity between any two points in the brain, reflecting the relatively arbitrary location of the surgical placement of intracranial electrodes. Using a group of eight epilepsy patients with intracranial electrodes, the connectivity from one method is compared to another method using all paired data points that are in common, yielding an overall correlation coefficient. This method is performed for all six paired-comparisons between the four methods. While these show statistically significant correlations, the magnitudes of the correlation are relatively modest (r^2 between 0.20 and 0.001). In summary, there are many pairs of points in the brain that correlate well using one measure yet correlate poorly using another measure. These experimental findings present a complicated picture regarding the measure or meaning of brain connectivity.

Keywords: intracranial electrodes, brain stimulation, functional MRI, structural connectivity, functional connectivity

INTRODUCTION

The importance of brain connectivity is self-evident given the underlying network structure of the brain. Structural MRI, which interrogates each point in the brain, is invaluable to science and medicine. The point-to-point relationships of connectivity imaging are equally as invaluable, if not more so, given the inherent network nature of brain functions. As such, connectivity imaging represents the next step in the continuing evolution of neuroimaging. However, unlike structural imaging, contemporary connectivity analyses have not yielded findings of relevance for treatment in individual patients.

There are many measures of connectivity, which could be dichotomized into functional and structural. Examples of structural connectivity are derived from invasive measures such as axonal tracing or nuclear tracing, with the prime non-invasive method of MRI using diffusion-weighted imaging (dMRI). Examples of functional connectivity include measures derived from scalp EEG, intracranial EEG, PET studies, cortical thickness studies, task-related fMRI, and resting state fMRI (rsfMRI). All these methods have advantages and disadvantages, related to spatial and temporal resolution, coverage, effectiveness, and invasiveness. Given numerous methodologies and metrics of connectivity (1, 2), it is natural to compare them with the hypothesis that if the metrics are sensitive to the underlying network architecture of the brain, then the connectivity measures should strongly correlate with each other. This inquiry raises the question about the exact definition of connectivity, and what could be considered the "gold standard."

The paper focuses on recent measurements obtained from a group of eight patients with medically intractable epilepsy, who underwent both invasive electroencephalographic (EEG) and evoked potentials mapping with implantable intracranial electrodes and advanced neuroimaging with MRI. Using these methods, a total of four modalities of connectivity were explored: structural connectivity using dMRI, functional connectivity using rsfMRI, functional connectivity using precise electrical stimulation and recording (cortico-cortical evoked potentials, CCEPs) from intracranial electrodes, and combined intracranial

Table 1 | Details of intracranial electrodes placed in eight patients.

Patient Number	Age	Implantation	Number of intracranial contacts	Number of CCEP stimulations	dMRI rsfMRI	DES-fMRI	Location of stimulation
1	45	SDG[a]	123	4	Y		Left Broca, Left Wernike, Ictal onset zone ×2
2	40	SEEG[b]	57	9	Y		Multiple bi-occipital and right temporal
3	19	SDG	106	7	Y		Left Broca, Wernike, ictal onset zone ×3
4	40	SEEG	104	5	Y		Multiple right frontoparietal
5	25	SEEG	120	1		Y	Left orbito-frontal
6	41	SEEG	130	1		Y	Right posterior cingulate
7	42	SEEG	160	1		Y	Right peri-insula
8	54	SEEG	130	1		Y	Right orbito-frontal

[a] *SDG: subdural grids.*

[b] *SEEG: stereoencephalography.*

stimulation and BOLD fMRI. These four modalities of connectivity are compared on a pairwise basis, and we show that although the comparisons reveal statistically significant correlations, the correlation values are modest. Furthermore, these methods, as commonly interpreted today, do not reach the same consensus. In other words, there are many pairs of points in the brain that correlate strongly using modality A, but correlate weakly using modality B, and visa versa. A possible future method to unify these differences may incorporate a mathematical model of brain function, which would permit the translation of one connectivity measure to another.

MATERIALS AND METHODS

Four different measures of connectivity are used in this study; all measured in epilepsy patients who underwent an invasive evaluation to better localize and map the extent of the epileptogenic zone (EZ). The four measures are functional connectivity derived from electrophysiological response to electrical stimulation (CCEPs); functional connectivity derived from low-frequency BOLD oscillations in the rsfMRI; functional connectivity derived from simultaneous direct electrical stimulation and BOLD functional MRI (DES-fMRI); and structural connectivity derived from dMRI using high-angular resolution diffusion imaging (HARDI).

After obtaining IRB approval, a total of eight patients were enrolled. All patients were recruited from the Cleveland Clinic Epilepsy Center with a diagnosis of intractable focal epilepsy, and underwent an intensive evaluation culminating in the placement of intracranial electrodes. All patients underwent CCEP stimulation, with multiple locations of stimulation, including the Broca's speech region, and the presumed EZ. The first four patients had HARDI and rsfMRI performed prior to implantation, and the last four had HARDI and rsfMRI performed after implantation. These measurements were performed as a "piggy back" during their standard clinical care, and did not interfere with their clinical care. **Table 1** lists some clinical characteristics of the patients and the different modalities that were measured.

CORTICO-CORTICAL EVOKED POTENTIALs

All CCEP stimulations used a GRASS used current-controlled Grass Technologies S88 and SUI-7 units (Astro-Med), with the following parameters: 1 Hz unipolar pulses with alternating polarity between pulses, 0.3 ms pulsewidth, with variable current (4–15 mA), applied across an adjacent electrode pair. An optical current isolator was used to ensure that the patient was isolated from ground. For each CCEP stimulation location shown in **Table 1**, between 16 and 60 (typically around 45) stimulating pulses were sent from the chosen electrode pair, and waveform responses were recorded from all other implanted contacts, at a 1 kHz recording rate. Four patients also had CCEP performed while simultaneously undergoing MRI, and for these patients a stimulation frequency of at least 10 Hz was required to elicit a robust BOLD response (3). The CCEP voltage waveforms obtained at each electrode were averaged, discarding any outliers that were usually due to motion and other artifacts. Because of the alternating polarity of each pulse, most of the stimulus artifact was removed, and average waveforms could be reliable seen as early as 5 ms after the stimulus. A scalar baseline was subtracted from each waveform, derived from an average of the waveform during a 40 ms window obtained just before the stimulus. There are many methods to "score" the strength of the averaged CCEP waveform, which can be used as the measure of electrophysiological connectivity. Typically, these methods use the average voltage during a time window after stimulus. Other methods can use the slope, latency, integral, magnitude, and other features of the voltage waveform. For this paper, the chosen time window depended on the other modality used to compare CCEP connectivity: for comparison with structural connectivity, a 5 ms window starting 10 ms after the stimulus was used to reflect the rapid first-pass excitation of distal cortex; for comparison with resting state connectivity a 100 ms window starting at 20 ms was used to reflect the longer timescale of an integrative process.

RESTING STATE fMRI

For all studies, rsfMRI was performed on a 3T Siemens Trio (Siemens Medical Solutions, Erlangen, Germany), using a whole-brain EPI sequence: 132 repetitions of 31 4-mm thick axial slices; TE/TR, 29 ms/2,800 ms; matrix, 128 × 128; FOV, 256 mm × 256 mm; receive bandwidth, 250 kHz. EPI data were unwarped using a field map prior to coregistration to the unwarped diffusion acquisition space (described below in Section Structural connectivity), which was used to cross-compare the different measures. Patients were instructed to rest with their eyes closed and refrain from any voluntary motion. The data were corrected for motion, adaptive physiologic noise sources (4, 5), and second-order motion (6). The data were interpolated to the DWI space (see below). Functional connectivity maps of the brain were produced using a seed approach, yielding a pairwise temporal correlation coefficient to every other brain voxel. The seed was selected to be the site of stimulation. The time waveforms used in the correlation were the average waveforms of the 27 voxels of a voxel and its nearest neighbors, excluding any CSF-containing voxels.

DIRECT ELECTRICAL STIMULATION AND FUNCTIONAL MRI

Direct electrical stimulation and functional MRI (DES-fMRI) is a recently developed modality (3) in which simultaneous fMRI is acquired during stimulation of a single intracranial electrode. The procedure was conducted in an intraoperative MRI suite with the patients under general anesthesia. Using appropriate stimulation frequencies and currents (typically around 20 Hz and 4–8 mA), robust BOLD activation could be generated both proximal and distal to the electrodes. Typically, the activation occurred in patterns that reflect the underlying network. Both positive and "negative" activation could be triggered. Activation could also be induced by white matter stimulation. Using this method, the connectivity metric between the stimulation point S and another point P can be defined as the degree of BOLD change or its statistical significance at point P. Thus, the usual 3D BOLD maps can be viewed as a connectivity map. Prior to DES-fMRI the patients had a comparable CCEP stimulation performed outside of the MRI with all electrodes in place and recording the stimulation's response, thereby measuring electrophysiological connectivity. By co-localizing the electrode location to the DES-fMRI, a comparison could be directly made between electrophysiological connectivity and DES-fMRI connectivity.

STRUCTURAL CONNECTIVITY

High-angular resolution diffusion imaging images were obtained on a Siemens Trio (Siemens Medical Solutions, Erlangen, Germany) with a standard 12-channel head coil. The HARDI acquisition provided whole-brain coverage with 2.5 mm isotropic voxels (256 mm × 256 mm FOV, 102 × 102 matrix, 48 slices. TE = 77 ms, TR = 6500 ms, BW = 1442 Hz/pixel, partial Fourier factor = 5/8, 61 non-collinear diffusion-weighting gradients with robust ordering with $b = 1000\ \mathrm{s/mm^2}$ and 7 $b = 0$ volumes, two averages). Warping effects were addressed by using static image-based unwarping (7) on the diffusion data prior to diffusivity calculation. Motion correction was performed with an iterative algorithm (8) that updated gradient vectors (9). Fiber orientation distributions were calculated in each voxel by spherical deconvolution (10) with user-independent optimized regularization (11). Local transition probabilities were calculated by integrating over the solid angle of a vector connecting each voxel with its 26 neighbors.

The cross-modal comparison performed in this project places additional demands on metrics to measure structural connectivity. For example, since intracranial electrode contacts can be placed in any arbitrary place in the brain, the task of comparing structural to electrophysiological connectivity requires that the structural metric be able to assess or "score" a connection between any two points in the brain. Since these two points may not necessarily both lie along a large fiber track, deterministic methods will fail and probabilistic methods are favored. A further demand is that the "seed" and/or "target" points may lie on the cortical surface, in a region of low FA that hinders the reliable start to a trajectory. One difficulty with probabilistic methods is that they can be computationally inefficient, if they adopt a method of randomly forming a path and discarding it if it fails to reach a target. To account for this difficulty a partial differential equation (PDE) approach was developed that is the solution of a probabilistic method assuming an infinite number of trials, akin to the underlying relationship between a PDE and Monte Carlo solution to classes of differential equations (12). Details of this method are presented in the Data Sheet 1 in Supplementary Material.

COREGISTRATION

The processes of coregistration of the electrode positions to the MRI voxels started with a thin section head CT following implantation of electrodes. Then using in-house techniques, all electrode contact positions were identified and recorded (13). The CT scan was then registered to the anatomical scan (T1-weighted MPRAGE) obtained prior to surgery, and the positions of all electrodes translated into the MRI-space. All image registration was affine and performed using FSL FLIRT (14, 15). Segmentation was performed on the T1 MPRAGE images using the Freesurfer package (http://surfer.nmr.mgh.harvard.edu/), whose parcelation maps were interpolated into the dMRI space.

PAIRED CORRELATION AND STATISTICAL MEASURES

For each of the four modalities, as summarized in **Table 2**, using a single location as a "seed," a large set of connectivity values can be computed to targets outside of the seed: for the CCEP modality the targets are the other recording electrodes (which can number up to 200), and for each target a connectivity value can be computed; for the other modalities the targets are the remaining voxels occupying cortical gray matter, which can number up to 5000–10,000. For a given patient with an intracranial electrode used for CCEP stimulation, all four measures of connectivity can be computed using the stimulation location as a common seed. This permits a cross-comparison between the modalities; specifically the connectivity from the seed to any target point can be compared between the four modalities. The comparison can be made for all targets in the form of a two-dimensional scatter plot, with each axis representing the magnitude of a modality's connectivity. One measure

Table 2 | Summary of the four measures of connectivity used for comparisons in epilepsy patients who underwent evaluation with intracranial electrodes.

	Category	Method	Measure of connectivity
1	Electrophysiological-stimulated	CCEP	Mean voltage during short time window
2	Functional-passive	Resting state fMRI	Temporal correlation coefficient, seed-based approach
3	Functional-stimulated	DES-fMRI	*t*-score from a BOLD activation map
4	Structural-passive	dMRI	Product of local connectivities along pathway determined from PDE approach

of the consistency between two modalities is the Pearson correlation coefficient, such that a value of 1 is a perfect correlation and 0 is no correlation. A p-value for the correlation coefficient is also obtained. These values were computed using Interactive Data Language (IDL, Exelis, Boulder CO, USA).

Aside from AFNI (22), FSL, and Freesurfer routines, all software routines were developed in house using the Interactive Data Language (IDL, Exelis, Boulder CO, USA). All IRB and HIPPA requirements were strictly followed.

RESULTS

CORTICO-CORTICAL EVOKED POTENTIALs

Robust distal and proximal activation is easily elicited with this technique. The top panel of **Figure 1** shows a typical example of one complete electrode recording obtained in the parietal lobe of a patient with a large subdural grid array (#1), who was stimulated in the frontal Broca's regions (as determined earlier by speech arrest using higher currents and frequencies). A series of 46 CCEP recordings are seen via their stimulation artifact (tall alternating spikes), occurring over a recording duration of 50 s. The middle panel of **Figure 1** shows an overlay of the 46 CCEP recordings from the same electrode mapped to a common stimulation time point, with the red line showing the mean signal. This plot reveals the degree of variability typical in these electrophysiological experiments. The white line in the bottom panel of **Figure 1** shows the mean signal from an electrode in the parietal lobe known to be associated with language (as determined earlier using speech arrest obtained after stimulation at higher currents and frequencies). The observation of speech arrest and the robust CCEP signal implies that both the stimulation and recording points lie on a portion of the language network, i.e., the presumed Broca's and Wernicke's area. The overlaid red line was obtained from an adjacent electrode about 10 mm distant, which appears markedly different, showing minimal evoked potential. The difference in these two graphs across 10 mm indicates the spatial scale across which markedly different EP connectivities can be measured using this technique.

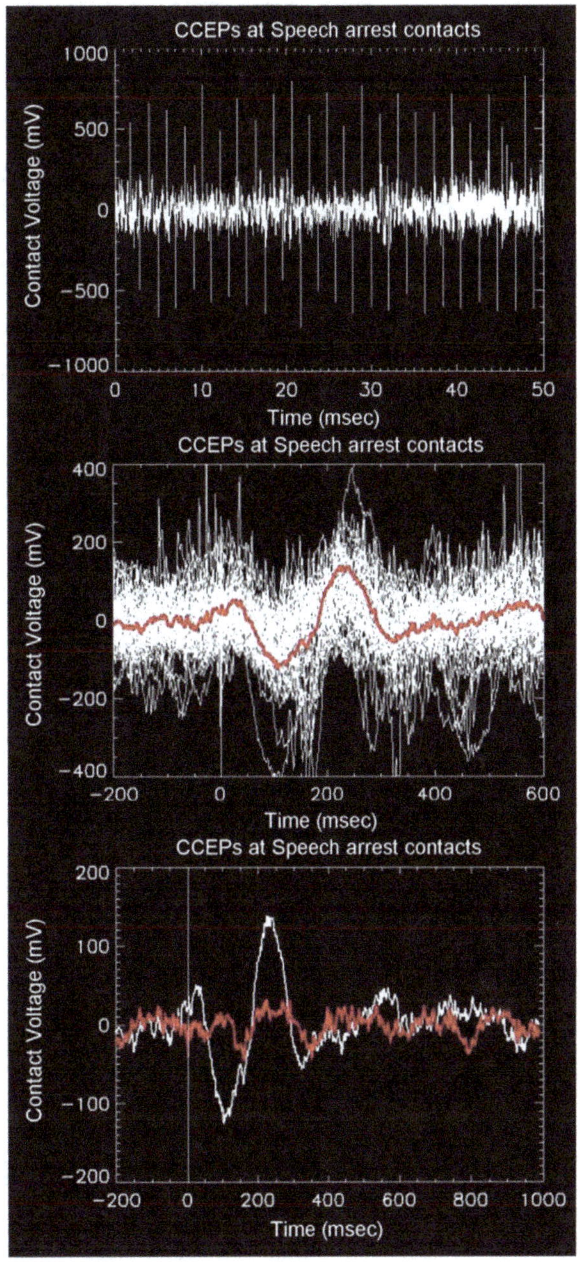

FIGURE 1 | Top: example of raw data recorded from one intracranial electrode (in this case overlaying the presumed Wernicke's area in the left angular gyrus) in response to stimulation from left Broca's region. There are a total of 46 alternating unipolar stimulations seen as spikes from stimulation artifact. The middle panel shows the overlay of all 46 waveforms as referenced to a common stimulation time. The red line shows the average of the waveforms, with a prominent downward peak at 100 ms, followed by an upward peak at 230 ms. The bottom panel shows the same average waveform overlaid with the waveform obtained from one adjacent electrode 10 mm away, showing strong spatial variability from distal stimulation.

Figure 2 shows an inflated surface reconstruction with an overlay of the CCEP response, obtained over a grid array of 120 electrodes. The electrical stimulation was applied to the left inferior frontal gyrus at $t = 0$ ms for a duration of 0.3 ms, at the location shown by the two small white circles in the first image. Red colors represent positive voltage and blue are negative, using a threshold

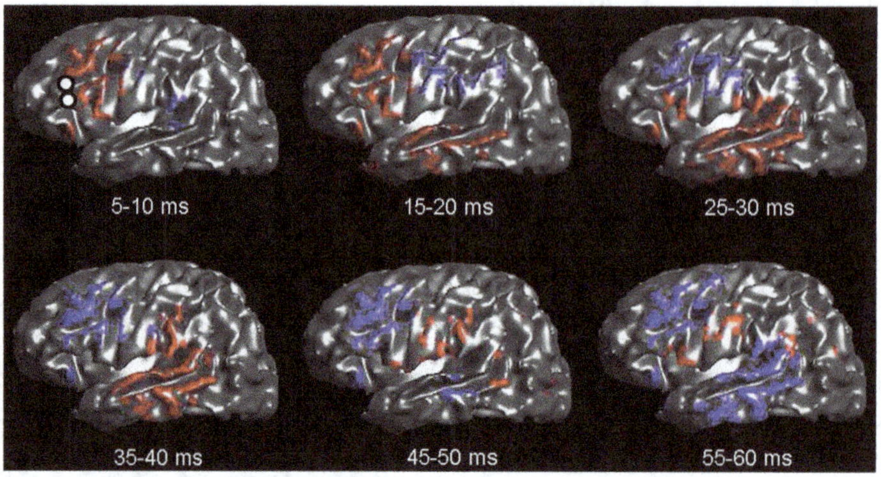

FIGURE 2 | Voltage patterns recorded from left-sided subdural grids in response to a CCEP stimulation at left Broca's region (whose electrode-pair is shown as two white circles in the first image). The underlay is the inflated brain. Voltages are taken as the average during a 5 ms window. Red represents positive voltages greater than 50 mV; blue represents voltages less than −50 mV. A total of six images are shown with mean voltages taken from the displayed time intervals. Note the rapid evolution of voltage spread, which qualitatively follows the expected connection along the arcuate fasciculus.

of $\pm 50\,\mu V$, respectively. The displayed time periods are the times during which the voltage was averaged. The figure shows the relatively rapid evolution of the pattern of response during the first 50 ms: a very early negative response is seen around the supramarginal gyrus, followed by intense activation in the temporal lobe which reverses polarity by 50 ms. Other temporal patterns can be seen, and altogether reveals the complex nature of globally evoked potentials stimulated by a point source.

RESTING STATE fMRI

Figure 3 shows an example of resting state connectivity as revealed from the temporal correlation coefficients using a seed method. Using the same patient in **Figure 2**, the seed point was taken as the stimulation location in the inferior frontal lobe, at the functional location of Broca's area as determined by earlier speech arrest. The green-yellow color indicates a positive correlation value greater than 0.5. The seed points are shown by the white circles, representing the locations of the stimulation electrode pair. The image reveals the widespread network of correlated resting-state fluctuations, which roughly correspond to the presumed distal language regions of the superior and inferior temporal gyri. We define our second measure of connectivity as the magnitude of the correlation coefficient. Due to the inherent three-dimensional nature of MRI, a complete map of connectivity can be produced and compared with other measures.

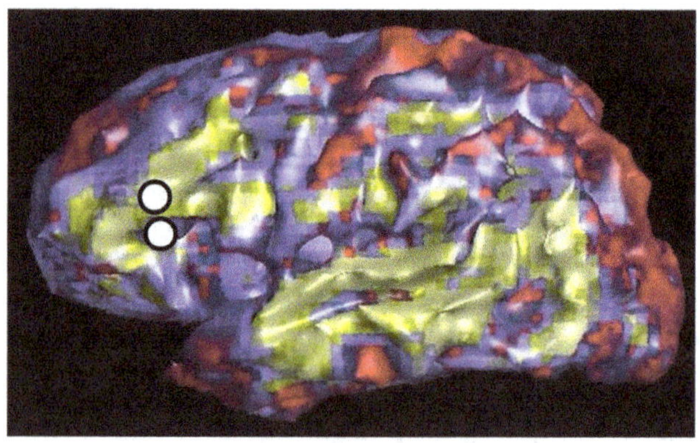

FIGURE 3 | Resting state connectivity map of left hemisphere, using seed-based approach with seed located at left Broca's region as indicated by two white circles. These are the same locations used for CCEP stimulation in **Figure 2**. The color scale reflects the value of the temporal correlation coefficient, with green-yellow representing any value greater than 0.5. Qualitatively there is strong correlation from Broca's region to other expected language areas in the left temporal lobe.

DIRECT ELECTRICAL STIMULATION AND FUNCTIONAL MRI

The major results of the DES-fMRI experiments has been recently reported (3), and was performed safely and successfully in four patients using the methods described above. **Figure 4** shows an example from one patient (#5 in **Table 1**) who was stimulated in the left orbito-frontal region, as shown by the small black asterisk highlighted by the magenta arrow. The overlaid color represents the magnitude of the statistical map (t-score) as indicated by the color bar. This image reveals many of the salient features from all patients: (1) robust BOLD activation can be induced; (2) activation is seen both proximally (e.g., adjacent insula and hippocampus) and distally (e.g., opposite hemisphere); (4) the patterns of activation are suggestive of underlying networks, e.g., the strong linear activation along the limbic system of the cingulate gyrus; and (5) robust deactivation (or "negative" activation) is seen, which also appears to conform to underlying networks. We hypothesize for this research that the magnitude of the t-score is our third measure of connectivity. Due to the inherent three-dimensional nature of MRI, a complete

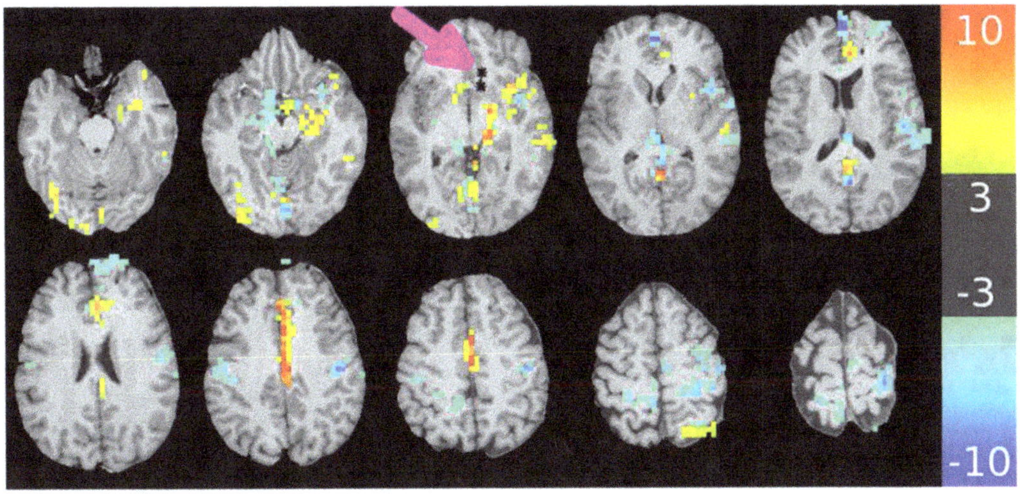

FIGURE 4 | Map of BOLD response in brain due to stimulation of an electrode-contact pair shown as asterisks indicated by the magenta arrow. The color bar to the right shows the value of the *t*-statistic, using a threshold magnitude of 3. Among the features represented are activation both proximal and distal to the contacts (including contralateral side); activation along known anatomic features such as the left cingulate gyrus; and strong negative activation as seen in the bilateral sensorimotor regions. The stimulation used a 32 s block design with an alternating unipolar 8 mA pulse at 20 Hz. The TR was 2 s, over four blocks for a 5 min acquisition. The patient was under general anesthesia (3).

map of connectivity can be produced and compared with other measures.

dMRI CONNECTIVITY

Figure 5 shows an example of the PDE method of tractography, using for the seed the mid-pons, and for the target the entire neocortex. A total of 200,000 tracks are produced, but for clarity only the 14,000 connecting to the precentral gyrus are displayed, which is an anterior view showing the resulting cortico-spinal tracks. Each pathway is color-coded by the magnitude of the pathway-score described in the methods. Note the method successfully tracks to all portions of the precentral gyrus, and is not affected by problems from crossing fibers from the corpus callosum or the superior longitudinal fasciculus. As expected, there is relatively strong connectivity to the upper and lower extremities, and lower connectivity to the bulbar region. The collective pathway follows the expected twisting-ribbon geometry of the known cortico-spinal tract.

By applying this method to the invasive patients, using as the seed the location of the stimulating electrodes and using as the target the remaining neocortex, a full cortical map can be produced wherein every cortical voxel obtains a value related to the pathway score. We assume for this research that the magnitude of the pathways-score is our fourth measure of connectivity. Again, due to the inherent three-dimensional nature of MRI, a complete map of connectivity can be produced and compared with other measures.

Figure 6 is an example of the dMRI method applied to the same patient in **Figures 2** and **3**, using as a seed the left Broca's region and then tracking to and scoring all remaining gray matter voxels. The white circles again represent the location of the stimulating electrodes, which were identified to stimulate Broca's region. The

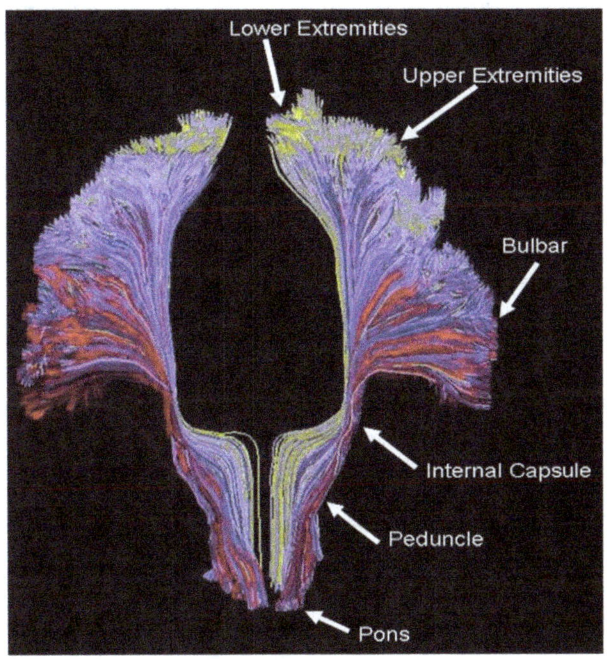

FIGURE 5 | Example of tractography using the method developed for this work, using as a seed the cortical spinal tract at the level of the central pons, and displaying all tracts connecting that location to all voxels located in the precentral gyrus. Each path is color-coded by the strength of the global connectivity score as described in the Data Sheet 1 in Supplementary Material (yellow-green represents high structural connectivity; blue is intermediate; red is low). The method recapitulates the known set of pathways connecting both medial and lateral aspects of the precentral gyrus, and is not significantly affected by crossing fibers from the transcallosal and superior longitudinal fasciculus.

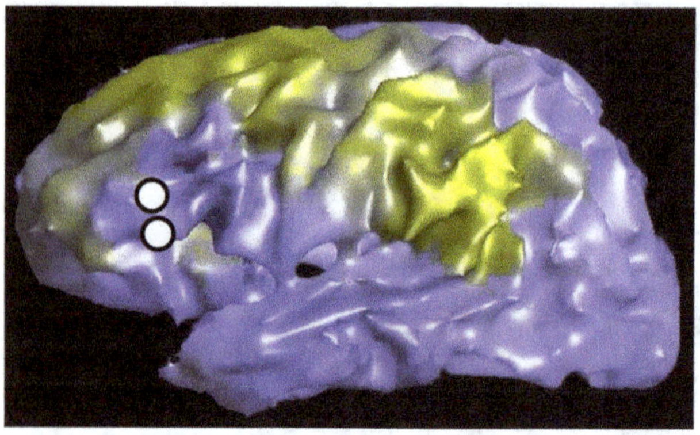

FIGURE 6 | Left lateral view of structural connectivity, using the electrode locations (white circles) stimulating Broca's region as a seed and connecting to all other cortical gray matter voxels. This is the same patient shown in **Figures 2** and **3**. The green color indicates higher structural connectivity, whereas blue color indicates lower structural connectivity.

color scale is normalized so that yellow-green is a higher pathway-score than blue. The pattern shows increased connectivity to the presumed language regions of the parietal lobe, in addition to connections in the frontal lobe. This procedure was repeated for all stimulation sites in patients #1–4. Since all cortical voxels can be scored, complete comparisons can be made to the other methods that compute a connectivity value at all cortical voxels, namely rsfMRI and DES-fMRI. CCEP is the only method of the four presented that computes a connectivity score at a relatively small number (100–200) of locations.

CROSS-CORRELATIONS

After applying these four methods of computing connectivity to a common seed location in an epilepsy patient with intracranial electrodes, a paired comparison can be made between any two selected methods. **Figure 7** displays the six different paired comparisons possible from four methods, each shown as a two-dimensional scatter plot with each axis representing the connectivity value of a selected method. The data from different seed locations are superimposed on each plot. In addition, all available data from the eight patients are also superimposed on each plot. For each plot, the Pearson correlation coefficient r^2 and its associated p-value are computed from the entire ensemble of displayed data points. These numbers are printed at the top and also listed in **Table 3**. Hypothesizing that the value of the correlation coefficient is a measure of the consistency between two methods of connectivity, there is a wide range of correspondence ranging from 0.001 to 0.20. All of the correlations show statistical significance, even for the lowest values, and is likely due to the enormous number of data points available for comparison. The lowest correlations are associated with rsfMRI, which the highest are related to CCEPs.

DISCUSSION

Although the four measures of connectivity show statistically significant correlation coefficients, the most striking observation for a given pair-correlation is the large scatter of points, particularly on the measures that permit inclusion of all voxels in the brain. That is, for a given pair of measures, there are many pairs of voxels in the brain that show a high level correlation using method A, with a low correlation using method B; and visa versa. While the statistically significant trend is scientifically useful for group comparisons, any possible medical applications to an individual patient require more robust metrics or another paradigm for understanding these discrepancies. There are many possible causes for the low correlation values, some may be intrinsic to the brain and its function, while others are technical and methodological, both of which are now discussed.

One likely contributor to the discrepancy in the pair correlation is the failure to correctly co-localize a point in MRI space with the source of an EEG signal. One reason is technical, that the co-registered position of the electrode as determined by CT is not correctly co-located to the corresponding point on the MRI. The error can be due to either the CT or MRI: brain shift occurring during the presence of implanted electrodes during CT, or warping of the MRI due to field gradients, particularly at the brain's base. Another reason is the exact location of the voltage source. That is, although the subtraction of an adjacent electrode-contact pair measures a given signal, there exists some uncertainty about the exact location of the source of the signal with respect to the paired contacts. If it is a point source, it is likely that the distance from the source to the electrode pair is comparable to the distance between the electrode contacts. For example, if the contacts are separated by 5 mm, that could represent a distance of two voxels from the imaged locations of the electrodes. This possibility is complicated by the reality that most sources will be distributed, likely over a spatial scale at least as large as 5 mm. One approach to address this consideration is to incorporate a source model of the CCEP waveforms (16) rather than directly use the electric signals that come from the equipment. However, source modeling is complex and introduces its own assumptions and uncertainties.

In addition to robust positive BOLD activation seen during stimulated fMRI, there are network-like regions of "negative" activation, or relative deactivation. This phenomenon is often seen with task-related paradigms and sometimes is attributed to the design, for example where the "rest" cycle is not truly at rest. However, in our DES-fMRI experiments the patient is anesthetized and the negative BOLD patterns appear as a consequence of positive stimulation. It is uncertain if this negative activation is the result of direct point-to-point action potentials from the stimulated region to the negatively activated cortex, or the result of positive stimulation to secondary cortex that in turn deactivates cortex. Regardless, it raises the question of how a shower of signals delivered to cortex results in relative deactivation. One possible explanation is that there is tremendous neuronal processing that occurs in a segment of cortex before electrical responses that synchronize sufficiently to produce a macroscopic voltage capable of detection with intracranial or extracranial electrodes. For example, it is known that an area at least 10 cm^2 of synchronized cortex is required for detection by a scalp electrode (17). The vast number of neurons required for this ensemble response is likely much more than the number initially stimulated by an incoming wave of action potentials. Thus, between the moment of initial stimulation and macroscopic signal detection there must be a computational buildup with tremendous intra-cortical processing. Although initially stimulated in a

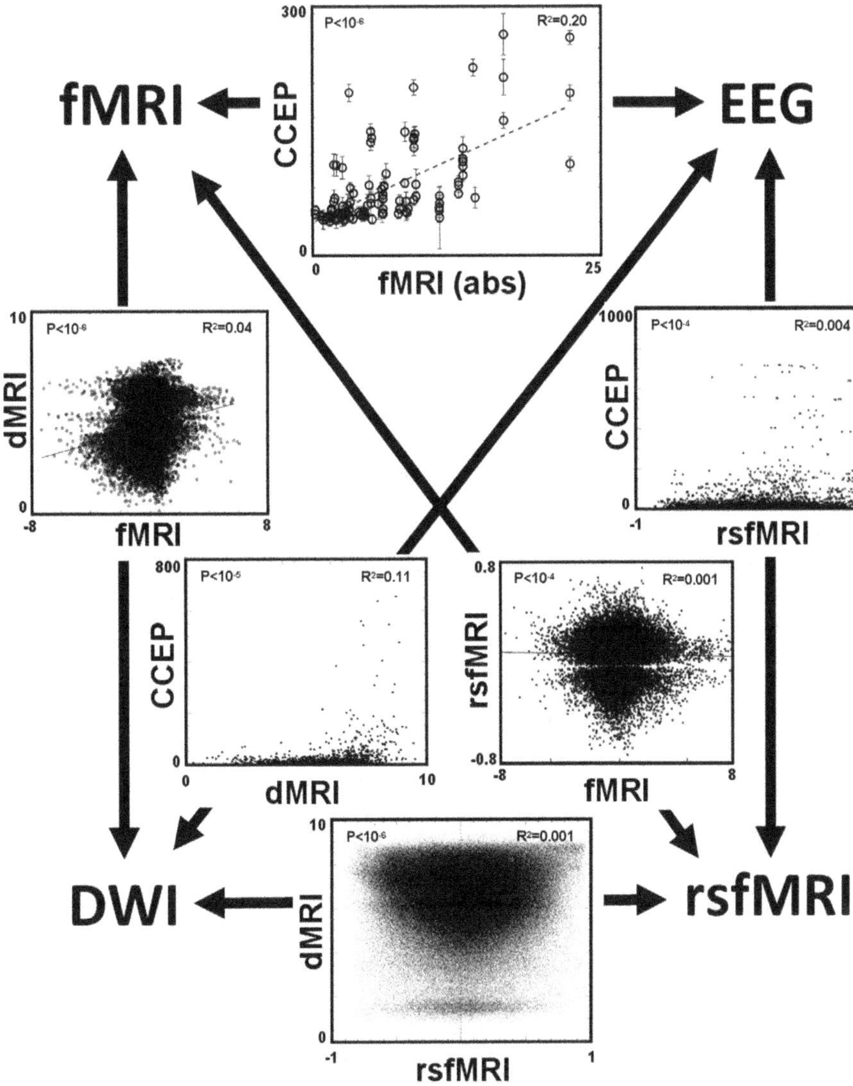

FIGURE 7 | The main result is displayed as a set of six paired comparisons from four different methods of measuring connectivity. Each square shows a two-dimensional scatter plot of points using the methods labeled along the axes. The data are a compilation from all eight patients. For data comparing the CCEP method, a point is plotted for each electrode contact. For the other comparisons a point is plotted for each cortical voxel, thus these plots have a higher density of points. The units of the CCEPs scale in μV; the units of the rsfMRI are the Pearson correlation coefficient typically ranging from −1 to 1; the units of fMRI are the statistical *t*-score (using the absolute value when compared with CCEP); and the units of the dMRI are arbitrary with 0 representing negligible structural connectivity and 10 representing strong structural connectivity. The value of the Pearson correlation coefficient r^2 computed from the data within each plot is printed in the top right corner; its associated *p*-value is printed in the top left corner.

positive sense by a relative small number of neurons, this intracortical processing could proceed in either increased or decreased tone, that is, either positive or negative reaction.

Another uncertainty likely contributing to the poor correlation regarding comparisons with CCEP signals is the scalar metric derived from the signal and used for comparison. One detail is which time window of the CCEP signal is most appropriate for comparison? For example, regarding comparison with structural connectivity may best compare with the early time course of the signal, perhaps a time scale comparable to the axonal transit time, say between 5 and 15 ms. On the contrary, regarding comparison with resting state connectivity or DES-fMRI, which likely elicit and more steady-state ensemble reaction of brain activity, a better comparison with structural activity might be to average the signal intensity over a much longer period of time, perhaps 0.1–1.0 s.

A source of variability leading to poor correlation may be the manner of electrical stimulation, particularly with the variables of current and frequency. Regarding current, larger currents will stimulate a larger volume of tissue, which may alter the distal patterns of response (18). Experimentally it is difficult to know the optimum current since the current is raised until a desired effect is noticed, whose threshold can vary in different brain regions. Similarly, the 1 Hz stimulation frequency of CCEP may elicit a different network of activation than at a higher – and more

Table 3 | Paired comparison of four methods for brain connectivity.

	CCEP	DES-fMRI	rsfMRI	dMRI
CCEP		$r^2 = 0.20$ $<10^{-5}$	$r^2 = 0.004$ $<10^{-4}$	$r^2 = 0.11$ $<10^{-5}$
DES-fMRI			$r^2 = 0.001$ $<10^{-4}$	$r^2 = 0.04$ $<10^{-6}$
rsfMRI				$r^2 = 0.001$ $<10^{-6}$
dMRI				

The top number is the Pearson correlation coefficient r^2, and the number below is the associated p-value.

physiologic – frequency. These are all experimental values worthy of exploration in future studies.

All data were derived from patients with long-standing and intractable epilepsy, whose brains feature foci of abnormal cortical excitability. These foci likely correspond to the nodes of some network, which raises the possibility of associated abnormal connectivity. This variation could contribute to the scatter seen with an ensemble of paired correlations.

In addition to the large scatter of paired correlations between two given modalities, there is strong variation of the overall correlation between the various pairs of modalities, for example the correlation between CCEP and DES-fMRI is the largest at $r^2 = 0.20$, while that between DES-fMRI and rsfMRI (and dMRI and rsfMRI) is the weakest at $r^2 = 0.001$. This difference may reflect the underlying scale of the modality: at one extreme dMRI reflects simple node-to-node connectivity between any two cortical points, whereas rsfMRI connectivity reflects a more "ensemble" of brain activity including the effects of feedback circuits containing multiple nodes. Thus the correlation coefficient may be highest between modalities featuring simple node-to-node connectivity (for example dMRI, and CCEPS derived from early time measurements), and lowest between any modality compared with rsfMRI. The initial expectancy that different measures of connectivity are mutually consistent may be misguided, for example a strong correlation between structural and functional connectivity, and that a pathway to better understanding one measure of connectivity it a detailed analysis of its difference to other measures.

While the *quantitative* comparison of the different connectivity measures is poor, often the qualitative patterns of the maps can seem similar. For example, the lateral surface images in **Figures 2**, **3**, and **6** are from the same patient for the modalities of CCEPs, rsfMRI, and dMRI connectivity, where the seed for each modality is the left Broca's area. While detailed pair-correlations of voxel-to-voxel scatter plots show the typical finding of a significant but weak correlation, the overall patterns of correlation compare well qualitatively to the eye. This could raise the possibility that coarse features of connectivity are similar, but there are errors in the details.

The practical clinical question arises about how such sophisticated comparisons, metrics, or models could be used to benefit patients with epilepsy. For example, how might knowledge of a network directly help the clinician? The ultimate goal is identification of the EZ, wherein removal of that tissue inhibits the electrophysiological cascade that erupts into a seizure. Assuming the EZ is one node in a network, an alternative approach could be resection of non-EZ node in the network such that its removal interrupts any epileptogenic circuitry that contributes to seizure generation. One of the major problems in the process of the presurgical localization of the EZ through scalp EEG recordings is the issue of false localization of a surface activity that is the result of a network/subcortical spread from a distant focus (in a different gyrus, lobe and at times hemisphere) (19). Optimizing non-invasive measures of connectivities would undoubtedly assist in the identification of the correct focus and would therefore result in the optimization of the surgical results through the resection of the source of the electrical activity rather than a non-needed resection of the wrong falsely localized "focus." Another approach to how epilepsy might benefit from an accurate relation of the different measures of connectivity is discussed in **Figure 8**. The data in **Figure 8** illustrate the more comprehensive nature of DES-fMRI for the mapping of all the nodes of a particular epileptic network as fMRI measures BOLD changes in the whole brain while depth or subdural electrodes measure a much more restricted part of the cortex that is based on a hypothesis that is generated from less than optimal non-invasive methods as discussed above.

One possible approach is to compare activated networks that are indigenously and spontaneously activated by interictal discharges to those stimulated externally. A technical problem to surmount is that, at a sufficiently small spatial scale, the exact location of depth electrode contacts can be relatively random with respect to the exact location of the EZ. But if sufficiently close, stimulation of the electrode contacts involving the EZ might activate the same spatial network as indigenous activation from an interictal discharge. If these patterns can be observed, for example using the full 3D capability of BOLD imaging, then overlap of the two maps can serve as verification that the location of stimulation by an electrode is the same location as the EZ. In effect, the BOLD pattern revealed by an interictal discharge could serve as a fingerprint regarding the origin of activation (the epileptic focus). In the far future, an enticing strategy would be any new method that can elicit an interictal discharge, or a seizure, which can be turned on and off as desired, and thereby forms the "task" in a BOLD fMRI experiment. This might be accomplished using a pharmacological method to "stress" the system, or modulate the thresholds to uncover epileptic activities in a controlled fashion.

Another approach is to examine the local vs. distal patterns of activation. The hypothesis could be that local cortical activation in the region of the EZ is augmented by the underlying disease and seizure history. Similar to a spreading depression, and propagated by innumerable interneurons along the cortical layers, local activation could appear different than distal stimulation elicited by long range white matter fiber tracks in terms of both amplitude and speed. For example, the mono-synaptic character of long range connections may proceed at a faster rate than polysynaptic connections within the cortical layers. (20) The presence of disease could alter this comparison whereby local activation proceeds abnormally quickly with abnormally high magnitude. The concept of altered local reactivity is supported

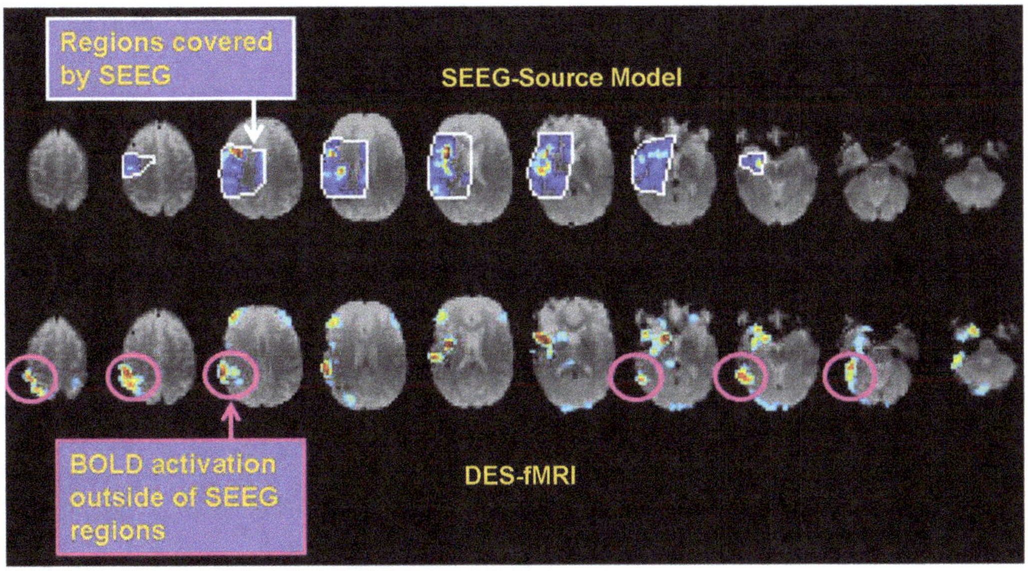

FIGURE 8 | Example of the possible clinical utility derived from accurate correspondence of different connectivity measures. While EEG or CCEP measures may form a gold standard, the drawback is limited brain coverage. The use of an EEG source model may improve local coverage between electrodes, but fails to adequately compute electrophysiological activity further outside these regions. The top row of images shows the EEG source model (computed using Brainstorm) from stimulation of an electrode in the right insular region in a patient with 12 right-sided stereotactically placed EEG depth electrodes (not shown). Visualization of the brain's response to stimulation appears more continuous in the regions of reliable computation (region bounded by white line), and may offer superior comparison to other methods of connectivity. Note the region of reliable results is only covers a minority of the entire brain. The bottom row shows the corresponding DES-fMRI BOLD connectivity map derived from stimulation of the same electrode-pair as the top row. While there is qualitative correspondence of the connectivity maps in the region of the temporal lobe and insula, the DES-fMRI map encompasses the entire brain and reveals strong areas of activation outside the coverage of SEEG electrodes, namely in the right parietal lobe. Establishing a reliable relation between these two measures of connectivity could synergistically enhance the coverage of invasive electrodes.

by electrophysiological observations to local electrodes upon stimulation of the EZ, wherein the magnitude of local electrodes is exaggerated (21).

One potential avenue of failure represented in **Figure 7** may result from an ill-posed assumption, namely that the correct comparison between different modalities is a simple pairwise correlation between them. Perhaps a better metric for one modality may incorporate information from other modalities. For example, functional connectivity could be informed from structural connectivity and thereby correct or exclude comparisons that that are not structurally connected. Further, functional connectivity between any pair of points may be influenced more by a multinodal network that connects them rather than a single point-to-point connection. This possibility suggests the future importance of a complete brain model that incorporates all the measurable modalities. Such a model can, in effect, translate between the metrics of different modalities. The ultimate goal would be a sufficiently sophisticated model that could conceivably model an individual brain. Such a model could not practically occur at the microscopic spatial scale of neurons, but at the mesoscopic scale of the imaging voxel. The challenge is finding a method to reliably inform the model, i.e., set all the innumerable parameters with information obtained from a non-invasive modality. Such a modality would need to be sufficiently content-rich to inform a large model. One possibility would be long-term resting state fMRI, informed by structural imaging from dMRI methods. This development would represent the next step in the evolution of neuroimaging, in which the imaging biomarker moves from being the images themselves, to a mathematical brain model that is informed by images.

CONCLUSION

A significant next step in the future of imaging brain function is connectivity; however, there are many different metrics for connectivity. This work presents experimental observations with cross-comparisons of four methods produced from eight epilepsy patients with intracranial electrodes. The major result is that although the four methods show statistically significant paired-consistency as computed by a non-zero correlation value, the magnitude of the correlations is relatively poor. Thus there is less cross-modal consensus than might be expected with a simple view of brain connectivity. For example, using two modalities A and B, there are many regions of the brain that show strong connectivity using A but low connectivity using B; and visa versa. The reason for the discrepancies is likely inherent to fundamental differences in the different modalities, thus the objective of a strong simple pairwise correlation is ill-posed. However, we envision that strong correlations can be recovered with the use of an intermediary mathematical model of the brain that can translate the connectivity between different modalities.

REFERENCES

1. Honey CJ, Sporns O, Cammoun L, Gigandet X, Thiran JP, Meuli R, et al. Predicting human resting-state functional connectivity from structural connectivity. *Proc Natl Acad Sci U S A* (2009) **106**(6):2035–40. doi:10.1073/pnas.0811168106
2. Skudlarski P, Jagannathan K, Calhoun VD, Hampson M, Skudlarska BA, Pearlson G. Measuring brain connectivity: diffusion tensor imaging validates resting state temporal correlations. *Neuroimage* (2008) **43**(3):554–61. doi:10.1016/j.neuroimage.2008.07.063
3. Jones SE, Zhang M, Avitsian R, Bhattachya P, Bulacio J, Cendes F, et al. Functional MRI networks induced by intracranial stimulation may help defining the epileptogenic zone. *Brain Connect* (2014) **4**(4):286–98. doi:10.1089/brain.2014.0225
4. Beall EB, Lowe MJ. Isolating physiologic noise sources with independently determined spatial measures. *Neuroimage* (2007) **37**(4):1286–300. doi:10.1016/j.neuroimage.2007.07.004
5. Beall EB, Lowe MJ. The non-separability of physiologic noise in functional connectivity MRI with spatial ICA at 3T. *J Neurosci Methods* (2010) **191**(2):263–76. doi:10.1016/j.jneumeth.2010.06.024
6. Bullmore ET, Brammer MJ, Rabe-Hesketh S, Curtis VA, Morris RG, Williams SC, et al. Methods for diagnosis and treatment of stimulus-correlated motion in generic brain activation studies using fMRI. *Hum Brain Mapp* (1999) **7**(1):38–48. doi:10.1002/(SICI)1097-0193(1999)7:1<38::AID-HBM4>3.3.CO;2-H
7. Holland D, Kuperman JM, Dale AM. Efficient correction of inhomogeneous static magnetic field-induced distortion in echo planar imaging. *Neuroimage* (2010) **50**(1):175. doi:10.1016/j.neuroimage.2009.11.044
8. Sakaie KE, Lowe MJ. Quantitative assessment of motion correction for high angular resolution diffusion imaging. *Magn Reson Imaging* (2010) **28**:290–6. doi:10.1016/j.mri.2009.07.004
9. Leemans A, Jones DK. The B-matrix must be rotated when correcting for subject motion in DTI data. *Magn Reson Med* (2009) **61**:1336–49. doi:10.1002/mrm.21890
10. Tournier JD, Calamante F, Gadian DG, Connelly A. Direct estimation of the fiber orientation density function from diffusion-weighted MRI data using spherical deconvolution. *Neuroimage* (2004) **23**(3):1176–85. doi:10.1016/j.neuroimage.2004.07.037
11. Sakaie KE, Lowe MJ. An objective method for regularization of fiber orientation distributions derived from diffusion-weighted MRI. *Neuroimage* (2007) **34**:169–76. doi:10.1016/j.neuroimage.2006.08.034
12. Zhang M, Sakaie KE, Jones SE. Logical foundations and fast implementation of probabilistic tractography. *IEEE Trans Med Imaging* (2013) **32**(8):1397–410. doi:10.1109/TMI.2013.2257179
13. Matsumoto R, Nair DR, LaPresto E, Najm I, Bingaman W, Shibasaki H, et al. Functional connectivity in the human language system: a cortico-cortical evoked potential study. *Brain* (2004) **127**(Pt 10):2316–30. doi:10.1093/brain/awh246
14. Jenkinson M, Smith SM. A global optimisation method for robust affine registration of brain images. *Med Image Anal* (2001) **5**:143–56. doi:10.1016/S1361-8415(01)00036-6
15. Jenkinson M, Bannister PR, Brady JM, Smith SM. Improved optimisation for the robust and accurate linear registration and motion correction of brain images. *Neuroimage* (2002) **17**:825–41. doi:10.1006/nimg.2002.1132
16. Cosandier-Rimélé D, Merlet I, Badier JM, Chauvel P, Wendling F. The neuronal sources of EEG: modeling of simultaneous scalp and intracerebral recordings in epilepsy. *Neuroimage* (2008) **42**(1):135–46. doi:10.1016/j.neuroimage.2008.04.185
17. Tao JX, Baldwin M, Ray A, Hawes-Ebersole S, Ebersole JS. The impact of cerebral source area and synchrony on recording scalp electroencephalography ictal patterns. *Epilepsia* (2007) **48**(11):2167–76. doi:10.1111/j.1528-1167.2007.01224.x
18. Ranck JB. Which elements are excited in electrical stimulation of mammalian central nervous system: a review. *Brain Res* (1975) **98**:417–40. doi:10.1016/0006-8993(75)90364-9
19. Wang ZI, Jin K, Kakisaka Y, Mosher JC, Bingaman WE, Kotagal P, et al. Imag(in)ing seizure propagation: MEG-guided interpretation of epileptic activity from a deep source. *Hum Brain Mapp* (2012) **33**(12):2797–801. doi:10.1002/hbm.21401
20. Muller L, Destexhe A. Propagating waves in thalamus, cortex and the thalamocortical system: experiments and models. *J Physiol Paris* (2012) **106**(5–6):222–38. doi:10.1016/j.jphysparis.2012.06.005
21. Iwasaki M, Enatsu R, Matsumoto R, Novak E, Thankappen B, Piao Z, et al. Accentuated cortico-cortical evoked potentials in neocortical epilepsy in areas of ictal onset. *Epileptic Disord* (2010) **12**(4):292–302. doi:10.1684/epd.2010.0334
22. Cox RW, Hyde JS. Software tools for analysis and visualization of fMRI data. *NMR Biomed* (1997) **10**:171–8. doi:10.1002/(SICI)1099-1492(199706/08)10:4/5<171::AID-NBM453>3.0.CO;2-L

10

A critical role for network structure in seizure onset: A computational modeling approach

George Petkov[1†], Marc Goodfellow[1†], Mark P. Richardson[2] and John R. Terry[1*]

[1] College of Engineering, Mathematics and Physical Sciences, University of Exeter, Exeter, UK
[2] Institute of Psychiatry, King's College London, London, UK

Correspondence:
John R. Terry, College of Engineering, Mathematics and Physical Sciences, University of Exeter, Exeter, Devon EX4 4QF, UK
e-mail: j.terry@exeter.ac.uk

[†]Denotes an equal contribution as first author.

Recent clinical work has implicated network structure as critically important in the initiation of seizures in people with idiopathic generalized epilepsies. In line with this idea, functional networks derived from the electroencephalogram (EEG) at rest have been shown to be significantly different in people with generalized epilepsy compared to controls. In particular, the mean node degree of networks from the epilepsy cohort was found to be statistically significantly higher than those of controls. However, the mechanisms by which these network differences can support recurrent transitions into seizures remain unclear. In this study, we use a computational model of the transition into seizure dynamics to explore the dynamic consequences of these differences in functional networks. We demonstrate that networks with higher mean node degree are more prone to generating seizure dynamics in the model and therefore suggest a mechanism by which increased mean node degree of brain networks can cause heightened ictogenicity.

Keywords: network dynamics, epilepsy, dynamical systems, graph theory, EEG

INTRODUCTION

Epilepsy is a serious neurological disorder characterized by the propensity of the brain to generate spontaneous and recurrent seizures. Traditionally, seizures have been defined as "a transient occurrence of signs and/or symptoms due to abnormal, excessive, or synchronous neural activity in the brain" (1). Very recently, the international league against epilepsy (ILAE) has further refined the definition of epilepsy (2) whereby an individual is now proposed to have epilepsy if one of the following conditions is met:

1. Experiencing two unprovoked seizures more than 24 h apart.
2. Experiencing a single unprovoked (or reflex) seizure with a probability of further seizures similar to the general risk of recurrence (~60%) if two unprovoked seizures had occurred.
3. An epilepsy syndrome is diagnosed.

It is important to note that epilepsy is a general term to capture over forty, often diverse, syndromes. However, in each case, the generation of clinical signs and symptoms are presumed to require large regions of the brain to be subject to abnormal dynamics and the initiation, recruitment, and spreading of such dynamics is facilitated by the network of synaptic connections between neurons and between regions of the brain. This is reflected in the recognition of the ILAE that many epilepsy syndromes are associated with disruptions to either global or local brain networks (3).

However, a precise definition of global and local brain networks is surprisingly non-trivial. In the global case, one can consider large-scale structural networks as defined by white matter tracts of axons that connect distal brain regions. These networks can be estimated non-invasively using diffusion imaging. An alternative is to examine the statistical inter-relationship between time series recorded at different locations in the brain, thus, defining a "functional" rather than a structural network. While to some extent, functional networks are constrained by the structural architecture of the brain, they also carry contributions from the dynamics of brain activity (4). We recently studied functional networks derived from scalp electroencephalogram (EEG) at rest and demonstrated significant differences between functional networks of people with idiopathic generalized epilepsy (IGE), their first-degree relatives, and healthy controls (5). Significant differences across a number of graph theory measures highlighted abnormalities in both the epilepsy cohort and their first-degree relatives. The most significant of these was that the mean node degree of networks inferred from both people with IGE and their relatives was much greater than that of controls, but that no differences were found between patients and their relatives. This observation suggests that differences between patients and controls cannot be attributed to medication, and thus, altered functional networks are associated with a propensity to generate recurrent seizures (i.e., epilepsy). However, abnormalities in these networks alone are not sufficient to generate seizures (since they are present in the relatives of people with IGE, whom themselves are seizures free) suggesting that the interplay between functional network structure and the dynamics supported by them must play an important role in seizure generating capability (ictogenicity).

The use of mathematical modeling to attempt to address this and related questions has grown substantially in the past few years. Particularly at the macroscopic scale, where the average response of a mass of neurons is represented by systems of differential equations, several studies have derived insight into the potential dynamic mechanisms that enable seizures associated with spike-wave discharges to emerge spontaneously from background activity (6–10). Lopes da Silva et al. (11) proposed a scenario in which the spontaneous transitions between background activity and seizure states arise due to bistability, i.e., that the background state and seizure state "coexist" and random inputs can perturb the brain from one state to another. This can be interpreted in terms of either state being able to be reached without a change in underlying constants or slowly varying parameters of the system. This type of model was used to demonstrate that the emergence of either focal or generalized seizure like events could occur due to either specific network disruptions or to alterations in excitability within apparently normal network structures (12).

Motivated by a desire to understand the fundamental mechanisms of seizure transitions more clearly, the concept of bistability has formed the basis of more abstract models of the brain, for example, the so-called Z^6 model (13), which provides a phenomenological representation of the critical features of more realistic physiological models. These abstract models, which we might consider to represent a normal form of the more detailed physiological representations, have recently been extended to study the role that explicit network structures have in facilitating transitions into seizure activity (14, 15).

Here, we build on this previous modeling work to further understand the role of network topology in the generation of transitions into seizure dynamics. In order to understand the potential consequence on ictogenecity of the differences in network structure highlighted by Chowdhury et al. (5), we artificially construct networks that preserve the values of mean node degree for each subject. When these networks are used as the connectivity structure for a bistable dynamic network model, we observe that networks with higher mean node degree transition more readily to a seizure state. We therefore suggest a mechanism by which increased mean node degree of brain networks can cause increased ictogenicity.

MATERIALS AND METHODS

MATHEMATICAL MODEL

Since we focus on the role that network structure plays in transitions between background and seizure states, we do not consider a detailed model of each node in a network. Instead, the foundation of our present work is a network of abstract models that are designed to capture a bistable transition between a "background" state and a high-amplitude "seizure" state [see, e.g., Kalitzin et al. (16)]:

$$\frac{d}{dt}Z = \left(a|Z|^4 + b|Z|^2 + C\right) Z + \varepsilon(t), \quad (1)$$

where $Z = x + iy$ is a complex variable (function of time); (a, b) are real constant coefficients, and $C = c + i\omega$ is a constant complex coefficient. The term $\varepsilon(t)$ is the complex input to the system, which incorporates a white noise component to mimic the effects of exogenous fluctuations.

A network model, where each node has as its basis the system described in Eq. 1 is then constructed:

$$\frac{d}{dt}Z_i = \left(a|Z_i|^4 + b|Z_i|^2 + c + i\omega\right) Z_i + \sum_{j=1}^{N} G_{ij}Z_j + \varepsilon_i(t) \quad (2)$$

Here, we consider the dynamics of N units, with linear interaction through an adjacency matrix G, where white noise is generated independently for each node within the network. In the current work, G is scaled by a factor of 0.1 to preserve transitions between states.

Model parameters are based upon our previous work (16) so that each node lies within the bistable regime. This allows transitions to occur between the steady state (SS), and limit cycle (LC) attractors, where the LC is considered to represent seizure dynamics.

CLINICAL EEG RECORDINGS AND CONSTRUCTION OF FUNCTIONAL NETWORKS

The network measures that form the basis of this study were inferred from clinical EEG recordings as described in Ref. (5). In brief, these recordings consisted of 19 channel scalp EEG obtained using standard 10–20 placing with an average reference, and sampled at 256 Hz. The recordings were band-passed between 1 and 70 Hz, and notch-filtered between 48 and 52 Hz to exclude mains frequency interference. The subjects from whom the EEG recordings were taken are divided into two main groups: 35 people with heterogeneous IGE and 40 healthy controls. From each EEG recording, one artifact-free, eyes-closed, 20 s segment was extracted representing a "resting state" or "background" EEG activity. Chowdhury et al. (5) found significant differences between controls and patients in the 6 and 9 Hz "low alpha" frequency band, and we therefore focus on that band here. The Hilbert transform was applied to the band-pass filtered EEG to generate instantaneous phase and amplitude estimates. For each electrode pair, the phase-locking factor [PLF, also known as phase-locking value (17) or mean phase coherence (18)] was calculated as follows:

$$C_1 = c_{ij} = \frac{1}{N_s}\left|\sum_{k=1}^{N_s} e^{i\Delta\phi_{ij}(t_k)}\right| \quad (3)$$

where $\Delta\phi_{ij}(t_k)$ is the instantaneous phase difference between signals i and j at the time point t_k. The $\Delta\phi_{ij}(t_k)$ were reconstructed from the original signals using the Hilbert transform.

This yields a value between 0 and 1 reflecting the strength of synchronous activity between each pair of signals. Functional networks were then constructed using electrode locations as nodes and PLF values as connectivity weights. Since the PLF measure is symmetrical, the resulting functional connectivity networks are undirected.

NETWORK MEASURES

The derived functional networks were quantified using the following graph theory measures: mean degree (MD), degree variance (DV), and local clustering coefficient (CC). The degree of a node is defined as the sum of the weights of the edges incident to that particular node. The MD and DV are defined as the average and the variance, respectively, of degrees over all nodes in the network. The local CC of a node in a network measures how close its neighbors are to a complete network (graph).

GENERATION OF ARTIFICIAL NETWORKS

We note that the networks used for connectivity in the model in this study were not directly inferred from patient data, rather "surrogate" networks were prepared, which preserved properties of the networks studied in Chowdhury et al. (5). Each matrix was originally based on the functional connectivity matrix inferred from the aforementioned EEG data. An undirected binary network with the equivalent value of MD as the original matrix was constructed by applying a set of thresholds to the original, and choosing the threshold for which MD was preserved. Further a computational algorithm was applied (19) in order to randomize the matrix, preserving the degree vector and therefore the MD value. In brief, the algorithm randomly swaps nodes and recalculates the degree vector, checking for disparity. For each original matrix, we constructed 30 artificial random binary matrices with the same MD value as the original weighted connectivity matrix. We verified that the spectrum of the artificial patient and control derived networks was different, confirming a difference in topology of the artificial networks.

MEASURE OF BRAIN NETWORK ICTOGENICITY

We measured the "ictogenicity" of each network by performing simulations using the network as the connectivity matrix for the mathematical model. Since we calculated this measure of ictogenicity from model simulations, we could define an appropriate model state that captured transitions between the non-seizure and seizure dynamics of the model. In the current work, the model seizure state was defined as a solution with local maxima and minima having magnitude >0.5.

For each simulation, of the model Eq. 2, we calculated the time that each node spent in a *LC*, normalized to the simulation time. Averaging over all the nodes, we obtain the probability of any node to be in a *LC and we refer to this probability as the brain network ictogenicity* (BNI).

STATISTICAL ANALYSIS

For comparison of quantitative network measures between groups, we used a non-parametric Kruskal–Wallis one-way ANOVA test. Results are declared significant for $p < 0.05$. For *post hoc* pairwise comparisons between groups, a Bonferroni corrected multiple comparison test was performed with significance level of 0.05.

RESULTS

FUNCTIONAL NETWORKS

Chowdhury et al. (5) reported that the MD of functional networks derived from people with epilepsy was higher than controls. In **Figure 1**, we show the distribution of MD for both epilepsy and control subjects included in that study. In this study, we focus on the dynamic consequences of changes in node degree independent of specific network topology and connectivity weights. We remove a layer of complexity from these networks by transforming them into binary (unweighted) networks, while preserving the MD of networks extracted from the EEG data. **Figure 1** demonstrates the match in value of mean node degree between the original networks and the artificially derived alternatives (see Materials and Methods).

Since the MD is accurately preserved in our artificial networks, the significant difference in MD between patients and controls is also maintained, as shown in **Figure 2**. The use of binary, rather than weighted networks leads our artificial networks to have higher DV than the original networks, as demonstrated in **Figures 2B,E**. A further reason for this difference is that the networks in Chowdhury et al. (5) were normalized to the DV value of 500 surrogate random networks, while in the present case of binary networks such normalization is not possible. However, **Figures 2B,E** show that a significant difference in DV between epilepsy and control subject derived networks is preserved.

Figures 2C,F demonstrate a lack of significant difference in CC between artificial "control" and "epilepsy" networks, in contrast to the EEG derived networks. This demonstrates that our artificially generated networks have removed some specific topological features of the original data, including those related to clustering.

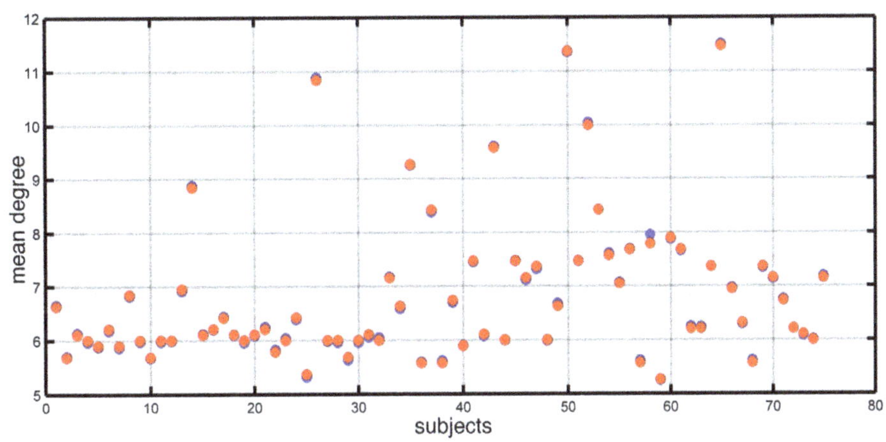

FIGURE 1 | Mean node degree values for each subject (blue dots) and each corresponding artificially constructed binary network (red dots).

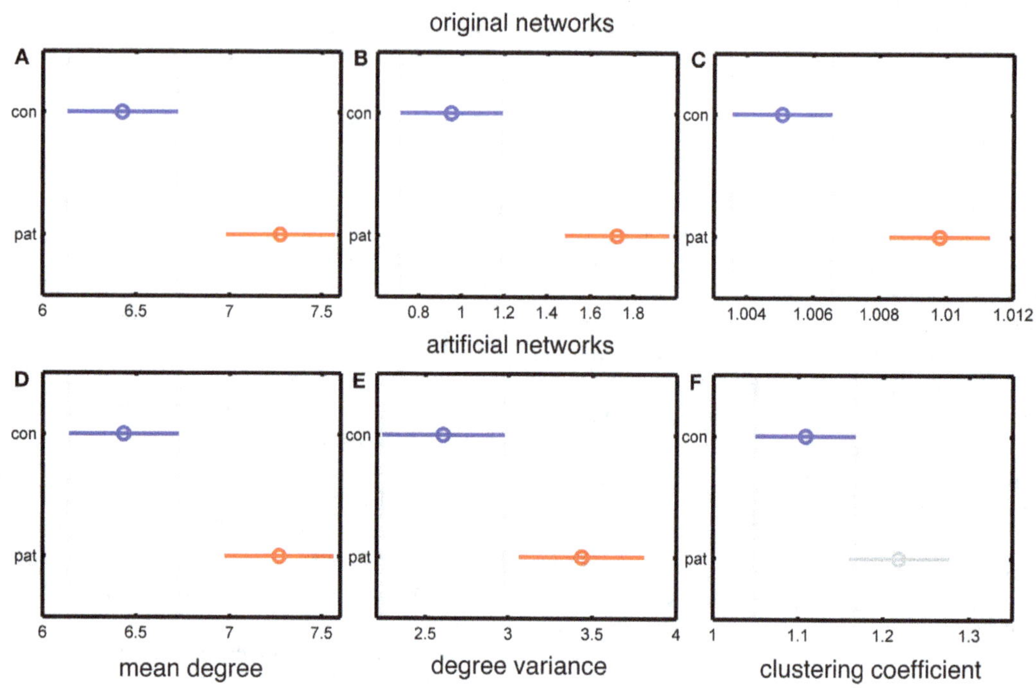

FIGURE 2 | Statistical analysis of the differences between the group mean values of people with epilepsy and healthy controls based on the MD, DV, and CC measures of the connectivity matrices. (A–C) represent data from original networks, whereas **(D–F)** represent data for artificial networks. **(A,D)** show MD, **(B,E)** show DV, and **(C,F)** show CC. The *y*-axis of each panel separates the two groups (control and patients), and the *x*-axis represents the group values of the corresponding network measure. The results are color coded blue for the control group and red for the epilepsy group (except for panel **F**, in which the epilepsy group is colored grey to indicate a lack of statistically significant difference). The horizontal line and the circle show the variance and the mean value of the corresponding network measure. The mean values are considered as statistically significant different if there is no overlap between the lines within a panel.

MODELING RESULTS

For each value of MD extracted from the epilepsy and control cohorts, 30 artificial networks were generated, preserving the MD. These networks were used as the connectivity scheme in the bistable model as described in Section "Materials and Methods." For all simulations of our network model Eq. 2, we fixed model parameters corresponding to the bistable phase space of a single node $\{a, b, c, \omega\} = \{-1, 2, -0.9, 1 + \delta\omega\}$, where $\delta\omega$ is a random number distributed equally in the interval $[-0.2, 0.2]$. This choice is made to avoid artificial phase locking because of the equal phase velocities within our multi-unit configuration. For each network, 30 simulations were performed with random initial conditions. The resulting dynamics were quantified according to the BNI measure described in Section "Materials and Methods." An example of the calculation of BNI and the effect of changes in node degree is given in **Figure 3**.

Four different kinds of dynamics can be seen in **Figure 3**. In **Figure 3A**, the model spends a large portion of the simulation time in the "background" attractor before transitioning to the seizure state. Thus, the BNI measurement is low. In contrast, the trajectory of the model in **Figures 3B–D** moves more quickly into the "seizure" attractor, and so BNI is higher. In addition, in **Figure 3C**, one of the nodes has not transitioned to the trajectory corresponding to the LC attractor in a single node. Rather, this node is being driven around the corresponding fixed point and therefore the BNI in this case is lower. It is clear that in this model, BNI provides a measure of how quickly the trajectory of the system performs an "escape" from the background to the seizure attractor.

Figure 4 shows BNI calculated from all simulations for artificial networks derived from the patient and control networks. It can be seen that BNI is significantly higher in the patient versus the control networks, and thus, networks with an increased node degree are shown to have a greater tendency toward seizure activity in this model.

DISCUSSION

In this study, we used mathematical modeling to investigate the link between the structure of brain networks and their propensity to generate seizure dynamics. Building upon previous studies, we used human EEG data to generate artificial networks preserving MD values, and thus, "isolating" this property for investigation. When networks with high MD were used as connectivity matrices in a model of seizure transitions, we observed significantly more time in the seizure state, as compared to networks with lower MD. We therefore provide evidence for a link between certain properties of network structure (here the MD) and the potential to generate seizure dynamics.

From the network perspective, MD and DV reflect how well connected the nodes within a graph are. Thus, networks with high MD and low DV would tend toward being fully connected, whereas

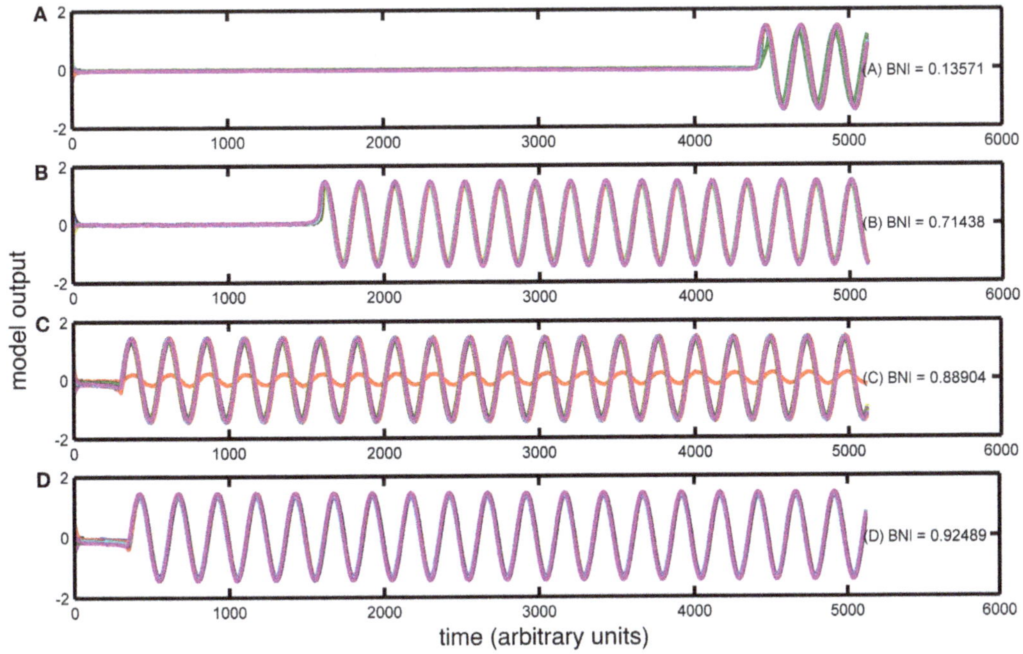

FIGURE 3 | Trajectories of four simulations with the Z^6 model over different artificially created networks. The figure contains **(A–D)** four simulations with different BNI values (as indicated). The *x*-axis of each panel represents the simulation time (arbitrary units) and the *y*-axis represents the amplitude of the simulated signal. In each case, all 19 channels are overlaid in different colors.

networks with high MD and high DV will have an increased number of "hub-like" nodes. Our randomized networks in the patient group displayed higher MD and DV than controls and therefore fall predominantly into this latter category. This suggests that "hub-like" nodes can more easily drive the rest of the network into the seizure state if they themselves enter that state.

Previous modeling studies in the context of temporal lobe seizures and the hippocampus have suggested a role for hub-like connectivity in generating hyper-excitability (20). Such structures have also been shown to be critical for dementia (21), a condition with which epilepsy is comorbid (22), as well as other pathologies of the brain (23). In a related study, Clemens et al. (24) performed a resting EEG derived, functional connectivity network analysis of people with juvenile myoclonic epilepsy (JME) and control subjects. They found no statistically significant differences in measures of local and global efficiency of the derived networks, where "efficiency" relates to the length of the shortest paths between nodes. We should therefore aim to elucidate exactly which topological features of networks can contribute to the generation of seizure dynamics. In future work, we will explore in more detail the dynamic role of centrality, efficiency, and other features of network topology (25) on seizure generation in our model.

The model employed in this study provides an abstract representation of the epileptic brain. It preserves the potential for transitions between "background" and "seizure" dynamics as postulated in the bistable perspective of generalized seizures (11). This simplified approach allows one to focus upon the role that network structure plays in the propensity for dynamic transitions. Indeed, this approach has been used with success in terms of estimating transition frequencies (26), exploring the key dynamic components for intermittent transitions (15) and examining the role of specific connection topologies in small networks (14). An interesting extension to the current work would be to assess the interplay between intrinsic node dynamics and network structure. This could be achieved by using abstract models with richer bifurcation structures (15, 27), or by employing neural mass models of specific epileptiform dynamics (8, 10, 28, 29).

We built artificial networks preserving MD so as to focus on the implications of changes in this property, with respect to the process of transitions from SS to LC. Precise analysis of the model Eq. 2 leads to the conclusion that the behavior of the system in these terms may depend on several factors such as (a) noise level, (b) initial conditions, (c) connection strength, and (d) network topology. As the main goal was to examine the influence of network topology, we removed the influence of all other factors by setting appropriate noise levels, randomly sampling initial conditions, and using binary instead of weighted networks. In future work, we will consider the effects of adding larger variance noise into the model, in order to facilitate recurrent transitions. In addition, we can expand upon the approach by analyzing weighted networks. We envisage that the addition of these kinds of heterogeneities will lead to a richer repertoire of model dynamics, and therefore, might be useful in further stratifying the effect of network topology on dynamic transitions.

Benjamin et al. (14) examined escape times into seizure dynamics in a similar model applied to networks with a small number of nodes. In that case, it was possible to derive analytic expressions

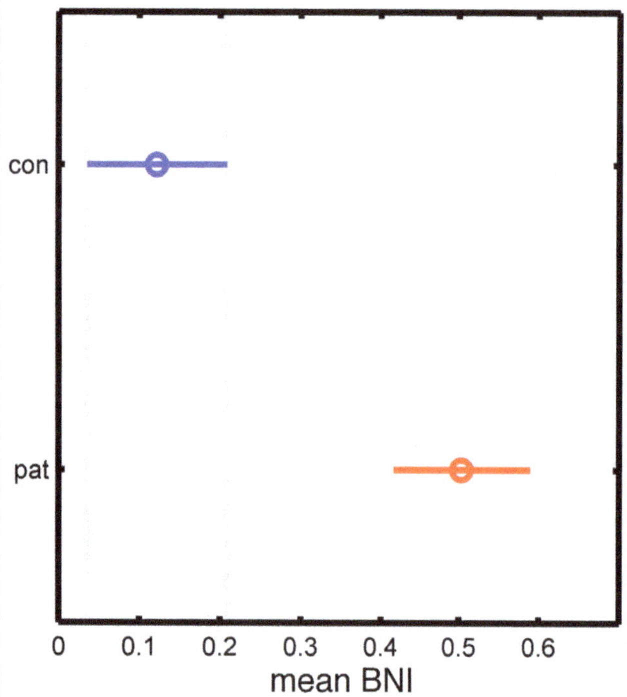

FIGURE 4 | Statistical analysis of the significant differences between control and patient groups based on the mean BNI measure. The *y*-axis separates the two groups, while the *x*-axis represents the mean BNI value. The horizontal line and the circle represent the variance and the mean value of BNI, respectively.

for escape times depending on the topology of networks. However, the complexity of this problem grows significantly as larger networks are considered. Here, in order to link directly with clinical data, we used a model with 19 nodes to represent EEG sensor space. Rather than focusing on explicit network structure, we were able to correlate changes in BNI with properties of the network, e.g., the MD. This provides an avenue to explore the seizure generating potential of more complex networks and could be extended in future work to include other graph theoretic measures, such as the CC, which has also been shown to vary significantly between people with IGE and controls (5, 27).

We used functional connectivity as the basis for the networks applied to our model, reflecting the nature of the available clinical data. This approach means that our model is not a direct representation of brain regions interacting over large scales via axonal connections, though such a model can be built in a patient specific way using diffusion data (29, 30). Rather, our model provides an abstract representation of the resting state of the brain, as projected onto the level of EEG. Networks derived from this projection are thought to be constrained by structural connectivity, though they are not a direct reflection of it (4). Functional networks by definition represent nodes that are evolving similarly, and therefore, capture a potentially important means by which information can be exchanged between brain regions (31). We should therefore consider that the "connections" of such networks can facilitate the emergence of pathological dynamics through synchronization, and we demonstrate here that this can lead to greater seizure generating potential in the epileptic brain.

On the other hand, functional networks can be viewed more simply as transformations of time series data recorded from subjects, i.e., as mappings from multivariate time series onto a static topological network that reflects a combination of structural and dynamic contributions for that instance of time. From this perspective, our modeling approach gives us a tool with which to interrogate data from people with epilepsy and compare these with control subjects. We therefore aim to explore further whether properties of the BNI derived from functional networks can be used as a marker in the clinical setting. We postulate that in some instances BNI may be able to distinguish between networks that appear similar when examined by traditional graph theoretic measures.

ACKNOWLEDGMENTS

The authors acknowledge the financial support of the Medical Research Council (MRC) via Programme Grant MR/K013998/01.

REFERENCES

1. Fisher RS, van Emde Boas W, Blume W, Elger C, Genton P, Lee P, et al. Epileptic seizures and epilepsy: definitions proposed by the international league against epilepsy (ILAE) and the international bureau for epilepsy (IBE). *Epilepsia* (2005) **46**(4):470–2. doi:10.1111/j.0013-9580.2005.66104.x
2. Fisher RS, Acevedo C, Arzimanoglou A, Bogacz A, Cross JH, Elger CE, et al. ILAE official report: a practical clinical definition of epilepsy. *Epilepsia* (2014) **55**(4):475–82. doi:10.1111/epi.12550
3. Berg AT, Berkovic SF, Brodie MJ, Buchhalter J, Cross JH, van Emde Boas W, et al. Revised terminology and concepts for organization of seizures and epilepsies: report of the ILAE commission on classification and terminology, 2005-2009. *Epilepsia* (2010) **51**(4):676–85. doi:10.1111/j.1528-1167.2010.02522.x
4. Honey CJ, Sporns O, Cammoun L, Gigandet X, Thiran JP, Meuli R, et al. Predicting human resting-state functional connectivity from structural connectivity. *Proc Natl Acad Sci U S A* (2009) **106**(6):2035–40. doi:10.1073/pnas.0811168106
5. Chowdhury FA, Woldman W, FitzGerald TH, Elwes RD, Nashef L, Terry JR, et al. Revealing a brain network endophenotype in families with idiopathic generalised epilepsy. *PLoS One* (2014) **9**(10):e110136. doi:10.1371/journal.pone.0110136
6. Breakspear M, Roberts JA, Terry JR, Rodrigues S, Mahant N, Robinson PA. A unifying explanation of primary generalized seizures through nonlinear brain modeling and bifurcation analysis. *Cereb Cortex* (2006) **16**(9):1296–313. doi:10.1093/cercor/bhj072
7. Suffczynski P, Kalitzin S, Lopes da Silva FH. Dynamics of non-convulsive epileptic phenomena modeled by a bistable neuronal network. *Neuroscience* (2004) **126**(2):467–84. doi:10.1016/j.neuroscience.2004.03.014
8. Goodfellow M, Schindler K, Baier G. Intermittent spike-wave dynamics in a heterogeneous, spatially extended neural mass model. *Neuroimage* (2011) **55**(3):920–32. doi:10.1016/j.neuroimage.2010.12.074
9. Marten F, Rodrigues S, Benjamin O, Richardson MP, Terry JR. Onset of polyspike complexes in a mean-field model of human electroencephalography and its application to absence epilepsy. *Philos Trans A Math Phys Eng Sci* (2009) **367**(1891):1145–61. doi:10.1098/rsta.2008.0255
10. Blenkinsop A, Valentin A, Richardson MP, Terry JR. The dynamic evolution of focal-onset epilepsies – combining theoretical and clinical observations. *Eur J Neurosci* (2012) **36**(2):2188–200. doi:10.1111/j.1460-9568.2012.08082.x
11. Lopes da Silva FH, Blanes W, Kalitzin SN, Parra J, Suffczynski P, Velis DN. Dynamical diseases of brain systems: different routes to epileptic seizures. *IEEE Trans Biomed Eng* (2003) **50**(5):540–8. doi:10.1109/TBME.2003.810703
12. Terry JR, Benjamin O, Richardson MP. Seizure generation: the role of nodes and networks. *Epilepsia* (2012) **53**(9):e166–9. doi:10.1111/j.1528-1167.2012.03560.x
13. Kalitzin S, Koppert M, Petkov G, Velis D, da Silva FL. Computational model prospective on the observation of proictal states in epileptic neuronal systems. *Epilepsy Behav* (2011) **22**(Suppl 1):S102–9. doi:10.1016/j.yebeh.2011.08.017

14. Benjamin O, Fitzgerald TH, Ashwin P, Tsaneva-Atanasova K, Chowdhury F, Richardson MP, et al. A phenomenological model of seizure initiation suggests network structure may explain seizure frequency in idiopathic generalised epilepsy. *J Math Neurosci* (2012) **2**(1):1. doi:10.1186/2190-8567-2-1
15. Goodfellow M, Glendinning P. Mechanisms of intermittent state transitions in a coupled heterogeneous oscillator model of epilepsy. *J Math Neurosci* (2013) **3**(1):17. doi:10.1186/2190-8567-3-17
16. Kalitzin S, Koppert M, Petkov G, da Silva FL. Multiple oscillatory states in models of collective neuronal dynamics. *Int J Neural Syst* (2014) **24**(6):1450020. doi:10.1142/S0129065714500208
17. Lachaux JP, Rodriguez E, Martinerie J, Varela FJ. Measuring phase synchrony in brain signals. *Hum Brain Mapp* (1999) **8**(4):194–208. doi:10.1002/(SICI)1097-0193(1999)8:4<194::AID-HBM4>3.0.CO;2-C
18. Mormann F, Lehnertz K, David P, Elger CE. Mean phase coherence as a measure for phase synchronization and its application to the EEG of epilepsy patients. *Physica D* (2000) **144**(3–4):358–69. doi:10.1016/S0167-2789(00)00087-7
19. Maslov S, Sneppen K. Specificity and stability in topology of protein networks. *Science* (2002) **296**(5569):910–3. doi:10.1126/science.1065103
20. Morgan RJ, Soltesz I. Nonrandom connectivity of the epileptic dentate gyrus predicts a major role for neuronal hubs in seizures. *Proc Natl Acad Sci U S A* (2008) **105**(16):6179–84. doi:10.1073/pnas.0801372105
21. de Haan W, Mott K, van Straaten EC, Scheltens P, Stam CJ. Activity dependent degeneration explains hub vulnerability in Alzheimer's disease. *PLoS Comput Biol* (2012) **8**(8):e1002582. doi:10.1371/journal.pcbi.1002582
22. Noebels J. A perfect storm: converging paths of epilepsy and Alzheimer's dementia intersect in the hippocampal formation. *Epilepsia* (2011) **52**(Suppl 1):39–46. doi:10.1111/j.1528-1167.2010.02909.x
23. Guye M, Bettus G, Bartolomei F, Cozzone PJ. Graph theoretical analysis of structural and functional connectivity MRI in normal and pathological brain networks. *MAGMA* (2010) **23**(5–6):409–21. doi:10.1007/s10334-010-0205-z
24. Clemens B, Puskas S, Besenyei M, Spisak T, Opposits G, Hollody K, et al. Neurophysiology of juvenile myoclonic epilepsy: EEG-based network and graph analysis of the interictal and immediate preictal states. *Epilepsy Res* (2013) **106**(3):357–69. doi:10.1016/j.eplepsyres.2013.06.017
25. Strogatz SH. Exploring complex networks. *Nature* (2001) **410**(6825):268–76. doi:10.1038/35065725
26. Suffczynski P, Lopes da Silva FH, Parra J, Velis DN, Bouwman BM, van Rijn CM, et al. Dynamics of epileptic phenomena determined from statistics of ictaltransitions. *IEEE Trans Biomed Eng* (2006) **53**(3):524–32. doi:10.1109/TBME.2005.869800
27. Schmidt H, Petkov G, Richardson MP, Terry JR. Dynamics on networks: the role of local dynamics and global networks on the emergence of hypersynchronous neural activity. *PLoS Comput Biol* (2014) **10**(11):e1003947. doi:10.1371/journal.pcbi.1003947
28. Nevado-Holgado AJ, Marten F, Richardson MP, Terry JR. Characterising the dynamics of EEG waveforms as the path through parameter space of a neural mass model: application to epilepsy seizure evolution. *Neuroimage* (2012) **59**(3):2374–92. doi:10.1016/j.neuroimage.2011.08.111
29. Jirsa VK, Stacey WC, Quilichini PP, Ivanov AI, Bernard C. On the nature of seizure dynamics. *Brain* (2014) **137**(Pt 8):2210–30. doi:10.1093/brain/awu133
30. Ritter P, Schirner M, McIntosh AR, Jirsa VK. The virtual brain integrates computational modeling and multimodal neuroimaging. *Brain Connect* (2013) **3**(2):121–45. doi:10.1089/brain.2012.0120
31. Engel AK, Fries P, Singer W. Dynamic predictions: oscillations and synchrony in top-down processing. *Nat Rev Neurosci* (2001) **2**(10):704–16. doi:10.1038/35094565

11

Specific resting-state brain networks in mesial temporal lobe epilepsy

Mona Maneshi[1]*, Shahabeddin Vahdat[2], Firas Fahoum[1], Christophe Grova[1,3] and Jean Gotman[1]

[1] Montreal Neurological Institute and Hospital, McGill University, Montreal, QC, Canada
[2] Functional Neuroimaging Unit, Centre de Recherche de l'Institut Universitaire de Gériatrie de Montréal, Montreal, QC, Canada
[3] Multimodal Functional Imaging Laboratory, Department of Biomedical Engineering, McGill University, Montreal, QC, Canada

***Correspondence:**
Mona Maneshi, Montreal Neurological Institute and Hospital, McGill University, 3801 University Street, Room 009d, Montréal, QC H3A 2B4, Canada
e-mail: mona.maneshi@mail.mcgill.ca

We studied with functional magnetic resonance imaging (fMRI) differences in resting-state networks between patients with mesial temporal lobe epilepsy (MTLE) and healthy subjects. To avoid any *a priori* hypothesis, we use a data-driven analysis assessing differences between groups independently of structures involved. Shared and specific independent component analysis (SSICA) is an exploratory method based on independent component analysis, which performs between-group network comparison. It extracts and classifies components (networks) in those common between groups and those specific to one group. Resting fMRI data were collected from 10 healthy subjects and 10 MTLE patients. SSICA was applied multiple times with altered initializations and different numbers of specific components. This resulted in many components specific to patients and to controls. Spatial clustering identified the reliable resting-state networks among all specific components in each group. For each reliable specific network, power spectrum analysis was performed on reconstructed time-series to estimate connectivity in each group and differences between groups. Two reliable networks, corresponding to statistically significant clusters robustly detected with clustering were labeled as specific to MTLE and one as specific to the control group. The most reliable MTLE network included hippocampus and amygdala bilaterally. The other MTLE network included the postcentral gyri and temporal poles. The control-specific network included bilateral precuneus, anterior cingulate, thalamus, and parahippocampal gyrus. Results indicated that the two MTLE networks show increased connectivity in patients, whereas the control-specific network shows decreased connectivity in patients. Our findings complement results from seed-based connectivity analysis (1). The pattern of changes in connectivity between mesial temporal lobe structures and other areas may help us understand the cognitive impairments often reported in patients with MTLE.

Keywords: temporal lobe epilepsy, independent component analysis, resting-state fMRI, brain networks, functional connectivity

INTRODUCTION

Mesial temporal lobe epilepsy (MTLE) is a common form of human focal epilepsy, with hippocampal sclerosis a common underlying pathology (2). Although seizures in MTLE heavily involve the temporal lobes, it is now clear that there are more anatomically widespread functional disturbances (3). In addition, it appears that structural and metabolic abnormalities in this population are not limited to the period of seizure occurrence and probably affect the periods with no epileptic discharges, i.e., the resting-state periods.

A method to investigate how different parts of the brain interact with each other is to measure the intrinsic function of the brain at resting-state using functional magnetic resonance imaging (fMRI). Because this approach does not require subjects to perform a specific task, it is attractive for clinical studies. In MTLE, studies have shown changes in functional connectivity of the temporal or mesial structures with other brain areas (1, 4–6), and reported impaired resting-state networks including the perceptual, attention, and default mode networks (DMN) (1, 7–10). Studies combining fMRI resting-state functional connectivity and diffusion tensor imaging (7, 11) suggest that functional connectivity changes in MTLE are affected by loss in gray matter volume and white matter integrity in the temporal lobe.

Independent component analysis (ICA) is a popular method to analyze resting-state fMRI data since it provides a network view of the changes in brain activity, by decomposing the data into statistical independent spatial components, each component being associated with a time-course (12). The main limitation of ICA is its nature, which does not generalize simply to drawing conclusions about groups of subjects. Despite this issue, a number of group-ICA approaches have been proposed (13, 14). These approaches differ in terms of data organization prior to the ICA analysis, types of available output, and the statistical approaches. However, there are challenges concerning most of the available group-ICA approaches, extensively discussed by Vahdat et al. (15), which cause ambiguity in the classification and detection of components at the group level.

We recently proposed a new ICA-based method to address the limitations of the current ICA approaches in the situation of multi-groups/multi-conditions comparisons (15). The method, called "shared and specific independent component analysis" or "SSICA," systematically performs between-group network comparisons. It extracts and classifies components (networks) into two categories: those that are common to groups and those that are specific to one of the groups. This is done by adding a constraint to the FastICA (16) algorithm to simultaneously deal with the data of multiple groups within one ICA estimation.

Here we studied, using fMRI, group-specific differences in resting-state networks between patients with unilateral MTLE and healthy control subjects. For this purpose, we considered the SSICA, since it does not require any *a priori* hypothesis, and therefore, can assess differences between the groups independently of the involved structures. Moreover, we were interested in finding the most reliable resting-state networks among all the components that are extracted as specific, and also in estimating functional connectivity in each group and exploring its changes across groups.

MATERIALS AND METHODS

SUBJECTS

Ten patients with unilateral MTLE (aged 29 ± 11 years, 3 males, 7 right MTLE) were selected from our EEG–fMRI dataset of patients scanned at 3-T. These patients were a subset whose fMRI data fulfilled our criteria for selecting patients, as explained below. All patients were taking medication at the time of study and they did not stop it for the purpose of scanning. The study was approved by the research ethics board of the Montreal Neurological Institute and Hospital and subjects participated in the research after giving written informed consent. Patients' inclusion criteria were: (a) having a unilateral mesial temporal epileptic focus according to the clinical information (history of febrile seizures, seizure types, and EEG and MRI findings), (b) no large structural or postsurgical lesion in order to ensure the accurate coregistration with the average standard space, (c) having at least two fMRI runs with no interictal epileptic discharges (IEDs) proven by the simultaneous EEG recording, (d) wakefulness proven by EEG recording during these runs, and (e) motion of <1 mm as determined by the realignment of the preprocessing (see "fMRI Preprocessing," preprocessing step 5). **Table 1** gives the demographic and clinical characteristics of all patients. Ten healthy controls (aged 32 ± 9 years, 5 males) were scanned using the same fMRI protocol, fulfilling inclusion criteria (d) and (e). There was no significant difference between the age distributions of the two groups (sign test, $p > 0.05$). Subjects were asked to keep their eyes closed during the scan and were instructed to refrain from any structured thoughts and from falling asleep.

EEG ACQUISITION

The EEG acquisition was performed using 25 MR compatible electrodes (Ag/AgCl) placed on the scalp using the 10–20 (21 usual electrodes without Fpz and Oz, reference at FCz) and 10–10 (F9, T9, P9, F10, T10, and P10) electrode placement system, as described elsewhere (17). Two electrodes located on the back recorded the electrocardiogram (ECG). To minimize movement artifacts and for the patient's comfort, the head was immobilized using a pillow filled with foam microspheres (Siemens, Germany). Data were transmitted from a BrainAmp amplifier (Brain Products, Munich, Germany, 5 kHz sampling rate) via an optic fiber cable to the EEG monitoring computer located outside the scanner room.

fMRI ACQUISITION

Functional images were continuously acquired using a 3-T MR scanner (Siemens Trio, Germany). A T1-weighted anatomical acquisition was first done (1 mm slice thickness, 256 × 256 matrix, TE = 9.2 ms, TR = 22 ms, and flip angle 30°). Four to seven fMRI runs, each recording 200 volumes, were acquired for each patient and 2–4 runs for each healthy control. TLE patients selected for this study had at least two runs with no epileptic discharges seen on EEG. In order to have the same number of runs for all subjects, only two runs for every patient and control subject were selected. For patients, fMRI data were collected with two EPI acquisition protocols: (I) 5 scans done before July 2008: voxel dimensions 5 mm × 5 mm × 5mm, 25 slices, 64 × 64 matrix, TE = 30 ms, TR = 1750 ms, and flip angle 90°, (II) 5 scans after July 2008: voxel dimensions 3.7 mm × 3.7 mm × 3.7 mm, 33 slices, 64 × 64 matrix, TE = 25 ms, TR = 1900 ms, and flip angle 70°. All the healthy controls were scanned with protocol (II).

EEG PROCESSING

The brain vision analyzer software (Brain Products, Munich, Germany) was used for off-line correction of the gradient artifact and filtering of the EEG signal. This software uses the method described by Allen and colleagues (18). A 50-Hz low-pass filter was also applied to remove remaining high-frequency artifact. The ballistocardiogram (BCG) artifact was removed by ICA (19, 20). A neurologist reviewed the EEG recordings and made sure that the selected runs in patients were free of epileptic discharges and that the patients and controls were awake during these runs.

fMRI PREPROCESSING

Regular preprocessing was performed using FMRIB software library (FSL), www.fmrib.ox.ac.uk, Oxford, UK, FSL version 4.1 (21, 22). The following preprocessing steps were applied: (1) flipping of patients' data to make a homogeneous left MTLE group (10 cases) and increase the sample size, (2) removal of the first two volumes of each scan to allow for equilibrium magnetization, (3) slice timing correction using Fourier-space time-series phase-shifting, (4) non-brain tissue removal (23), (5) motion correction using a six-parameter linear transformation using a maximization of the correlation ratio (default settings of FSL) (24), (6) intensity normalization of all volumes of each run as implemented in FSL (7) spatial smoothing using a Gaussian kernel with 6 mm full width at half maximum (FWHM), and (8) high-pass temporal filtering with cut off frequency of 0.01 Hz. To achieve the transformation between the low-resolution functional data and the average standard space [MNI152: average T1 brain image constructed from 152 normal subjects (25)], we performed two transformations. The

Table 1 | Patients' clinical data.

Patient	Gender	Age/ onset of epilepsy	Epilepsy type	History of febrile seizures	Seizure types	Interictal EEG	Ictal EEG	MRI	Anti-epileptic medications
1	F	20/15	R MTLE	No	Psychic aura, LOC, and postictal fatigue	R T spikes ≫ L T spikes	N/A	R hippocampal and parahippocampal lesion	VPA, LEV, and PB
2	F	36/7	R MTLE	Yes	Epigastric aura, LOC, oral automatism, and R hand automatism	R T spikes	R T	R HA	CBZ
3	M	29/14	L MTLE	No	Aura of déjà vu, LOC, oral automatism, and rare GTCS	L T spikes and L T slow waves	L T	Non-lesional	CBZ
4	F	46/32	L MTLE	Yes	Olfactory aura, L hand automatism, R hand dystonia, and postictal dysphasia	L T spikes ≫ R T spikes	N/A	L HA and HS	TPM and OXC
5	M	18/17	R MTLE	No	Aura of déjà vu, LOC, and rare GTCS	L T spikes and L T slow waves	N/A	R T DNET and R HA	GBP and CLB
6	F	40/39	R MTLE	Yes	Olfactory aura, sensation of coldness, bad odor, LOC, and oral automatisms	R T spikes	R T	Non-lesional	CBZ and CLB
7	F	27/6	R MTLE	Yes	Epigastric aura, warm sensation, fear, tachycardia, postictal confusion, and rare GTCS	R T spikes and sharp waves	R T	R mesial temporal atrophy	CBZ and CLB
8	M	19/14	L MTLE	No	Epigastric aura, LOC, L hand automatism, and R hand dystonia	L T spikes	N/A	L HA and HS	CBZ, CLB, and LTG
9	F	16/5	R MTLE	Yes	Aura of déjà vu, LOC, and manual automatism	R T spikes and R T rhythmic slow waves	N/A	R HA and HS	VPA, CLB, LEV, and TPM
10	F	40/1	R MTLE	Yes	Epigastric aura, nausea, and LOC	R T spikes and R T slow waves	N/A	R HA and HS	VPA, LEV, and PB

MTLE, mesial temporal lobe epilepsy; R, right; L, left; T, temporal; M, male; F, female; HA, hippocampal atrophy per MRI; HS, hippocampal hyperintensity per MRI; DNET, dysembryoplastic neuroepithelial tumor; VPA, valproate; CLB, clobazam; LEV, levetiracetam; CBZ, carbamazepine; LTG, lamotrigine; GBP, gabapentin; TPM, topiramate, OXC, oxcarbazepine, PB, phenobarbital; LOC, loss of consciousness; GTCS, generalized tonic clonic seizures.

first was from the low-resolution EPI image to the T1-weighted structural image (using 7 degrees of freedom affine transformation), and the second was from T1-weighted structural image to the average standard space (using a 12 degrees of freedom linear affine transformation, voxel size $= 2\text{ mm} \times 2\text{ mm} \times 2\text{ mm}$). Data were then sub-sampled to 4 mm isotropic space to limit the computational burden.

SSICA METHOD

Shared and specific independent component analysis employs a three-step data reduction and whitening procedure prior to its simultaneous ICA analysis and network-classification (see Supplementary Material; **Figure 1** for details). Here, the size of each subject's preprocessed data was reduced from 2×198 to 50 time-points by performing the first principal component analysis (PCA). We chose 50 time-points since it explained at least 90% of data variability in each subject's dataset. In total 30 components (shared and specific together) were extracted in both groups. This was done on the aggregate reduced data of both groups, where the size of each group's concatenated data was reduced from (10×50) to $(30\text{-}K2)$ for group-1 and $(30\text{-}K1)$ for group-2; where $K1$ and $K2$ are the maximum number of specific components in group-1 and group-2. In order to test the stability of our results with respect to the total number of extracted components, we did additional analyses by extracting 40 and 50 components at the group level.

Shared and specific independent component analysis was applied several times with different numbers of extracted specific components. We chose to extract up to three specific components per group $[K1 \text{ and } K2 = (0, 1, 2, \text{and } 3)]$, as allowing more specific components only resulted in repetition or combination of already-extracted specific components (i.e., it did not introduce any new component). Therefore, we considered four possible values for the

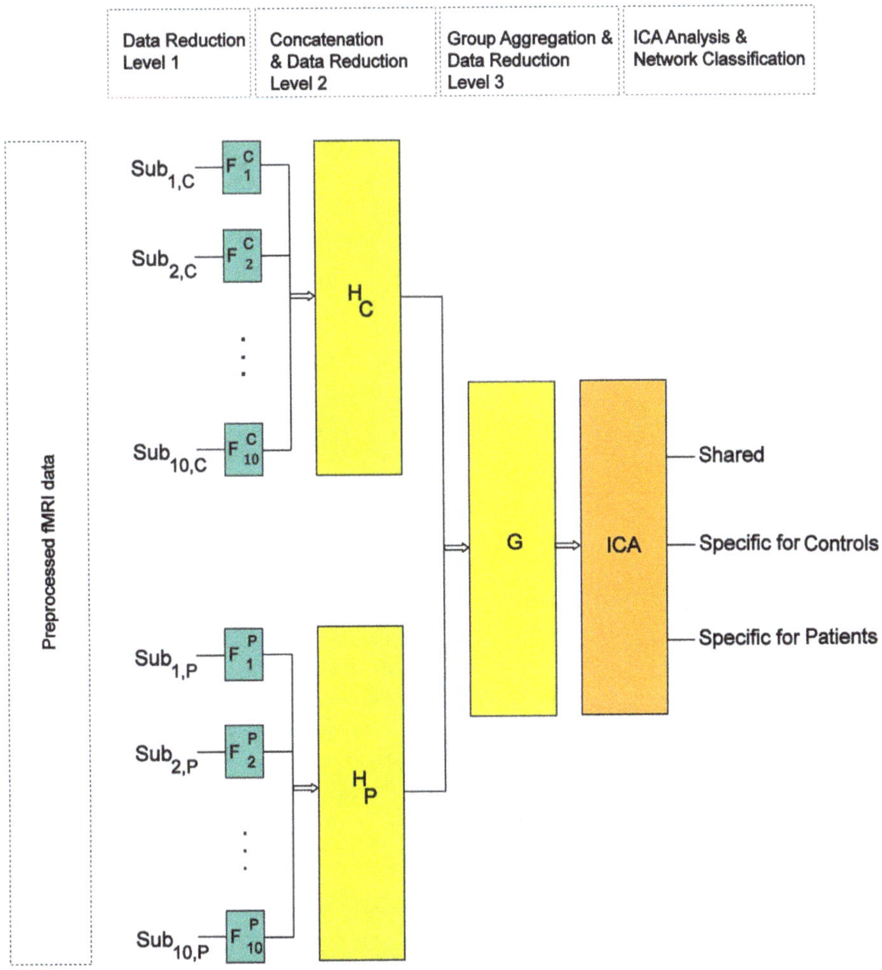

FIGURE 1 | Schematic of the SSICA algorithm. There are three levels of data whitening and reduction. F, H, and G, respectively represent the transformation matrices at the first (subject), second (within-group), and the third (between-group) levels of data reduction.

number of specific components, and for each run of the SSICA, we assigned one of these values to the number of extracted specific components in each group (e.g., 0 for group-1 and 1 for group-2, 0 for group-1 and 2 for group-2, 0 for group-1 and 3 for group-2, and so on). Consequently, the number of possible combinations with repetition was 4 × 4, equal to 16. Excluding the condition where 0 specific networks are extracted in both groups, we ended up with 15 cases. We repeated the whole procedure five times to account for the effect of the ICA initialization, which introduces stochastic behaviors of ICA algorithms and could play an important role in algorithmic instability (26). So in total 15 × 5 = 75 SSICA estimations were considered for further analysis. The number of extracted specific components for patients with MTLE was 118, while for controls 39 specific components were extracted. It should be noted that the outputs of SSICA are spatial Z-score maps.

SPATIAL CLUSTERING ANALYSIS

The remaining important issue was to find the most reliable specific components among all the specific components in each group. To do so, the following analysis based on the clustering method proposed by Hyvarinen and Ramkumar (27) was performed. In their method, the null hypothesis models the case where the components for different subjects/sessions have no similarity at all, other than what would be expected by chance (randomness). They introduced a null distribution, which embodies the two possible sources of such randomness (scenario I. complete failure of the ICA algorithm and scenario II. the underlying components are completely different for each subject). For constructing the null distribution, instead of using an explicit model of multivariate distribution, they proposed a model where parameters can be directly estimated from the observed data. Using the p-values computed for the similarities between sets of components, they proposed a hierarchical clustering procedure, where median was used as the linkage strategy and determined the pairwise distance between components. Correcting for multiple testing, this clustering method controls the false positive rate (FPR) for the formation of clusters, and the false discovery rate (FDR) for adding new elements to clusters.

As implemented in the clustering package ISCTEST, for each group, our input to the clustering algorithm was a three-dimensional tensor containing k 2-D matrices (k being the total number of specific components extracted in that group), where each 2-D matrix was an extracted specific component's spatial map. We set the FPR and FDR to the conservative value of 10% as recommended by Hyvarinen and Ramkumar (27) in the context of real fMRI. The outputs of this analysis were several clusters of specific components, which had the highest within-cluster similarities and the lowest between-clusters similarities (simple spatial correlation was used as the similarity metric). Then, all the components within each cluster were averaged to obtain a representation of that cluster. Results were then overlaid on standard MNI152 at 1 mm resolution for visualization purposes. The thresholded Z-maps ($Z > 2.3$) were labeled according to the Harvard–Oxford cortical and subcortical (28), and Juelich histological atlases (29).

FUNCTIONAL CONNECTIVITY ESTIMATION

In this part of the analysis, we were interested to estimate the functional connectivity of each reliable specific resting-state network and to compare it between groups. Here, we defined functional connectivity of a network based on the power of its corresponding time-course in the frequency band of the resting-state BOLD signal (0.01–0.1 Hz). For each reliable specific network and each subject (patient or control), we used the subject's fMRI data and the network's spatial map in a general linear model (GLM) to find one associated time-course per network and subject. We then used power spectrum analysis (with the standard Hamming window as implemented in MATLAB) to assess the power of this estimated time-course within the 0.01–0.1 Hz frequency band. For each group and each reliable specific network, power was averaged across subjects within that group to calculate the functional connectivity of that network.

RESULTS

Following the clustering algorithm described above, two significant clusters of components were detected specific to the MTLE group and one specific to the control group. These clusters respectively included 111, 6, and 23 specific components (in total there were 118 specific components in the MTLE and 39 in the control group). Setting FPR and FDR thresholds of the clustering analysis at 10%, 1 component in patients and 16 in controls were not included into any significant cluster. The three reliable specific networks, corresponding to these three clusters, are illustrated in **Figures 2A–C**. As explained before, all the components within each cluster were averaged to obtain the representation of that cluster (the reliable specific network).

Our result in **Figure 2A** demonstrates that the most reliable MTLE-specific network comprises bilateral hippocampi, amygdalae, and inferior temporal gyri (more on the side of focus). The other reliable MTLE-specific network comprises the postcentral gyri and bilateral temporal pole, with more involvement on the healthy side (**Figure 2B**). Results in **Figure 2C** demonstrate that the reliable control-specific network, comprising precuneus, anterior cingulate, thalamus, brainstem, and parahippocampal gyrus. For the cases where 40 or 50 components were extracted at the group level, we found very similar results as when 30 components were extracted.

Results of power spectrum analysis on the temporal dynamics of the detected resting-state networks show that the two MTLE-specific networks show increased functional connectivity in the patients compared to the controls (**Figures 3A,B**), whereas the control-specific network shows decreased functional connectivity in patients (**Figure 3C**). This explains why we chose to illustrate the MTLE-specific networks (**Figures 2A,B**) in red and the control-specific network (**Figure 2C**) in blue.

DISCUSSION

We used an ICA-based analysis to study resting-state brain activity in patients with MTLE and investigated the resting-state networks specific to them when compared to healthy controls. Following the framework proposed in SSICA, we assume that the specific networks are those that differ when comparing both groups; either a normal network identified in controls, which is less or more

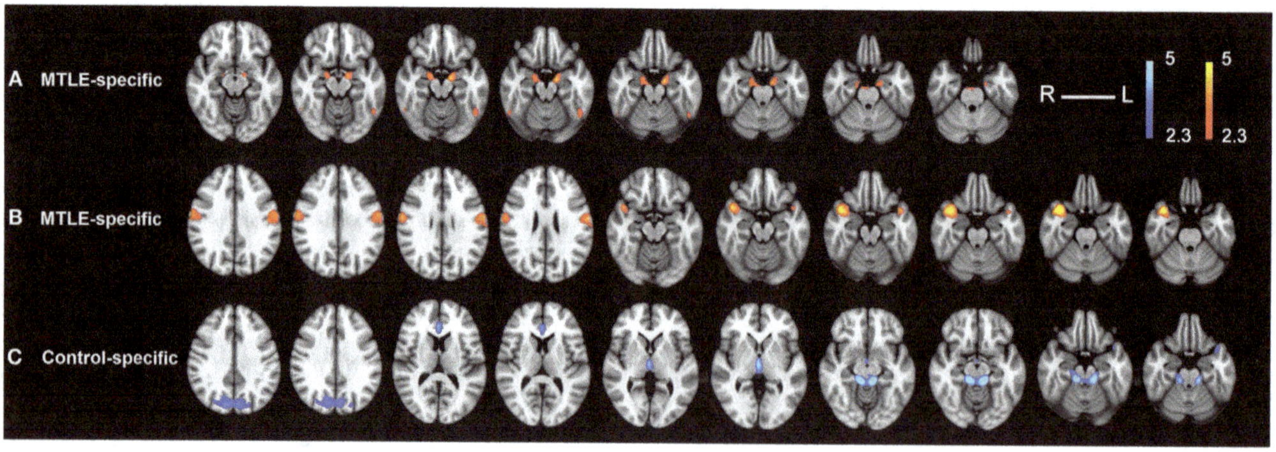

FIGURE 2 | The three detected reliable specific resting-state networks. Reliable resting-state networks specific to the MTLE group **(A,B)**, reliable resting-state networks specific to the control group **(C)**. Note that this result is showing the average of spatial maps within each reliable cluster. Z-values range between 2.3 and 5 in both cases. To be compatible with the results in **Figure 3**, we chose to illustrate the MTLE-specific networks **(A,B)** in red and the control-specific network **(C)** in blue.

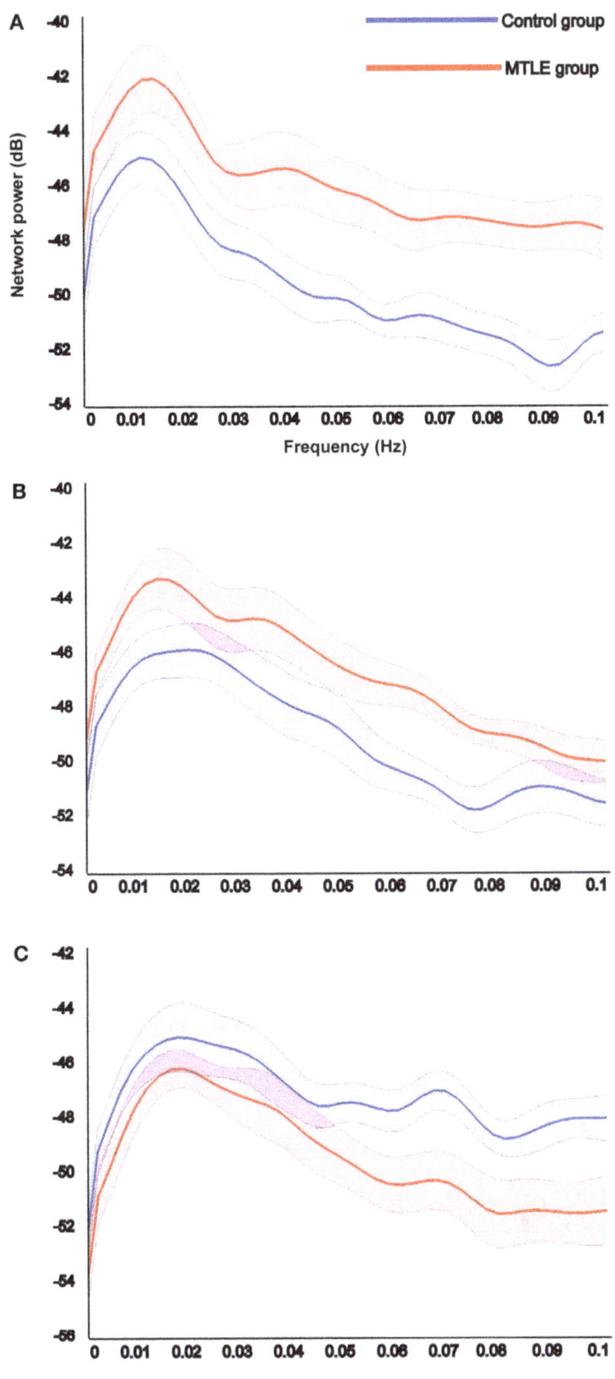

FIGURE 3 | Results of the power spectrum analysis on the temporal dynamics of each detected specific resting-state networks. The reliable resting-state networks specific to the MTLE group show increased functional connectivity in patients compared to controls **(A,B)**, whereas the reliable resting-state network specific to the controls shows the opposite **(C)**. *X*-axis shows the frequency in Hertz and *Y*-axis indicates the power in decibel. Shaded area shows standard error of the mean.

present in patients, or a pathological network that only exists in the patients. The SSICA requires as input the number of networks specific to each group but the true value of this number is not known *a priori*. We therefore ran the SSICA multiple times, with different maximum numbers of specific components, providing us with a large number of components specific to the patients and to the controls (we also ran SSICA with multiple initializations to increase statistical performance and decrease sensitivity to initial conditions). A subsequent clustering analysis on the specific components estimated in each group resulted in the detection of two reliable resting-state networks specific to the MTLE group and one specific to the control group. To explore changes of functional connectivity across groups, power spectrum analysis was performed. This analysis demonstrated that the two reliable MTLE-specific networks show increased functional connectivity in the MTLE group compared to the healthy control group, whereas the one control-specific network shows the opposite.

In a previous seed-based functional connectivity study by our group, Pittau et al. (1) demonstrated that amygdala and hippocampus on the affected and to a lesser extent, on the healthy side are functionally less connected with contralateral homologous structure. Our results demonstrated that the most reliable MTLE-specific network includes bilateral hippocampus and amygdala, more on the side of the focus and comprises regions where functional connectivity, measured through power of network, is higher in patients than in controls.

Even though at first sight this result may seem to be contradiction with the finding of Pittau's study, we believe that this difference is originating from dissimilar strategies for functional connectivity estimation. The difference can be explained as follows: one may assume that as a result of sporadic epileptic discharges, the BOLD signal extracted from the seeds in the affected areas, specifically the hippocampus and amygdala, show more variability compared to the signal from the same areas in healthy controls. Since in the context of SSICA functional connectivity of a resting-state network is defined based on the power of its corresponding time course, this extra variability of the BOLD signal within the MTLE group could result in its extraction as a specific network. However, as a result of the same variability, the correlation between the BOLD signals extracted from the affected and the healthy hippocampus and amygdala could be reduced and therefore, decreased functional connectivity will be detected using seed-based analysis.

Bettus et al. also reported complementary but inconsistent information on functional connectivity in TLE measured by BOLD signal and by intracerebral EEG (iEEG). In their study, using both modalities, functional connectivity was estimated during the interictal period in epileptic and in non-affected regions. Functional connectivity measured from the iEEG signal was reported to be higher in affected regions compared to non-affected areas, whereas an opposite pattern was found for functional connectivity measured from the BOLD signal (4). Using regional homogeneity (ReHo) as an index of ongoing activity, Zeng et al. also reported increased synchronized brain activity, in MTLE patients relative to controls, in some regions including ipsilateral parahippocampal gyrus (30).

Our other finding was that the second most reliable MTLE-specific network shows increased functional connectivity in patients compared to controls between the postcentral gyri and bilateral temporal poles. As also suggested by Maccotta et al. (31), we believe that as a result of recurrent seizures, structural degeneration and decreased connection density, or a combination of both, some neural connections may be facilitated, which in turn lead to elevation of functional connectivity within MTLE-specific networks. In this regard, Holmes et al. investigated the gray matter concentration in left TLE at the voxel level and found decrease in patients in a network comprised of left hippocampus and left postcentral gyrus (32). In a quantitative MRI study, Coste et al. (33) demonstrated that in refractory TLE, the temporal pole is frequently atrophic ipsilateral to seizure onset. Labate et al. (34), using cortical thickness for assessment of neuropathologic changes, demonstrated progressive neocortical atrophy in intractable MTLE patients, which likely represents seizure-induced damage. The involvement of neocortical regions, such as sensorimotor cortex, in the pathophysiology of TLE has also been reported by other authors (35, 36).

Finally, we found that the reliable control-specific network, comprised of precuneus, anterior cingulate, thalamus, brainstem, and parahippocampal gyrus, shows decreased functional connectivity in patients compared to controls. We find this result consistent and complementary to the findings of Pittau et al. (1), which demonstrated that in MTLE patients compared to controls, amygdala and hippocampus on the affected and to a lesser extent on the contralateral side are functionally less connected with the dopaminergic mesolimbic network and the DMN. We believe that in MTLE, the amount of correlation between the BOLD signals extracted from seeds in the affected areas and remote regions will be reduced since distant regions do not necessarily show BOLD changes related to epileptic discharges. Moreover, as the BOLD signals extracted from regions beyond the affected structures in TLE do not necessarily have more variation in patients compared to controls, the control-specific network shows less power in patients compared to controls. In a recent study by McCormick et al. (37), patients with MTLE showed reduced resting-state functional connectivity from the posterior cingulate cortex to the epileptogenic hippocampus. Zeng et al. (30) also reported decreased ReHo in DMN, including precuneus and posterior cingulate gyrus, bilateral inferior lateral parietal and mesial prefrontal cortex. In addition, Liao et al. (7) showed that in MTLE patients compared to controls, functional and structural connectivity of the bilateral mesial temporal lobes were significantly decreased with the posterior cingulate cortex and with precuneus and suggested that in MTLE, the decreased connection density in several areas in the DMN might be responsible for decreased functional connectivity within this network.

It is important to note that a causal relationship cannot be inferred from the current analysis and our results simply reflect the state of the brain of patients with MTLE, which may relate to structural abnormalities, long-standing epilepsy, or medication, a combination of these, or a common cause for this type of epilepsy. The fact that patients were on different medications may be considered as a confounding factor between patients and controls in our analysis. Unfortunately, it is almost impossible to dissociate the long term effect of medication from the effect of disease when studying patients with a long duration of epilepsy since the vast majority of patients take a combination of different medications since the onset of their disease.

Given the number of patients, this study did not allow us to investigate the correlation between the functional connectivity of the two detected reliable MTLE-specific resting-state networks and the duration of epilepsy. However, it would be interesting for future studies to investigate those networks that show greater alterations in functional connectivity in patients with a longer history of disease. In addition, given the small number of subjects in each group of MTLE patients, we could not study the two groups separately and therefore were not able to investigate whether there are different mechanisms underlying left and right MTLE.

We want to reemphasize that although SSICA and seed-based functional connectivity analysis measure different aspects of brain activity organization and sometimes give apparently inconsistent results, they may complement each other and provide more information about the underlying processes resulting in changes of functional connectivity.

ACKNOWLEDGMENT

We used the grant MOP-38079 from the Canadian Institutes of Health Research.

REFERENCES

1. Pittau F, Grova C, Moeller F, Dubeau F, Gotman J. Patterns of altered functional connectivity in mesial temporal lobe epilepsy. *Epilepsia* (2012) **53**:1013–23. doi:10.1111/j.1528-1167.2012.03464.x
2. Engel J. Mesial temporal lobe epilepsy: what have we learned? *Neuroscientist* (2001) **7**:340–52. doi:10.1177/107385840100700410
3. Bell B, Lin JJ, Seidenberg M, Hermann B. The neurobiology of cognitive disorders in temporal lobe epilepsy. *Nat Rev Neurol* (2011) **7**:154–64. doi:10.1038/nrneurol.2011.3
4. Bettus G, Ranjeva JP, Wendling F, Bénar CG, Confort-Gouny S, Régis J, et al. Interictal functional connectivity of human epileptic networks assessed by intracerebral EEG and BOLD signal fluctuations. *PLoS One* (2011) **6**:e20071. doi:10.1371/journal.pone.0020071
5. Pereira FR, Alessio A, Sercheli MS, Pedro T, Bilevicius E, Rondina JM, et al. Asymmetrical hippocampal connectivity in mesial temporal lobe epilepsy: evidence from resting state fMRI. *BMC Neurosci* (2010) **11**:66. doi:10.1186/1471-2202-11-66
6. Waites AB, Briellmann RS, Saling MM, Abbott DF, Jackson GD. Functional connectivity networks are disrupted in left temporal lobe epilepsy. *Ann Neurol* (2006) **59**:335–43. doi:10.1002/ana.20733
7. Liao W, Zhang Z, Pan Z, Mantini D, Ding J, Duan X, et al. Default mode network abnormalities in mesial temporal lobe epilepsy: a study combining fMRI and DTI. *Hum Brain Mapp* (2011) **32**:883–95. doi:10.1002/hbm.21076
8. Zhang Z, Lu G, Zhong Y, Tan Q, Liao W, Chen Z, et al. Impaired perceptual networks in temporal lobe epilepsy revealed by resting fMRI. *J Neurol* (2009) **256**:1705–13. doi:10.1007/s00415-009-5187-2
9. Zhang Z, Lu G, Zhong Y, Tan Q, Yang Z, Liao W, et al. Impaired attention network in temporal lobe epilepsy: a resting fMRI study. *Neurosci Lett* (2009) **458**:97–101. doi:10.1016/j.neulet.2009.04.040
10. Zhang Z, Lu G, Zhong Y, Tan Q, Liao W, Wang Z, et al. Altered spontaneous neuronal activity of the default-mode network in mesial temporal lobe epilepsy. *Brain Res* (2010) **1323**:152–60. doi:10.1016/j.brainres.2010.01.042

11. Voets NL, Beckmann CF, Cole DM, Hong S, Bernasconi A, Bernasconi N. Structural substrates for resting network disruption in temporal lobe epilepsy. *Brain* (2012) **135**:2350–7. doi:10.1093/brain/aws137
12. Comon P. Independent component analysis, a new concept? *Signal Process* (1994) **36**:287–314. doi:10.1016/0165-1684(94)90029-9
13. Beckmann CF, Smith SM. Tensorial extensions of independent component analysis for multisubject fMRI analysis. *Neuroimage* (2005) **25**:294–311. doi:10.1016/j.neuroimage.2004.10.043
14. Calhoun VD, Adali T, Pearlson GD, Pekar JJ. A method for making group inferences from functional MRI data using independent component analysis. *Hum Brain Mapp* (2001) **14**:140–51. doi:10.1002/hbm.1048
15. Vahdat S, Maneshi M, Grova C, Gotman J, Milner TE. Shared and specific independent components analysis for between-group comparison. *Neural Comput* (2012) **24**:3052–90. doi:10.1162/NECO_a_00355
16. Hyvarinen A. Fast and robust fixed-point algorithms for independent component analysis. *IEEE Trans Neural Netw* (1999) **10**:626–34. doi:10.1109/72.761722
17. Moeller F, Tyvaert L, Nguyen D, LeVan P, Bouthillier A, Kobayashi E, et al. EEG-fMRI: adding to standard evaluations of patients with non lesional frontal lobe epilepsy. *Neurology* (2009) **73**(23):2023–30. doi:10.1212/WNL.0b013e3181c55d17
18. Allen PJ, Josephs O, Turner R. A method for removing imaging artifact from continuous EEG recorded during functional MRI. *Neuroimage* (2000) **12**:230–9. doi:10.1006/nimg.2000.0599
19. Bénar C, Aghakhani Y, Wang Y, Izenberg A, Al-Asmi A, Dubeau F, et al. Quality of EEG in simultaneous EEG-fMRI for epilepsy. *Clin Neurophysiol* (2003) **114**:569–80. doi:10.1016/S1388-2457(02)00383-8
20. Srivastava G, Crottaz-Herbette S, Lau KM, Glover GH, Menon V. ICA-based procedures for removing ballistocardiogram artifacts from EEG data acquired in the MRI scanner. *Neuroimage* (2005) **24**:50–60. doi:10.1016/j.neuroimage.2004.09.041
21. Smith SM, Jenkinson M, Woolrich MW, Beckmann CF, Behrens TE, Johansen-Berg H, et al. Advances in functional and structural MR image analysis and implementation as FSL. *Neuroimage* (2004) **23**(Suppl 1):S208–19. doi:10.1016/j.neuroimage.2004.07.051
22. Woolrich MW, Jbabdi S, Patenaude B, Chappell M, Makni S, Behrens T, et al. Bayesian analysis of neuroimaging data in FSL. *Neuroimage* (2009) **45**:S173–86. doi:10.1016/j.neuroimage.2008.10.055
23. Smith SM. Fast robust automated brain extraction. *Hum Brain Mapp* (2002) **17**:143–55. doi:10.1002/hbm.10062
24. Jenkinson M, Bannister P, Brady M, Smith S. Improved optimization for the robust and accurate linear registration and motion correction of brain images. *Neuroimage* (2002) **17**:825–41. doi:10.1006/nimg.2002.1132
25. Collins DL, Neelin P, Peters TM, Evans AC. Automatic 3D intersubject registration of MR volumetric data in standardized Talairach space. *J Comput Assist Tomogr* (1994) **18**:192–205. doi:10.1097/00004728-199403000-00005
26. Himberg J, Hyvarinen A, Esposito F. Validating the independent components of neuroimaging time series via clustering and visualization. *Neuroimage* (2004) **22**:1214–22. doi:10.1016/j.neuroimage.2004.03.027
27. Hyvarinen A, Ramkumar P. Testing independent component patterns by inter-subject or inter-session consistency. *Front Hum Neurosci* (2013) **7**:94. doi:10.3389/fnhum.2013.00094
28. Desikan RS, Ségonne F, Fischl B, Quinn BT, Dickerson BC, Blacker D, et al. An automated labeling system for subdividing the human cerebral cortex on MRI scans into gyral based regions of interest. *Neuroimage* (2006) **31**:968–80. doi:10.1016/j.neuroimage.2006.01.021
29. Eickhoff SB, Stephan KE, Mohlberg H, Grefkes C, Fink GR, Amunts K, et al. A new SPM toolbox for combining probabilistic cytoarchitectonic maps and functional imaging data. *Neuroimage* (2005) **25**:1325–35. doi:10.1016/j.neuroimage.2004.12.034
30. Zeng H, Pizarro R, Nair VA, La C, Prabhakaran V. Alterations in regional homogeneity of resting-state brain activity in mesial temporal lobe epilepsy. *Epilepsia* (2013) **54**:658–66. doi:10.1111/epi.12066
31. Maccotta L, He BJ, Snyder AZ, Eisenman LN, Benzinger TL, Ances BM, et al. Impaired and facilitated functional networks in temporal lobe epilepsy. *Neuroimage Clin* (2013) **2**:862–72. doi:10.1016/j.nicl.2013.06.011
32. Holmes MJ, Yang X, Landman BA, Ding Z, Kang H, Abou-Khalil B, et al. Functional networks in temporal-lobe epilepsy: a voxel-wise study of resting-state functional connectivity and gray-matter concentration. *Brain Connect* (2013) **3**:22–30. doi:10.1089/brain.2012.0103
33. Coste S, Ryvlin P, Hermier M, Ostrowsky K, Adeleine P, Froment JC, et al. Temporopolar changes in temporal lobe epilepsy: a quantitative MRI-based study. *Neurology* (2002) **59**:855–61. doi:10.1212/WNL.59.6.855
34. Labate A, Cerasa A, Aguglia U, Mumoli L, Quattrone A, Gambardella A. Neocortical thinning in "benign" mesial temporal lobe epilepsy. *Epilepsia* (2011) **52**:712–7. doi:10.1111/j.1528-1167.2011.03038.x
35. Bonilha L, Rorden C, Castellano G, Pereira F, Rio PA, Cendes F, et al. Voxel-based morphometry reveals gray matter network atrophy in refractory medial temporal lobe epilepsy. *Arch Neurol* (2004) **61**:1379–84. doi:10.1001/archneur.61.9.1379
36. Henry TR, Mazziotta JC, Engel J Jr. Interictal metabolic anatomy of mesial temporal lobe epilepsy. *Arch Neurol* (1993) **50**:582–9. doi:10.1001/archneur.1993.00540060022011
37. McCormick C, Quraan M, Cohn M, Valiante TA, McAndrews MP. Default mode network connectivity indicates episodic memory capacity in mesial temporal lobe epilepsy. *Epilepsia* (2013) **54**:809–18. doi:10.1111/epi.12098
38. Lang S. *Calculus of Several Variables*. New York, NY: Springer-Verlag (1987).

12

Detection of abnormal resting-state networks in individual patients suffering from focal epilepsy: An initial step toward individual connectivity assessment

Christian L. Dansereau [1,2,3]***, Pierre Bellec*** [3,4]***, Kangjoo Lee*** [1,2]***, Francesca Pittau*** [2]***, Jean Gotman*** [2] ***and Christophe Grova*** [1,2,5]*******

[1] *Multimodal Functional Imaging Lab, Biomedical Engineering Department, McGill University, Montreal, QC, Canada*

[2] *Neurology and Neurosurgery Department, Montreal Neurological Institute, McGill University, Montreal, QC, Canada*

[3] *Centre de Recherche de l'Institut Universitaire de Gériatrie de Montréal, Functional Neuroimaging Unit, Université de Montréal, Montreal, QC, Canada*

[4] *Department of Computer Science and Operations Research, University of Montreal, Montreal, Quebec, Canada*

[5] *Physics Department, PERFORM Center, Concordia University, Montreal, QC, Canada*

****Correspondence:***
Christophe Grova, Physics Department, PERFORM Center, Concordia University, Loyola Campus - Office SP 365.12, 7141 Sherbrooke Street West, Montreal, QC H4B 1R6, Canada
e-mail: christophe.grova@concordia.ca

The spatial coherence of spontaneous slow fluctuations in the blood-oxygen-level dependent (BOLD) signal at rest is routinely used to characterize the underlying resting-state networks (RSNs). Studies have demonstrated that these patterns are organized in space and highly reproducible from subject to subject. Moreover, RSNs reorganizations have been suggested in pathological conditions. Comparisons of RSNs organization have been performed between groups of subjects but have rarely been applied at the individual level, a step required for clinical application. Defining the notion of modularity as the organization of brain activity in stable networks, we propose Detection of Abnormal Networks in Individuals (DANI) to identify modularity changes at the individual level. The stability of each RSN was estimated using a spatial clustering method: Bootstrap Analysis of Stable Clusters (BASC) (Bellec et al., 2010). Our contributions consisted in (i) providing functional maps of the most stable cores of each networks and (ii) in detecting "abnormal" individual changes in networks organization when compared to a population of healthy controls. DANI was first evaluated using realistic simulated data, showing that focussing on a conservative core size (50% most stable regions) improved the sensitivity to detect modularity changes. DANI was then applied to resting state fMRI data of six patients with focal epilepsy who underwent multimodal assessment using simultaneous EEG/fMRI acquisition followed by surgery. Only patient with a seizure free outcome were selected and the resected area was identified using a post-operative MRI. DANI automatically detected abnormal changes in 5 out of 6 patients, with excellent sensitivity, showing for each of them at least one "abnormal" lateralized network closely related to the epileptic focus. For each patient, we also detected some distant networks as abnormal, suggesting some remote reorganization in the epileptic brain.

Keywords: functional connectivity, resting state fMRI, focal epilepsy, single subject design, outlier detection

INTRODUCTION

Connectivity analysis in resting-state functional magnetic resonance imaging (rs-fMRI) is a promising tool to study neurological disorders. So far, rs-fMRI has been applied mainly at the level of groups of patients, as for instance in mental disorders (Broyd et al., 2009), in Alzheimer's disease (Goveas et al., 2011; Damoiseaux et al., 2012; Jacobs et al., 2013) and also in epilepsy (Bernhardt et al., 2013; Constable et al., 2013; Lang et al., 2014). However, a large amount of inter-patient variability is typically observed in any neurological disorder. In some applications, patient-specific features are the only clinically useful information. A prominent example is the multimodal investigation of patient with drug-resistant epilepsy, which aims at identifying an epileptogenic focus that could be surgically resected (Stefan et al., 2011; De Ciantis and Lemieux, 2013). The main goal of this study is to develop a method to capture inter-individual variations in resting-state networks (RSNs), and assess its potential usefulness in patients with focal epilepsy.

Usually, the analysis of patient-specific epileptogenic focus is based on analysing brain activity at the time of epileptic discharges. However, epileptic discharges are spontaneous and rare events that may not occur during time-limited standard neuroimaging investigations, such as simultaneous electro-encephalography/functional magnetic resonance imaging (EEG/fMRI) (Gotman and Pittau, 2011) or magneto-encephalography (MEG) (Stefan et al., 2011) explorations. When studying resting-state activity in the absence of epileptic discharges, some group-level studies have demonstrated rs-fMRI connectivity patterns specific to idiopathic generalized epilepsy (IGE) (Luo et al., 2011; Maneshi et al., 2012) and temporal lobe epilepsy (TLE) (Waites et al., 2006; Liao et al., 2011; Pittau et al., 2012b). For example, using seed regions in the epileptic focus, group comparison between TLE patients and age-matched healthy controls, we found significant decreases in connectivity between homologous mesio-temporal structures and also with the dopaminergic mesolimbic and with the default mode network (Pittau et al., 2012b). For IGE patients, we found significant increases and decreases in FC when using seeds in the attention network (Maneshi et al., 2012). The few studies, which have investigated FC changes at the individual level in patients with epilepsy, did report some reorganization of functional networks, notably in terms of their laterality (Negishi et al., 2011; Stufflebeam et al., 2011; Luo et al., 2014). Taken together, these results support our main hypothesis that resting-state fMRI connectivity could identify clinically relevant information in individual patients suffering from epilepsy.

Resting-state functional connectivity captures the spatial correlations of spontaneous fluctuations in the blood-oxygen-level dependent (BOLD) fMRI signal (Biswal et al., 1995). Maps of functional connectivity, i.e., temporal correlations of fMRI time series across brain regions, reveal highly organized spatial RSNs. These maps were found to be reproducible at the individual (Himberg et al., 2004; Shehzad et al., 2009) and at the group levels (Damoiseaux et al., 2006). Each RSN is a combination of multiple brain regions, not necessarily spatially contiguous, which share similar low frequency BOLD signal fluctuations (Fox and Raichle, 2007). These networks capture some aspects of the functional organization of the brain (Yeo et al., 2011). Many methods have been proposed to identify RSNs, including mainly variants of independent component analysis (ICA) (Smith, 2012) and cluster analysis (Yeo et al., 2011), see Smith et al. (2013) for a review. Initial applications of these techniques have focussed on group level analysis, (e.g., Damoiseaux et al., 2006), and it is only recently that their capacity to establish a correspondence between group and individual RSNs has been a topic of active research. Techniques available to address this problem include back-reconstruction in ICA (Calhoun et al., 2009) and dual-regression ICA (Beckmann et al., 2009). Here, we decided to build on a technique called Bootstrap Analysis of Stable Clusters (BASC) (Bellec et al., 2010), because of two of its unique features. First, the technique offers a statistical framework to assess the stability of RSNs at the individual and at the group level, by replicating a cluster analysis many times after small perturbations of the original dataset. This quantification of stability is an asset to establish whether atypical RSN organization observed in an individual can simply be attributed to statistical noise or reflects biological individual characteristics. Second, BASC explicitly looks at the modular organization of the brain, i.e., the ability to identify clusters based on the relative strength of intra-network vs. inter-network connectivity, independently of the absolute value of connectivity measures (see Alexander-Bloch et al., 2012 for a discussion of the distinction between connectivity and modularity). Dual-regression and back-reconstruction ICA, by contrast, perform a regression of temporal dynamics, which is sensitive to the absolute magnitude of connectivity. Absolute measures of functional connectivity are particularly sensitive to physiological noise, in particular motion (Power et al., 2012). We hypothesized that modularity would be more robust to physiological noise than absolute measures of connectivity.

To the best of our knowledge, none of the standard data-driven techniques for RSN mapping (ICA, clustering) has been evaluated at the individual level. They have rather been used to detect changes between two groups. The objective of this study was thus to develop and validate a statistical methodology, entitled "Detection of Abnormal resting state Networks in Individuals," (DANI) aiming at identifying RSNs with atypical, or outlier, spatial distribution, when compared to a population of controls. The outlier RSNs were characterized by differences in stability and spatial extent with respect to a typical RSN distribution. We also extended BASC to include the notion of core of stability, defined as the most stable regions of a network. Because every RSN includes regions with fairly unstable cluster assignment, we hypothesized that focussing on RSN cores rather than on full networks would translate into improved characterisation of individual biological variability. In the first part of the paper, we assessed the ability of DANI to identify atypical and individual modular organization on a battery of simulated datasets.

Evaluation of RSN mapping for real individual fMRI datasets is challenging because of the lack of ground truth. The quality of individual mapping has been mainly assessed by test-retest reliability studies (Shehzad et al., 2009; Zuo et al., 2010) but test-retest reliability in itself does not indicate if reliable features are clinically meaningful. Concerning patients with epilepsy, the seizure outcome after surgery remains the gold standard to validate a technique. For this reason, in the second part of this study, DANI was applied to resting state fMRI data of six patients with focal epilepsy who underwent multimodal assessment using simultaneous EEG/fMRI acquisition followed by surgery.

MATERIALS AND METHODS

SUBJECT SELECTION

We selected healthy control subjects who underwent simultaneous EEG/fMRI acquisitions (Gotman et al., 2004), with the following inclusion criteria:

(i) Right-handed.
(ii) EEG/fMRI runs during which the subject was awake: EEG stage W according to Iber and American Academy of Sleep Medicine (2007).
(iii) EEG/fMRI runs involving only minimal motion (less than 1 mm translation and 1° rotation between volumes).

Based on these criteria, we selected 25 right-handed healthy control subjects The mean age was 32.8 years, ranging from 18 to 55. Written informed consent was obtained according to the guidelines and approval of the Montreal Neurological Institute research ethics review board. Note that this database of healthy controls acquired in our laboratory was the same as the one considered in our previous study (Pittau et al., 2012b).

SIMULTANEOUS EEG/fMRI ACQUISITION

EEG was continuously recorded as described in Gotman et al. (2004) inside a 3T MRI scanner (Siemens, Trio, Germany). The EEG acquisition was performed with 25 MR compatible electrodes (Ag/AgCl) placed on the scalp using the 10–20 (reference at FCz) and the 10–10 (F9, T9, P9, F10, T10, and P10) placement systems. Two electrodes were placed on the back to record the electrocardiogram. The head of the subject was immobilized with a pillow filled with foam microspheres (Siemens, Germany) to minimize movement artifacts and for subject's comfort. Data were transmitted from a BrainAmp amplifier (Brain Products, Munich, Germany, 5 kHz sampling rate) to the EEG monitor located outside the scanner room via an optical fiber cable.

A T1-weighted anatomic acquisition was first done (1 mm slice thickness, 256 × 256 matrix; echo time $TE = 7.4$ ms and repetition time $TR = 23$ ms; flip angle 30°). This scan was used for co-registration purposes and to superimpose the functional images on the anatomy. Functional data were acquired in runs of 6 min using a T2*-weighted EPI sequence (64 × 64 matrix; 33 slices, 3.7 × 3.7 × 3.7 mm, $TE = 25$ ms, $TR = 1.9$ s; flip angle 90°). Subjects were instructed not to move and stay with eyes closed, resting. Three runs were selected during wakefulness, with less than 1 mm of variation between two volumes for the three axes in translation and less then 1° of variation between two volumes for the three axes in rotation.

fMRI DATA PREPROCESSING

The fMRI database was preprocessed using the Neuroimaging Analysis Kit (NIAK) release 0.7[1] (Bellec et al., 2011). Each fMRI dataset was corrected for inter-slice difference in acquisition time. Parameters of a rigid-body motion transformation were estimated for each time frame. Rigid-body motion was estimated within as well as between runs. The median volume of one selected fMRI run for each subject was coregistered with the individual anatomical T1 scan with Minctracc (Collins and Evans, 1997), using a rigid transformation. The T1 MRI of each subject was itself non-linearly co-registered to the Montreal Neurological Institute (MNI) stereotaxic template (Fonov et al., 2011), using CIVET pipeline (Zijdenbos et al., 2002). We used the MNI symmetric template, generated from the ICBM152 sample of 152 young adults, after 40 iterations of non-linear co-registration. The rigid-body fMRI-to-T1 transform and the non-linear T1-to-stereotaxic transform were all combined, and the functional volumes were resampled in the MNI space at a 3 mm isotropic resolution. The "scrubbing" method proposed by Power et al. (2012) was used to remove the volumes with excessive motion, i.e., all frames showing a displacement greater than 0.5 mm were removed. On average, 4% of the frames were thus removed using this "scrubbing" method. The following nuisance parameters were regressed out from the time series at each voxel: slow time drifts (basis of discrete cosines with a 0.01 Hz high-pass cut-off), average signals in conservative masks of the white matter and the lateral ventricles as well as the first principal components (accounting for 95% variance) of the six rigid-body motion parameters and their squares (Lund et al., 2006; Giove et al., 2009). The fMRI volumes were finally spatially smoothed with a 6 mm isotropic Gaussian blurring kernel. A more detailed description of the pipeline can be found on NIAK website (http://www.nitrc.org/projects/niak/).

To reduce the computational burden of the analysis, the spatial dimension of the individual fMRI dataset was reduced using a region-growing algorithm. The spatial dimension was selected arbitrarily by setting the maximal size where the growing process stopped: we chose a threshold of 800 mm^3 resulting in $R = 739$ regions. The regions were built to maximize the homogeneity of the time series within the regions, i.e., the average correlation between the time series associated with any pair of voxels of the region. The region growing was applied on the time series concatenated across all subjects (after transformation to zero mean and unit variance), such that the homogeneity was maximized on average for all subjects, ensuring the use of small homogeneous and identical regions for all subjects. Because of the temporal concatenation of time series, we had to limit the memory demand, and the region-growing was thus applied sequentially and independently within each of the 116 anatomical areas of the AAL atlas (Tzourio-Mazoyer et al., 2002). See Bellec et al. (2006) for evaluation and further details regarding the implementation of this region-growing algorithm. Overall, this process reduced the dataset Y of each subject into a $(T \times R)$ data array, where T is the number of time samples and R is the number of regions.

The analysis of neuroimaging databases typically involves a large number of inter-connected steps. We used the Pipeline System for Octave and Matlab PSOM (Bellec et al., 2012) to execute processes in parallel on a cluster of workstations.

FULL BRAIN FUNCTIONAL CONNECTIVITY ANALYSIS USING BASC

Starting from preprocessed resting state fMRI data, we used the clustering method entitled BASC (Bellec et al., 2010) to quantify FC patterns at the individual and at the group level. BASC models FC between distant regions using spatial clustering of BOLD time courses. The key idea of BASC is to associate spatial clustering with Bootstrap resampling (Efron and Tibshirani, 1993) to assess the stability of such clustering among several replications, thus leading to a statistical measure of stability of the FC patterns. Since all the analyses were first done at the individual level and then across subjects at a group level, BASC offers a unique possibility to compare individual-level and group-level identifications of RSNs.

BASC analysis at the individual level

For each data matrix Y obtained at the individual level, FC was quantified using a spatial k-means clustering. Each clustering estimated an $R \times R$ binary adjacency matrix, setting a value of 1 when two regions were associated to the same cluster, and 0 otherwise. To assess the statistical stability of this clustering, the data matrix Y $(T \times R)$ was resampled using circular block bootstrap of the BOLD time-series, and a k-means clustering was then applied on each of the $B = 300$ replications. The average of all the B adjacency matrices resulted in a stability matrix $\hat{I}_i$ ($i = 1, \ldots, C$, being the subject index) representing the likelihood to cluster together the time-series of two regions.

[1]NIAK website: http://www.nitrc.org/projects/niak.

BASC analysis at the group level

A similar process was considered to assess FC patterns at the inter-subject group level. To do so, the individual stability matrices of all the subjects $\hat{I}_i$ $(i = 1, \ldots, C)$ were first averaged in order to generate a first group stability matrix. In a second step, a hierarchical clustering was applied using the Euclidean distance between columns of this group stability matrix as a similarity index to identify the columns with similar stability profiles. A threshold was then applied to cut the tree at L number of clusters, thus providing a binarised group level adjacency matrix (matrix exhibiting a 1 when two regions were associated within the same cluster, 0 otherwise). In order to take into account the statistical stability of such a clustering at the group level, standard bootstrap resampling among the C subjects was applied 1000 times and the same hierarchical clustering procedure was applied on each bootstrap sample.

By averaging the resulting 1000 binary adjacency matrices at the group level, we obtained the stability matrix at the group level $\hat{G}$ representing the likelihood to cluster together pairs of regions, while taking into account both single subject and group inherent variability of the data.

PARTITION OF THE BRAIN INTO FUNCTIONAL RSN

To identify Consistent Resting State Networks (CRSNs) at the group level, the stability matrix $\hat{G}$ was converted into a partition of the whole brain, grouping regions that have been frequently associated within the same cluster, i.e., regions exhibiting high FC stability in $\hat{G}$ through bootstrap resampling. To do so, a last hierarchical clustering was applied on $\hat{G}$ to identify brain regions depicting similar stability profiles. Here again, the Euclidean distance between columns of $\hat{G}$ was used as a similarity index to identify the columns with similar stability profiles. A threshold was then applied to cut the tree at the desired number of clusters. We decided to threshold the dendrogram in $N = 12$ clusters, thus ensuring that we did not miss any important CRSN. Indeed, the literature usually refers to 7–10 CRSNs in healthy subjects (Damoiseaux et al., 2006; Smith et al., 2009). Note that for $N =$ 12 CRSNs, we estimated $k = 13$ for the individual level k-means clustering and $L = 14$ to threshold each group level hierarchical clustering. These thresholds were estimated by optimizing a stability contrast as proposed in Bellec et al. (2010). This is a two-pass procedure, a first pass consisted in a fast ($B = 30$ bootstrap samples) exploration of a large grid of scales to find the scales (k(N), L(N), N) maximizing the stability of the clustering, as measured with a modified silhouette criterion of the group stability matrix, constraining k and L values within a close neighborhood of N. Local maxima of the modified silhouette (as a function of N) were then automatically identified. We chose to focus here on the local maximum found for $N = 12$, as this level of RSN decomposition was most similar to the ones traditionally reported in the literature (Damoiseaux et al., 2006). For such a scale of $N = 12$, the optimal parameters of $k = 13$ and $L = 14$ have been estimated. Following the scale selection procedure, the individual stability matrices for $N = 12$ were estimated a second time with a larger number of bootstrap samples ($B = 300$).

Let us define as $P(r)$ for $r \in [1, R]$ a vector representing the resulting partition obtained after thresholding the hierarchical clustering of $\hat{G}$ in N clusters. When two regions are associated within the same cluster, they are associated to the same label in P (**Figure 1A**).

DETECTION OF ABNORMAL NETWORKS IN INDIVIDUALS (DANI)

BASC allows estimating stability of FC patterns at the individual level and at the group level, what we will call modules. The objective of DANI is to detect, at the individual level, possible modifications of those modules that could be considered as deviant or outliers when compared to a population of controls.

BASC extension: from stability matrices to trimmed stability maps

Starting from the stability matrices estimated at the individual level $\hat{I}_i$ or at the group level $\hat{G}$ using BASC, our first contribution was to propose a method to improve the visualization of spatially FC information represented in these stability matrices. Therefore, we propose to convert a stability matrix into a series of N **stability maps**. Each of these maps is generated using information provided by one of the N clusters of the partition P. Consequently, the stability maps are reporting for each region the amount of stability estimated for one particular cluster of the partition. We will refer to each of these spatial maps as a network.

This procedure to estimate "**trimmed stability maps**" is applied on each cluster of the partition. It aims at generating 3D stability maps with enhanced contrast and increased consistency across runs. To do so, the rows of each cluster of the partition matrix P were first reordered in decreasing order of average stability. We then considered a percentage μ of most stable rows, representing the stability cores. The stability profile was then estimated by averaging only these "most stable rows." The resulting *3D trimmed stability map* obtained from this procedure is illustrated in **Figure 1C**. It yielded greater contrast than when simply averaging all the rows of the cluster (**Figure 1B**). We performed simulations varying the values of the parameter μ of 25, 50, and 75% to assess the impact of such threshold on the sensitivity of our detection method. It is important to mention that, whereas only rows corresponding to a particular cluster of P are selected, stability values from all R regions are actually averaged to generate stability maps. Consequently regions not belonging to that specific cluster may also exhibit some non-null stability values.

The 3D trimmed stability maps estimated at the group level from the stability matrix $\hat{G}$ represent the CRSNs. These CRSNs were considered as our reference when characterizing the functional organization of RS brain activity over a population of healthy controls.

The 3D trimmed stability maps, estimated at the individual level from the stability matrices $\hat{I}_i$, characterized the amount of stability assessed for each subject, within each of the CRSNs identified at the group level. Since all maps were estimated within the same referential space, comparison between maps estimated at the individual level and at the group level became feasible. Estimating all trimmed stability maps from the same partition is a strong constraint but it was necessary to provide consistency across subjects. While providing the similar basis for comparison, this method allowed flexibility to adapt to the particularities of each individual.

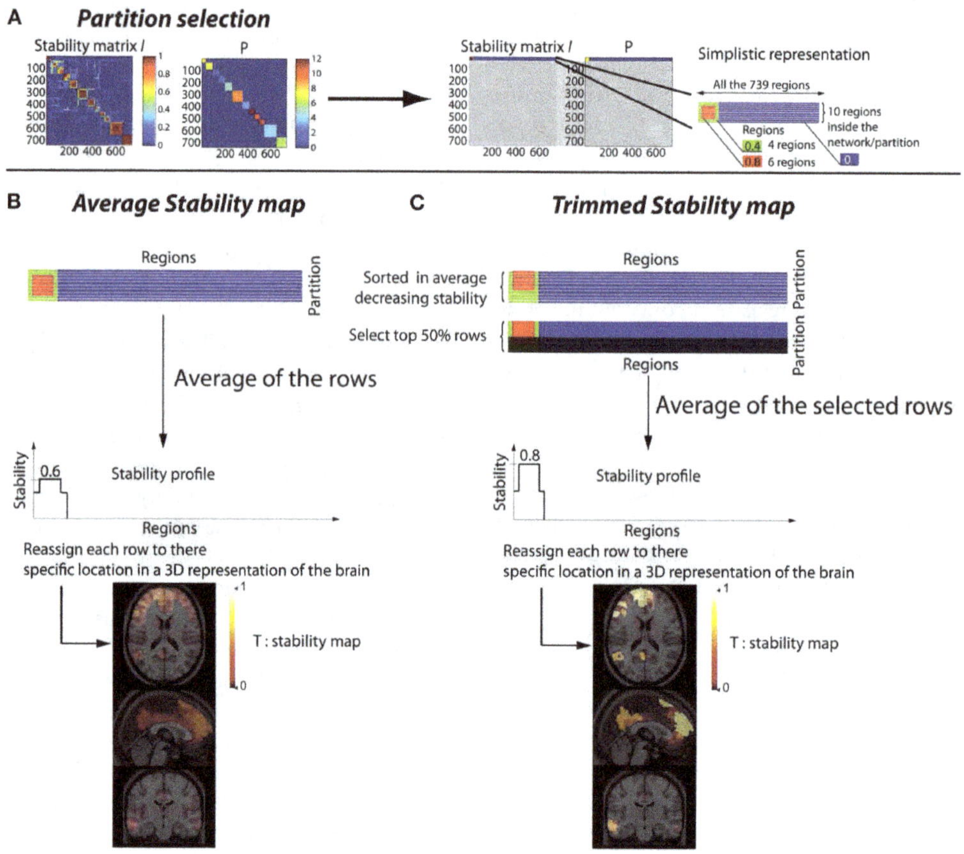

FIGURE 1 | Methodology to convert a stability matrix into a spatial stability map for each network. The same process is applied for each cluster of the partition *P*, thus every stability map was constrained by the corresponding CRSN. **(A)** Simplistic representation in which the first cluster of the partition *P* was selected on the stability matrix. **(B)** Averaged stability map obtained by averaging all the rows inside a network partition, resulting in a diffuse and low contrast representation of the network. **(C)** Trimmed stability map obtained by averaging the 50% rows showing the largest stability values, resulting in a representation of the network with greater contrast.

Detection of abnormal modifications of functional connectivity

Let us define as $CI_n^c(r)$ the $R \times N \times C$ matrix containing the trimmed stability values of the region r $(r = 1 \ldots R)$ for the network n $(n = 1 \ldots N)$ and for the healthy control subject c $(c = 1 \ldots C)$. For a specific target subject to be tested with DANI, let us denote T_n the vector of size R containing the trimmed stability values for the network n $(n = 1 \ldots N)$ for this particular subject. The objective of DANI is to identify automatically which of the trimmed stability maps T_n could be considered as outliers when compared to the trimmed stability maps of all controls $(CI_n^c, c = 1 \ldots C)$. The first step was to detect networks exhibiting variations in stability when compared to controls maps. The second step was to quantify whether these variations were statistically significant.

Detecting stability variations in the functional network organization. When performing a region-based comparison of an individual map T_n with all CI_n^c maps $(c = 1 \ldots C)$ from a population of controls, it was not possible to use a standard Z-score. Indeed, each map quantifies stability in FC within a network, i.e., estimated from a predefined cluster of the partition P. Consequently these maps are not continuous through the whole brain volume (see **Figure 1C**). Whereas some regions outside the corresponding cluster may exhibit non-null stability values, many other voxels exhibit stability values very close or equal to zero. Consequently, estimating a voxel-based mean and a standard deviation both close to zero among the controls would lead to unstable Z-score values. Indeed, one can obtain large Z-values, even though the local stability was very close to zero. This issue can cause problems of interpretation since it will attract attention to a non-stable area of rare occurrence.

To address this issue, instead of computing Z-scores, we propose to use a binary mask, denoted $Zmask_n$, to highlight brain regions depicting significant differences in stability for the target subject and the network n when compared to the population of C controls. These masks were defined as follows:

$$Zmask_n(r) = \left[\left| T_n(r) - \overline{CI_n(r)} \right| > 3.17 \times std\left(CI_n(r)\right) \right] \quad (1)$$

Where r denotes the region within the brain volume $(r = 1 \ldots R)$, $\overline{CI_n(r)}$ and $std(CI_n(r))$ refer to the mean and the standard deviation maps estimated over all CI_n^c maps $(c = 1 \ldots C)$, for the network n $(n = 1 \ldots N)$. 3.17 was chosen as the Z-threshold considered for a non-corrected significant level of $p < 0.001$.

Note that $Zmask_n$ will identify any significant change in the target subject, whether it consisted in an increase or a decrease of stability.

Combined map assessing the amount of stability within the detected $Zmask_n$. Since stability values estimated using BASC are statistical measurements, i.e., a probability to belong to a specific network, we created a map exhibiting these stability values within brain regions showing significant differences between the target subject and the population of controls. To do so, we applied the $Zmask_n$ to the difference between the individual subject-map T_n and the mean stability map $\overline{CI_n(r)}$ from all the controls (see **Figure S1**).

$$Cmap_n(r) = Zmask_n(r) \times \left[T_n(r) - \overline{CI_n(r)}\right] \qquad (2)$$

Where r denotes the region within the brain volume. Using $Cmap_n$ instead of Z-scores maps will avoid biasing the interpretation toward brain regions showing large Z-score values and very low stability values. Note that **Figure 2** is showing a graphical summary of all the steps included in this pipeline.

Thresholding the combined map $Cmap_n$

In order to identify outliers when investigating changes in stability for a particular target subject, the null hypothesis distribution of $Cmap_n$ values was assessed by applying Equation (2) on each of the C subjects of the control database and for each of the N networks. Therefore, we estimated the distribution of so-called "stability changes" likely to occur within a healthy control population. When pooling values from all $C = 25$ controls and $N = 12$ networks, we obtained 0.1 and 99.9 percentile values of -0.34 and 0.34, respectively. Therefore, in order to consider only stability changes likely to be the most significant at the individual level, all $Cmap_n$ values between -0.34 and 0.34 were threshold and subsequently set to zero for the next analyses.

Analysis of the most salient findings for a specific individual

As mentioned earlier, stability measurements considered in this study constitute already statistical measurements. Therefore, we propose to consider first the most salient findings identified for every target subject, i.e., for every patient with epilepsy selected for this particular study. Consequently, for each of the six selected patients, we carefully inspected all the $N = 12$ $Cmap_n$ and only the maps exhibiting a maximum stability increase greater than 0.5 or a minimum stability decrease lower than -0.5 were reported. Since the 0.1 and 99.9 percentiles of stability changes measured over the control database were, respectively -0.34 and 0.34, the threshold of 0.5 was chosen arbitrarily in order to investigate only the most salient findings.

Automatic detection of modularity changes for a specific individual

In addition to the inspection of all $Cmap_n$ results, we also propose a statistical analysis to automatically detect significant changes in modularity. To do so, we proposed a new metric assessing, for each individual network of each target subject, the strength and spatial extent of stability interaction when compared to other CRSNs.

Let us define $W_n(r)$ a 3D spatial map estimating which of the N CRSNs defined in the partition $P(r)$ were involved in local modifications detected using $Zmask_n(r)$:

$$W_n(r) = P(r) \times Zmask_n(r) \qquad (3)$$

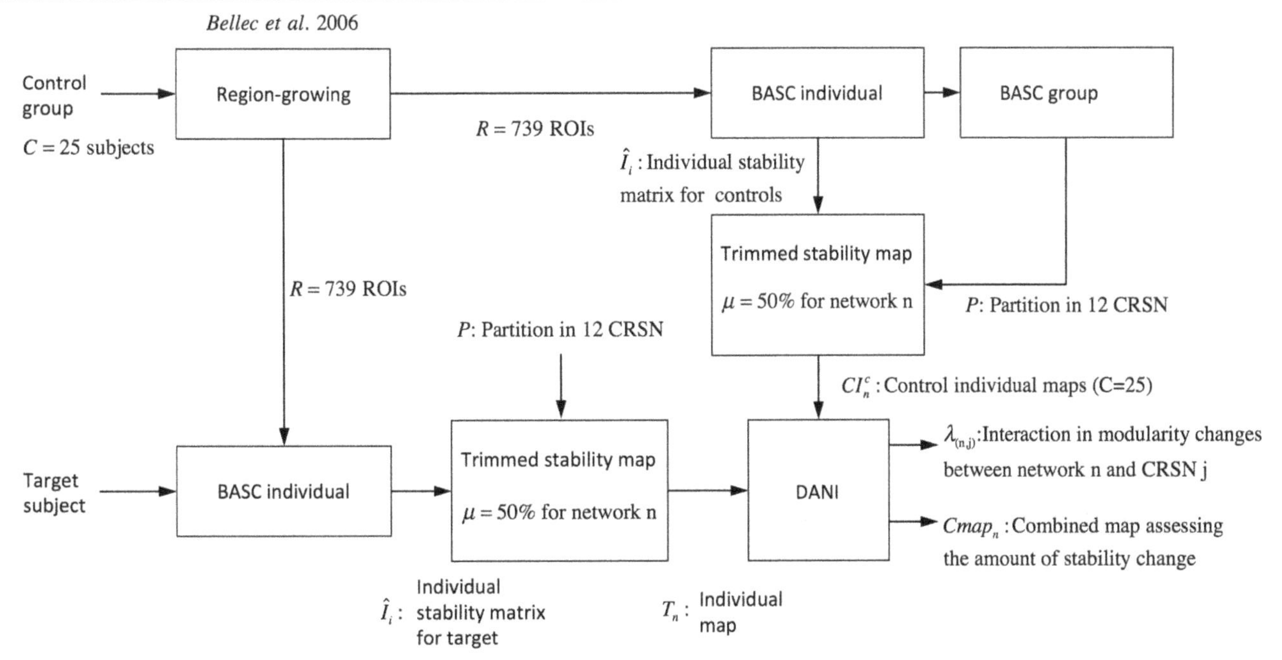

FIGURE 2 | Pipeline summarizing the steps involved in DANI method starting from the preprocessed fMRI images of the control population and the preprocessed images of the target subject on which DANI was applied.

This operation simply consists in applying the binary mask $Zmask_n$ to the partition P. We then introduce the metric $\lambda_{n,j}$, for $n = 1 \ldots N$ and $j = 1 \ldots N$, assessing the interaction between local changes of stability of the nth individual network ($Cmap_n$) with the jth CRSN (i.e., voxels where $(W_n(r) == j)$):

$$\lambda_{n,j} = \sum_r ((W_n(r) == j) \times |Cmap_n(r)|) \quad (4)$$

$\lambda_{n,j}$ quantifies the amount of stability change with which the jth CRSN contributes to the nth network of the target subject to be evaluated. As a summation, this metric is sensitive to both the strength and the spatial extent of the stability changes. It is important to mention that this metric is estimated only within $Zmask_n$, therefore only significant changes in stability are accounted for and only within regions belonging to the jth CRSN.

Therefore the $N \times N$ matrix $\lambda_{n,j}$ provides an overview of all local changes in FC of a target subject when compared to all N CRSNs extracted from the control database.

Using the interaction metric $\lambda_{n,j}$, outlier detection was applied in order to detect abnormal networks, i.e., interactions that are very unlikely to occur for a specific subject. Since the a priori null distribution of this metric is not known, a non-parametric test was considered. To estimate the null hypothesis distribution, a $N \times N$ matrix $\lambda_{n,j}$ was first estimated for each of the C subjects of the control database. The null distribution for each network n and CRSN j was then estimated using a generalized jackknife approach (Sharot, 1976). To do so, 2/3rd of the control sample was randomly selected to calculate the mean and standard deviation and one target sample was randomly selected among the remaining 1/3rd to compute the metric $\lambda_{n,j}$ under the null hypothesis. The procedure was perform 10,000 times using the $C = 25$ controls to characterize the null distribution H0 for each network n and CRSN j. The values of the metric $\lambda_{n,j}$ estimated for the target subject were then compared to the corresponding H0 distribution and p-values were estimated.

VALIDATION OF DANI USING REALISTIC SIMULATED DATA

The objective of this section is to further evaluate DANI using simulated data obtained within a fully controlled realistic environment, thus providing a gold-standard to assess the performance of the method.

Generation of simulated data

We evaluated the performance of DANI by adding different levels of structured signal to perturb the underlying "network" organization of real resting state fMRI state data. This structured signal actually consisted in the average time series of all regions belonging to the visual network (CRSN #4) of another control subject. We also evaluated the influence, on DANI detection properties, of the core size parameter μ considered when estimating the trimmed stability map.

The simulated Signal-to-Noise Ratio (SNR) was defined as follows:

$$SNR_{dB} = 20log_{10}\left(\frac{RMS_{data}}{RMS_{simul}}\right) \quad (5)$$

Where RMS is the root mean square amplitude of the time-series corresponding to the region where the perturbation was applied. We refer to RMS_{data} as the root mean square of the original fMRI time-series of the subject and as RMS_{simul} as the root mean square of the time-series introduced to perturb the system.

Perturbation with structured signal. To force the fusion of two networks and assess the ability of DANI to detect it, structured signal was added on specific parts of two networks within resting state fMRI data of one control subject. Regions belonging to parts of the right hemisphere of the sensory-motor network (CRSN #9) and the auditory network (CRSN #3) were selected as the area to be perturbed (denoted area A). Structured signal was estimated as the average time series of all regions belonging to the visual network (CRSN #4) of another control subject. We then assessed, at what SNR_{dB} level, DANI could detect the fusion of these two parts of the perturbed networks, varying SNR_{dB} from −25 to 25 dB by steps of 1 dB. Small SNR_{dB} values then corresponded to the addition of a large amount of structured signal to corrupt an area involving some regions of the sensory-motor and auditory networks (**Figure S2**).

Validation metric

To quantify the performance of DANI when applied on these simulated data, we first estimated the trimmed stability map of the sensory-motor (**Figure 4**, CRSN #9) and the auditory (**Figure 4**, CRSN #3) networks, using a specific core size parameter μ. For each of these two CRSNs, we evaluated the resulting estimated stability values inside and outside the perturbed zone on which structured signal was added, but limited to the boundaries of the CRSN of interest. Let us define as I_{n_0} the average of all stability values inside the perturbed zone A for a specific network n_0.

$$I_{n_0} = \frac{1}{card(A)} \sum_{r \in A} T_{n_0}(r) \quad (6)$$

Where $card(A)$ refers to the number of voxels belonging to the perturbed zone A and T_{n_0} is the trimmed stability map of the target subject for the network n_0.

Let us define as A' the area of the specific CRSN n_0 located outside the perturbed zone , we introduced the metric O_{n_0} as the average of all the stability values outside the perturbed zone A but within a specific network n_0.

$$O_{n_0} = \frac{1}{card(A')} \sum_{r \in A'} T_{n_0}(r) \quad (7)$$

The validation metrics I_{n_0} and O_{n_0} were evaluated for different SNR_{dB} levels over two different perturbed networks, namely the sensory motor network and the auditory network. **Figure 3** presents a schematic overview of this validation pipeline.

An increase in I_{n_0} would therefore be interpreted as the occurrence of a more stable and consistent network within the targeted region, whereas a decrease in I_{n_0} would be interpreted as a lost of the affected region in favor of another network. On the other hand, a decrease in O_{n_0} would mean that the outside of the original network is no longer associated with the new organization,

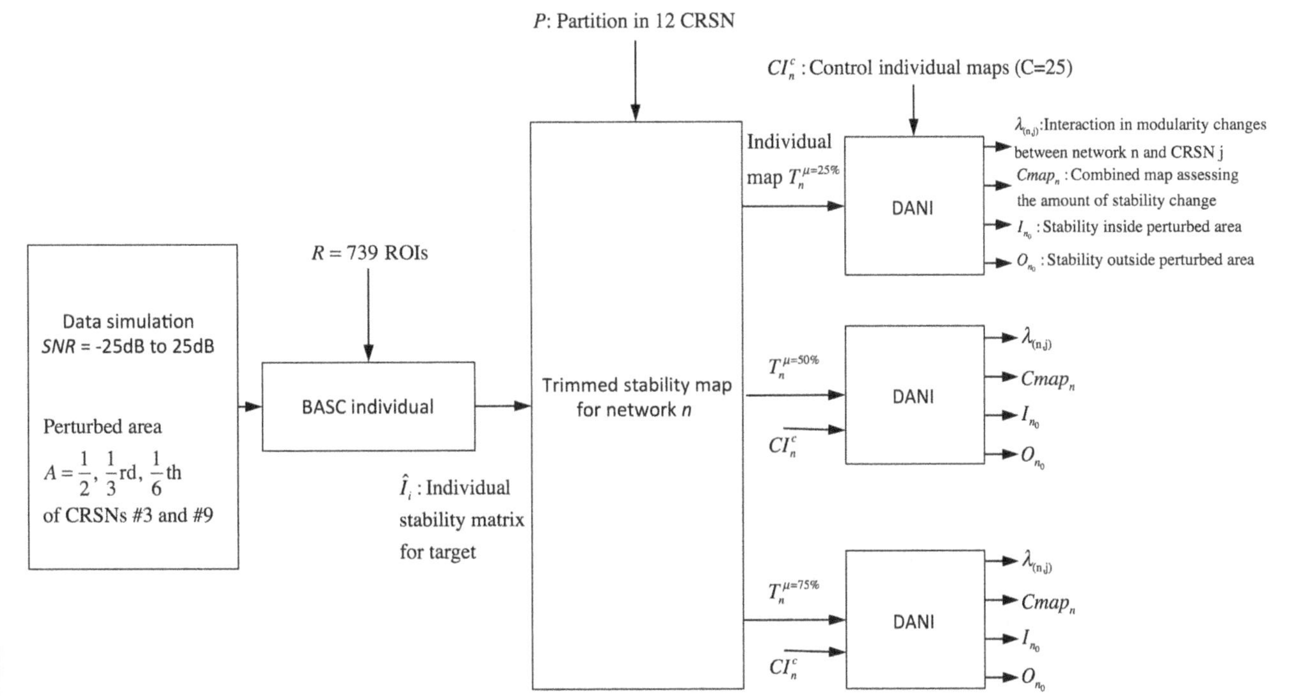

FIGURE 3 | Pipeline summarizing the validation procedure: the input is the preprocessed fMRI data perturbed within a region of size A (A = 1/2, 1/3, and 1/6 of the targeted networks) at a specific SNR_{dB} and the outputs are the metrics $Cmap_n$, $\lambda_{n,j}$, I_{n0} and O_{n0}. Simulations were performed considering 3 core sizes (μ = 25, 50, and 75%) for the estimation of the trimmed stability maps.

whereas a stable O_{n_0} value would mean that the integrity of the original network was preserved.

Validation parameters

DANI performance was evaluated by varying the following parameters:

- The SNR_{dB} at which the structured signal was added ranged from -25 to 25 dB by steps of 1 dB.
- The size of the perturbed zone A varied from 1/2, 1/3rd, and 1/6th of the sensory-motor network and the auditory network.
- The core size parameter μ considered when estimating the trimmed stability maps varied from 25, 50, and 75% of the most stable rows in a given cluster.

EVALUATION OF DANI ON CLINICAL DATA

This section describes the application of DANI on resting state fMRI data of patients with focal epilepsy, who underwent multimodal assessment using simultaneous EEG/fMRI acquisition followed by surgery.

Subject selection criteria for clinical evaluation

Among a population of patients with history suggestive of drug-resistant focal epilepsy (1989; Berg et al., 2010), we selected patients who underwent surgery after simultaneous EEG/fMRI investigation (Gotman et al., 2004), with at least 12 months follow-up. Candidates underwent routine presurgical evaluation, whereas EEG/fMRI was performed independently of other modalities and not considered for placing intracranial electrodes or for surgical decision.

Besides general criteria mentioned in Section Subject Selection, we included the following additional inclusion criteria:

(i) Seizure free patients with at least 12 months follow up. The location of the resection was obtained from postsurgical morphological MRI data.
(ii) Patients who had at least two runs of EEG/fMRI showing epileptic discharges, for which the BOLD response to epileptic discharges was evaluated as either fully concordant or partially concordant with the location of the resection, following the methodology proposed in An et al. (2013).
(iii) Patients who had also at least two runs of EEG/fMRI with no or small numbers of epileptic discharges on scalp EEG in order to investigate functional connectivity patterns independently from the occurrence of epileptic discharges.

Six patients were selected for this study: patients 1 and 2 had right orbito frontal epilepsy. Whereas the anatomical MRI was evaluated as non-lesional, a small focal cortical dysplasia (FCD) was confirmed by pathology. Patients 3 and 4 had, respectively left and right mesio-temporal lobe epilepsy (MTLE) with hippocampal sclerosis. Patients 5 and 6 had, respectively left and right frontal lobe epilepsy (FLE) with the presence of a FCD detected on the MRI and confirmed by pathology (see **Table 1** for further details).

Table 1 | Patients' clinical data.

Numbers	Age/Gender	Anat MRI	Syndrome (Etiology)	Resection	Pathology	Follow up
1	16/F	Normal	R FLE (NL)	R OF	FCD IIa	24
2	38/M	Normal	R FLE (NL)	R OF	FCD IIb	12
3	20/M	L MTS	L TLE (MTS)	L ant TL	Gliosis	12
4	39/F	R MTS	R TLE (MTS)	R ant TL	Neuronal loss and gliosis	24
5	26/F	L 2nd F gyrus FCD	L FLE (FCD)	L 2nd and 3rd F gyrus	FCD IIb	12
6	15/M	R F psagittal FCD	R FLE (FCD)	R 1st F gyrus	FCD IIb	36

R, Right; L, Left; FLE, Frontal Lobe Epilepsy; NL, Non-Lesional; OF, Orbito-Frontal; FCD, Focal Cortical Dysplasia; MTS, Mesio-Temporal Sclerosis; TLE, Temporal Lobe Epilepsy.

Estimation of the BOLD response to epileptic discharges

The analysis of BOLD response to epileptic discharges detected on scalp EEG was identical to the method considered in previous studies from our group (Bagshaw et al., 2004; Gotman and Pittau, 2011; An et al., 2013; Heers et al., 2014). fMRI data were preprocessed following a similar methodology than the one presented in Section fMRI Data Preprocessing. After correcting EEG data from MR gradient artifact (Allen et al., 2000) and ballistocardiogram artifact (Benar et al., 2003), EEG was reviewed by an expert epileptologist (FP) and epileptic discharges were marked. Timing and duration of each discharge were considered to generate regressors and convolved with four hemodynamic response functions (HRFs) peaking at 3, 5, 7, and 9 s, in order to model inherent variability of HRF in patients with epilepsy (Bagshaw et al., 2004). Motion parameters were modeled as confounds and all regressors were included in the same general linear model. A combined *t*-map was created by taking, at each voxel, the maximum t value from the four *t*-maps based on four HRFs. To be significant, a response required five contiguous voxels having a *t*-value > 3.17 ($p < 0.05$ using Bonferroni correction to take into account the four HRFs analyses).

Multimodal assessment

Postsurgical morphological MRI data consisted either in 3D high resolution T1 weighted MRI (1 mm isotropic resolution) or T2 weighted axial or coronal slices (in plane resolution: 0.46 mm, slice thickness: 5 mm). Postsurgical MRI data were co-registered to the high resolution anatomical MRI acquired during the EEG/fMRI session, by maximizing normalized mutual information (Studholme et al., 1999), assuming an affine geometrical transformation between the two volumes. Using the inverse transformations of the rigid-body fMRI-to-T1 transform and the nonlinear T1-to-stereotaxic transform introduced in Section fMRI Data Preprocessing, DANI results, i.e., the combined maps of stability changes $Cmap_n$ for all $n = 1 \ldots N$ networks, were resampled in the native space of the anatomical MRI of each patient. Therefore, DANI results, BOLD responses to epileptic discharges and postsurgical MRI data could be compared on a voxel/voxel basis with the native MRI space of every patient.

RESULTS

CONSISTENT RESTING STATE NETWORKS

The resulting trimmed stability maps obtained from group level BASC analysis of the 25 healthy controls, resulting in the identification of 12 CRSNs, are presented in **Figure 4**. These CRSNs were used as the reference functional networks to detect possible abnormal networks in patients.

VALIDATION OF DANI USING SIMULATED DATA

Figure 5 shows the impact on DANI results when adding structured signals to perturb resting state fMRI data from parts of the sensory-motor and the auditory CRSNs and when varying the core size parameter μ, i.e., the percentage of stability considered when estimating trimmed stability maps. The left column of the Figure represents the average stability inside the target zone as a function of SNR_{dB}, the middle column shows the average stability estimated outside of the target zone as a function of SNR_{dB} and the third column shows the resulting trimmed stability maps for both networks at $SNR_{dB} = -25\ dB$, i.e., at the highest perturbation level. Overall, DANI was able to identify changes around 7 dB regardless of the size of the target zone and with all core sizes. When adding perturbation in half (**Figure 5A**), 1/3rd (**Figure 5B**) and 1/6th (**Figure 5C**) of the two networks, choosing a core size μ of 25% drastically enhanced the stability within the target region (left column), whereas at the same time the resulting stability outside the target was significantly reduced, down to zero for the auditory network, meaning that this network was lost and completely taken over by its fusion with the sensory-motor network. Resulting trimmed stability maps obtained when most intense perturbation was added ($SNR_{dB} = -25dB$) are confirming this trend, since mainly the fused perturbed network was detected for both networks (**Figure 5**. right column). On the other hand, using a core size μ of 75%, only moderate changes could be detected from stability profiles especially when perturbation was added on 1/6th of the two networks (**Figure 5C**), yielding a poor stability contrast between regions of interest. This trend was also confirmed on the resulting trimmed stability maps obtained at $SNR_{dB} = -25\ dB$ (**Figure 5** right column). Finally, choosing a core size μ of 50% provided a good trade-off yielding good sensitivity to detect the new fused network (**Figure 5** left column), while providing accurate stability measures within the remaining sections of the non-perturbed networks (**Figure 5** middle). This trade-off corresponding to an ideal detection contrast obtained at $\mu = 50\%$ is illustrated on the resulted trimmed stability maps obtained at $SNR_{dB} = -25\ dB$ (**Figure 5** right column).

When perturbing a large target zone involving half of both networks (**Figure 5A**), DANI detected one large fused network at the detriment of the two original ones. The remaining non-perturbed

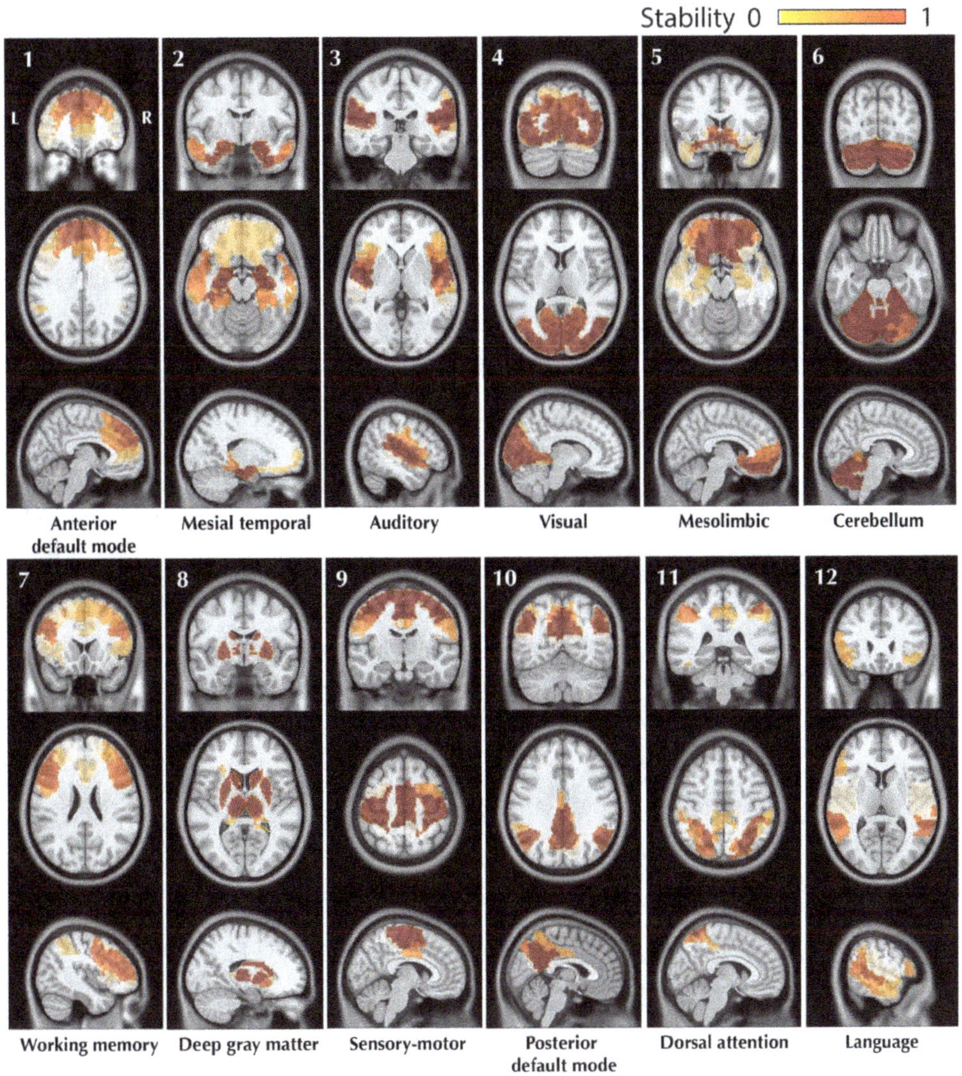

FIGURE 4 | Visual representation of the 12 CRSNs identified using BASC group level analysis of 25 healthy control subjects. For each CRSN: 3 slices (coronal, axial, sagittal) are shown superimposed on an anatomical MRI template (MNI152). Labeling of each network was done visually based on previously reported CRSNs in the literature. The figure shows the usual networks: Default Mode Network (1,10), Auditory (3), Visual (4), Sensory-Motor (9), Attention (7,11) and Language(12). BASC also identified 4 other networks, less often reported, but characterized by high statistical stability: Mesio- Temporal (2), Mesolimbic (5), Cerebellum (6) and Deep Gray Matter (8).

areas of the original networks were no longer classified as being part of the network and a new fused network was detected. We observed a different behavior when perturbing 1/3rd of the two networks (**Figure 5B**) instead of completely merging the two networks together, DANI partially merged them. When perturbing only a small region (1/6th of both networks, **Figure 5C**), the perturbed part of the sensory-motor network was associated with the auditory network, resulting in the detection of a smaller sensory-motor network and a larger auditory network.

EVALUATION OF DANI ON CLINICAL DATA

Results from both statistical analyses applied on DANI clinical results are reported in **Table 2**. For every patient and for every network n, the maximum and minimum values of $Cmap_n$ were first reported. Networks exhibiting salient stability increases, associated with a maximum value larger than 0.5, are indicated in red font. Note that no network exhibited salient stability decreases associated with a minimum value lower than −0.5. The second analysis consisted in an automatic detection of modularity changes using a non-parametric approach (see Section Automatic detection of modularity changes for a specific individual). Networks identified in a significant interaction, i.e., rejecting the null hypothesis $\lambda_{n,j} = 0$ with $p < 0.001$, were reported using a bold font and a "∗" sign in **Table 2**.

Note that results for each patient are represented using $Cmap_n$, measuring, for each network n, only the significant differences in stability observed for the target individual patient when compared to the population of controls. This is the reason why remote regions from the underlying CRSN partition could be detected in those maps, whereas main regions associated with the

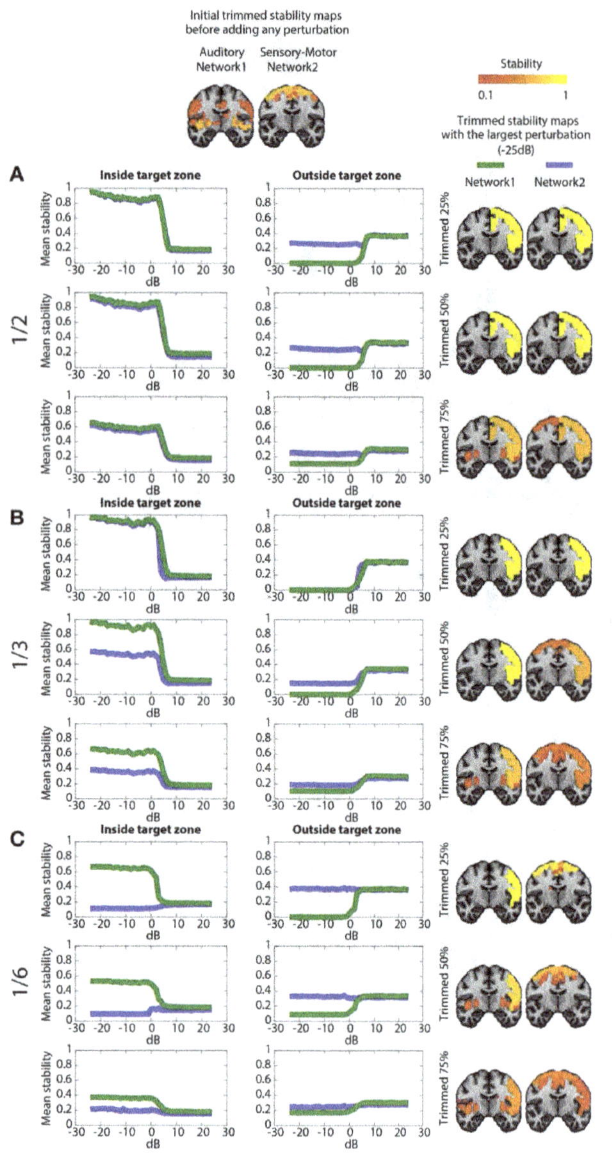

FIGURE 5 | Evaluation of DANI using simulated data. The first line shows the initial trimmed stability maps T_n obtained for the Auditory network (network 1) and the Sensory-Motor network (network 2) before adding any perturbution. Graphs present the average stability inside I_{n_0} (left column) outside O_{n_0} (middle column) the perturbed area as a function of SNR_{dB} values ranging from −25 dB to +25 dB, for both the Auditory (green) and the Sensory-Motor (blue) networks. The right column shows the resulting trimmed stability maps T_n obtained when adding the largest perturbation at $SNR_{dB} = -25dB$. **(A)** perturbation zone involving 1/2 of both Auditory and Sensory-Motor networks, **(B)** perturbation zone involving 1/3rd of both Auditory and Sensory-Motor networks, **(C)** perturbation zone involving 1/6th of both Auditory and Sensory-Motor networks. In each case, results obtained when varying the core size parameter μ at 25, 50, and 75% are presented.

underlying CRSN partition might not be present if no significant stability changes were detected. All $Cmap_n$ have been thresholded above the 99.9% percentile (resp. below the 0.1% percentile) measured over the control population, i.e., above 0.34 and below −0.34.

Main results obtained for patient 1 with right orbito-frontal epilepsy are presented in **Figure 6**. A BOLD activation to epileptic discharges was found in the right orbito-frontal focus and was fully concordant with the location of the resection (patient seizure free at 24 months). Whereas the anatomical MRI was evaluated as non-lesional, pathology confirmed a FCD within the focus. The networks that showed most salient stability increases in $Cmap_n$ were the Mesio-Temporal, Mesolimbic, Cerebellum and Dorsal Attention networks. All these networks except the Dorsal Attention were also involved in significant interactions of modularity changes ($p < 0.001$). $Cmap_n$ for the Mesolimbic network, containing the focus, showed increases in stability within the whole Mesolimbic network, involving notably the focus and showing increase in stability within most bilateral regions of this network. Increase stability suggest that, when compared to a population of controls, these regions are more reliably connected together for this specific patient. A local maximum in $Cmap_n$ was found within the right frontal pole, actually in a close neighborhood around the focus. $Cmap_n$ for the MesioTemporal network showed large increases in stability (up to 0.74, i.e., 74% more stable than within the control population) within bilateral mesial and lateral temporal regions and the Cerebellum. Connections between the Mesolimbic and Mesiotemporal networks are well-known propagation pathways in epilepsy. $Cmap_n$ for the Cerebellum network showed increases in stability within bilateral mesial and lateral temporal regions, involving notably both temporal poles. $Cmap_n$ for the Dorsal Attention network shows stability increases within itself, involving as well some regions of the posterior Default Mode Network (DMN) (results not shown).

Main results obtained for patient 2 with right orbito-frontal epilepsy are presented in **Figure 7**. A BOLD activation fully concordant with the resected area in the right orbito-frontal region was also observed for this patient. The MRI was evaluated as non-lesional and a FCD was identified by pathology analysis. Most salient stability increases in $Cmap_n$ were found for the Mesolimbic, Cerebellum, and the Dorsal Attention networks. On the other hand, the Sensori-Motor network, the posterior DMN and the Dorsal Attention network were also involved in significant interactions of modularity changes. $Cmap_n$ for the Mesolimbic network showed stability increases within the right frontal pole (lateralized on the side of the focus), bilateral heads of the caudate nuclei and bilateral insulae regions, suggesting notably increase stability in several regions surrounding the focus. $Cmap_n$ for the Cerebellum network showed stability increases in some regions of the Cerebellum, with some involvement of bilateral temporal structures. $Cmap_n$ for the Dorsal Attention network shows large stability increases within itself, involving as well some regions of the posterior DMN and a right anterior frontal region (also lateralized on the side of the focus). A very similar pattern was found for $Cmap_n$ of the posterior DMN network (results not shown). $Cmap_n$ for the Sensory Motor network identified increase in stability with itself, involving as well some frontal more anterior regions, far from the focus (results not shown).

Main results obtained for patient 3 with left MTLE and hippocampal sclerosis are presented in **Figure 8**. BOLD activations to epileptic discharges were found within the left mesio-temporal

Table 2 | Analysis of the most salient findings detected by DANI.

Network numbers	S1	S2	S3	S4	S5	S6
1. Ant. DMN	−0.16/0.44	−0.24/0.27	−0.21/0.43	**−0.20/0.35***	−0.19/0.43	−0.16/0.49
2. Mesio-Temporal	**−0.10/0.74***	−0.10/0.38	−/−	−0.10/0.70	−0.08/0.52	−0.10/0.54
3. Auditory	−0.28/0.22	−0.24/0.35	−0.26/0.30	−0.30/0.38	−0.29/0.38	−0.30/0.50
4. Visual	−0.18/0.37	−0.33/0.40	**−0.24/0.57***	**−/0.46***	−0.22/0.20	**−0.26/0.70***
5. Mesolimbic	**−0.48/0.58***	−/0.56	−/0.53	−/0.51	−/0.40	**−/0.59***
6. Cerebellum	**−0.34/0.64***	−0.41/0.54	**−0.48/0.59***	**−0.49/0.48***	−0.35/0.60	−0.47/**0.72***
7. Working Memory	−0.17/0.30	−0.15/0.24	−0.16/0.33	−0.17/0.34	−0.17/0.41	−0.16/0.33
8. Deep Gray Matter	−0.29/0.29	−0.28/0.39	−0.26/0.37	−0.26/0.43	−0.22/0.50	−0.32/0.39
9. Sensory Motor	−0.16/0.49	**−0.30/0.43***	−0.18/0.32	**−0.17/0.55***	−0.18/0.57	−0.16/0.60
10. Post. DMN	−0.22/0.40	**−0.30/0.47***	−0.30/0.48	−0.30/0.43	−0.36/0.49	−0.27/0.47
11. Dorsal attention	−0.13/0.50	**−0.22/0.58***	**−0.17/0.56***	−0.25/0.43	−0.23/0.51	−0.23/0.49
12. Language	−0.17/0.30	−0.14/0.14	**−0.16/0.41***	−0.17/0.26	−0.15/0.40	−0.15/0.30

For each of the 12 networks and for each patient, we are reporting the global maximum and minimum value of stability changes identified in $Cmap_n$. Networks exhibiting the most salient increases in stability, i.e., more than 0.5, were indicated in red font (no salient findings showing a minimum decrease in stability lower than −0.5 were found). Network involved in significant interactions of modularity changes with other CRSN at $p < 0.001$ (cf. Section Automatic detection of modularity changes for a specific individual) were indicated with a "" and in bold font. ("-" indicates that no negative values were found in $Cmap_n$).*

focus, involving as well the left temporal neocortex. BOLD results were classified as fully concordant with the location of the resection involving the anterior part of the temporal lobe. Most salient stability changes in $Cmap_n$ were found for the Visual, Mesolimbic, Cerebellum and Dorsal Attention networks. The Visual, Cerebellum, Dorsal Attention and also the Language networks have been identified within significant interaction in modularity changes. Very widespread stability increases have been identified within $Cmap_n$ of the Visual network, involving mainly the secondary-association visual areas including the fusiform gyri bilaterally, and not the primary visual areas. Stability increases were also found in the left hippocampus, bilateral thalami, putamen, insulae, cerebellum and some regions of the Dorsal Attention network. Interestingly, $Cmap_n$ of the Mesolimbic network showed a well-localized and lateralized left temporo-lateral stability increase, closely related to the focus. $Cmap_n$ of the Cerebellum network exhibited some reorganization resulting in stability increases and decreases within the cerebellum itself. $Cmap_n$ of the Dorsal Attention network suggests stability increases within itself, involving also some regions of the posterior DMN (results not shown). $Cmap_n$ of the Language network shows increase in stability in bilateral temporo-posterior regions at the temporo-occipital junction, involving also bilateral fusiform gyri. Increase stability in bilateral thalami was also identified (results not shown).

Main results obtained for patient 4 with right MTLE and hippocampal sclerosis are presented in **Figure 9**. BOLD activation to epileptic discharge was found in the right mesio-temporal structures, fully concordant with the location of the resection. Most salient stability changes in $Cmap_n$ were found for the Mesio-Temporal, Mesolimbic and Sensory Motor networks, whereas significant interaction in modularity changes were found for the anterior DMN, the Visual, the Cerebellum and the Sensory Motor networks. The largest stability increases in $Cmap_n$ were found for the MesioTemporal network (maximum of 0.7), involving mainly the right mesio-temporal focus, as well as left mesial and lateral temporal regions and bilateral cerebellum. $Cmap_n$ of the Mesolimbic network shows stability increases in the fronto-mesial and polar regions on the side of the focus. $Cmap_n$ for the Cerebellum network shows very interestingly a lateralized stability increase in the right temporal region, very close to the focus, and a bilateral stability decrease within the cerebellum itself. Slight stability increases within regions of the Mesolimbic and Dorsal Attention networks were also observed. Note that even if Cerebellum $Cmap_n$ was not considered among the most salient findings, the maximum stability increase of 0.48 was very close to our arbitrary threshold of 0.5. Within $Cmap_n$ of the Visual network, we identified a bilateral stability increase within secondary-association visual areas including the fusiform gyri and within the right insula (lateralized on the side of the focus, results not shown). $Cmap_n$ of the Sensory Motor network exhibited stability increases withing itself involving also some regions of the posterior DMN and Visual network, bilaterally (results not shown). $Cmap_n$ of the anterior DMN showed a small focal stability increase in the supplementary motor area (results not shown).

Main results obtained for patient 5 with left frontal FCD are presented in **Figure 10**. The resection was circumscribed to the lesional area and a BOLD deactivation response to epileptic discharges had a maximum t-value (negative value) at the anterior edge of the resection. Even if the overlapping voxels were only few, the fact that they contained the maximum t-value allowed us classifying this case as "partially concordant." Most salient stability increases in $Cmap_n$ involved MesioTemporal, Cerebellum, Deep Gray Matter, Sensory Motor and Dorsal Attention networks, whereas no significant interactions of modularity changes could be detected. None of these changes were really spatially concordant with the left frontal focus or lateralized to the side of the focus. $Cmap_n$ of the Deep Gray Matter network exhibited increase stability within itself also

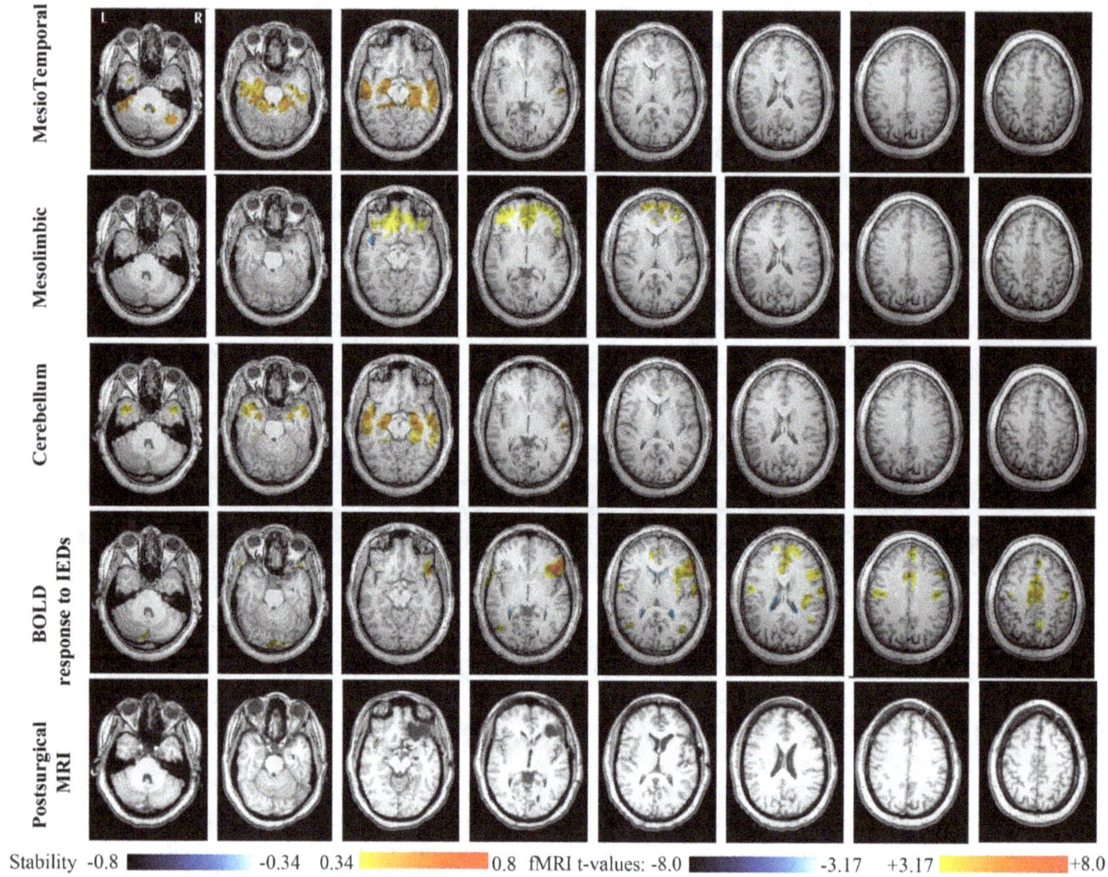

FIGURE 6 | Evaluation of DANI on Patient 1 with right Orbito-Frontal epilepsy. Results are presenting most salient stability changes observed in $Cmap_n$ followed by a t-map of the BOLD response to epileptic discharges and a postsurgical T1 MRI, all resampled in the native anatomical MRI space of the patient. Most salient stability changes observed for $Cmap_n$ of Mesio-Temporal, Mesolimbic, and Cerebellum networks are presented. These three networks were also involved in significant interactions of modularity changes at $p < 0.001$. $Cmap_n$ are presented between 0.34 and 0.8 (resp. −0.34 and −0.8) and BOLD *t*-map between 3.17 and 8.0 (resp. −3.17 and −8.0) using a yellow–red colormap (resp. white–blue colormap).

involving bilateral insulae. $Cmap_n$ of the Sensory-Motor network shows increase stability within itself and also involving regions of the posterior DMN. $Cmap_n$ of the Dorsal Attention network shows increase stability within itself and in some bilateral lateral and mesial frontal regions of the anterior DMN. $Cmap_n$ of the MesioTemporal network shows increase in stability in bilateral Cerebellum regions and $Cmap_n$ of the Cerebellum shows increase in stability in bilateral temporal (results not shown).

Main results obtained for patient 6 with right frontal FCD are presented in **Figure 11**. The resection was circumscribed to the lesional area. The BOLD response to epileptic discharges was really noisy. The cluster of BOLD activation showing a maximum *t*-value in the right central region is partially concordant with the edge of resection, but the presence of motion artifacts cannot let us classify this case as "concordant." Most salient stability changes in $Cmap_n$ involved MesioTemporal, Auditory, Visual, Mesolimbic, Cerebellum, and Sensory Motor networks. Among these networks, the Visual, Mesolimbic and Cerebellum networks were also involved in significant interactions of modularity changes. $Cmap_n$ of the visual network shows stability increase within secondary-association visual areas including the fusiform gyri. $Cmap_n$ of the Cerebellum network exhibited local stability increases and decreases within the Cerebellum but also a very focal and very intense right postcentral stability increase (maximum increase of 0.72), partially concordant with BOLD activation and lateralized to the side of the lesion. $Cmap_n$ of the Sensory Motor network shows increase stability within itself and involving some more posterior parietal bilateral regions. $Cmap_n$ of the Mesolimbic network shows increase stability within bilateral temporal regions, $Cmap_n$ of the Mesio-Temporal network shows increase stability in bilateral temporal and anterior cingulate region (part of the Mesolimbic network) and $Cmap_n$ of the auditory network shows bilateral increase in stability within itself and within Thalami (results not shown). Since BOLD results to epileptic discharges were really contaminated by motion artifacts, similar artifact could have also biased DANI results in this case, although we carefully removed all the frames showing a displacement of more than 0.5 mm as suggested by Power et al. (2012).

Even though we reported mainly the concordance of the stability changes detected using DANI and the BOLD responses to epileptic discharges with the resected area, it is important to point

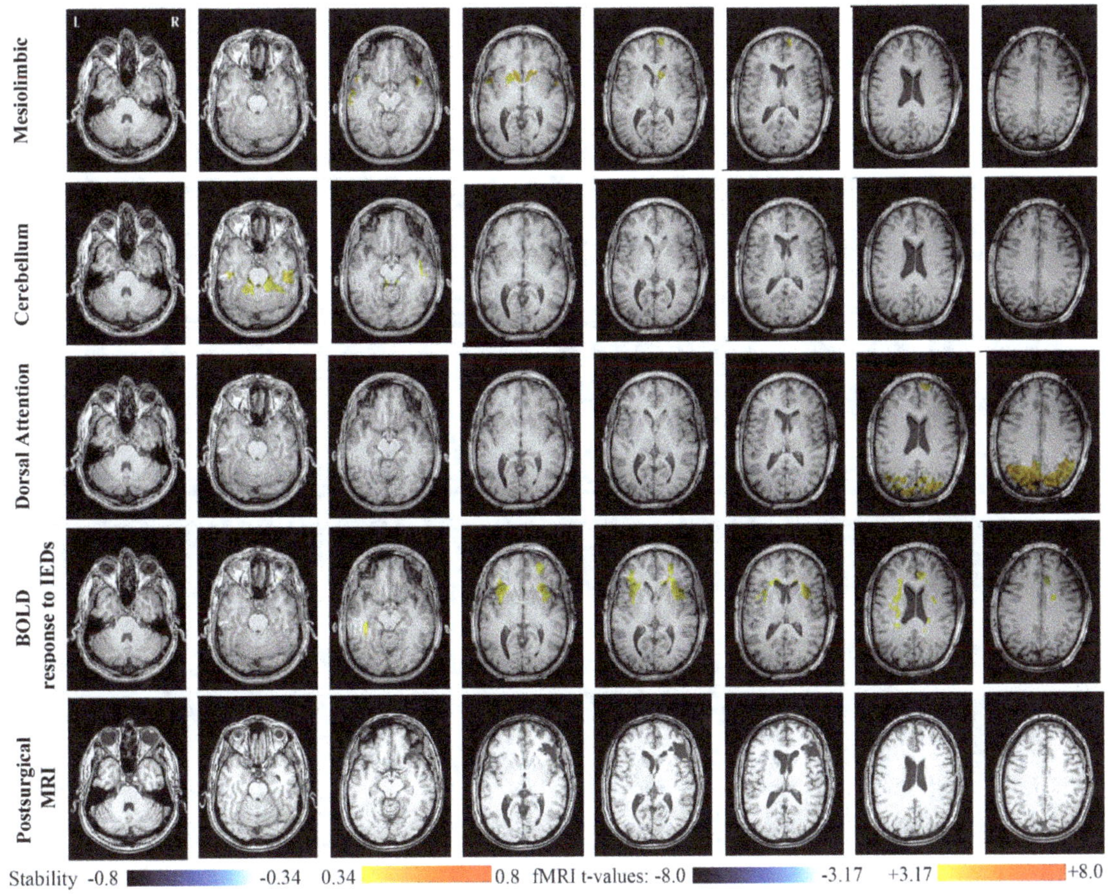

FIGURE 7 | Evaluation of DANI on Patient 2 with right Orbito-Frontal epilepsy. Results are presenting most salient stability changes observed in $Cmap_n$ followed by a t-map of the BOLD response to epileptic discharges and a postsurgical T1 MRI, all resampled in the native anatomical MRI space of the patient. Most salient stability changes observed for $Cmap_n$ of Mesolimbic, Cerebellum, and Dorsal Attention networks are presented. The Dorsal Attention network was also involved in significant interactions of modularity changes at $p < 0.001$. Same colormap conventions than in **Figure 6**.

out that for most patients both results, i.e., DANI and BOLD responses to epileptic discharges, were not only showing significant changes closely related to the presumed epileptic focus, but were also exhibiting more complex connectivity patterns reorganization extending to some more distant regions.

DISCUSSION

The advantage of our proposed method DANI is the ability to identify atypical and individual modular organization of FC for one specific individual. Besides extending BASC (Bellec et al., 2010) to produce trimmed stability maps focussing on the core of the networks, we reproduced the main CRSNs in agreement with previous studies, using the group level BASC analysis on 25 healthy controls (Raichle et al., 2001; Damoiseaux et al., 2006; Fox and Raichle, 2007; Smith et al., 2009). We notably reproduced group level BASC results presented in Bellec et al. (2010), using another database of 25 healthy controls. The trimmed stability maps, representing at the group or at the individual the statistically most stable networks allows focussing on RSN cores rather than on full networks. Our evaluation using simulated data demonstrated than an optimal sensitivity contrast was obtained when choosing a core size μ of 50%. Using these maps, we were able to characterize individual variability with a good compromise between flexibility and consistency. This approach provides consistency across subjects while allowing for flexibility to adapt the networks at the individual level. The combined maps $Cmap_n$ exhibiting significant changes in stability, allowed us to avoid the problem of large and unstable Z-scores in regions where the mean and standard deviation of stability in the controls were close to zero. In order to detect abnormal networks statistically stable at the level of individuals, we proposed DANI, which involves the following steps: (i) generation of trimmed stability maps of each network at the individual level, (ii) assessment of significant stability variations in FC using $Cmap_n$, (iii) nonparametric test to automatically detect significant interactions of modularity changes with other CRSNs.

DANI was first evaluated using realistic simulated data. Our results demonstrate that detecting modular changes over various spatial extents was possible. DANI is sensitive to changes caused by the addition of structured signal to modify modular

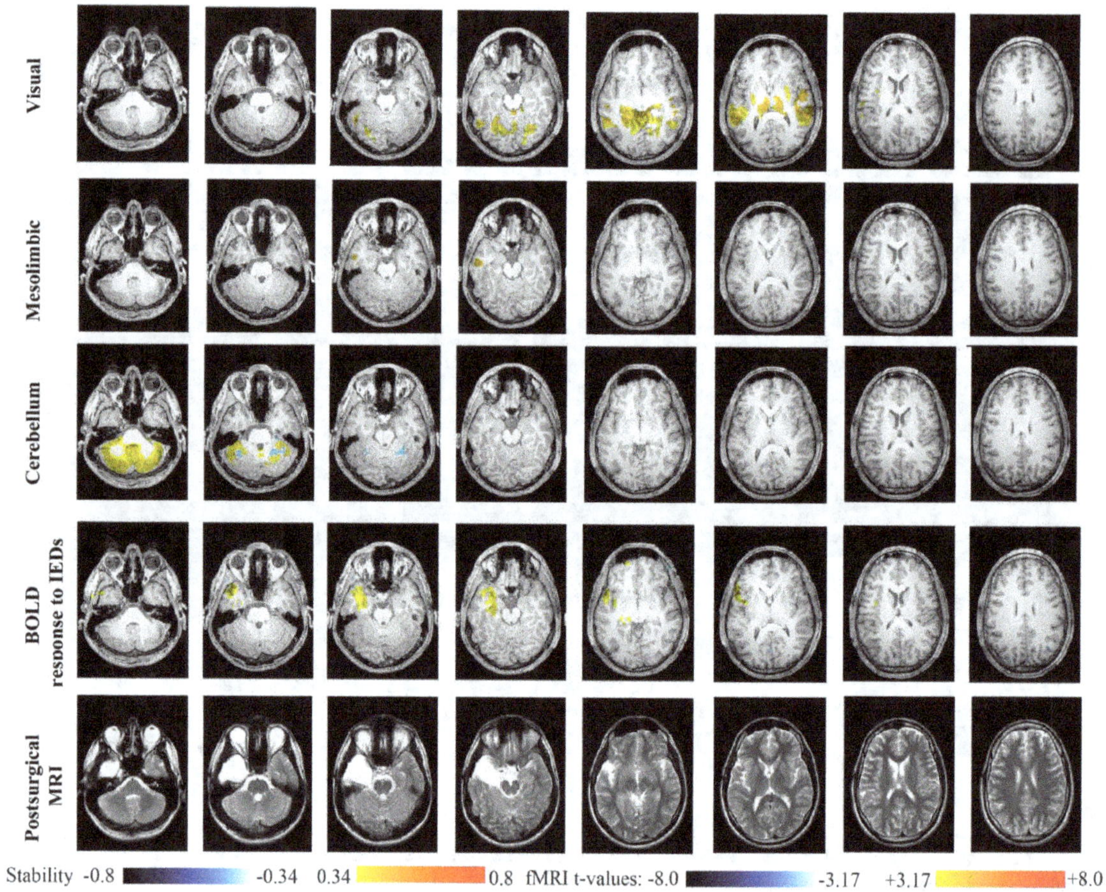

FIGURE 8 | Evaluation of DANI on Patient 3 with left MTLE. Results are presenting most salient stability changes observed in $Cmap_n$ followed by a t-map of the BOLD response to epileptic discharges and a postsurgical T2 MRI, all resampled in the native anatomical MRI space of the patient. Most salient stability changes observed for $Cmap_n$ of Visual, Mesolimbic and Cerebellum networks are presented. The Visual and Cerebellum networks were also involved in significant interactions of modularity changes at $p < 0.001$. Same colormap conventions than in **Figure 6**.

structures. Whatever was the size of the simulated perturbation, DANI detected changes in modularity up to an energy ratio of 7 dB between the original signal and the simulated signal. The criterion to choose an optimal core size μ for the trimmed map is to be sensitive to small changes without completely changing the modular structure, when the affected regions were representing a substantial fraction of the original module. A core size μ of 50% of the most stable regions in each cluster has proven to be a good candidate to meet this criterion. We showed that when the perturbed area was spatially limited (1/6th of the networks), the modular reorganization tended to associate that perturbed zone with one of the two original networks (the auditory network), while removing it from the other one (the somato-sensory network). When increasing the size of that perturbation zone, the new perturbed zone started to overcome the stability of the two original networks, resulting in the extinction of one or both of the original networks.

We acknowledge the fact that the proposed method includes a series of parameters that have to be set, for which the default (recommended) values are summarized in **Table 3**. First of all, BASC and DANI have been applied on a parcellation of the brain in $R = 739$ ROIs. These ROIs were obtained using a region-growing algorithm proposed in Bellec et al. (2006), in order to ensure homogeneity, over all control subjects, of the measurements on small functional units or parcels. Although a target subject to be evaluated using DANI might exhibit slightly different functional parcels in theory, we believe that those changes will be reflected in the stability strengths of the regions in question. We therefore think that this approach should allow sufficient flexibility to capture individual changes while maintaining a good consistency across subjects. Moreover, the main reason for applying BASC and DANI on a parcellation of the brain was for dimensionality reduction purposes, in order to limit the computational burden of the proposed method. A potential improvement not explored in this study would be to apply BASC and DANI directly at the voxel-level instead of the parcel-level. This interesting modification of the method was out of the scope of the present study. Secondly, the overall analysis was proposed using a scale of $N = 12$ CRSNs, in order to be in agreement with the literature describing those CRSNs (Damoiseaux et al., 2006; Smith et al., 2009). However, in BASC, Bellec et al. (2010) suggested and evaluated an optimization strategy to estimate the parameters k, L

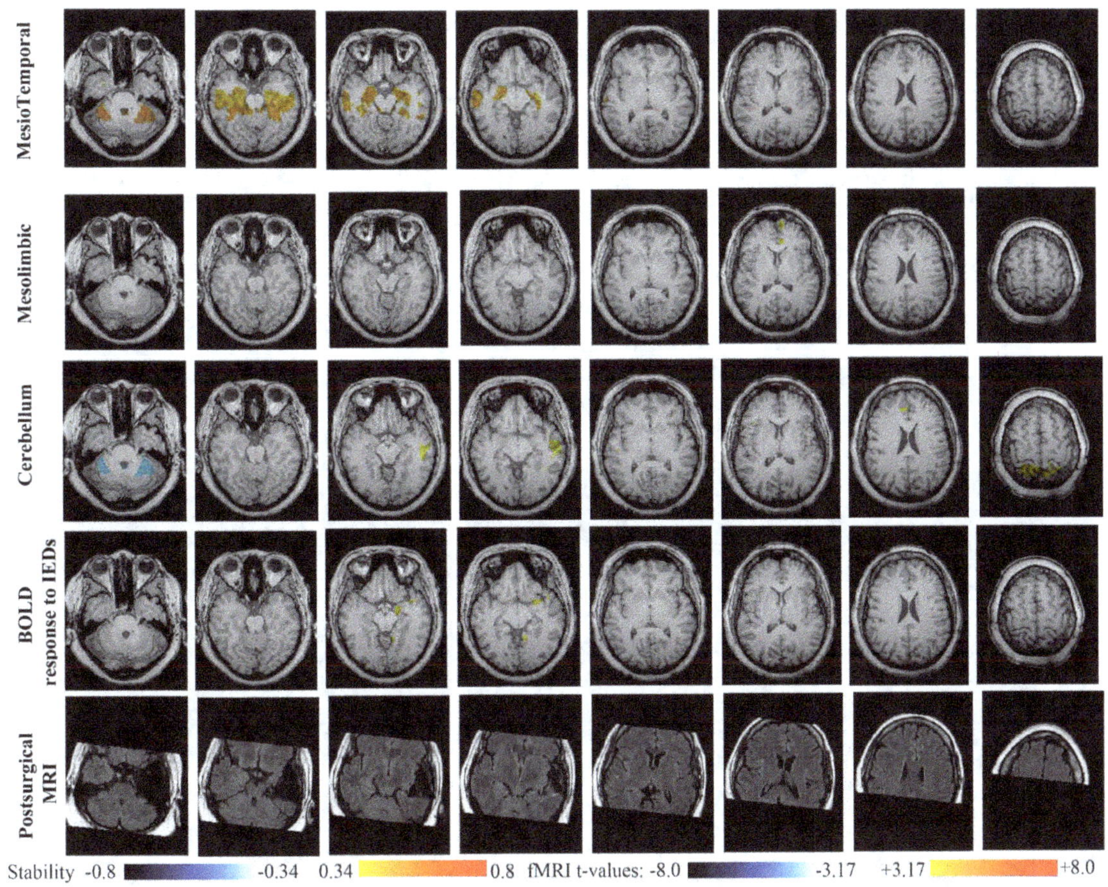

FIGURE 9 | Evaluation of DANI on Patient 4 with right MTLE. Results are presenting most salient stability changes observed in $Cmap_n$ followed by a *t*-map of the BOLD response to epileptic discharges and a postsurgical FLAIR MRI, all resampled in the native anatomical MRI space of the patient. Most salient stability changes observed for $Cmap_n$ of Mesio-Temporal and Mesolimbic networks are presented. We also present $Cmap_n$ of the Cerebellum network (max. stability increase of 0.48), since it was involved in significant interactions of modularity changes at $p < 0.001$. Same colormap conventions than in **Figure 6**.

and *N* for different scales of interest. In this context, it would be highly relevant in a future study to investigate how the choice of such a scale could impact the sensitivity and specificity of DANI results. Finally, when presenting these preliminary results on 6 patients with focal epilepsy, we focussed our interest on the most salient findings only (cf. $Zmask_n$ threshold at 3.17 ($p < 0.001$ non-corrected), $Cmap_n$ threshold at 0.34 (99.9% percentile over the control population and maximum $Cmap_n$ showing more than 50% of stability changes). It would be relevant to investigate furthermore in a future study, the specificity of the method when applied on a larger dataset of controls and patients as well as the reproducibility of the results, using test/re-test reliability for instance.

DANI was then evaluated on resting state fMRI data from six patients with focal epilepsy who underwent simultaneous EEG/fMRI acquisition followed by surgery. Only patients with a seizure free outcome and at least 12 months follow up were selected. For all patients, the BOLD responses to epileptic discharges were evaluated as fully or partially concordant with the location of the resection, following the methodology proposed by An et al. (2013). Interpretation of BOLD responses for patient 5 and 6 was more difficult (details hereunder). The most significant BOLD responses (maximum positive or negative *t*-values) were considered to assess the level of concordance between BOLD results and the location of the resection. Whereas we acknowledge that BOLD responses are also often found distant from the presumed focus (e.g., patients 1, 2, and 6), we previously demonstrated that considering the most significant BOLD results provided best agreement with the presumed focus and EEG results (Pittau et al., 2012a; Heers et al., 2014). Overall DANI identified clearly several outlier networks for each patient. These changes in the stability of FC patterns were salient, showing increases in stability larger than 0.5, whereas the 99.9% percentile of stability increase measured over the healthy controls database was 0.34. For 5 out of 6 patient, "abnormal" or outlier networks closely related to the epileptogenic focus were detected. We also found reorganizations of some remote networks distant from the focus (e.g., Dorsal Attention network and posterior DMN). These results suggest large reorganization of FC patterns, extended far the from the focus. Similar findings

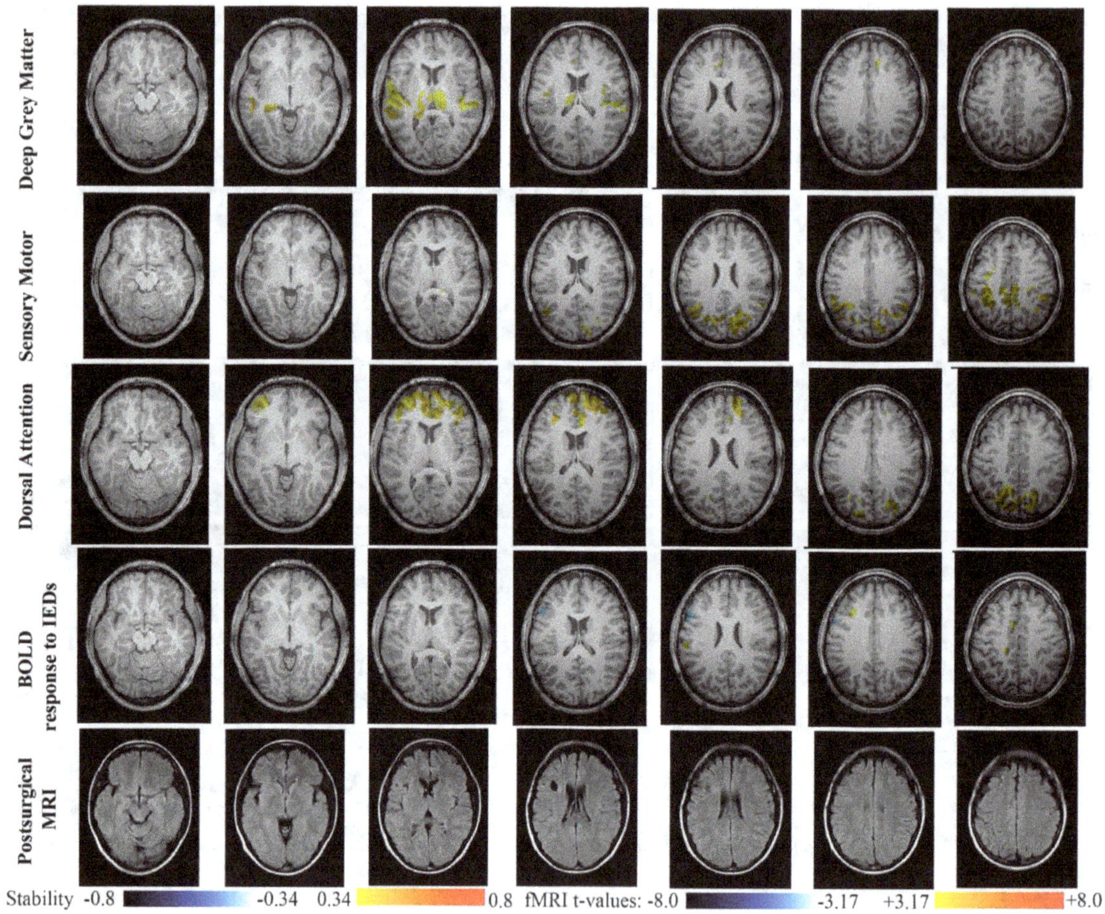

FIGURE 10 | Evaluation of DANI on Patient 5 with left frontal FCD. Results are presenting most salient stability changes observed in $Cmap_n$ followed by a *t*-map of the BOLD response to epileptic discharges and a postsurgical FLAIR MRI, all resampled in the native anatomical MRI space of the patient. Most salient stability changes observed for $Cmap_n$ of Deep Gray Matter, Sensory Motor, and Dorsal Attention networks are presented. No networks were involved in significant interactions of modularity changes at $p < 0.001$. Same colormap conventions than in **Figure 6**.

have been suggested in group analysis of MTLE patients (see Bernhardt et al., 2013; for a recent review), but also in the few studies including individual level analysis of patients with epilepsy (Negishi et al., 2011; Stufflebeam et al., 2011; Luo et al., 2014). Whereas CRSNs observed in healthy controls are usually bilateral, we identified for 5 out of 6 patients at least one abnormal network exhibiting increase in stability lateralized on the side of the focus. Despite widespread involvement of several networks, the importance of laterality in FC patterns of patients with epilepsy has been suggested as a key feature by several studies (Bettus et al., 2009; Negishi et al., 2011; Constable et al., 2013; Luo et al., 2014). For instance, Negishi et al. (2011) proposed to use patient specific BOLD responses to epileptic discharges to define seeds for a seed-based FC analysis. They found that poor surgical outcome was associated with a low degree of laterality of FC maps. The potential clinical impact of providing accurate and sensitive FC analysis during presurgical investigation in the context of neurooncology, epilepsy surgery, and deep brain stimulation has been recently reviewed by Lang et al. (2014), pointing out the importance of developing methods dedicated to single subject analysis of FC patterns.

For patients 1 and 2 who had right orbito-frontal epilepsy, DANI detected specific reorganization within the Mesolimbic, Mesio-Temporal and Cerebellum networks. The right orbito-frontal focus belongs to the Mesolimbic network, which exhibited stability increases in the Mesolimbic and Mesio-Temporal networks. Interaction between these two networks was not surprising. Concerning the involvement of the cerebellum, BOLD responses in cerebellum regions during frontal epileptic discharges have been suggested by Fahoum et al. (2012). Several studies have demonstrated the interaction among brain regions belonging to the Mesolimbic and Mesio-Temporal networks. This topic has been recently reviewed for TLE (Cataldi et al., 2013), but it is much more difficult to establish connectivity starting from the orbito-frontal region. Whereas the epileptogenic network in TLE is relatively well-characterized (Spencer, 2002) and encompasses orbito-frontal regions, it is not clear which brain regions should be part of the orbito-frontal network in epilepsy. Nevertheless, intracranial EEG studies in orbito-frontal epilepsy showed that epileptic discharges from the orbito-frontal focus have the tendency to spread toward the mesial temporal structures (Munari et al., 1995; Smith et al., 2004).

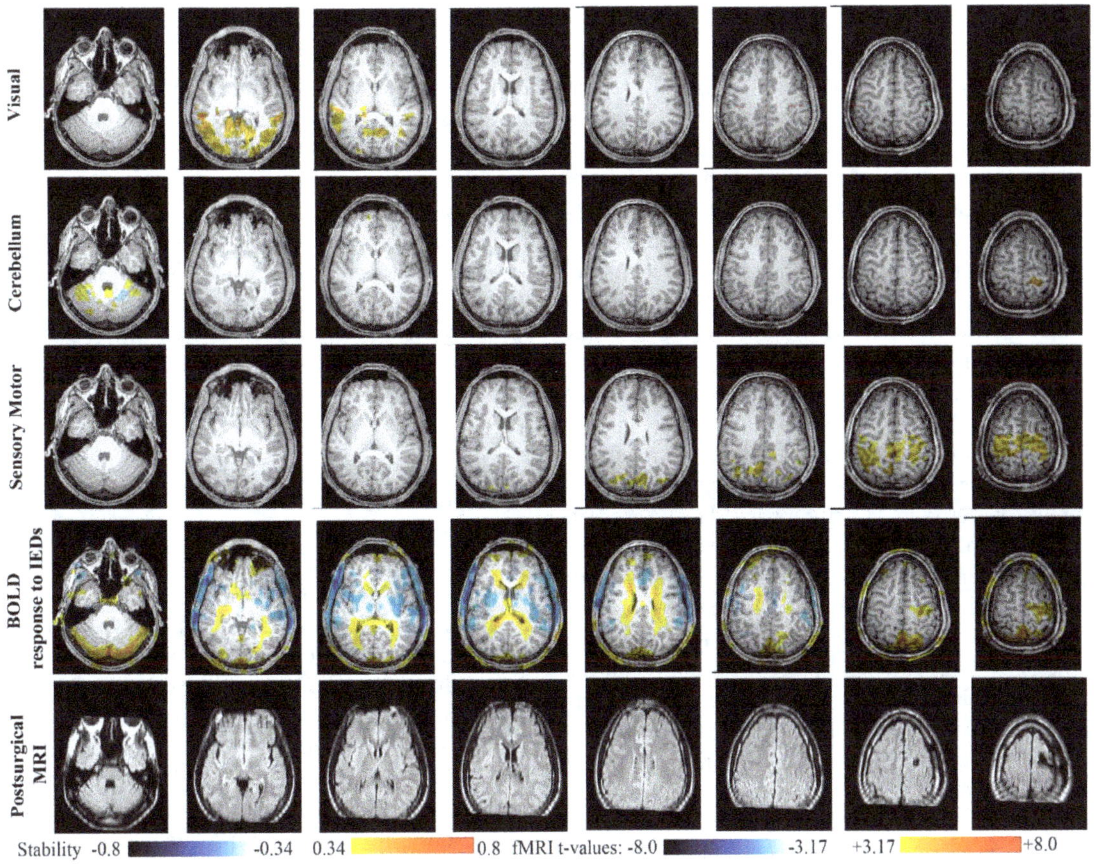

FIGURE 11 | Evaluation of DANI on Patient 6 with right frontal FCD. Results are presenting most salient stability changes observed in $Cmap_n$ followed by a t-map of the BOLD response to epileptic discharges and a postsurgical FLAIR MRI, all resampled in the native anatomical MRI space of the patient. Most salient stability changes observed for $Cmap_n$ of Visual, Cerebellum, and Sensory Motor networks are presented. The Visual and Cerebellum networks were also involved in significant interactions of modularity changes at $p < 0.001$. Same colormap conventions than in **Figure 6**.

Table 3 | Parameters used in the method.

Symbol	Description	Value(s)	Default
-	Maximal size of a region in the region-growing process	800 mm^3	800–1000 mm^3
R	Number of regions	739	This was obtained by the region-growing on all controls
k	Individual level clustering threshold	13	Estimated using BASC
L	Group level hierarchical clustering threshold	14	Estimated using BASC
N	Final clustering threshold at the group level	12	Selected scale in agreement with most literature on CRSNs
μ	Core size for estimating the trimmed stability maps	25%, 50%, 75%	50% according to our simulations
-	$Zmask_n$ threshold to identify the mask of significant stability changes ($p < 0.001$, non-corrected)	3.17	3.17
-	$Cmap_n$ threshold (combined map assessing the amount of stability change), selected as the 99.9% percentile estimated over the control population	0.34	
-	Threshold for the detection of most salient findings: max $\|Cmap_n\|$ > threshold	0.5	0.5
-	Significant level testing for interaction of modularity changes between network n and CRSN j: $\lambda_{n,j}$ (non-parametric test)	$p < 0.001$	$p < 0.001$

List of the parameters that are referred in the method with their respective values as well as the default recommended values.

For patients 3 and 4 with, respectively left and right MTLE and hippocampal sclerosis, the most salient findings identified using DANI involved mainly the Visual, the Mesolimbic and the Cerebellum networks, as well as the Mesio-Temporal network (patient 4 only). As stated before, the connection and propagation pathways between the Mesio-Temporal and the Mesolimbic regions have been clearly identified in MTLE patients (Spencer, 2002) and associated changes in FC involving these networks in MTLE patients have been identified by our group Pittau et al. (2012b) and carefully reviewed in Cataldi et al. (2013) and Bernhardt et al. (2013). The involvement of BOLD activation in the mid-cingulate gyri, at the time of temporal lobe discharges, has been demonstrated by Fahoum et al. (2012). Importantly, DANI identified clearly lateralizing results, as for instance a left temporal increase in stability observed for patient 3 within the Mesolimbic $Cmap_n$, and a right temporal increase in stability observed for patient 4 within the Cerebellum $Cmap_n$. The importance of laterality patterns in FC studies in MTLE has been suggested in Bettus et al. (2009) showing increased connectivity between temporal regions contralateral to the focus and in Pittau et al. (2012b) showing decreased connectivity between ipsilateral and contralateral temporo-mesial regions. Interestingly, the Visual network $Cmap_n$ was detected by DANI for both patients. Stability increases consisted mainly in lateral parts of this network, containing the fusiform gyri. These regions are secondary-association visual and memory areas and are connected to the posterior part of mesial and lateral part of the temporal lobes. Note that for patient 3, stability increases in Visual network $Cmap_n$ were also found in subcortical sutructures (thalamus and putamen).

Overall results obtained for patients 5 and 6 were less obvious to interpret. Differently from the first four cases, some concerns were raised regarding the BOLD responses to epileptic discharges: case 5 had a deactivation only partially concordant with the location of the resection; in case 6 the whole BOLD response was affected by motion artifacts, and only a part of the activation was found in "partial" agreement with the resected area. In both cases, the lesion consisted in a relatively focal dysplasia clearly identified on structural MRI data and the resection was circumscribed to the lesion. Some interesting findings were observed for patient 6, showing some partial concordance between a right postcentral increase in stability observed for the Cerebellum network $Cmap_n$, stability increase within the sensory motor network, a right central BOLD activation and a right precentral lesion. However, the fact that a small resection allowed these patients to become seizure free suggests that the network reorganization was less spread spatially, despite clear involvement of the sensory-motor network for patient 6.

For 4 out of 6 patients, DANI detected the Dorsal Attention network as abnormal, showing mainly stability increases within itself but also in posterior and anterior DMN regions and Mesolimbic regions. Overall, these network reorganizations were bilateral and distant from the focus. Whereas an involvement of DMN is well-known for patients with temporal and extratemporal lobe epilepsy (Laufs et al., 2007; Kobayashi et al., 2009; Fahoum et al., 2012), the attention network has been less studied, especially in patients with extratemporal lobe epilepsy, probably because of the difficulty of finding homogeneous groups for this type of epilepsy. Nevertheless, the involvement of the dorsal attention network has been demonstrated as impaired in patients with TLE (Zhang et al., 2009), frontal epilepsy (Fahoum et al., 2012) as well as in patients with epileptic syndromes (Vaudano et al., 2014).

In the last decade connectivity studies have shed light to several aspects of the epileptic brain. However, clinical applications (for diagnostic or prognostic purposes) of each method, including our proposed method DANI, require further validations before being consistently applied to the clinical management of the single patient. Moreover, it is important to remember that each diagnostic technique has to be integrated with all the other clinical and diagnostic data of the individual patient.

CONCLUSION

We proposed DANI as a new method to capture inter-individual variations in RSNs, and assess its performance in realistic simulations and its potential usefulness in patients. DANI is based on an extension of the BASC method to extract FC networks, allowing the assessment of statistical stability in RSNs at the individual level. Our results suggest that the ability of the method to capture modular changes is affected by the core size used to obtain the trimmed map. BASC is indeed sensitive to modular changes within the FC structure of a subject and DANI is able to detect small perturbations of those modules as well as the fusion of areas of various sizes with good sensitivity. The evaluation of the method on subjects with epilepsy identified in most cases (5/6) abnormal networks exhibiting significant changes in FC stability closely related and lateralized to the epileptogenic focus. These results are encouraging since the findings are supported by other modalities and were obtained without any prior on the disease. DANI also showed the involvement of distant networks, not containing the focus, suggesting remote reorganization. Although the fact that focal epilepsies affect distant networks is more and more recognized (Richardson, 2012), it is still premature to evaluate whether significant changes in FC are linked to effects of the discharge of the individual patient, or to other effects more remotely associated to the epilepsy of the patient (e.g., effect of medication, neuropsychological impairment). Clinical studies involving more patients and a specific comparison with the epileptogenic network of each patient will be required to investigate these issues.

ACKNOWLEDGMENTS

This work was supported by the Natural Sciences and Engineering Research Council of Canada Discovery Grant Program (Christophe Grova) and the Canadian Institutes of Health Research MOP 38079, #130442 (Jean Gotman). Christophe Grova was also supported by a salary award from the Fonds de Recherche en Santé du Québec (FRSQ). We would like to thank Dr. D. An for providing help in patients selection and Natalja Zazubovits for EEG/fMRI data acquisition. We would like to thank the neurologists Dr. F. Dubeau and Dr. E. Kobayashi as well as the neurosurgeons Dr. J. Hall and Dr. A. Olivier for providing clinical information and post-operative MRI data on the selected patients.

SUPPLEMENTARY MATERIAL

Figure S1 | Data workflow used to generate the combined significant stability-map $Cmap_n$ comparing, for one particular network, the trimmed stability map of one subject vs. the population of controls. A binary mask $Zmask_n$ assessing significant changes in local stability is first estimated. This binary mask is then applied to the subject trimmed stability map centered using the mean stability of all controls. $Cmap_n$ allows the identification of most stable regions showing significant changes in stability when compared to the average of controls. In this example, $Cmap_n$ of the auditory network identified an increase in stability in bilateral Thalami. Note that the most posterior region also identified in $Zmask_n$ was not detected in $Cmap_n$, because it was associated with very low stability values.

Figure S2 | Method used to combine some structured noise time-series with the original fMRI signal of the sensory-motor and auditory network time-series. This process is repeated for each region of these two networks located inside the red area corresponding to the simulated perturbed zone. The structured noise consisted in the averaged time-series of the visual network of an independent control, thus introducing additional correlations between the auditory and sensory-motor networks.

REFERENCES

1. (1989). Proposal for revised classification of epilepsies and epileptic syndromes. Commission on classification and Terminology of the International League Against Epilepsy. *Epilepsia* 30, 389–399. doi: 10.1111/j.1528-1157.1989.tb05316.x
2. Alexander-Bloch, A., Lambiotte, R., Roberts, B., Giedd, J., Gogtay, N., and Bullmore, E. (2012). The discovery of population differences in network community structure: new methods and applications to brain functional networks in schizophrenia. *NeuroImage* 59, 3889–3900. doi: 10.1016/j.neuroimage.2011.11.035
3. Allen, P. J., Josephs, O., and Turner, R. (2000). A method for removing imaging artifact from continuous EEG recorded during functional MRI. *Neuroimage* 12, 230–239. doi: 10.1006/nimg.2000.0599
4. An, D., Fahoum, F., Hall, J., Olivier, A., Gotman, J., and Dubeau, F. (2013). Electroencephalography/functional magnetic resonance imaging responses help predict surgical outcome in focal epilepsy. *Epilepsia* 54, 2184–2194. doi: 10.1111/epi.12434
5. Bagshaw, A. P., Aghakhani, Y., Benar, C. G., Kobayashi, E., Hawco, C., Dubeau, F., et al. (2004). EEG-fMRI of focal epileptic spikes: analysis with multiple haemodynamic functions and comparison with gadolinium-enhanced MR angiograms. *Hum. Brain Mapp.* 22, 179–192. doi: 10.1002/hbm.20024
6. Beckmann, C. F., Mackay, C. E., Filippini, N., and Smith S. M. (2009). "Group comparison of resting-state FMRI data using multi-subject ICA and dual regres- sion," in *Proceedings of the 15th International Conference on Organization for Human Brain Mapping* (San Francisco, CA).
7. Bellec, P., Carbonell, F. M., Perlbarg, V., Lepage, C., Lyttelton, O., Fonov, V., et al. (2011). "A neuroimaging analysis kit for Matlab and Octave," in *Proceedings of the 17th International Conference on Functional Mapping of the Human Brain* (Quebec).
8. Bellec, P., Lavoie-Courchesne, S., Dickinson, P., Lerch, J. P., Zijdenbos, A. P., and Evans, A. C. (2012). The pipeline system for Octave and Matlab (PSOM): a lightweight scripting framework and execution engine for scientific workflows. *Front. Neuroinform.* 6:7. doi: 10.3389/fninf.2012.00007
9. Bellec, P., Perlbarg, V., Jbabdi, S., Pelegrini-Issac, M., Anton, J. L., Doyon, J., et al. (2006). Identification of large-scale networks in the brain using fMRI. *NeuroImage* 29, 1231–1243. doi: 10.1016/j.neuroimage.2005.08.044
10. Bellec, P., Rosa-Neto, P., Lyttelton, O. C., Benali, H., and Evans, A. C. (2010). Multi- level bootstrap analysis of stable clusters in resting-state fMRI. *NeuroImage* 51, 1126–1139. doi: 10.1016/j.neuroimage.2010.02.082
11. Benar, C., Aghakhani, Y., Wang, Y., Izenberg, A., Al-Asmi, A., Dubeau, F., et al. (2003). Quality of EEG in simultaneous EEG-fMRI for epilepsy. *Clin. Neurophysiol.* 114, 569–580. doi: 10.1016/S1388-2457(02)00383-8
12. Berg, A. T., Berkovic, S. F., Brodie, M. J., Buchhalter, J., Cross, J. H., Van Emde Boas, W., et al. (2010). Revised terminology and concepts for organization of seizures and epilepsies: report of the ILAE Commission on Classification and Terminology, 2005–2009. *Epilepsia* 51, 676–685. doi: 10.1111/j.1528- 1167.2010.02522.x
13. Bernhardt, B. C., Hong, S., Bernasconi, A., and Bernasconi, N. (2013). Imaging structural and functional brain networks in temporal lobe epilepsy. *Front. Hum. Neurosci.* 7:624. doi: 10.3389/fnhum.2013.00624
14. Bettus, G., Guedj, E., Joyeux, F., Confort-Gouny, S., Soulier, E., Laguitton, V., et al. (2009). Decreased basal fMRI functional connectivity in epileptogenic networks and contralateral compensatory mechanisms. *Hum. Brain Mapp.* 30, 1580–1591. doi: 10.1002/hbm.20625
15. Biswal, B., Yetkin, F. Z., Haughton, V. M., and Hyde, J. S. (1995). Functional con- nectivity in the motor cortex of resting human brain using echo-planar MRI. *Magn. Reson. Med.* 34, 537–541. doi: 10.1002/mrm.1910340409
16. Broyd, S. J., Demanuele, C., Debener, S., Helps, S. K., James, C. J., and Sonuga-Barke, E. J. (2009). Default-mode brain dysfunction in mental dis- orders: a systematic review. *Neurosci. Biobehav. Rev.* 33, 279–296. doi: 10.1016/j.neubiorev.2008.09.002
17. Calhoun, V. D., Liu, J., and Adali, T. (2009). A review of group ICA for fMRI data and ICA for joint inference of imaging, genetic, and ERP data. *NeuroImage* 45, S163–S172. doi: 10.1016/j.neuroimage.2008.10.057
18. Cataldi, M., Avoli, M., and De Villers-Sidani, E. (2013). Resting state networks in temporal lobe epilepsy. *Epilepsia* 54, 2048–2059. doi: 10.1111/epi.12400
19. Collins, D. L., and Evans, A. C. (1997). Animal: validation and applications of non- linear registration-based segmentation. *Int. J. Pattern Recognit. Artif. Intell.* 11, 1271–1294. doi: 10.1142/S0218001497000597
20. Constable, R. T., Scheinost, D., Finn, E. S., Shen, X., Hampson, M., Winstanley, F. S., et al. (2013). Potential use and challenges of functional connectivity mapping in intractable epilepsy. *Front. Neurol.* 4:39. doi: 10.3389/fneur.2013.00039
21. Damoiseaux, J. S., Prater, K. E., Miller, B. L., and Greicius, M. D. (2012). Functional connectivity tracks clinical deterioration in Alzheimer's disease. *Neurobiol. Aging* 33, 828 e819–828 830. doi: 10.1016/j.neurobiolaging.2011.06.024
22. Damoiseaux, J. S., Rombouts, S. A., Barkhof, F., Scheltens, P., Stam, C. J., Smith, S. M., et al. (2006). Consistent resting-state networks across healthy subjects. *Proc. Natl. Acad. Sci. U.S.A.* 103, 13848–13853. doi: 10.1073/pnas.0601417103
23. De Ciantis, A., and Lemieux, L. (2013). Localisation of epileptic foci using novel imaging modalities. *Curr. Opin. Neurol.* 26, 368–373. doi: 10.1097/WCO.0b013e328363372c
24. Efron, B., and Tibshirani, R. (1993). *An Introduction to the Bootstrap*. New York, NY: Chapman & Hall.
25. Fahoum, F., Lopes, R., Pittau, F., Dubeau, F., and Gotman, J. (2012). Widespread epileptic networks in focal epilepsies: EEG-fMRI study. *Epilepsia* 53, 1618–1627. doi: 10.1111/j.1528-1167.2012.03533.x
26. Fonov, V., Evans, A. C., Botteron, K., Almli, C. R., Mckinstry, R. C., Collins, D. L., et al. (2011). Unbiased average age-appropriate atlases for pediatric studies. *Neuroimage* 54, 313–327. doi: 10.1016/j.neuroimage.2010.07.033
27. Fox, M. D., and Raichle, M. E. (2007). Spontaneous fluctuations in brain activity observed with functional magnetic resonance imaging. *Nat. Rev. Neurosci.* 8, 700–711. doi: 10.1038/nrn2201
28. Giove, F., Gili, T., Iacovella, V., Macaluso, E., and Maraviglia, B. (2009). Images-based suppression of unwanted global signals in resting-state func- tional connectivity studies. *Magn. Reson. Imaging* 27, 1058–1064. doi: 10.1016/j.mri.2009.06.004
29. Gotman, J., Benar, C. G., and Dubeau, F. (2004). Combining EEG and FMRI in epilepsy: methodological challenges and clinical results. *J. Clin. Neurophysiol.* 21, 229–240. doi: 10.1097/01.WNP.0000139658.92878.2A
30. Gotman, J., and Pittau, F. (2011). Combining EEG and fMRI in the study of epileptic discharges. *Epilepsia* 52(Suppl. 4), 38–42. doi: 10.1111/j.1528- 1167.2011.03151.x
31. Goveas, J. S., Xie, C., Ward, B. D., Wu, Z., Li, W., Franczak, M., et al. (2011). Recovery of hippocampal network connectivity correlates with cogni- tive improvement in mild Alzheimer's disease patients treated with

donepezil assessed by resting-state fMRI. *J. Magn. Reson. Imaging* 34, 764–773. doi: 10.1002/jmri.22662
32. Heers, M., Hedrich, T., An, D., Dubeau, F., Gotman, J., Grova, C., et al. (2014).
33. Spatial correlation of hemodynamic changes related to interictal epileptic dis- charges with electric and magnetic source imaging. *Hum. Brain Mapp.* 35, 4396–4414. doi: 10.1002/hbm.22482
34. Himberg, J., Hyvarinen, A., and Esposito, F. (2004). Validating the independent components of neuroimaging time series via clustering and visualization. *Neuroimage* 22, 1214–1222. doi: 10.1016/j.neuroimage.2004.03.027
35. Iber, C., and American Academy of Sleep Medicine. (2007). *The AASM Manual for the Scoring of Sleep and Associated Events: Rules, Terminology, and Technical Specifications.* Westchester, IL: American Academy of Sleep Medicine.
36. Jacobs, H. I., Radua, J., Luckmann, H. C., and Sack, A. T. (2013). Meta-analysis of functional network alterations in Alzheimer's disease: toward a network biomarker. *Neurosci. Biobehav. Rev.* 37, 753–765. doi: 10.1016/j.neubiorev.2013.03.009
37. Kobayashi, E., Grova, C., Tyvaert, L., Dubeau, F., and Gotman, J. (2009). Structures involved at the time of temporal lobe spikes revealed by interindividual group analysis of EEG/fMRI data. *Epilepsia* 50, 2549–2556. doi: 10.1111/j.1528- 1167.2009.02180.x
38. Lang, S., Duncan, N., and Northoff, G. (2014). Resting-state functional mag- netic resonance imaging: review of neurosurgical applications. *Neurosurgery* 74, 453–464. discussion: 464–455.
39. Laufs, H., Hamandi, K., Salek-Haddadi, A., Kleinschmidt, A. K., Duncan, J. S., and Lemieux, L. (2007). Temporal lobe interictal epileptic discharges affect cerebral activity in "default mode" brain regions. *Hum. Brain Mapp.* 28, 1023–1032. doi: 10.1002/hbm.20323
40. Liao, W., Zhang, Z., Pan, Z., Mantini, D., Ding, J., Duan, X., et al. (2011). Default mode network abnormalities in mesial temporal lobe epilepsy: a study combin- ing fMRI and DTI. *Hum. Brain Mapp.* 32, 883–895. doi: 10.1002/hbm.21076
41. Lund, T. E., Madsen, K. H., Sidaros, K., Luo, W.-L., and Nichols, T. E. (2006). Non- white noise in fMRI: Does modelling have an impact? *NeuroImage* 29, 54–66. doi: 10.1016/j.neuroimage.2005.07.005
42. Luo, C., An, D., Yao, D., and Gotman, J. (2014). Patient-specific connectivity pattern of epileptic network in frontal lobe epilepsy. *Neuroimage Clin.* 4, 668–675. doi: 10.1016/j.nicl.2014.04.006
43. Luo, C., Li, Q., Lai, Y., Xia, Y., Qin, Y., Liao, W., et al. (2011). Altered functional connectivity in default mode network in absence epilepsy: a resting-state fMRI study. *Hum. Brain Mapp.* 32, 438–449. doi: 10.1002/hbm.21034
44. Maneshi, M., Moeller, F., Fahoum, F., Gotman, J., and Grova, C. (2012). Resting- state connectivity of the sustained attention network correlates with dis- ease duration in idiopathic generalized epilepsy. *PLoS ONE* 7:e50359. doi: 10.1371/journal.pone.0050359
45. Munari, C., Tassi, L., Di Leo, M., Kahane, P., Hoffmann, D., Francione, S., et al. (1995). Video-stereo-electroencephalographic investigation of orbitofrontal cortex. Ictal electroclinical patterns. *Adv. Neurol.* 66, 273–295.
46. Negishi, M., Martuzzi, R., Novotny, E. J., Spencer, D. D., and Constable, R. T. (2011). Functional MRI connectivity as a predictor of the surgical outcome of epilepsy. *Epilepsia* 52, 1733–1740. doi: 10.1111/j.1528-1167.2011.03191.x
47. Pittau, F., Dubeau, F., and Gotman, J. (2012a). Contribution of EEG/fMRI to the definition of the epileptic focus. *Neurology* 78, 1479–1487. doi: 10.1212/WNL.0b013e3182553bf7
48. Pittau, F., Grova, C., Moeller, F., Dubeau, F., and Gotman, J. (2012b). Patterns of altered functional connectivity in mesial temporal lobe epilepsy. *Epilepsia* 53, 1013–1023. doi: 10.1111/j.1528-1167.2012.03464.x
49. Power, J. D., Barnes, K. A., Snyder, A. Z., Schlaggar, B. L., and Petersen, S.
50. E. (2012). Spurious but systematic correlations in functional connectivity MRI networks arise from subject motion. *NeuroImage* 59, 2142–2154. doi: 10.1016/j.neuroimage.2011.10.018
51. Raichle, M. E., Macleod, A. M., Snyder, A. Z., Powers, W. J., Gusnard, D. A., and Shulman, G. L. (2001). A default mode of brain function. *Proc. Natl. Acad. Sci. U.S.A.* 98, 676–682. doi: 10.1073/pnas.98.2.676
52. Richardson, M. P. (2012). Large scale brain models of epilepsy: dynamics meets connectomics. *J. Neurol. Neurosurg. Psychiatry* 83, 1238–1248. doi: 10.1136/jnnp-2011-301944
53. Sharot, T. (1976). The generalized jackknife: finite samples and subsample sizes. *J. Am. Stat. Assoc.* 71, 451–454. doi: 10.1080/01621459.1976.10480367
54. Shehzad, Z., Kelly, A. M., Reiss, P. T., Gee, D. G., Gotimer, K., Uddin, L. Q., et al. (2009). The resting brain: unconstrained yet reliable. *Cereb. Cortex* 19, 2209–2229. doi: 10.1093/cercor/bhn256
55. Smith, J. R., Sillay, K., Winkler, P., King, D. W., and Loring, D. W. (2004). Orbitofrontal epilepsy: electroclinical analysis of surgical cases and literature review. *Stereotact. Funct. Neurosurg.* 82, 20–25. doi: 10.1159/000076656
56. Smith, S. M. (2012). The future of FMRI connectivity. *Neuroimage* 62, 1257–1266. doi: 10.1016/j.neuroimage.2012.01.022
57. Smith, S. M., Fox, P. T., Miller, K. L., Glahn, D. C., Fox, P. M., Mackay, C. E., et al. (2009). Correspondence of the brain's functional architecture dur- ing activation and rest. *Proc. Natl. Acad. Sci. U.S.A.* 106, 13040–13045. doi: 10.1073/pnas.0905267106
58. Smith, S. M., Vidaurre, D., Beckmann, C. F., Glasser, M. F., Jenkinson, M., Miller, K. L., et al. (2013). Functional connectomics from resting-state fMRI. *Trends Cogn. Sci.* 17, 666–682. doi: 10.1016/j.tics.2013.09.016
59. Spencer, S. S. (2002). Neural networks in human epilepsy: evidence of and implications for treatment. *Epilepsia* 43, 219–227. doi: 10.1046/j.1528- 1157.2002.26901.x
60. Stefan, H., Rampp, S., and Knowlton, R. C. (2011). Magnetoencephalography adds to the surgical evaluation process. *Epilepsy Behav.* 20, 172–177. doi: 10.1016/j.yebeh.2010.09.011
61. Studholme, C., Hill, D. L. G., and Hawkes, D. J. (1999). An overlap invariant entropy measure of 3d medical image alignment. *Pattern Recognit.* 32, 71–86. doi: 10.1016/S0031-3203(98)00091-0
62. Stufflebeam, S. M., Liu, H., Sepulcre, J., Tanaka, N., Buckner, R. L., and Madsen, J. R. (2011). Localization of focal epileptic discharges using functional con- nectivity magnetic resonance imaging. *J. Neurosurg.* 114, 1693–1697. doi: 10.3171/2011.1.JNS10482
63. Tzourio-Mazoyer, N., Landeau, B., Papathanassiou, D., Crivello, F., Etard, O., Delcroix, N., et al. (2002). Automated anatomical labeling of activa- tions in SPM using a macroscopic anatomical parcellation of the MNI MRI single-subject brain. *NeuroImage* 15, 273–289. doi: 10.1006/nimg. 2001.0978
64. Vaudano, A. E., Ruggieri, A., Vignoli, A., Avanzini, P., Benuzzi, F., Gessaroli, G., et al. (2014). Epilepsy-related brain networks in ring chromosome
65. 20 syndrome: an EEG-fMRI study. *Epilepsia* 55, 403–413. doi: 10.1111/epi.12539
66. Waites, A. B., Briellmann, R. S., Saling, M. M., Abbott, D. F., and Jackson, G. D. (2006). Functional connectivity networks are disrupted in left temporal lobe epilepsy. *Ann. Neurol.* 59, 335–343. doi: 10.1002/ana.20733
67. Yeo, B. T., Krienen, F. M., Sepulcre, J., Sabuncu, M. R., Lashkari, D., Hollinshead, M., et al. (2011). The organization of the human cerebral cortex estimated by intrinsic functional connectivity. *J. Neurophysiol.* 106, 1125–1165. doi: 10.1152/jn.00338.2011
68. Zhang, Z., Lu, G., Zhong, Y., Tan, Q., Liao, W., Chen, Z., et al. (2009). Impaired perceptual networks in temporal lobe epilepsy revealed by resting fMRI. *J. Neurol.* 256, 1705–1713. doi: 10.1007/s00415-009-5187-2
69. Zijdenbos, A. P., Forghani, R., and Evans, A. C. (2002). Automatic "pipeline" anal- ysis of 3-D MRI data for clinical trials: application to multiple sclerosis. *IEEE Trans. Med. Imaging* 21, 1280–1291. doi: 10.1109/TMI.2002.806283
70. Zuo, X. N., Kelly, C., Adelstein, J. S., Klein, D. F., Castellanos, F. X., and Milham, M. P. (2010). Reliable intrinsic connectivity networks: test-retest evaluation using ICA and dual regression approach. *Neuroimage* 49, 2163–2177. doi: 10.1016/j.neuroimage.2009.10.080

13

Negative BOLD in default-mode structures measured with EEG-MREG is larger in temporal than extra-temporal epileptic spikes

Julia Jacobs[1,2]*, Antonia Menzel[1], Georgia Ramantani[2], Katharina Körbl[1], Jakob Assländer[3], Andreas Schulze-Bonhage[2], Jürgen Hennig[3] and Pierre LeVan[3]

[1] *Department of Neuropediatrics and Muscular Diseases, University Medical Center Freiburg, Freiburg, Germany*
[2] *Epilepsy Center, University Medical Center Freiburg, Freiburg, Germany*
[3] *Medical Physics, Freiburg, Germany*

***Correspondence:**
Julia Jacobs, Department of Neuropediatrics and Muscular Diseases, University Medical Center Freiburg, Mathildenstrasse 1, 79106 Freiburg, Germany
e-mail: julia.jacobs@gmx.de

Introduction: EEG-fMRI detects BOLD changes associated with epileptic interictal discharges (IED) and can identify epileptogenic networks in epilepsy patients. Besides positive BOLD changes, negative BOLD changes have sometimes been observed in the default-mode network, particularly using group analysis. A new fast fMRI sequence called MREG (Magnetic Resonance Encephalography) shows increased sensitivity to detect IED-related BOLD changes compared to the conventional EPI sequence, including frequent occurrence of negative BOLD responses in the DMN. The present study quantifies the concordance between the DMN and negative BOLD related to IEDs of temporal and extra-temporal origin.

Methods: Focal epilepsy patients underwent simultaneous EEG-MREG. Areas of overlap were calculated between DMN regions, defined as precuneus, posterior cingulate, bilateral inferior parietal and mesial prefrontal cortices according to a standardized atlas, and significant negative BOLD changes revealed by an event-related analysis based on the timings of IED seen on EEG. Correlation between IED number/lobe of origin and the overlap were calculated.

Results: 15 patients were analyzed, some showing IED over more than one location resulting in 30 different IED types. The average overlap between negative BOLD and DMN was significantly larger in temporal ($23.7 \pm 19.6\,cm^3$) than extra-temporal IEDs ($7.4 \pm 5.1\,cm^3$, $p = 0.008$). There was no significant correlation between the number of IEDs and the overlap between DMN structures and negative BOLD areas.

Discussion: MREG results in an increased sensitivity to detect negative BOLD responses related to focal IED in single patients, with responses often occurring in DMN regions. In patients with high overlap with the DMN, this suggests that epileptic IEDs may be associated with a brief decrease in attention and cognitive ability. Interestingly this observation was not dependent on the frequency of IED but more common in IED of temporal origin.

Keywords: fast fMRI, default mode, epileptic spikes, refractory epilepsy, EEG-fMRI

INTRODUCTION

EEG-fMRI is a non-invasive method to identify epileptic networks activated by IEDs in patients with focal and generalized epilepsy (Gotman et al., 2006; Grouiller et al., 2011). In focal epilepsy, IED-related positive BOLD changes are found in the area of IED origin in the majority of patients (Moeller et al., 2008; Tyvaert et al., 2008). Moreover, positive BOLD changes could be found within or in the vicinity of epileptogenic lesions such as focal cortical dysplasia, nodular heterotopia and mesial temporal sclerosis (Kobayashi et al., 2006b; Jacobs et al., 2007). Zijlmans and colleagues showed that EEG-fMRI can be a useful additional diagnostic tool in the presurgical evaluation of patients with refractory epilepsy by improving the identification of patients suitable for surgery (Zijlmans et al., 2007). This observation was confirmed by a study providing evidence that the surgical removal of the area with the strongest positive BOLD is correlated with a good post-surgical seizure outcome (Thornton et al., 2010; An et al., 2013). Thus, there is strong evidence that BOLD changes related to epileptic spikes are able to identify epileptic networks

Abbreviations: BOLD, Blood Oxygenation Level Dependent; DMN, default mode network; EPI, Echo Planar Imaging; fMRI, functional magnetic resonance imaging; IED, inter-ictal epileptic discharge; MREG, Magnetic-Resonance-Encephalography; TLE, Temporal Lobe Epilepsy.

and EEG-fMRI has a large potential as a diagnostic tool in epilepsy.

Additionally to positive BOLD changes, negative BOLD changes also called deactivations are observed related to IEDs (Archer et al., 2003; Jacobs et al., 2007; Moeller et al., 2008; An et al., 2013). Mechanisms of negative BOLD changes are less well understood in general and their interpretation is subject to debate in patients with epilepsy. Some negative BOLD changes have been observed as focal changes with a close relationship with the spike origin (Jacobs et al., 2007, 2009), but in the majority of cases they are rather widespread and distant (Kobayashi et al., 2006b; Laufs et al., 2007).

An improved understanding of negative BOLD responses is important to facilitate the interpretation of BOLD responses in a clinical setting. Moreover negative BOLD responses may provide additional information about the effect of IEDs on the patient's brain. Many of the observed negative BOLD responses occur in the precuneus, posterior cingulate, bilateral inferior parietal and mesial prefrontal cortices, structures which are known to be part of the default mode network (DMN) (Archer et al., 2003; Gotman et al., 2005). This network was first described in PET studies. Its structures are most active during periods of relaxed wakefulness and their activity is reduced during specific tasks (Mazoyer et al., 2001; Raichle et al., 2001). Strong changes within the DMN have been shown in patients during coma and anesthesia supporting its importance for consciousness (Laureys et al., 2004).

In epilepsy, the strongest negative BOLD in the DMN was observed during absence seizures in idiopathic generalized epilepsy (Moeller et al., 2008; Berman et al., 2010) or following generalized epileptic discharges (Gotman et al., 2005). In patients with focal epilepsy, group analyses reliably detect changes in the DMN (Laufs et al., 2007) and several studies report on negative BOLD in the DMN in some of their individual patients (Fahoum et al., 2012, 2013). In contrast to absence seizures, a change of consciousness is usually not observed in association with focal interictal spikes. Some studies however suggest that focal IEDs in around 50% of patients are associated with a transitory cogitive impairment (TCI) (Binnie, 2003). In focal IED this impairment is especially visible during complex tasks and has most often been shown during studies assessing language or working memory (Hutt and Gilbert, 1980; Aarts et al., 1984). In line with the idea that IEDs can affect cognition the negative BOLD in DMN related to interictal spikes has been interpreted as an indication that focal IEDs may interfere with networks of normal attention (Gotman et al., 2005; Laufs et al., 2007). Interestingly, the observed changes were more prominent during spikes of temporal than extra-temporal origin (Jacobs et al., 2009), which is in line with the more prominent alteration of consiousness during temporal than neocortical seizures. The interference level caused by focal IEDs is probably below the threshold necessary for clinical observation of altered consiousness, but it may still have a long-term influence on the cognitive performance of affected patients.

Recently a number of fast fMRI sequences have been developed (Lin et al., 2006; Feinberg et al., 2010; Posse, 2012). Magnetic Resonance Encephalography is one which allows whole-brain imaging with a temporal resolution of 100 ms (Zahneisen et al., 2012; Assländer et al., 2013). The increased temporal resolution not only improves the tracking of fast artifacts and brain activity, but it also increases sensitivity of functional imaging by recording an increased number of images during each hemodynamic response. Our group could demonstrate that this results in a higher sensitivity to detect IED-associated BOLD changes in focal epilepsy (Jacobs et al., 2014). Moreover, the increased sensitivity resulted in a frequent detection of negative BOLD changes in the DMN even without performing group analysis. It is thus possible to assess the alterations in the DMN associated with IEDs for every single patient, which may be the key to a better understanding of the clinical importance of this phenomenon. The present study aims to quantify negative BOLD in the DMN with the hypothesis that the amount of interference may be dependent on the region of IED generation or the frequency of IEDs observed in each patient.

MATERIALS AND METHODS

PATIENTS

Patients with focal epilepsies who were admitted to the Epilepsy Centre Freiburg were included in this study. All patients signed informed consent and the study was approved by the Research Ethics Committee of the University of Freiburg.

EEG-fMRI data were only acquired in patients who fulfilled the following criteria:

(1) ability to stay calmly in the MRI scanner over a period of 1 h and
(2) frequent IEDs (>10 in 60 min) recorded on routine EEG outside the scanner.

All patients underwent scanning with the EEG-MREG sequence for 20–40 min depending on ability to cooperate.

DATA ACQUISITION

A 64-channel scalp EEG was continuously recorded inside the MRI scanner (3-Tesla Trio Tim, Siemens Healthcare, Erlangen, Germany) with a reference located between Fz and Cz. Sintered Ag/AgCl ring electrodes were attached using a "BrainCap" (Easycap, Herrsching, Germany), which is part of the MR-compatible EEG recording system "BrainAmp-MR" (Brain Products, Munich, Germany). Electrode impedances were kept below 15 kΩ. An electrode was placed perivertebrally on the left for acquisition of the electrocardiogram. Data was transmitted from the amplifier (5 kHz sampling rate synchronized with the 10 MHz scanner clock, 0.016–250 Hz band-pass filter) via an optic fiber cable to a computer located outside the scanner room (Mandelkow et al., 2006). During the whole measurement, the patient's respiration and ECG were monitored with the physiological monitoring unit (pneumatic breathing belt, ECG electrodes) of the MRI scanner (3-Tesla Trio Tim, Siemens Healthcare, Erlangen, Germany).

A 3D, T1-weighted anatomical acquisition (MPRAGE, $TR = 2200$ ms, $TE = 2.15$ ms, FOV = 256 mm, 256×256 matrix, 160 sagittal slices, 1 mm slice thickness) was performed for co-registration with the functional images. This was followed by the fMRI acquisition using 3D MREG. Acquisition was performed with the following parameters ($TR = 100$ ms, $TE = 20$ ms, FOV = 192–256 mm, 64 × 64 × 64 matrix, flip angle = 15°, 12,800 volumes, total acquisition time 21:20 min (Zahneisen et al., 2012).

EEG PROCESSING

Gradient artifacts were corrected offline by an averaged artifact subtraction method (Allen et al., 2000). The pulse artifact was then also corrected using averaged artifact subtraction (Allen et al., 1998), followed by an Independent Component Analysis-based procedure to remove residual noise (Srivastava et al., 2005; Debener et al., 2007).

IEDs were marked by two independent reviewers (Julia Jacobs and Katharina Körbl) and were classified into distinct types for each patient according to spatial distribution and morphology (if more than one type was present), verifying that they were similar to epileptic discharges recorded in routine EEG outside the scanner. IED-like transients occurring in a window of 150–500 ms following the QRS complex in the ECG were not marked to avoid including residual ballistocardiographic (BCG) artifact in the analysis (Flanagan et al., 2009; Ertl et al., 2010). EEG quality was considered as appropriate if it allowed the identification of IED types seen in the routine clinical EEG. All IEDs were classified according to their focal distribution at the time of the scan, according to whether they derived from temporal or extra-temporal origin.

MREG ANALYSIS

fMRI images were reconstructed from the raw MREG data (Hugger et al., 2011) and then motion corrected and smoothed (Gaussian kernel, FWHM = 6 mm) using FSL software (http://fsl.fmrib.ox.ac.uk/fsl/fslwiki/) (Smith et al., 2004). Data was then analyzed as an event-related design in the general linear model (GLM) framework using fMRIstat software (Worsley et al., 2002). The noise term in the GLM was modeled as a 5th-order autoregressive (AR) process to account for additional autocorrelations originating from the higher temporal resolution (Worsley et al., 2002; Posse, 2012). The order of the AR model had been determined in a recent study on patients with epilepsy (Jacobs et al., 2014).

IEDs with distinct spatial distribution were analyzed as separate regressors. Motion parameters obtained from the motion correction step and cardio-respiratory regressors based the synchronized recording of the physiological unit of the MRI scanner (Glover et al., 2000) were used as confounds in the model. Four separate event-related analyses were conducted, using HRFs consisting of a single gamma function peaking at 3, 5, 7, or 9 s after the event. This allowed some variation in the latency of the BOLD response while retaining information about its expected shape (Bagshaw et al., 2004). A BOLD response was considered statistically significant if it was significant in any of the 4 analyses. For visualization purposes, a single combined map was thus generated from the highest absolute value for each voxel among the four t-maps. Significant responses were defined as 7 or more contiguous voxels with $|t| > 3.5$ ($p = 0.05$), corrected for multiple comparisons (Worsley et al., 2002) at the cluster level (Friston et al., 1993) with an additional Bonferroni correction due to the 4 analyses.

OVERLAP BETWEEN THE DEFAULT-MODE NETWORK AND NEGATIVE BOLD

The following brain regions were considered to be part of the default-mode network: precuneus, posterior cingulate, bilateral inferior parietal and mesial prefrontal cortices (Raichle et al., 2001; Gotman et al., 2005; Laufs et al., 2007). A spatial template of the default-mode network was thus created from those regions as defined in the automatic anatomical labeling (AAL) atlas (Tzourio-Mazoyer et al., 2002). According to the names given in the AAL atlas the following regions were included in the analysis:

- medial prefrontal regions: frontal superior orbital, frontal superior medial, frontal medial orbital, rectus, cingulum anterior
- lateral inferior parietal regions: parietal inferior, angular, supramarginal
- posterior cingulate: *cingulum posterior*
- precuneus: *precuneus*

The atlas was co-registered to each patient's anatomical image, resulting in individual default-mode network templates on which clusters of significant IED-related negative BOLD responses were overlaid.

For each patient, the volume of the default-mode templates, regions of significant negative BOLD responses, and overlap between the two were used to generate the following two measures:

- Percentage of the overall negative BOLD associated with a given IED type, which is located within the structures of the default-mode network
- Percentage of default-mode structures covered by significant negative BOLD changes

The calculated percentages of overlap were then correlated with the number of IED for each IED type using a Spearman correlation. Percentage of overlap was compared for temporal vs. extra-temporal IED using a t-test. Significance level for both tests was $p < 0.05$.

RESULTS

PATIENTS

Fifteen consecutive patients were included. Six patients showed one, four patients two, four patients three and one patient four distinct IED types. Thus, a total of 30 distinct IED types could be analyzed in this study, 12 of which were classified as temporal IED. Clinical details of all patients are given in **Table 1**.

OCCURRENCE OF NEGATIVE BOLD RESPONSES

Details about all IED types and resulting BOLD responses are given in **Table 2**. The average size of AAL DMN template for each individual patient was 182.5 ± 14.9 cm³. The average size of brain areas showing significant negative BOLD responses was 109.2 ± 96.5 cm³. The average overlap between

Table 1 | Clinical information.

Patient	Age	m/f	Age of Onset	Epilepsy classification	Seizure types	MRI	AED
1	26	m	7y	Structural	CPS	Hypothalamic harmatoma	LEV, OXC, LCM
2	36	m	7y	Structural TLE	CPS	MTS R	LTG, LCM
3	17	m	13y	Unclear	SPS/CPS GTCS	Normal	LTG, OXC
4	17	f	16y	Structural TLE	CPS	Unclear mass in the L superior T gyrus	OXC
5	27	m	11y	Structural FLE	SPS/CPS GTCS	Surgical cavity F L	LEV, OXC
6	12	m	9y	Structural FLE	CPS	Caveroma F R	none
7	9	m	4y	Structural FLE	SPS/CPS	Extensive R polymicrogyria	LEV, VPA
8	28	f	11y	FLE of unclear origine	SPS/CPS GTCS	Unclear lesion F R, including insular cortex.	LTG, LCM
9	71	m	70y	Structural TLE	CPS	Cystic tumor mesio-temporal L	VPA
10	31	f	31y	TLE	CPS	Normal	OXC
11	60	m	40y	Structural TLE	CPS	Defect /sclerosis T pole L.	OXC
12	23	m	14y	Structural TLE	SPS, CPS	FCD T L	LTG
13	40	f	23y	Bilateral TLE	CPS, GTCS	Malrotation HC R	LTG
14	14	f	7y	Structural FLE	CPS	FCD F R	VPA, OXC
15	16	m	1y	Structural PLE	CPS	Tuberous sclerosis	LEV, ZNS

AED, antiepileptic drugs; C, central; CPS, complex partial seizures; FCD, focal cortical dysplasia; f, female; F, frontal; FLE, frontal lobe epilepsy; GTCS, generalized tonic clonic seizures; HC, hippocampus; m, male; L, left; LCM, lacosamide; LEV, levetirazetam; LTG, lamotrigine; O, occipital; OXC, oxcarbazepin; P, parietal; PLE, parietal lobe epilepsy; R, right; SPS, simple partial seizures; y, years; T, temporal; TLE, temporal lobe epilepsy; VPA, valproate; ZNS, zonisamide.

both areas was $12.3 \pm 14.3\,cm^3$. The large variation in overlap mainly results from the strongly varying amount of negative BOLD seen in different patients and distinct IED types.

The average size of negative BOLD in temporal IED was with $154.9 \pm 126.1\,cm^3$ was significantly larger than in extra-temporal with $78.7 \pm 56.4\,cm^3$ ($p = 0.01$, **Figure 1A**). The average size of overlap between both regions was significantly larger in temporal IEDs with $23.7 \pm 19.6\,cm^3$ than for extra-temporal IEDs with $7.4 \pm 5.1\,cm^3$ ($p = 0.008$, **Figure 1B**).

PERCENTAGE OF OVERALL NEGATIVE BOLD RESPONSES FOUND IN DMN

The average percentage of overall negative BOLD responses found within the DMN structures was $11.2 \pm 6.1\%$. Again a large variation was seen between IED types. Seventeen patients showed between 10 and 20% overlap and 3 patients more than 20% overlap (see **Table 2**, for examples see **Figures 2, 3**).

There was no significant correlation between the number of single IED per IED type and the amount of overlap. There was no significant difference between IEDs of temporal ($11.5 \pm 5\%$) and extra-temporal origin ($10.9 \pm 6.6\%$) (**Figure 4A**).

PERCENTAGE OF DMN COVERED BY NEGATIVE BOLD:

The average percentage of DMN structures covered by negative BOLD was $6.7 \pm 7\,cm^3$. Three patients showed between 10 and 20% overlap and two patients more than 20% overlap (see **Table 2**, for examples see **Figures 1, 2**).

There was no significant correlation between the number of IEDs per IED type and the amount DMN structures covered by negative BOLD. There was a significantly larger area of DMN structures covered by negative BOLD for IED with temporal origin ($10.4 \pm 10.3\%$) that IED of extra-temporal origin ($4.2 \pm 2.9\%$, $p = 0.01$) (**Figure 4B**).

COMPARISON OF TEMPORAL AND NON-TEMPORAL IEDs

Six patients had both temporal and extra-temporal IEDs (for details see **Table 2**), in one patient three comparisons, in three patients two comparisons and in two patients one comparison between temporal and extra-temporal IEDs were possible. In regard to the percentage of DMN structures covered by negative BOLD the statistical comparison just within the single patients shows a trend toward temporal IED causing larger overlap than extra-temporal ones ($p = 0.07$). For the percentage of negative BOLD lying within DMN structures no significant difference can been seen as for the overall group ($p = 0.2$).

DISCUSSION

The present study confirms the observation that a high number of patients with focal epilepsy show alterations in the DMN during focal IED occurrence. This observation is mainly possible due to the use of MREG which increases the sensitivity of event-related fMRI for IEDs. The amount of negative BOLD in the DMN was highly variable between distinct types of IED and stronger in IEDs generated in the temporal lobe. This suggests that different IEDs may affect attention and consciousness to variable degrees and it may be of clinical interest for patients with epilepsies to identify those subtypes with a large effect on important networks such as the DMN.

METHODOLOGICAL ISSUES

The present analysis of single patients was to a large extent only possible as a result of the increased sensitivity of the MREG sequence (Zahneisen et al., 2012; Assländer et al., 2013). During the analysis, statistical methods were carefully adapted to correct for the increase of autocorrelations and multiple comparisons. In EEG-fMRI in epilepsy, the definition of a gold standard to which all BOLD changes can be compared is difficult and the most valid is probably comparing BOLD changes with activity

Table 2 | Summary of IED types and overlap between DMN and negative BOLD.

Patient #	IED type	IED topography	Location T vs. Ex-T	# of IED	% of neg BOLD in DMN	% of DMN covered by neg. BOLD
1	1	TP right	T	6	11	6
2	2	F T right	T	4	12	14
	3	T right	T	1	19	9
3	4	F right	EX-T	7	10	5
	5	PO Left	EX-T	2	15	6
	6	F left	EX-T	13	11	3
4	7	T right	T	1	18	4
	8	P right	Ex-T	2	21	7
	9	F right	Ex-T	3	9	6
5	10	C left	Ex-T	46	17	5
	11	T left	T	8	16	32
	12	F pole left	Ex-T	9	10	2
	13	F right	Ex-T	3	10	4
6	14	T left	T	2	12	7
7	15	F pole right	Ex-T	1	0	0
	16	FP right	Ex-T	1	24	2
8	17	F left	Ex-T	3	3	2
	18	FP right	Ex-T	21	4	5
	19	T right	T	2	5	0
9	20	F pole left	Ex-T	2	6	5
	21	F left	Ex-T	2	6	4
	22	T right	T	2	3	2
10	23	T right	T	1	6	2
11	24	FT left	T	2	10	5
	25	CP right	Ex-T	1	7	0
12	26	FT left	T	10	10	14
13	27	T right	T	3	15	29
	28	P right	Ex-T	12	14	2
14	29	F pole right	Ex-T	1	21	13
15	30	F pole right	Ex-T	4	8	5
Mean and SD					11.2 ± 6.2	6.7 ± 8

C, central; DMN, default mode network; Ex-T, extra-temporal; F, frontal, IED, interitcal epileptic discharge; P, parietal; pos, positive; neg, negative; SD, standard deviation; T, temporal.

from intracranial EEG (Pittau et al., 2011) or surgical removal and postsurgical outcome (Thornton et al., 2010). However, BOLD changes detected by MREG have so far only been compared with the lobe of spike origin or the localization of lesion (Jacobs et al., 2014), as the method is still quite recent; additional data acquisitions will need to be performed to allow a valid comparison with other measures.

As with all EEG-fMRI studies, it is important to exclude sources of artifact which may result in incorrect BOLD responses. One advantage of MREG is the ability to measure un-aliased physiological artifacts such as respiration and ECG, which could then be corrected as part of our analysis (LeVan et al., 2012).

A second potential source for mistakes during EEG-fMRI is the false detection of motion artifacts such as the ballistocardiogram as IED (Flanagan et al., 2009; Jansen et al., 2012). The first step to avoid this mistake is the thorough correction of EEG artifacts, which has been performed with all currently available methods in the present study (Allen et al., 1998; Debener et al., 2007). Moreover, Van Houdt and coworkers could show that a more robust identification of IED results from reviewing the EEGs by more than one reviewer, as we performed in our analysis (Van Houdt et al., 2010) MREG increases sensitivity to a point where BOLD changes related to artifacts may also be more likely to be detected, which is why we felt that IED selection should be rather specific than sensitive.

In the present study IEDs occurring during the time window of the ballistocardiogram were not included in the analysis. This measure likely resulted in the exclusion of true IEDs and thus in a decreased sensitivity of the identified BOLD responses (Flanagan et al., 2009). However, this was considered a more benign effect compared to the potential inclusion of non-epileptiform motion events among true IEDs, which may result in not only a decreased sensitivity for the identification of IED-related BOLD responses, but also possibly causing spurious negative BOLD in the DMN (Flanagan et al., 2009). Due to the use of MREG as fMRI sequence and its high sensitivity for the detection of IED related BOLD changes (Jacobs et al., 2014), which may compensate the loss of sensitivity, as well as for the sake of our primary goal to analyze negative BOLD in DMN structures, it thus appears to be more reasonable to exclude events coinciding with movements such as the BCG. The development of better monitoring of patient motion is likely to greatly facilitate the distinction of true and motion-related epileptiform events (Masterton et al., 2007; Flanagan et al., 2009; LeVan et al., 2013).

ORIGIN OF NEGATIVE BOLD RESPONSES

It should be pointed out that we did not preselect patients in regard to whether they showed any negative BOLD for this analysis. Therefore, it is not surprising that the area covered by negative BOLD varied between zero and 380 cubic-centimeters depending on patient and spike type. The underlying physiological mechanism of negative BOLD is largely unknown. One theory has suggested that it might result from a "vascular steal" phenomenon, which implies that neighboring areas of increased blood flow and BOLD cause a decreased blood flow and negative BOLD (Harel et al., 2002). In previous as well as the current study this explanation seems rather unlikely as we could not observe any correlation between positive and negative BOLD as well as no spatial relationship (Kobayashi et al., 2006a; Jacobs et al., 2014). Other authors suggest that the neurovascular coupling necessary to observe the well-known positive BOLD effect might be impaired in some regions of patients with epilepsy, which could result in a lack of blood flow increase caused by high deoxyhemoglobin levels (Fink et al., 1996; Bruehl et al., 1998). A study of Stefanovic and colleagues however found convincing evidence for intact neurovascular coupling in patients with epilepsy (Stefanovic et al., 2005). Impaired neuro-vascular coupling is thus unlikely to explain the presence of negative BOLD changes either in the DMN or elsewhere, as described before as well as in our study.

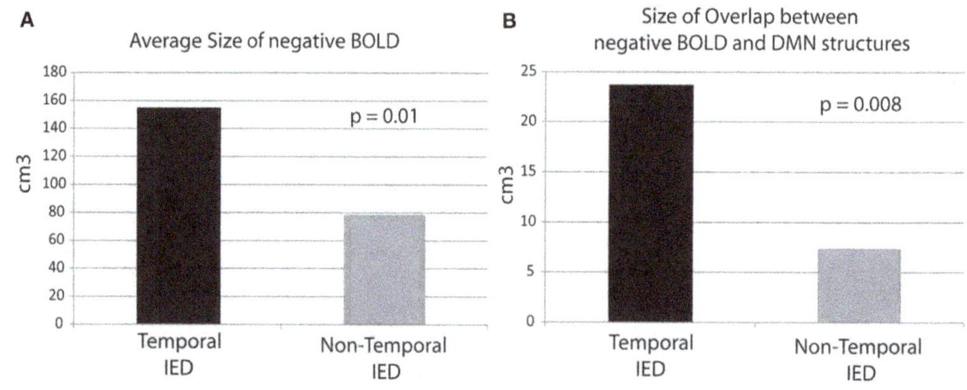

FIGURE 1 | Average size of overlap in cubic-centimeters between the negative BOLD and DMN structures in temporal and extra-temporal IED. The average size of negative BOLD as well as the overlap is significantly larger for temporal than extra-temporal IED. **(A)** Average size areas covered by negative BOLD. **(B)** Average size of overlap between DMN and negative BOLD.

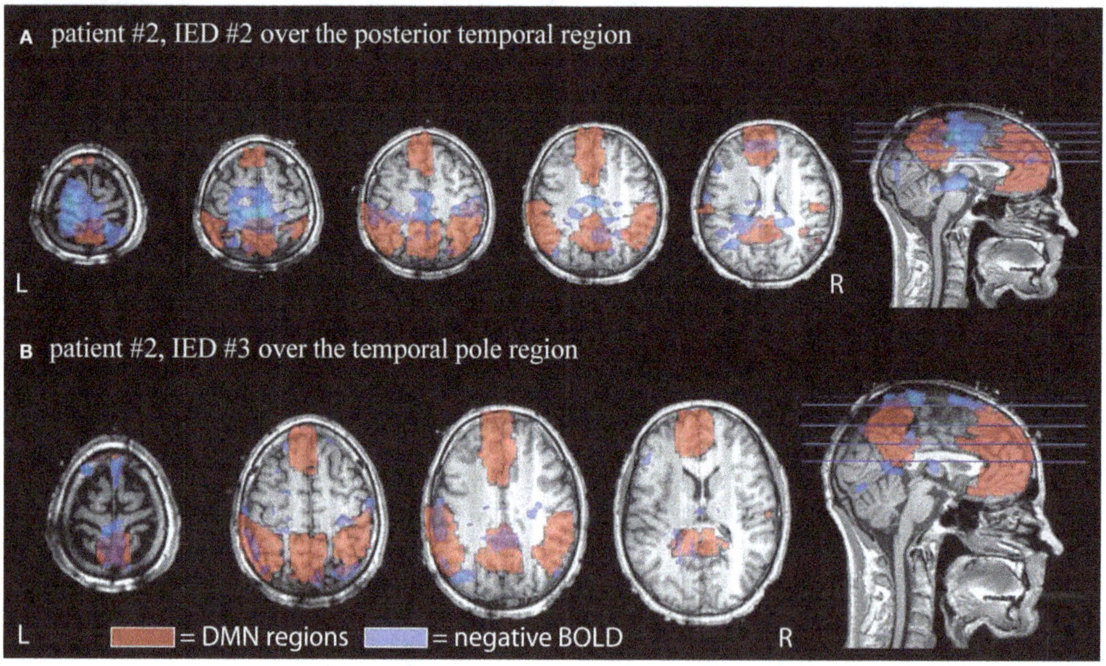

FIGURE 2 | Example of the overlap between negative BOLD responses and DMN regions. Patient # 2 had two different IED generated over the anterior and posterior region of temporal structures. DMN regions according to the AAL atlas are shown in red, negative BOLD in blue. **(A)** Shows the overlap for IED # 2 which occurred 4 times during the scan. 12% of the negative BOLD was located within the DMN and 14% of the DMN were covered by negative BOLD. **(B)** Shows the response to IED # 2 which only occurred once during the scan time. 19% of negative BOLD was located within DMN regions and 9% of DMN was covered by negative BOLD.

Another possible explanation for the occurrence of negative BOLD might be a decreased neuronal activity at the time of IEDs in these regions. This explanation is in line with the observation of increased concentrations of the inhibitory transmitter GABA in regions of negative BOLD (Chatton et al., 2003; Stefanovic et al., 2004). If negative BOLD reflects increased inhibition, negative BOLD related to IEDs is suggestive of areas with increased inhibition associated with IED. While IEDs are considered excitatory phenomena, inhibition directly after the IED has often been described (Urrestarazu et al., 2006). This observation of postspike inhibition is in line with results from EEG-fMRI, in which negative focal BOLD changes in the epileptic focus were often preceded by a positive BOLD in the same area (Jacobs et al., 2009). Thus, negative BOLD could also been seen as an undershoot phenomenon or a post-spike period of inhibition. Whether this interpretation can explain negative BOLD in the DMN however is rather questionable as no earlier positive responses were observed in the same

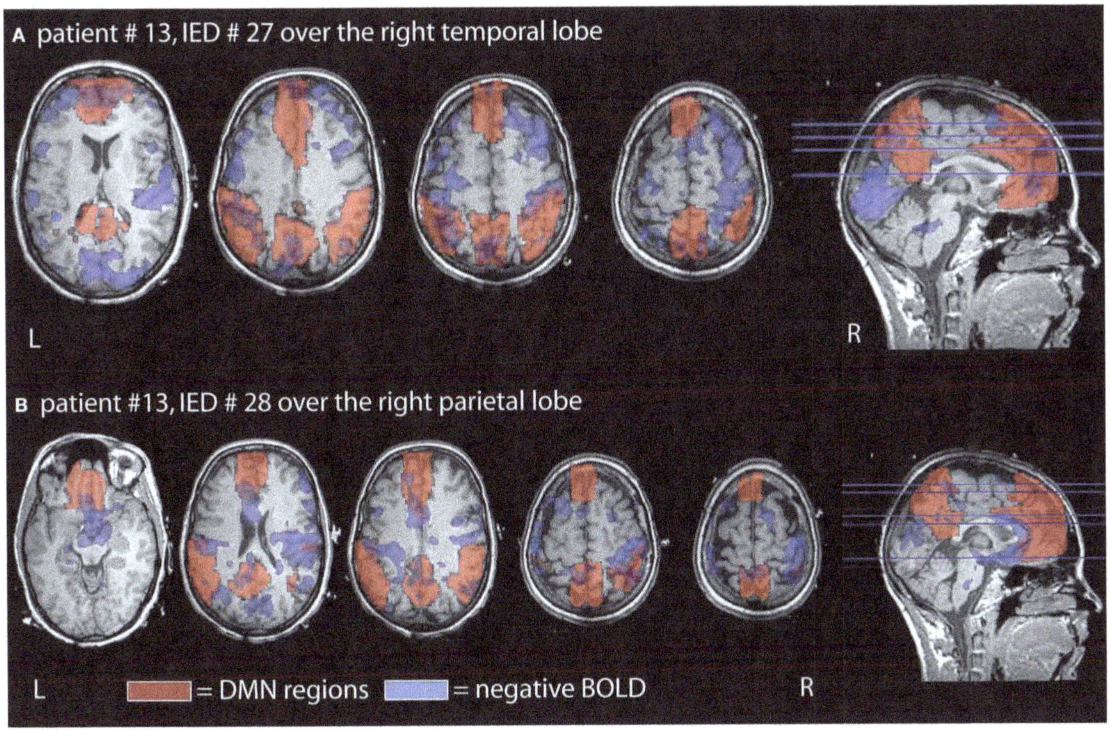

FIGURE 3 | Example of the overlap between negative BOLD responses and DMN regions. Patient # 13 had two different IED one generated over the right temporal and the other over the right parietal region. **(A)** Demonstrates that overlap for the temporal IED with 15% of the negative BOLD located within the DMN and 29% of the DMN covered by negative BOLD. In agreement with our findings the overlap is larger than in the parietal IED of the same patient even if the temporal IEDs only occurred 3 times, while the parietal time was seen 12 times during the measurement. **(B)** Shows the negative BOLD changes related to the parietal IED. 14% of the negative BOLD are located in the DMN region and 2% of the DMN are covered by negative BOLD.

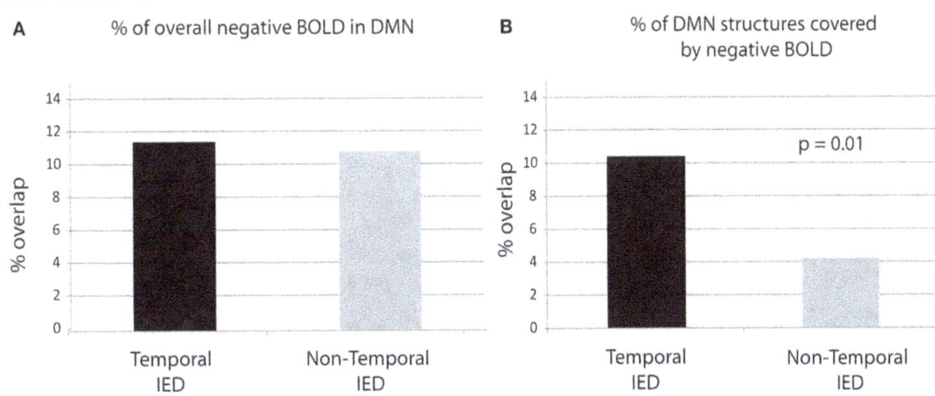

FIGURE 4 | Percentage of overlap between negative BOLD and DMN structures. The percentage of DMN structures covered by negative BOLD is significantly higher in temporal than extra-temporal IED. Panel **(A)** display of the negative BOLD lying within regions of the DMN. Panel **(B)** display of the percentage of DMN covered by negative BOLD.

regions (Gotman et al., 2005; Jacobs et al., 2014). Nevertheless, one could imagine that DMN structures or the connections between them are inhibited during an IED. Independent of mechanisms of negative BOLD the most important finding of this and previous studies is that DMN structures can be related to IED occurrence and that this effect is largely variable.

INTERACTIONS BETWEEN DEFAULT MODE NETWORK AND EPILEPSY

The DMN was originally discovered as a network of structures which are active or show positive BOLD during periods of rest in contrast to the actual activity under examination (Shulman et al., 1997; Mazoyer et al., 2001). Its functional role is not completely understood yet, but it is strongly activated during biographical memory retrieval, envisioning the future and conceiving the perspectives of others, while its activity is reduced during periods in which the brain focuses on external stimuli (Dosenbach et al., 2006). Changes in the structures and functional connectivity of the DMN as well as reduced activation of the network has been described in several brain diseases such as Alzheimer's dementia, schizophrenia and autism disorders (Greene et al., 2001; Lustig et al., 2003; Buckner et al., 2005; Fox et al., 2005). During interictal and ictal epileptic activity, studies so far mostly reported negative BOLD changes in the DMN (Gotman et al., 2006; Laufs et al., 2007). Negative BOLD in the DMN in studies with healthy subjects have been interpreted as a decreased activity in the DMN when comparing tasks in which the DMN was highly active to those in which it was less active (Buckner et al., 2008). In line with this it has been hypothesized that the IEDs associated with negative BOLD in the DMN act like an external stimulus interrupting the function of the normal DMN (Cataldi et al., 2013). Fahoum and colleagues analyzed IED-related changes in the intracranial EEG in the DMN regions and observed a reduction of gamma power and increase of lower frequency EEG activity specific to these regions (Fahoum et al., 2013). Suppression in the gamma band is in line with brain activity usually observed after external stimulation such as visual stimuli (Ossandón et al., 2011). Thus, it seems that the IED have similar effects on the epileptic brain's DMN as repetitive external stimuli.

Our study confirmed previous observations that the degree to which IEDs affect the DMN is largely variable. While a clear correlation between cognitive decline and disruption of the DMN has been observed in Alzheimer's dementia (Broyd et al., 2009; Miao et al., 2011), the clinical importance of alterations in the DMN is still unknown in epilepsy. Some authors suggest that negative BOLD on the DMN directly reflects a short interruption of attention or consciousness during the epileptic events, while others suggest rather a long-term effect on cognition due to the repetitive interruption of the DMN by IEDs (Blumenfeld et al., 2004; Laufs et al., 2007; Fahoum et al., 2012).

The first hypothesis would suggest a short repetitive interruption of consciousness or normal function of the region generating the IED. Such loss of consciousness is especially observed in generalized epilepsies where trains of generalized spikes and waves lead to interrupted consciousness during absence seizures. These seizures are one of the very few seizure types which can be observed during EEG-fMRI as they occur frequently and without excessive motion. Absence seizures are associated with strong negative BOLD changes in the DMN (Blumenfeld, 2005; Moeller et al., 2008). Ictal EEG-fMRI in focal epilepsy is rare and only a few reports demonstrated DMN changes during these seizures (Blumenfeld and Taylor, 2003). Again during these focal seizures, reduction in DMN activity was mainly observed when loss of consciousness or secondary generalization occurred (Norden and Blumenfeld, 2002; Blumenfeld et al., 2009). EEG studies support this observation by showing neocortical slowing during the period of impaired consciousness in TLE (Blumenfeld et al., 2004; Englot et al., 2010). The association between decreased consciousness and DMN changes observed during ictal activity might also be true for focal IEDs with the only difference that focal IEDs are usually generated over too small brain areas to cause clinically visible alterations of consciousness.

Short impairments of cognitive function as described in TCI (Binnie, 2003) can only be detected using complex cognitive testing and do not refer to consciousness levels in general but the specific task at hand. Existing studies are biased like ours toward patients with frequent IEDs and limited to short test periods. However, it could be clearly shown that temporal, more precisely hippocampal, IEDs can lead to transient cognitive impairment by disrupting memory maintenance and retrieval (Kleen et al., 2013). While cognitive interruption during working memory has been associated with negative BOLD in the DMN during generalized IEDs (Chaudhary et al., 2013), it remains unclear whether transitory cognitive impairment related to focal, specifically temporal, IEDs would result in negative BOLD changes. Thus, the strongest evidence for the idea that negative BOLD in DMN reflects short interruptions of cognition or even consciousness comes from the observation that the DMN changes were stronger in TLE, which is usually associated with earlier and stronger impairment of consciousness than neocortical epilepsies (Laufs et al., 2007; Cataldi et al., 2013).

The rare and scarce occurrence of DMN changes in the analysis of single patients due to the low sensitivity of classical fMRI sequences has been a major challenge for such a study design. The fact that we saw negative BOLD changes in the DMN in all patients suggests that MREG will facilitate this type of investigation and hopefully enable us to answer the question whether focal IED have the potential to interrupt consciousness or cognition.

The alternative hypothesis suggests that negative BOLD in the DMN reflects negative long-term effect of IED on cognition. This would mean that IEDs associated with DMN changes reflect stronger long-term interference with cognition than IEDs which do not deactivate the DMN. Again this question could only be answered by having long-term studies correlating DMN deactivation and cognitive decline in patients with epilepsy, as has been done for Alzheimer's dementia (Broyd et al., 2009; Miao et al., 2011). In our study most patients had long-lasting refractory epilepsy as they were recruited from an epilepsy center specialized in pre-surgical diagnostics and epilepsy surgery. Cognitive decline and loss of specific cognitive function are well-known disabilities in epilepsy and recurrent uncontrolled seizure are correlated with more severe impairments (Carreño et al., 2008; Avanzini et al., 2013). It might therefore be that the frequent occurrence of negative BOLD of DMN network reflects the fact that most of our patients had more severe epilepsy and cognitive disability than the average population of patients with epilepsy. Nevertheless, most studies using EEG-fMRI in epilepsy are performed in large epilepsy centers and pre-surgical units (Moeller et al., 2009; Thornton et al., 2010). Thus, the frequent occurrence of negative BOLD in DMN is probably mostly reflecting increased sensitivity of MREG and again studies correlating cognitive performance and strength of DMN disruption are necessary to understand the clinical importance of our findings. As EEG-MREG is a non-invasive tool it might be even more interesting to investigate patients with new onset focal epilepsy to see whether changes in DMN during IED are prognostic for cognitive problems in these patients.

EFFECT OF FREQUENT SPIKING

IED are often believed to reflect the epileptic potential of the underlying tissue and are usually monitored in EEG recordings to assess treatment control. While it is certainly true that frequent inter-ictal activity is associated with severity of disease and cognitive decline in some epileptic syndromes such as continuous spike wave status (CSWS) in sleep (Pera et al., 2013), for most epilepsies there is no clinical correlation between frequency of IED and seizure frequency or cognitive decline (Spencer et al., 2008). Nevertheless, one could imagine that a frequent occurrence of IED disturbs the brain networks more extensively than rare occurrence, resulting in more prominent negative effects on attention and cognition. Our study did however not suggest any correlation between IED frequency and DMN changes. It has to be noted that our study was biased toward patients with regular IED occurrence on the EEG, as this was a necessary requirement for successful EEG-fMRI analysis in the time-limited framework of MR scanning. It is therefore not possible to draw conclusion about patients in whom rare or no IEDs are seen on the scalp EEG. Still IED numbers varied quite strongly between 1 and 46 IED within the 40-min measurement and no evidence was found suggesting that patients with high IED numbers showed more prominent DMN involvement. This suggests that DMN involvement is not dependent on the acute likelihood of epileptic tissue to generate spikes but rather on the anatomical structure generating the IED and its connections with other brain regions.

DMN INVOLVEMENT DURING TEMPORAL AND NEOCORTICAL IEDs

It was the aim of the present study to investigate the overlap between DMN and negative BOLD occurrence. As we hypothesized this overlap was larger in temporal than neocortical IEDs, as has been shown in previous group analysis (Laufs et al., 2007). Changes in the DMN in TLE have been investigated quite extensively. It seems unclear whether these are more of a structural or functional nature. The hippocampal formation itself is not only the generator of IEDs but also sometimes considered to be part of the DMN and it often shows extensive structural damage as part of the epilepsy syndrome. Thus, it has been debated whether reduced connectivity and activity of DMN might be a result of these structural changes rather than reflecting an ongoing interruption of DMN function (Liao et al., 2010, 2011). However, functional studies like ours which find negative BOLD at the time of IEDs in contrast to baseline activity underline the suggestion that the DMN undergoes a continuous functional alteration. The same is suggested by studies of functional connectivity which not only discovered decreased connectivity between DMN nodes but also hyper-connectivity between others in TLE (Zhang et al., 2010; Pittau et al., 2012).

Recently TLE is increasingly believed to be a network disease and permanent changes such as atrophy of brain regions have been described even far from the focus (Spencer, 2002; Bartolomei et al., 2005, 2008). EEG-fMRI analysis of patients with TLE support this observation, as positive as well as negative BOLD responses are rarely focal but often suggest involvement of subcortical and distant cortical regions (Laufs et al., 2007; Kobayashi et al., 2009). The present study focused on the analysis of negative BOLD responses and it is therefore remarkable that not only the overlap between DMN structures and negative BOLD was larger in temporal spikes but it was also the case for the overall extent of negative BOLD. Indeed, while the initial focus of the study was to investigate deactivations in DMN structures associated with IEDs, the large majority of negative BOLD responses actually occurred outside DMN regions. This finding might be interpreted as an indication that IED generated over temporal regions affect larger networks by fast propagation and that this effect might be predominantly inhibitory. Moreover not only the DMN but also other resting state networks such as the attention network and executive control network have been described to be impaired in TLE (Cataldi et al., 2013). The lack of significant difference in the percentage of negative BOLD in DMN regions between temporal and extratemporal spikes also indicates that deactivations are not necessarily specific to the DMN, and additionally may suggest a large variability within the temporal and extra-temporal groups. Therefore, our study suggests that additional investigation of the localization of negative BOLD responses outside the DMN might reveal other resting state that show interference by focal IEDs not only in TLE patients in general, but also at the individual patient level.

CONCLUSION

In the present study quantification of overlap between DMN regions and negative BOLD occurrence after focal IED revealed involvement of DMN structures to varying extent in all patients. MREG as a method of fast fMRI allows very sensitive detection of BOLD changes in the DMN structures. Interestingly the frequency of IEDs did not affect the occurrence of negative BOLD in the DMN, but the origin of IED did. Thus, preexisting network structures seem to be a relevant factor for the ability of an IED to interfere with the DMN. IED generated from the mesial temporal structures which are part of the DMN or their vicinity result in stronger interruption of the DMN activity. The clinical implications of these findings are unknown, but if spontaneous repetitive IEDs interrupt the resting state networks of the brain in similar but less directed way as external stimuli, a resulting impairment of consciousness and cognition are likely.

ACKNOWLEDGMENTS

This work was supported by the ERC grant agreement 232908 and the DFG cluster of excellence EXC-1086 BrainLinks-BrainTools. Julia Jacobs was supported by grant JA 1725/2-1 of the German Research Foundation.

REFERENCES

1. Aarts, J. H., Binnie, C. D., Smit, A. M., and Wilkins, A. J. (1984). Selective cognitive impairment during focal and generalized epileptiform EEG activity. *Brain* 107(Pt 1), 293–308. doi: 10.1093/brain/107.1.293
2. Allen, P. J., Josephs, O., and Turner, R. (2000). A method for removing imaging artifact from continuous EEG recorded during functional MRI. *Neuroimage* 12, 230–239. doi: 10.1006/nimg.2000.0599
3. Allen, P. J., Polizzi, G., Krakow, K., Fish, D. R., and Lemieux, L. (1998). Identification of EEG events in the MR scanner: the problem of pulse artifact and a method for its subtraction. *Neuroimage* 8, 229–239. doi: 10.1006/nimg.1998.0361
4. An, D., Fahoum, F., Hall, J., Olivier, A., Gotman, J., and Dubeau, F. (2013). Electroencephalography/functional magnetic resonance imaging responses help predict surgical outcome in focal epilepsy. *Epilepsia* 54, 2184–2194. doi: 10.1111/epi.12434

5. Archer, J. S., Abbott, D. F., Waites, A. B., and Jackson, G. D. (2003). fMRI "deactivation" of the posterior cingulate during generalized spike and wave. *Neuroimage* 20, 1915–1922. doi: 10.1016/S1053-8119(03)00294-5
6. Assländer, J., Zahneisen, B., Hugger, T., Reisert, M., Lee, H.-L., LeVan, P., et al. (2013). Single shot whole brain imaging using spherical stack of spirals trajec- tories. *Neuroimage* 73, 59–70. doi: 10.1016/j.neuroimage.2013.01.065
7. Avanzini, G., Depaulis, A., Tassinari, A., and de Curtis, M. (2013). Do seizures and epileptic activity worsen epilepsy and deteriorate cognitive function? *Epilepsia* 54(Suppl. 8), 14–21. doi: 10.1111/epi.12418
8. Bagshaw, A. P., Aghakhani, Y., Bénar, C.-G., Kobayashi, E., Hawco, C., Dubeau, F., et al. (2004). EEG-fMRI of focal epileptic spikes: analysis with multiple haemodynamic functions and comparison with gadolinium-enhanced MR angiograms. *Hum. Brain Mapp.* 22, 179–192. doi: 10.1002/hbm.20024
9. Bartolomei, F., Chauvel, P., and Wendling, F. (2008). Epileptogenicity of brain structures in human temporal lobe epilepsy: a quantified study from intrac- erebral EEG. *Brain* 131(Pt 7), 1818–1830. doi: 10.1093/brain/awn111
10. Bartolomei, F., Khalil, M., Wendling, F., Sontheimer, A., Régis, J., Ranjeva, J.-P., et al. (2005). Entorhinal cortex involvement in human mesial temporal lobe epilepsy: an electrophysiologic and volumetric study. *Epilepsia* 46, 677–687.doi: 10.1111/j.1528-1167.2005.43804.x
11. Berman, R., Negishi, M., Vestal, M., Spann, M., Chung, M. H., Bai, X., et al. (2010). Simultaneous EEG, fMRI, and behavior in typical childhood absence seizures. *Epilepsia* 51, 2011–2022. doi: 10.1111/j.1528-1167.2010.02652.x
12. Binnie, C. D. (2003). Cognitive impairment during epileptiform discharges: is it ever justifiable to treat the EEG? *Lancet Neurol.* 2, 725–730. doi: 10.1016/S1474- 4422(03)00584-2
13. Blumenfeld, H. (2005). Consciousness and epilepsy: why are patients with absence seizures absent? *Prog. Brain Res.* 150, 271–286. doi: 10.1016/S0079-6123(05)50020-7
14. Blumenfeld, H., Rivera, M., McNally, K. A., Davis, K., Spencer, D. D., and Spencer, S. S. (2004). Ictal neocortical slowing in temporal lobe epilepsy. *Neurology* 63, 1015–1021. doi: 10.1212/01.WNL.0000141086.91077.CD
15. Blumenfeld, H., and Taylor, J. (2003). Why do seizures cause loss of consciousness? *Neuroscientist* 9, 301–310. doi: 10.1177/1073858403255624
16. Blumenfeld, H., Varghese, G. I., Purcaro, M. J., Motelow, J. E., Enev, M., McNally, K. A., et al. (2009). Cortical and subcortical networks in human secondarily generalized tonic-clonic seizures. *Brain* 132(Pt 4), 999–1012. doi: 10.1093/brain/awp028
17. Broyd, S. J., Demanuele, C., Debener, S., Helps, S. K., James, C. J., and Sonuga-Barke, E. J. S. (2009). Default-mode brain dysfunction in mental disorders: a systematic review. *Neurosci. Biobehav. Rev.* 33, 279–296. doi: 10.1016/j.neubiorev.2008.09.002
18. Bruehl, C., Hagemann, G., and Witte, O. W. (1998). Uncoupling of blood flow and metabolism in focal epilepsy. *Epilepsia* 39, 1235–1242. doi: 10.1111/j.1528- 1157.1998.tb01320.x
19. Buckner, R. L., Andrews-Hanna, J. R., and Schacter, D. L. (2008). The brain's default network: anatomy, function, and relevance to disease. *Ann. N.Y. Acad. Sci.* 1124, 1–38. doi: 10.1196/annals.1440.011
20. Buckner, R. L., Snyder, A. Z., Shannon, B. J., LaRossa, G., Sachs, R., Fotenos, A. F., et al. (2005). Molecular, structural, and functional characterization of Alzheimer's disease: evidence for a relationship between default activity, amy- loid, and memory. *J. Neurosci.* 25, 7709–7717. doi: 10.1523/JNEUROSCI.2177- 05.2005
21. Carreño, M., Donaire, A., and Sánchez-Carpintero, R. (2008). Cognitive disorders associated with epilepsy: diagnosis and treatment. *Neurologist* 14(6 Suppl. 1), S26–S34. doi: 10.1097/01.nrl.0000340789.15295.8f
22. Cataldi, M., Avoli, M., and de Villers-Sidani, E. (2013). Resting state networks in temporal lobe epilepsy. *Epilepsia* 54, 2048–2059. doi: 10.1111/epi.12400
23. Chatton, J.-Y., Pellerin, L., and Magistretti, P. J. (2003). GABA uptake into astrocytes is not associated with significant metabolic cost: implications for brain imaging of inhibitory transmission. *Proc. Natl. Acad. Sci. U.S.A.* 100, 12456–12461. doi: 10.1073/pnas.2132096100
24. Chaudhary, U. J., Centeno, M., Carmichael, D. W., Vollmar, C., Rodionov, R., Bonelli, S., et al. (2013). Imaging the interaction: epileptic discharges, working memory, and behavior. *Hum. Brain Mapp.* 34, 2910–2917. doi: 10.1002/hbm.22115
25. Debener, S., Strobel, A., Sorger, B., Peters, J., Kranczioch, C., Engel, A. K., et al. (2007). Improved quality of auditory event-related potentials recorded simultaneously with 3-T fMRI: removal of the ballistocardiogram artefact. *Neuroimage* 34, 587–597. doi: 10.1016/j.neuroimage.2006.09.031
26. Dosenbach, N. U. F., Visscher, K. M., Palmer, E. D., Miezin, F. M., Wenger, K. K., Kang, H. C., et al. (2006). A core system for the implementation of task sets. *Neuron* 50, 799–812. doi: 10.1016/j.neuron.2006.04.031
27. Englot, D. J., Yang, L., Hamid, H., Danielson, N., Bai, X., Marfeo, A., et al. (2010).
28. Impaired consciousness in temporal lobe seizures: role of cortical slow activity. *Brain* 133(Pt 12), 3764–3777. doi: 10.1093/brain/awq316
29. Ertl, M., Kirsch, V., Leicht, G., Karch, S., Olbrich, S., Reiser, M., et al. (2010). Avoiding the ballistocardiogram (BCG) artifact of EEG data acquired simul- taneously with fMRI by pulse-triggered presentation of stimuli. *J. Neurosci. Methods* 186, 231–241. doi: 10.1016/j.jneumeth.2009.11.009
30. Fahoum, F., Lopes, R., Pittau, F., Dubeau, F., and Gotman, J. (2012). Widespread epileptic networks in focal epilepsies: EEG-fMRI study. *Epilepsia* 53,1618–1627. doi: 10.1111/j.1528-1167.2012.03533.x
31. Fahoum, F., Zelmann, R., Tyvaert, L., Dubeau, F., and Gotman, J. (2013). Epileptic discharges affect the default mode network—FMRI and intrac- erebral EEG evidence. *PLoS ONE* 8:e68038. doi: 10.1371/journal.pone.00 68038
32. Feinberg, D. A., Moeller, S., Smith, S. M., Auerbach, E., Ramanna, S., Gunther, M., et al. (2010). Multiplexed echo planar imaging for sub-second whole brain FMRI and fast diffusion imaging. *PLoS ONE* 5:e15710. doi: 10.1371/jour- nal.pone.0015710
33. Fink, G. R., Pawlik, G., Stefan, H., Pietrzyk, U., Wienhard, K., and Heiss, W. D. (1996). Temporal lobe epilepsy: evidence for interictal uncoupling of blood flow and glucose metabolism in temporomesial structures. *J. Neurol. Sci.* 137, 28–34. doi: 10.1016/0022-510X(95)00323-T
34. Flanagan, D., Abbott, D. F., and Jackson, G. D. (2009). How wrong can we be? The effect of inaccurate mark-up of EEG/fMRI studies in epilepsy. *Clin. Neurophysiol.* 120, 1637–1647. doi: 10.1016/j.clinph.2009.04.025
35. Fox, M. D., Snyder, A. Z., Vincent, J. L., Corbetta, M., Van Essen, D. C., and Raichle, M. E. (2005). The human brain is intrinsically organized into dynamic, anticor- related functional networks. *Proc. Natl. Acad. Sci. U.S.A.* 102, 9673–9678. doi: 10.1073/pnas.0504136102
36. Friston, K. J., Frith, C. D., and Frackowiak, R. S. (1993). Principal component anal- ysis learning algorithms: a neurobiological analysis. *Proc. Biol. Sci.* 254, 47–54. doi: 10.1098/rspb.1993.0125
37. Glover, G. H., Li, T. Q., and Ress, D. (2000). Image-based method for retrospec- tive correction of physiological motion effects in fMRI: RETROICOR. *Magn. Reson. Med.* 44, 162–167. doi: 10.1002/1522-2594(200007)44:1<162::AID- MRM23>3.0.CO;2-E
38. Gotman, J., Grova, C., Bagshaw, A., Kobayashi, E., Aghakhani, Y., and Dubeau, F. (2005). Generalized epileptic discharges show thalamocortical activation and suspension of the default state of the brain. *Proc. Natl. Acad. Sci. U.S.A.* 102, 15236–15240. doi: 10.1073/pnas.0504935102
39. Gotman, J., Kobayashi, E., Bagshaw, A. P., Bénar, C.-G., and Dubeau, F. (2006). Combining EEG and fMRI: a multimodal tool for epilepsy research. *J. Magn. Reson. Imaging* 23, 906–920. doi: 10.1002/jmri.20577
40. Greene, J. D., Sommerville, R. B., Nystrom, L. E., Darley, J. M., and Cohen, J. D. (2001). An fMRI investigation of emotional engagement in moral judgment. *Science* 293, 2105–2108. doi: 10.1126/science.1062872
41. Grouiller, F., Thornton, R. C., Groening, K., Spinelli, L., Duncan, J. S., Schaller, K., et al. (2011). With or without spikes: localization of focal epileptic activ- ity by simultaneous electroencephalography and functional magnetic resonance imaging. *Brain* 134(Pt 10), 2867–2886. doi: 10.1093/brain/awr156
42. Harel, N., Lee, S.-P., Nagaoka, T., Kim, D.-S., and Kim, S.-G. (2002). Origin of negative blood oxygenation level-dependent fMRI signals. *J. Cereb. Blood Flow Metab.* 22, 908–917. doi: 10.1097/00004647-200208000-00002
43. Hugger, T., Zahneisen, B., LeVan, P., Lee, K. J., Lee, H.-L., Zaitsev, M., et al. (2011). Fast undersampled functional magnetic resonance imaging using non- linear regularized parallel image reconstruction. *PLoS ONE* 6:e28822. doi: 10.1371/journal.pone.0028822
44. Hutt, S. J., and Gilbert, S. (1980). Effects of evoked spike-wave discharges upon short term memory in patients with epilepsy. *Cortex* 16, 445–457. doi: 10.1016/S0010-9452(80)80045-1
45. Jacobs, J., Kobayashi, E., Boor, R., Muhle, H., Stephan, W., Hawco, C., et al. (2007). Hemodynamic responses to interictal epileptiform discharges in children with symptomatic epilepsy. *Epilepsia* 48, 2068–2078. doi: 10.1111/j.1528- 1167.2007.01192.x
46. Jacobs, J., Levan, P., Moeller, F., Boor, R., Stephani, U., Gotman, J., et al. (2009). Hemodynamic changes preceding the interictal EEG spike in patients with focal epilepsy investigated using simultaneous EEG-fMRI. *Neuroimage* 45, 1220–1231. doi: 10.1016/j.neuroimage.2009.01.014

47. Jacobs, J., Stich, J., Zahneisen, B., Assländer, J., Ramantani, G., Schulze-Bonhage, A., et al. (2014). Fast fMRI provides high statistical power in the analysis of epileptic networks. *Neuroimage* 88, 282–294. doi: 10.1016/j.neuroimage.2013.10.018
48. Jansen, M., White, T. P., Mullinger, K. J., Liddle, E. B., Gowland, P. A., Francis, S. T., et al. (2012). Motion-related artefacts in EEG predict neuronally plau- sible patterns of activation in fMRI data. *Neuroimage* 59, 261–270. doi: 10.1016/j.neuroimage.2011.06.094
49. Kleen, J. K., Scott, R. C., Holmes, G. L., Roberts, D. W., Rundle, M. M., Testorf, M., et al. (2013). Hippocampal interictal epileptiform activity disrupts cognition in humans. *Neurology* 81, 18–24. doi: 10.1212/WNL.0b013e318297ee50
50. Kobayashi, E., Bagshaw, A. P., Grova, C., Dubeau, F., and Gotman, J. (2006a). Negative BOLD responses to epileptic spikes. *Hum. Brain Mapp.* 27, 488–497. doi: 10.1002/hbm.20193
51. Kobayashi, E., Bagshaw, A. P., Grova, C., Gotman, J., and Dubeau, F. (2006b). Grey matter heterotopia: what EEG-fMRI can tell us about epileptogenicity of neuronal migration disorders. *Brain* 129(Pt 2), 366–374.
52. Kobayashi, E., Grova, C., Tyvaert, L., Dubeau, F., and Gotman, J. (2009). Structures involved at the time of temporal lobe spikes revealed by interindividual group analysis of EEG/fMRI data. *Epilepsia* 50. 2549–2556. doi: 10.1111/j.1528- 1167.2009.02180.x
53. Laufs, H., Hamandi, K., Salek-Haddadi, A., Kleinschmidt, A. K., Duncan, J. S., and Lemieux, L. (2007). Temporal lobe interictal epileptic discharges affect cerebral activity in "default mode" brain regions. *Hum. Brain Mapp.* 28, 1023–1032. doi: 10.1002/hbm.20323
54. Laureys, S., Owen, A. M., and Schiff, N. D. (2004). Brain function in coma, vegetative state, and related disorders. *Lancet Neurol.* 3, 537–546. doi: 10.1016/S1474- 4422(04)00852-X
55. LeVan, P., Jacobs, J., Stich, J., Zahneisen, B., Hugger, T., Assländer, J., et al. (2012). "EEG-fMRI using the ultra-fast MREG sequence allows the single-trial local- ization of epileptic spikes," in *Proceedings of the 18th Annual Meeting of the Organization for Human Brain Mapping (OHBM)* (Beijing).
56. LeVan, P., Maclaren, J., Herbst, M., Sostheim, R., Zaitsev, M., and Hennig, J. (2013). Ballistocardiographic artifact removal from simultaneous EEG- fMRI using an optical motion-tracking system. *Neuroimage* 75, 1–11. doi: 10.1016/j.neuroimage.2013.02.039
57. Liao, W., Zhang, Z., Pan, Z., Mantini, D., Ding, J., Duan, X., et al. (2010). Altered functional connectivity and small-world in mesial temporal lobe epilepsy. *PLoS ONE* 5:e8525. doi: 10.1371/journal.pone.0008525
58. Liao, W., Zhang, Z., Pan, Z., Mantini, D., Ding, J., Duan, X., et al. (2011). Default mode network abnormalities in mesial temporal lobe epilepsy: a study combin- ing fMRI and DTI. *Hum. Brain Mapp.* 32, 883–895. doi: 10.1002/hbm.21076
59. Lin, F.-H., Wald, L. L., Ahlfors, S. P., Hämäläinen, M. S., Kwong, K. K., and Belliveau, J. W. (2006). Dynamic magnetic resonance inverse imaging of human brain function. *Magn. Reson. Med.* 56, 787–802. doi: 10.1002/mrm. 20997
60. Lustig, C., Snyder, A. Z., Bhakta, M., O'Brien, K. C., McAvoy, M., Raichle, M. E., et al. (2003). Functional deactivations: change with age and dementia of the Alzheimer type. *Proc. Natl. Acad. Sci. U.S.A.* 100, 14504–14509. doi: 10.1073/pnas.2235925100
61. Mandelkow, H., Halder, P., Boesiger, P., and Brandeis, D. (2006). Synchronization facilitates removal of MRI artefacts from concurrent EEG record- ings and increases usable bandwidth. *Neuroimage* 32, 1120–1126. doi: 10.1016/j.neuroimage.2006.04.231
62. Masterton, R. A. J., Abbott, D. F., Fleming, S. W., and Jackson, G. D. (2007). Measurement and reduction of motion and ballistocardiogram artefacts from simultaneous EEG and fMRI recordings. *Neuroimage* 37, 202–211. doi: 10.1016/j.neuroimage.2007.02.060
63. Mazoyer, B., Zago, L., Mellet, E., Bricogne, S., Etard, O., Houdé, O., et al. (2001). Cortical networks for working memory and executive functions sustain the conscious resting state in man. *Brain Res. Bull.* 54, 287–298. doi: 10.1016/S0361- 9230(00)00437-8
64. Miao, X., Wu, X., Li, R., Chen, K., and Yao, L. (2011). Altered connectivity pat- tern of hubs in default-mode network with Alzheimer's disease: an Granger causality modeling approach. *PLoS ONE* 6:e25546. doi: 10.1371/journal.pone. 0025546
65. Moeller, F., Siebner, H. R., Wolff, S., Muhle, H., Granert, O., Jansen, O., et al. (2008). Simultaneous EEG-fMRI in drug-naive children with newly diag- nosed absence epilepsy. *Epilepsia* 49, 1510–1519. doi: 10.1111/j.1528-1167.2008. 01626.x
66. Moeller, F., Tyvaert, L., Nguyen, D. K., LeVan, P., Bouthillier, A., Kobayashi, E., et al. (2009). EEG-fMRI: adding to standard evaluations of patients with nonlesional frontal lobe epilepsy. *Neurology* 73, 2023–2030. doi: 10.1212/WNL.0b013e3181c55d17
67. Norden, A. D., and Blumenfeld, H. (2002). The role of subcortical struc- tures in human epilepsy. *Epilepsy Behav.* 3, 219–231. doi: 10.1016/S1525- 5050(02)00029-X
68. Ossandón, T., Jerbi, K., Vidal, J. R., Bayle, D. J., Henaff, M.-A., Jung, J., et al. (2011). Transient suppression of broadband gamma power in the default-mode net- work is correlated with task complexity and subject performance. *J. Neurosci.* 31, 14521–14530. doi: 10.1523/JNEUROSCI.2483-11.2011
69. Pera, M. C., Brazzo, D., Altieri, N., Balottin, U., and Veggiotti, P. (2013). Long-term evolution of neuropsychological competences in encephalopathy with status epilepticus during sleep: a variable prognosis. *Epilepsia* 54(Suppl. 7), 77–85. doi: 10.1111/epi.12313
70. Pittau, F., Grova, C., Moeller, F., Dubeau, F., and Gotman, J. (2012). Patterns of altered functional connectivity in mesial temporal lobe epilepsy. *Epilepsia* 53, 1013–1023. doi: 10.1111/j.1528-1167.2012.03464.x
71. Pittau, F., Levan, P., Moeller, F., Gholipour, T., Haegelen, C., Zelmann, R., et al. (2011). Changes preceding interictal epileptic EEG abnormalities: compari- son between EEG/fMRI and intracerebral EEG. *Epilepsia* 52, 1120–1129. doi: 10.1111/j.1528-1167.2011.03072.x
72. Posse, S. (2012). Multi-echo acquisition. *Neuroimage* 62, 665–671. doi: 10.1016/j.neuroimage.2011.10.057
73. Raichle, M. E., MacLeod, A. M., Snyder, A. Z., Powers, W. J., Gusnard, D. A., and Shulman, G. L. (2001). A default mode of brain function. *Proc. Natl. Acad. Sci. U.S.A.* 98, 676–682. doi: 10.1073/pnas.98.2.676
74. Shulman, G. L., Fiez, J. A., Corbetta, M., Buckner, R. L., Miezin, F. M.,
75. Raichle, M. E., et al. (1997). Common Blood Flow Changes across Visual Tasks: II. Decreases in Cerebral Cortex. *J. Cogn. Neurosci.* 9, 648–663. doi: 10.1162/jocn.1997.9.5.648
76. Smith, S. M., Jenkinson, M., Woolrich, M. W., Beckmann, C. F., Behrens, T. E. J., Johansen-Berg, H., et al. (2004). Advances in functional and structural MR image analysis and implementation as FSL. *Neuroimage* 23(Suppl. 1), S208–S219. doi: 10.1016/j.neuroimage.2004.07.051
77. Spencer, S. S. (2002). When should temporal-lobe epilepsy be treated surgically? *Lancet Neurol.* 1, 375–382. doi: 10.1016/S1474-4422(02)00163-1
78. Spencer, S. S., Goncharova, I. I., Duckrow, R. B., Novotny, E. J., and Zaveri, H. P. (2008). Interictal spikes on intracranial recording: behavior, physiology, and implications. *Epilepsia* 49, 1881–1892. doi: 10.1111/j.1528-1167.2008.01641.x
79. Srivastava, G., Crottaz-Herbette, S., Lau, K. M., Glover, G. H., and Menon, V. (2005). ICA-based procedures for removing ballistocardiogram artifacts from EEG data acquired in the MRI scanner. *Neuroimage* 24, 50–60. doi: 10.1016/j.neuroimage.2004.09.041
80. Stefanovic, B., Warnking, J. M., Kobayashi, E., Bagshaw, A. P., Hawco, C., Dubeau, F., et al. (2005). Hemodynamic and metabolic responses to acti- vation, deactivation and epileptic discharges. *Neuroimage* 28, 205–215. doi: 10.1016/j.neuroimage.2005.05.038
81. Stefanovic, B., Warnking, J. M., and Pike, G. B. (2004). Hemodynamic and metabolic responses to neuronal inhibition. *Neuroimage* 22, 771–778. doi: 10.1016/j.neuroimage.2004.01.036
82. Thornton, R., Laufs, H., Rodionov, R., Cannadathu, S., Carmichael, D. W., Vulliemoz, S., et al. (2010). EEG correlated functional MRI and postoperative outcome in focal epilepsy. *J. Neurol. Neurosurg. Psychiatry* 81, 922–927. doi: 10.1136/jnnp.2009.196253
83. Tyvaert, L., Hawco, C., Kobayashi, E., LeVan, P., Dubeau, F., and Gotman, J. (2008). Different structures involved during ictal and interictal epileptic activity in malformations of cortical development: an EEG-fMRI study. *Brain* 131(Pt 8), 2042–2060. doi: 10.1093/brain/awn145
84. Tzourio-Mazoyer, N., Landeau, B., Papathanassiou, D., Crivello, F., Etard, O., Delcroix, N., et al. (2002). Automated anatomical labeling of activations in SPM using a macroscopic anatomical parcellation of the MNI MRI single-subject brain. *Neuroimage* 15, 273–289. doi: 10.1006/nimg.2001.0978
85. Urrestarazu, E., Jirsch, J. D., LeVan, P., Hall, J., Avoli, M., Dubeau, F., et al. (2006). High-frequency intracerebral EEG activity (100-500 Hz) following interictal spikes. *Epilepsia* 47, 1465–1476. doi: 10.1111/j.1528-1167.2006. 00618.x
86. Van Houdt, P. J., de Munck, J. C., Zijlmans, M., Huiskamp, G., Leijten, F. S. S., Boon, P. A. J. M., et al. (2010). Comparison of analytical strategies for EEG-correlated fMRI data in patients with epilepsy. *Magn. Reson. Imaging* 28, 1078–1086. doi: 10.1016/j.mri.2010.03.022
87. Worsley, K. J., Liao, C. H., Aston, J., Petre, V., Duncan, G. H., Morales,

F., et al. (2002). A general statistical analysis for fMRI data. *Neuroimage* 15, 1–15. doi: 10.1006/nimg.2001.0933

88. Zahneisen, B., Hugger, T., Lee, K. J., LeVan, P., Reisert, M., Lee, H.-L., et al. (2012). Single shot concentric shells trajectories for ultra fast fMRI. *Magn. Reson. Med.* 68, 484–494. doi: 10.1002/mrm.23256
89. Zhang, Z., Lu, G., Zhong, Y., Tan, Q., Liao, W., Wang, Z., et al. (2010). Altered spontaneous neuronal activity of the default-mode network in mesial temporal lobe epilepsy. *Brain Res.* 1323, 152–160. doi: 10.1016/j.brainres. 2010.01.042
90. Zijlmans, M., Huiskamp, G., Hersevoort, M., Seppenwoolde, J.-H., van Huffelen, A. C., and Leijten, F. S. S. (2007). EEG-fMRI in the preoperative work-up for epilepsy surgery. *Brain* 130(Pt9), 2343–2353. doi: 10.1093/brain/awm141

14

Sensitivity and specificity of interictal EEG-fMRI for detecting the ictal onset zone at different statistical thresholds

Simon Tousseyn[1,2]*, Patrick Dupont[1,2,3], Karolien Goffin[4], Stefan Sunaert[2,5] and Wim Van Paesschen[1,2]

[1] Laboratory for Epilepsy Research, UZ Leuven and KU Leuven, Leuven, Belgium
[2] Medical Imaging Research Center, UZ Leuven and KU Leuven, Leuven, Belgium
[3] Laboratory for Cognitive Neurology, UZ Leuven and KU Leuven, Leuven, Belgium
[4] Department of Nuclear Medicine, UZ Leuven and KU Leuven, Leuven, Belgium
[5] Radiology Department, UZ Leuven and KU Leuven, Leuven, Belgium

***Correspondence:**
Simon Tousseyn, Laboratory for Epilepsy Research, UZ Leuven and KU Leuven, Herestraat 49, Leuven 3000, Belgium
e-mail: simon.tousseyn@gmail.com

There is currently a lack of knowledge about electroencephalography (EEG)-functional magnetic resonance imaging (fMRI) specificity. Our aim was to define sensitivity and specificity of blood oxygen level dependent (BOLD) responses to interictal epileptic spikes during EEG-fMRI for detecting the ictal onset zone (IOZ). We studied 21 refractory focal epilepsy patients who had a well-defined IOZ after a full presurgical evaluation and interictal spikes during EEG-fMRI. Areas of spike-related BOLD changes overlapping the IOZ in patients were considered as true positives; if no overlap was found, they were treated as false-negatives. Matched healthy case-controls had undergone similar EEG-fMRI in order to determine true-negative and false-positive fractions. The spike-related regressor of the patient was used in the design matrix of the healthy case-control. Suprathreshold BOLD changes in the brain of controls were considered as false positives, absence of these changes as true negatives. Sensitivity and specificity were calculated for different statistical thresholds at the voxel level combined with different cluster size thresholds and represented in receiver operating characteristic (ROC)-curves. Additionally, we calculated the ROC-curves based on the cluster containing the maximal significant activation. We achieved a combination of 100% specificity and 62% sensitivity, using a *Z*-threshold in the interval 3.4–3.5 and cluster size threshold of 350 voxels. We could obtain higher sensitivity at the expense of specificity. Similar performance was found when using the cluster containing the maximal significant activation. Our data provide a guideline for different EEG-fMRI settings with their respective sensitivity and specificity for detecting the IOZ. The unique cluster containing the maximal significant BOLD activation was a sensitive and specific marker of the IOZ.

Keywords: EEG-fMRI, refractory focal epilepsy, presurgical evaluation, sensitivity and specificity, interictal

INTRODUCTION

The goal of the presurgical evaluation in refractory focal epilepsy is to define the epileptogenic zone, the area indispensable for the generation of epileptic seizures (1).

In the last decade, the value of simultaneous electroencephalography-functional magnetic resonance imaging (EEG-fMRI) as a localizing tool of the epileptogenic zone has been explored. In this technique, changes in blood oxygen level dependent (BOLD) contrast, related in a statistical way to interictal epileptic discharges or seizures, are displayed as spatial maps. Sensitivity of EEG-fMRI for localizing the epileptogenic zone has received a lot of attention, but specificity has largely been neglected (2), hampering the clinical implementation of EEG-fMRI in the presurgical evaluation of refractory focal epilepsy.

In order to address this issue, correlational studies of EEG-fMRI with a "gold standard" are crucial (3). Since the epileptogenic zone is a theoretical concept, the ictal onset zone (IOZ), the area from which seizures are generated, is a valuable alternative. The IOZ can be determined by ictal scalp/invasive EEG-registrations and/or ictal single photon emission computed tomography (SPECT) in concordance with other presurgical investigations (1).

Several validation studies assessed the sensitivity of spike-related EEG-fMRI using the results of ictal invasive EEG-registrations as indication of the IOZ (4–17). A major disadvantage of intracranial EEG is the limited spatial coverage and the necessity of an *a priori* hypothesis of the IOZ with possible non-localizing or misleading results (18, 19). The IOZ is then determined by arbitrary margins around contact points, active during seizure onset, but the technique is blind to uncovered areas, a particular problem when comparing with BOLD activity, as experienced by several authors (5, 8, 17, 20–23).

Ictal perfusion SPECT has the advantage of demonstrating dynamic seizure-related changes in cerebral perfusion on a whole brain scale, which offers ideal comparison with fMRI studies.

Several interictal EEG-fMRI studies used the results of ictal SPECT in their validation (5, 6, 9, 11, 12, 24–26). Due to its low temporal resolution, both the IOZ and seizure propagation pathways can be found (27–30). Therefore, combinations of imaging modalities [structural MRI, interictal and ictal SPECT and subtraction ictal SPECT co-registered to MRI (SISCOM), and interictal ^{18}F-fluorodeoxyglucose positron emission tomography (^{18}F-FDG PET)], which integrate the additional information of each independent modality, may provide superior information compared to the information provided by ictal SPECT alone (29).

More recently, spike-related EEG-fMRI results have been compared with postsurgical resection zone and epilepsy outcome (5, 9–12, 14, 16, 17, 21, 24, 26, 31, 32). After successful epilepsy surgery, sufficient brain tissue has been resected. However, the resection zone depends on the surgical approach (conservative versus extended resection) (33) and the accessibility and can overestimate the actual IOZ.

A much larger problem than the exact definition of the IOZ to define sensitivity of EEG-fMRI is the lack of knowledge about specificity of EEG-fMRI (2). The extent and pattern of the BOLD changes are dependent on the statistical threshold levels that are used. Less stringent threshold levels will not only induce more widespread and multifocal patterns but also more false-positive results.

At conventional statistical threshold levels [family-wise error (FWE) corrected $p < 0.05$ and uncorrected $p < 0.001$] both focal and multifocal, widespread BOLD responses have been described. Widespread BOLD signal clusters have been interpreted as representing widespread epileptic abnormalities with poor surgical prognosis if not completely included in the resection (10, 16, 21, 31). However, in the absence of knowledge about specificity of EEG-fMRI, the clinical significance of these different patterns remains uncertain. As mentioned by Chaudhary and colleagues in 2012, EEG-fMRI studies demonstrate "often complex BOLD patterns, raising the issue of specificity of the findings and the unknown clinical relevance of individual BOLD clusters" (34). In a paper of van Houdt and colleagues, this was rephrased as "there are currently no standards for the statistical thresholds in EEG-fMRI analysis" (17).

In this study, we propose an innovative approach to quantitatively define the effect of different statistical thresholds on sensitivity and specificity of spike-related BOLD changes for detecting the IOZ. We determined true-positive and false-negative BOLD fluctuations in patients, and false-positive and true-negative BOLD fluctuations in age- and gender-matched healthy case-controls.

MATERIALS AND METHODS

INCLUSION CRITERIA

This study was approved by an independent ethical standards committee on human experimentation of the University Hospitals Leuven and written informed consent was obtained from all participants.

Inclusion criteria were (i) consecutive adults who underwent a full presurgical evaluation for refractory focal epilepsy between August 2010 and November 2013, including seizure history, neurological and physical examination, neuropsychological assessment, interictal and ictal scalp EEG-recordings, video-analysis of seizures, high-resolution MRI of the brain, and in most patients SISCOM and interictal ^{18}F-FDG PET. In selected cases, intracranial EEG-recordings were performed; (ii) concordant data pointing to one epileptic focus using all available presurgical investigations, including a SISCOM or else successful outcome after epilepsy surgery [international league against epilepsy (ILAE) outcome classification 1–3 (1, completely seizure-free; 2, only auras; 3, one to three seizure days per year $\pm$ auras; 4, four seizure days per year to 50% reduction of baseline seizure days $\pm$ auras; 5, <50% reduction of baseline seizure days to 100% increase of baseline seizure days $\pm$ auras; 6, more than 100% increase of baseline seizure days $\pm$ auras)] (35); (iii) recording of interictal spikes during EEG-fMRI.

OPERATIONAL DEFINITION OF THE ICTAL ONSET ZONE

The IOZ was defined as follows:

(i) In patients with successful outcome after epilepsy surgery, we considered the manually outlined resected brain area as the IOZ.
(ii) In patients, awaiting surgery, refusing surgery, or ineligible for surgery due to proximity of the epileptogenic zone to eloquent regions, we determined the IOZ as the hypothetical resection zone, based on multidisciplinary clinical consensus using all non-invasive and invasive data except EEG-fMRI results. As the patients were selected for concordant localizing data, we ensured not to rely on a single testing modality. The volume of this IOZ was further restricted to the region of ictal hyperperfusion on SISCOM within this hypothetical resection area. The hyperperfusion was thresholded with a Z-score $= 1.5$. This threshold was shown to be optimal for localizing the epileptogenic zone (36).

EEG-fMRI ACQUISITION AND PROCESSING

Functional images were acquired using a whole brain single-shot T2* gradient-echo Echo Planar Imaging sequence in one of two 3 T MR scanners (Achieva TX with a 32-channel head coil and Intera Achieva with an eight-channel head coil, Philips Medical Systems, Best, The Netherlands); TE $= 33$ ms, TR $= 2.2$ or 2.5 s, voxel size 2.6 mm × 3 mm × 2.6 mm.

A 64- or 32-channel MR compatible EEG cap was used for simultaneous EEG-fMRI recordings with a BrainAmp amplifier (Brain Products, Munich, Germany; sampling rate 5 kHz). In patients admitted to the hospital, we used a 24-channel MR compatible electrode set (Yves EEG solutions, Newburyport, MA, USA) both in the telemetry unit and in the scanner with the BrainAmp amplifier. Patients were asked to rest with closed eyes.

The EEG was filtered offline (bandpass 1–50 Hz) and gradient artifacts were removed using the Bergen plug-in (Bergen fMRI Group, Bergen, Norway)[1] (37) for EEGLAB.[2] Pulse artifacts were subtracted with Brain Vision Analyzer software (Brain Products, Munich, Germany) (38).

[1] http://fmri.uib.no/tools/bergen_plugin.htm
[2] http://www.sccn.ucsd.edu/eeglab/

The fMRI data were analyzed with statistical parametric mapping (SPM), version 8 (Wellcome Department of Imaging Neuroscience, University College London, UK)[3]; running on MATLAB (MathWorks, Natick, MA, USA). Images were realigned, slice-time corrected, normalized into the Montreal Neurological Institute (MNI) space using the T1 MRI template available in SPM (voxel size: 2 mm × 2 mm × 2 mm), and spatially smoothed using an isotropic Gaussian kernel of 6 mm full width at half-maximum (FWHM).

Interictal spikes were visually marked by a neurologist (Simon Tousseyn) and discussed with a second neurologist (Wim Van Paesschen). Statistical analysis was performed using the general linear model approach. The regressor of the interictal spike was created using the timings of the event convolved with the canonical hemodynamic response function. Included as confounding covariates were (i) the six rigid-body motion correction parameters, (ii) the fMRI signal averaged over the lateral ventricles, and (iii) the fMRI signal averaged over a region centered in the white matter (39). When a sudden head movement (>1 mm translation) appeared, we added a dummy regressor, which was set to one for the corresponding scan as well as for the next three scans. The remainder of the regressor was set to 0. In case this sudden movement was present in different consecutive blocks, a dummy regressor was created for each block (40, 41).

A statistical Z-score map was obtained for the interictal spike event-related regressor. In case, a patient had more than one spike-type, only EEG-fMRI results corresponding to the most frequent spike-type, determined during video-telemetry, were used for the analysis.

[3]http://www.fil.ion.ucl.ac.uk/spm/

SENSITIVITY AND SPECIFICITY FOR LOCALIZING THE ICTAL ONSET ZONE

Sensitivity and specificity were calculated as follows: true-positive cases were defined as those patients in whom we found a suprathreshold cluster of a suprathreshold size overlapping the IOZ. Patients, in whom this was not the case, were considered false-negative cases. Epilepsy can be regarded as a network disorder (42, 43). This network concept implies interregional interactions between the IOZ and other sites. Based on this theory, we believe it is not appropriate to classify activations outside the IOZ, related to spikes in patients, as false positives. To determine false-positive and true-negative cases, we introduced age- and gender-matched healthy controls assigned to each patient in order to obtain a statistical map using the spike event-related regressor of that patient (corresponding to nonsense events for the control subject). False-positive cases were those controls who showed a suprathreshold cluster of a suprathreshold size somewhere in the brain while true-negative cases were those controls for whom this was not the case (see **Figure 1**). In a way, we treated the controls as a surrogate for the patient group, assuming that the results would have been the same if we had been able to look at those parts of the brain, which were not linked to the epileptic network. Each control underwent EEG-fMRI using the same session length as the corresponding patient. The spatial normalization step ensured that the number of voxels, which were analyzed, as well as the cluster size was similar between all patients and controls.

At a certain statistical threshold, sensitivity was defined as the proportion of true-positive cases within the patient group and

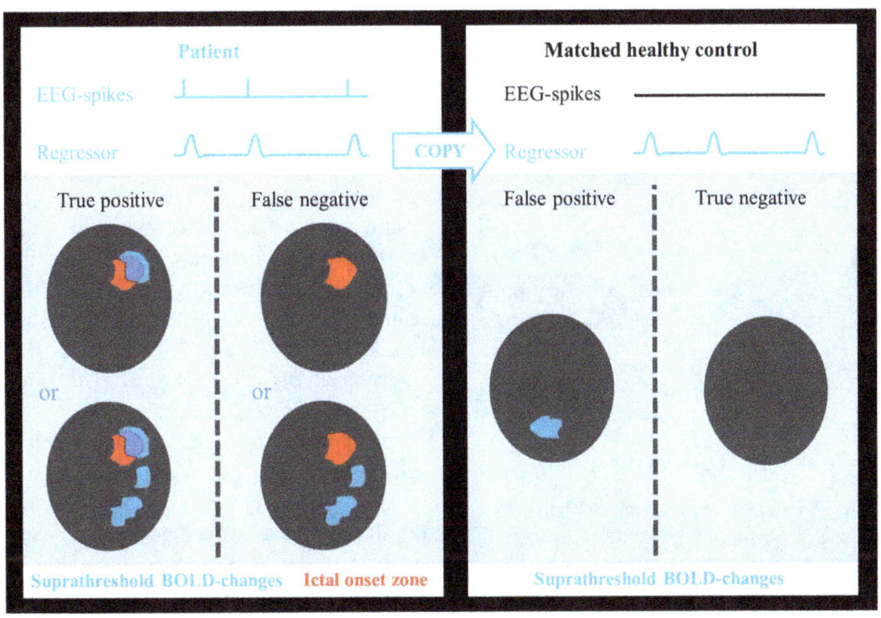

FIGURE 1 | Determination of test outcome. EEG-spikes = spike-time course based on manually indicated interictal spikes. Regressor = spike-time course of patient convolved with canonical hemodynamic response function. Areas of suprathreshold BOLD changes overlapping the ictal onset zone in patients were considered as true positives and if no overlap was found, they were treated as false negatives. Suprathreshold BOLD changes in any part of the brain in healthy controls were considered as false positives, absence of BOLD responses as true negatives.

the "surrogate" specificity as the proportion of true-negative cases within the control group (see **Figure 2**). Sensitivity and specificity were calculated for different statistical thresholds at the voxel level (*Z*, 0–13; step-size, 0.1). This was combined with different thresholds for the minimal cluster size up to 600 voxels (step-size, 50 voxels, voxel size, 2 mm × 2 mm × 2 mm). Six hundred voxels correspond to a brain volume of 4800 mm^3, comparable to the volumes of a hippocampus (44), or a focal cortical dysplasia (27). Based on these results, receiver operating characteristic (ROC)-curves were calculated. We performed the calculations for activations and deactivations, separately.

In an attempt to identify the most localizing cluster of BOLD changes, if widespread BOLD changes were present, several authors looked at the cluster containing the maximal significant activation or at the maximal significant activation voxel (45, 46). In an additional analysis, we calculated the ROC-curves based upon each of these selections.

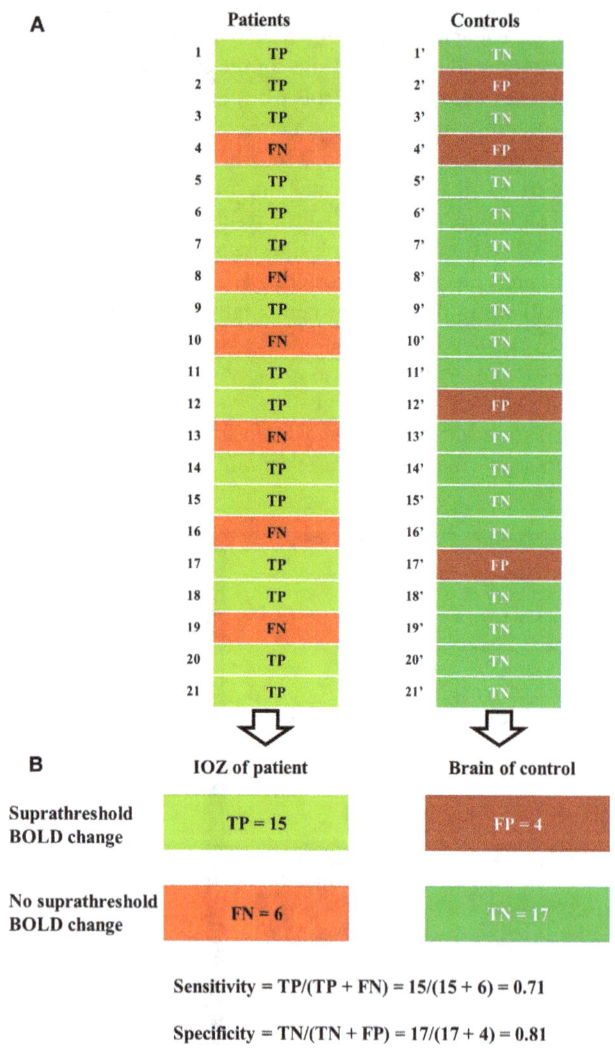

FIGURE 2 | Illustration of a contingency table. (A) For a certain statistical threshold, true-positive (TP) or false-negative (FN) cases are determined in patients, false-positive (FP) or true-negative (TN) cases in control subjects. **(B)** Sensitivity (number of true positives over the number of true positives and false negatives) was defined solely in the patient group and specificity (number of true negatives over the number of true negatives and false positives) solely in the control group.

RESULTS

STUDY POPULATION

Twenty-one consecutive patients (age: 36 ± 14 years, age at epilepsy onset: 12 ± 10 years, 16 women) met the inclusion criteria. Clinical data are presented in **Table 1**. Patients had a median seizure frequency of eight seizure days per month (range 0.5–30) and had failed 7 ± 4 antiepileptic drugs at the time of evaluation. Thirteen patients had temporal lobe epilepsy (TLE): six mesial TLE, seven lateral TLE, while seizure onset was extratemporal (ETLE) in the other eight patients. Structural imaging was normal in 3/21 patients. All ictal SPECT injections used for analysis in this study were performed during the ictal phase [median seizure duration, 84 s (range: 5–423); median time of initiation of ictal SPECT tracer injection, 17 s (range: 1–43)]. Intracranial EEG-recordings, available in five patients, were concordant with non-invasive investigations.

So far, eight patients underwent epilepsy surgery with a successful outcome [ILAE class 1 (completely seizure-free) in six cases, class 2 (only auras) in two cases] (35) (median follow-up time, 9 months; range, 2–27): temporal lobe resection (patients 3, 7, 17, and 18), frontal lesionectomy (patients 6 and 9), functional hemispherotomy (patient 12), and hippocampus/amygdala radiosurgery (patient 16).

Functional magnetic resonance imaging sessions lasted on average 49 ± 15 min. The median spike-rate during EEG-fMRI was 187 spikes/h (range: 8–2018). Twenty-one healthy case-controls (age, 36 ± 12 years; 16 women) underwent EEG-fMRI using the same session length.

SENSITIVITY AND SPECIFICITY FOR LOCALIZING THE ICTAL ONSET ZONE

Electroencephalography-functional magnetic resonance imaging BOLD activations corresponding to the statistical threshold of uncorrected $p < 0.001$ ($Z = 3.1$, no constraint on cluster size) resulted in 86% sensitivity (suprathreshold activations in the IOZ in 18 of the 21 patients) and 0% specificity (all controls had a suprathreshold detection in the brain). In contrast, when a significance level of FWE corrected $p < 0.05$ was used (corresponding to a *Z* between 4.9 and 5.1 in our study, no constraint on cluster size), sensitivity dropped to 62–57% but specificity increased to 95–100% (**Figures 3** and **4**).

We report the settings that give the highest sensitivity for maximal specificity. *Z*-score thresholds of 3.4 and 3.5 both resulted in 62% sensitivity and 100% specificity, using a minimal cluster size of 350 voxels (**Figure 3**). At these settings, 6 of the 13 patients (46%) with an overlap between a cluster of BOLD activation and the IOZ had at least one additional activation cluster in more remote areas, not overlapping the IOZ. Exclusion of these remote activations from resection did not preclude successful outcome in three of the eight operated patients (patients 3, 6, and 16). In patient 3, a dysembryoplastic neuroepithelial tumor (DNET) in the left temporal lobe was resected. Remote activations were

Table 1 | Clinical data of patients.

Patient	Gender/ age/ age at onset	Ictal onset zone	Etiology	Symptomatogenic zone	Structural MRI	SISCOM localization	Interictal ^{18}F-FDG PET hypometabolism	Scalp interictal spike localization§	Scalp ictal EEG localization	icEEG	Epilepsy surgery	ILAE outcome	Follow-up time after surgery (m)	Pathology	Spike-rate (spikes/h) during fMRI
1	F/48/3	R insula	Unknown	Insula	Normal	R insula	Not contributive	F4	R frontal	Concordant	Planned				384
2	F/38/12	R temporal	CNS infection	R temporal	Ischemic R temporoparieto-occipital lesion	R temporal	Not done	T4	R	Not done	Refusal				1171
3	F/23/9	L anterior temporal	DNET	L temporal	L temporal DNET	L temporal	L temporal	F7 T1	L temporal	Not done	Yes	2	27	DNET	187
4	F/56/8	R parietooccipito-temporal	Sturge-Weber	R temporal	Superficial angioma and hemiatrophy R posterior convexity	R parietooccipito-temporal	Not done	F8	R frontocentral	Not done	Planned				156
5	M/20/7	L temporopari-etal	Unknown	Temporal	L parietal gliosis after surgery	L temporopari-etal	Not done	T5	L posterotem-poral	Concordant	Overlap eloquent cx				15
6	F/34/15	R frontal	FCD	R extratemporal	R frontal FCD	R frontal	R frontal	Cz C4	R centroparietal	Concordant	Yes	2	22	Gliosis, neuronal loss, microglia activation	853
7	F/55/38	L anterior temporal	HS	L temporal	L HS	L temporal	L temporal	F7 T1	L temporal	Not done	Yes	1	27	HS	156
8	F/61/12	L frontal	FCD	L frontal	L frontal FCD	L frontal	Not done	C3 Cz	L frontocentral	Not done	Overlap eloquent cx				915
9	M/29/27	R frontal	FCD	R frontal	R frontal FCD	R frontal	Not done	F4	R frontocentral	Concordant	Yes	1	5	FCD	64
10	M/30/15	R temporal	Unknown	Temporal	Normal	R temporal	Not done	F8 T4	R temporal	Not done	Planned				733
11	F/23/2	L temporal	FCD	Temporal	L temporal FCD	L temporal	L temporal	F7 T1	L temporal	Not done	Refusal				181
12	F/23/9	L parietooccip-ital	Perinatal infarction	Extratemporal	L medial cerebral artery infarction	L parietal	L parietooccip-ital	O1	Midcentral	Not done	Yes	1	2	No significant abnormali-ties	398
13	F/33/6	L temporooc-cipital	FCD	L posterior quadrant	L posterior temporal FCD	L occipitotem-poral	L occipital	T3 T5	L posterior	Not done	Overlap eloquent cx				1613
14	M/16/7	R frontal	FCD	R frontoparietal	R mesial frontal FCD	R frontal	Frontoparietal	Cz	R and midcentral	Concordant	Overlap eloquent cx				2018
15	F/40/1	L parietal	FCD	Extratemporal	L parietal FCD	L parietal	Not done	Pz	L and midcentral	Not done	Overlap eloquent cx				589

(Continued)

Table 1 | Continued

Patient	Gender/ age/ age at onset	Ictal onset zone	Etiology	Symptomato-genic zone	Structural MRI	SISCOM localization	Interictal ^{18}F-FDG PET hypometa-bolism	Scalp interictal spike locali-zation$	Scalp ictal EEG localization	icEEG	Epilepsy surgery	ILAE out-come	Follow-up time after surgery (m)	Pathology	Spike-rate (spikes/h) during fMRI
16	F/43/12	L anterior temporal	HS	L temporal	L HS	L temporal	L temporal	F7T1	L temporal	Not done	Yes (radiosurgery)	1	10	Not available	73
17	F/30/14	R temporal	Ganglioglioma	R temporal	R temporal ganglioglioma	Not done	R temporal	F8	R temporal	Not done	Yes	1	8	Ganglioglioma	115
18	M/20/8	L anterior temporal	HS	Temporal	L HS	Not done	L temporal	F7T1	L temporofrontal	Not done	Yes	1	3	HS	8
19	F/45/19	R temporal	Unknown	R temporal	Normal	R temporal	R temporal	F8T2	R temporal	Not done	Refusal				168
20	F/56/32	R temporal	HS	R temporal	R HS	R temporal	R temporal	F8T2	R temporal	Not done	Refusal				602
21	F/30/0	L temporal	HS	L temporal	L HS	L temporal	L temporal	F7T1	L temporal	Not done	Planned				40

SISCOM, subtraction ictal SPECT co-registered to MRI; $ international 10–20 EEG-system (additional T1 and T2 electrodes); icEEG, intracranial EEG-recordings; ILAE outcome (35) for available follow-up, F, female; M, male; R, right; L, left; CNS, central nervous system; DNET, dysembryoplastic neuroepithelial tumor; FCD, focal cortical dysplasia; HS, hippocampal sclerosis; cx, cortex.

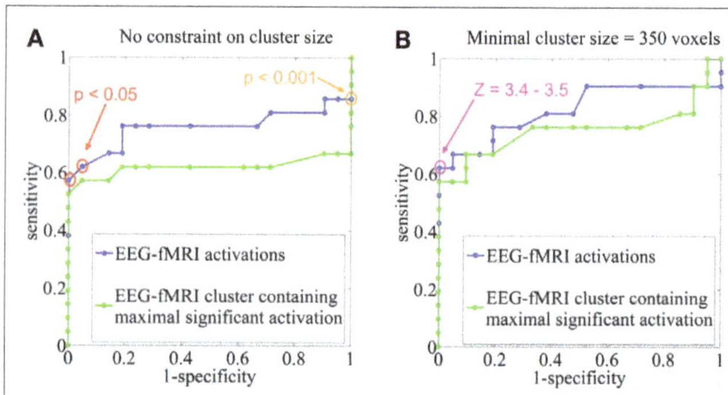

FIGURE 3 | Sensitivity and specificity. Receiver operating characteristic (ROC)-curves using different statistical Z-score thresholds at the voxel level (range, 0–13; step-size, 0.1) and **(A)** no constraint on cluster size, **(B)** a minimal cluster extent of 350 voxels. The results were based on all EEG-fMRI activations (blue) and upon the cluster containing the maximal significant activation only (green). The orange circle corresponds to the statistical threshold of uncorrected $p < 0.001$ ($Z = 3.1$), red circles to a significance level of FWE corrected $p < 0.05$ ($Z = 4.9$–5.1). The pink circle represents Z-score thresholds of 3.4 and 3.5. Note that not every change in Z-score threshold is associated with a change in sensitivity and specificity.

mainly located in mesial occipital areas. Patient 6, with a focal cortical dysplasia in the right primary motor cortex, had a contralateral cerebellar activation (**Figure 5**). Successful radiosurgery involved the left hippocampus in patient 16 with left hippocampal sclerosis. Additional BOLD activations were present in the left temporal neocortex.

In an additional analysis, we looked at the cluster containing the maximal significant BOLD activation. This resulted in similar sensitivity and specificity when using the same minimal cluster extent of 350 voxels (**Figure 3**). A sensitivity of 57% and a specificity of 100% were obtained for a broad range of Z-score thresholds from 3.2 to 3.5 (green areas in **Figure 5**). Interestingly, this combination of sensitivity and specificity could also be reached using other settings for minimal cluster size (from 250 voxels up to 600 voxels) but with a smaller range of corresponding Z-score thresholds. By using the cluster containing the maximal significant activation instead of all EEG-fMRI activations, we discarded the additional, non-localizing clusters (blue areas in **Figure 4**) distant from the IOZ with sacrificing minimal sensitivity (4.8%) at 100% specificity. Only 1 of 21 patients (4.8%) (patient 15) showed a BOLD activation cluster overlapping the IOZ, which did not contain the maximal significant activation (**Figure 5**).

Finally, when using the maximal significant activation voxel or when considering BOLD deactivations, an overall low performance was found.

DISCUSSION

Electroencephalography-functional magnetic resonance imaging has evolved from a research tool and is on the brink of becoming a clinical method to delineate the ictal onset in the presurgical evaluation of patients with refractory focal epilepsy. Before taking decisions based on EEG-fMRI, validation studies are a prerequisite. We felt that it was important to investigate sensitivity and specificity of interictal EEG-fMRI for localizing the IOZ, in those

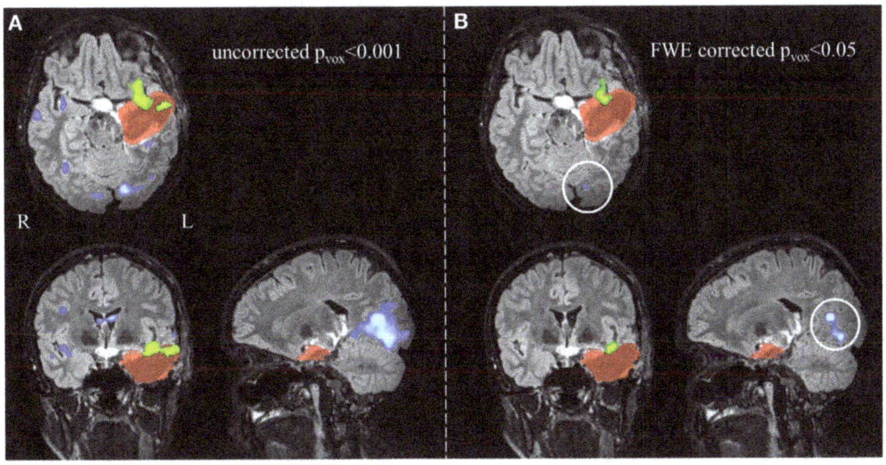

FIGURE 4 | Electroencephalography-functional magnetic resonance imaging activations are overlaid on representative slices of the postsurgical structural image of patient 3 (A) after thresholding at an uncorrected $p < 0.001$ ($Z = 3.1$, no constraint on cluster size) and (B) at a FWE corrected $p < 0.05$ ($Z = 5.1$, no constraint on cluster size). **(A)** The EEG-fMRI cluster containing the maximal significant activation (green colored) is overlapping the IOZ (red colored). Widespread additional suprathreshold activation clusters (blue colored) are present. At these settings, it is unclear whether these activations outside the IOZ represent false- or true-positive activations. **(B)** Using a more stringent statistical threshold (corresponding to 100% specificity), fewer activation clusters survive. The left occipital activation (white circle) is not a false-positive but a true-positive detection and is considered part of a spike-related network; R, right; L, left.

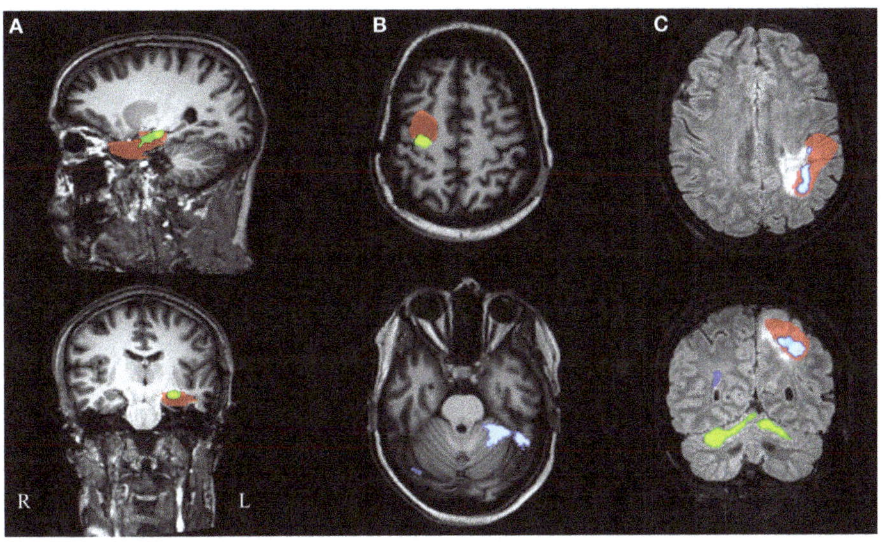

FIGURE 5 | Electroencephalography-functional magnetic resonance imaging results after thresholding at $Z = 3.5$ at the voxel level combined with a minimal cluster extent of 350 voxels are overlaid on representative slices of the structural MRI in three patients. **(A)** Patient 16 had only 1 suprathreshold activation. This cluster containing the maximal significant activation (green colored) was localized within the IOZ (red colored). **(B)** In patient 6, the cluster containing the maximal significant activation (green colored) was overlapping the IOZ, while an additional activation cluster (blue colored) was situated within the contralateral cerebellum. **(C)** Patient 15 was the only patient with a BOLD activation cluster (blue colored) overlapping the IOZ, which did not contain the maximal significant activation (green colored); R, right; L, left.

patients in whom spikes were visually detected during EEG-fMRI. A reliable test combines a high sensitivity with a high specificity.

SPECIFICITY

The setting of an appropriate statistical threshold in functional imaging is a critical point (6, 32, 46, 47). EEG-fMRI validation studies focused on sensitivity for detecting the IOZ, using "standard" statistical thresholds, but the specificity of these results is still largely unknown. fMRI responses exceeding the epileptogenic zone are often reported (17, 48, 49). A possible explanation may be the choice of a low statistical threshold resulting in false-positive responses (25) and understanding how to minimize these false positives would be of great interest (50). On the other hand, it is not excluded that hemodynamic changes outside the IOZ are related to an epileptic network. Hence, it would not be appropriate to consider hemodynamic changes, associated to spikes in patients and localized partially within and partially outside the IOZ, as false positives. To tackle this issue, we chose to determine false-positive and true-negative cases in age- and gender-matched healthy case-controls. The interictal spike event-related regressor of the patient was used in the design matrix of the healthy case-control (corresponding to nonsense events for this control subject). False-positive cases were those controls who showed a suprathreshold BOLD change in the brain while true-negative cases were those controls for whom this was not the case. As argued before, we treated controls as a surrogate for the patient group with the assumption that results would have been the same if we were able to look at those parts of the brain that were not linked to the epileptic network. The surrogate specificity was subsequently determined as the proportion of true-negative cases within the control group. A disadvantage of our approach is the unknown contribution of differences in noise level between patient and control datasets.

Alternatively, false-positive and true-negative rates could be established in the patient group after random annotation of spike onsets (2). Specificity would then equal the proportion of patients who lack a suprathreshold BOLD fluctuation in the brain, related to these nonsense events. The calculation of true-positive and false-negative rates could remain unchanged, based on real spike onsets. This approach holds two potential risks. In patients with high spike rates, coincidental correlation between regressors related to nonsense events and to real spikes becomes more likely, causing an overestimation of false-positive rates. This problem does not apply in healthy volunteers. A second risk is related to the poorly understood occurrence in time of epileptic spikes. It is not excluded that this occurrence follows a rhythmic pattern, which exhibits (whether or not coincidental) temporal similarities with activity fluctuations of normal physiological brain processes. In that case, random assignment of spike onsets would break this rhythmicity and potentially cause an underestimation of false-positive rates. When we copy the regressor-of-interest to healthy volunteers, this rhythmicity remains unmodified. Notwithstanding the concerns of the alternative method described above, permutation of original spike onsets led to similar sensitivity and specificity (see alternative approach, included as Supplementary Material).

To the best of our knowledge, only three papers formally addressed the topic of specificity of interictal EEG-fMRI in a quantitative way. First, Waites and colleagues used a non-parametric permutation approach in two patients with childhood absence epilepsy and one healthy control to investigate if interictal discharges lead to a BOLD response that is significantly different from chance (2). It was shown that "activations" (at a corrected $p < 0.05$), related to randomly assigned events, survived more often than expected by chance (i.e., more than 1 in 20). Second, Flanagan and colleagues evaluated the effect of including non-epileptic sharp EEG transients in the EEG-fMRI analysis of clear epileptic spikes (51). These events can result in physiologically plausible BOLD changes that survive a statistical threshold (in both the patient and control group). Third, An and colleagues determined sensitivity and specificity of EEG-fMRI through a different approach, using surgical outcome as "ground truth" (32). True-positive (concordance with resection zone and good surgical outcome) and false-negative (discordance with resection zone and good surgical outcome) fractions were determined in the patients, as were true-negative (discordance with resection zone and poor surgical outcome) and false-positive (concordance with resection zone and poor surgical outcome) fractions. However, poor surgical outcome could have several reasons (incorrect location of surgery, correct location but intra- or post-operative complications, partial resection of the epileptogenic zone, and no resectable epileptogenic zone), leading to equivocal interpretation of the results (52). This is the reason why we established sensitivity only in successfully operated or well-defined patients, taking the (effective or hypothetical) resection zone as central point (patients with poor surgical outcome were not included). On the other hand, specificity was defined in healthy case-controls, taking absence of epileptic activity as "ground truth."

Different statistical thresholds (uncorrected $p < 0.001$ and FWE corrected $p < 0.05$, for instance) can result in very divergent specificities and sensitivities. This information is crucial as these thresholds are commonly reported in EEG-fMRI validation studies. We argue that EEG-fMRI outcome studies should be reported with settings that have maximal specificity. However, when the purpose of EEG-fMRI is to guide the implantation of intracranial electrodes, a high sensitivity might be preferred (17).

THE CLUSTER CONTAINING THE MAXIMAL SIGNIFICANT ACTIVATION

The presence of multiple clusters of BOLD activation raises an important question: how can we identify the cluster overlapping the IOZ in a highly specific but often widespread interictal epileptic network without prior knowledge of the IOZ? The cluster, containing the maximal significant BOLD activation, with a minimal cluster size of 350 voxels, and with a broad range of Z-score thresholds from 3.2 to 3.5, had 57% sensitivity and 100% specificity for localizing the IOZ, similar to the accuracy of all EEG-fMRI activation clusters. The performance of this unique cluster was robust and did not critically depend on a single Z-score or cluster size threshold. Our findings confirm the observations that the cluster containing the maximal significant activation is important in the localization of the IOZ (45).

We considered two other aspects of the EEG-fMRI maps. First, the maximal significant activation voxel had a lower performance for localizing the IOZ compared with the cluster containing this voxel. In some patients, this voxel was localized at the border, but just outside the IOZ, while in others, it was found more remote. Hauf and colleagues (46) ascribed similar findings of distant fMRI peak activations to the effect of propagation. Second, deactivations were only infrequently found inside the IOZ, consistent with other reports (21, 53).

INVOLVEMENT OF REMOTE REGIONS: AN EPILEPTIC NETWORK

There is a bulk of evidence that so called "focal" epilepsies are not strictly localized to well-circumscribed focal brain areas, but constitute larger epileptic networks (42, 43). When using a setting of high specificity (100%), almost half the patients with an activation overlapping the IOZ had at least one additional activation cluster in more distant areas. These remote findings can be considered as true positives. Activations at a distance have been interpreted as an extended or multifocal IOZ (10, 21). However, the presence of these remote activations did not preclude successful surgical outcome in three operated patients in our study. Therefore, spike-related BOLD clusters distant to the IOZ could also represent areas of propagated activity, as suggested by different authors (6, 25, 54, 55).

VALIDITY OF THE ICTAL ONSET ZONE DEFINITION

Seizure freedom and good functional outcome are the ultimate goals of epilepsy surgery. So far, 8 of the 21 patients underwent successful surgery, and we considered the resection zone as IOZ. The extent of the resection zone depends on the surgical approach and can overestimate the actual IOZ. We have shown that only about one-quarter of resected brain tissue overlapped the structural lesion or SISCOM hyperperfusion cluster (27). However, after successful surgery, sufficient brain tissue has been resected.

Thirteen patients are awaiting surgery, refused surgery, or were ineligible for surgery due to proximity of the IOZ to eloquent regions. In this non-operated group, we chose to define the IOZ as the hypothetical resection zone, based on multidisciplinary clinical consensus and regardless of eloquent cortex. As already mentioned, a prerequisite for inclusion was concordance of all modalities, including electroclinical information, structural imaging, SISCOM, FDG PET, and intracranial EEG-recordings. Multimodal concordant seizure focus localizing data increase the likelihood of benefit from surgical treatment (56–58). To avoid a rater-dependent bias in the manual delineation, we restricted the volume of the IOZ to the region of ictal hyperperfusion within this hypothetical resection zone. In our center, ictal and interictal SPECT are part of the presurgical work-up. SISCOM has several advantages: (i) it samples the whole brain, which offers an ideal comparison with the results of EEG-fMRI, (ii) it displays relative changes in cerebral blood perfusion associated with neuronal metabolic activity, (iii) a SISCOM Z-threshold = 1.5 results in optimal localization of the IOZ (36), (iv) it is a non-invasive test, and (v) early ictal tracer injections, as achieved in most of our patients, are known to be related to correct localization of the IOZ (59).

LIMITATIONS

We stress that sensitivity and specificity calculations only apply to patients in whom spikes were found during EEG-fMRI. In two patients, more than one spike-type (based on topography) was found during fMRI. In these cases, we decided to determine the results driven by the most frequent spike-type during video-telemetry only, similar to Elshoff and colleagues (26). High correlations between the localization of the lobe producing the most active spiking and that of the IOZ have been found for temporal lobe epilepsies (60). Moreover, it was shown that the lobe producing the most active spiking correlated highly with the ultimately resected lobe harboring cortical dysplasia (61).

The number of successfully operated patients and their follow-up period is limited. To increase the group size, a surrogate for the effective resection zone was adopted in those patients who could not undergo surgery. This allowed us to study a representative and larger sample of patients with a well-defined IOZ after a presurgical evaluation. Studies including larger number of patients and control subjects will be required to fine-tune EEG-fMRI settings. Furthermore, this could allow subpopulations (TLE versus ETLE) to be studied, as sensitivity and specificity are presumably also dependent on brain localization.

CONCLUSION

High sensitivity and specificity of spike-related EEG-fMRI for the detection of the IOZ are crucial for the clinical implementation of the technique in the presurgical planning of refractory focal epilepsy. Our data provide a guideline for different EEG-fMRI settings with their respective sensitivity and specificity for detecting the IOZ. Using optimal settings, we found that the unique cluster containing the maximal significant BOLD activation was a sensitive (57%) and specific (100%) marker of the IOZ.

AUTHOR CONTRIBUTIONS

Substantial contributions to the conception or design of the work; or the acquisition, analysis, or interpretation of data for the work: Simon Tousseyn, Patrick Dupont, Karolien Goffin, Stefan Sunaert, and Wim Van Paesschen; drafting the work or revising it critically for important intellectual content: Simon Tousseyn, Patrick Dupont, Karolien Goffin, Stefan Sunaert, and Wim Van Paesschen; final approval of the version to be published: Simon Tousseyn, Patrick Dupont, Karolien Goffin, Stefan Sunaert, and Wim Van Paesschen; agreement to be accountable for all aspects of the work in ensuring that questions related to the accuracy or integrity of any part of the work are appropriately investigated and resolved: Simon Tousseyn, Patrick Dupont, Karolien Goffin, Stefan Sunaert, Wim Van Paesschen.

ACKNOWLEDGMENTS

We acknowledge discussions with Maarten De Vos, Borbola Hunyadi, Ronald Peeters, David Robben, Laura Seynaeve and Katrien Vanderperren. We thank Bart De Dobbelaer for software support. The authors are grateful to Guido Van Driel and the epilepsy monitoring team for helping to collect the EEG data. This study was funded by a grant for Applied Biomedical Research (TBM) no. 080658 from the Flemish government agency for Innovation by Science and Technology (IWT); grant no. G.048010N from Fonds Wetenschappelijk Onderzoek-Vlaanderen; grant no. IUAP EMF-B6772-p6/29 from Inter-University-Attraction-Pole; and Belspo IAP grant P7/11 and grant no. FPV10/008 from Excellentie-Financiering.

REFERENCES

1. Rosenow F, Lüders H. Presurgical evaluation of epilepsy. *Brain* (2001) **124**:1683–700. doi:10.1093/brain/124.9.1683
2. Waites AB, Shaw ME, Briellmann RS, Labate A, Abbott DF, Jackson GD. How reliable are fMRI-EEG studies of epilepsy? A nonparametric approach to analysis validation and optimization. *Neuroimage* (2005) **24**:192–9. doi:10.1016/j.neuroimage.2004.09.005

3. Laufs H, Duncan JS. Electroencephalography/functional MRI in human epilepsy: what it currently can and cannot do. *Curr Opin Neurol* (2007) **20**:417–23. doi:10.1097/WCO.0b013e3282202b92
4. Krakow K, Woermann FG, Symms MR, Allen PJ, Lemieux L, Barker GJ, et al. EEG-triggered functional MRI of interictal epileptiform activity in patients with partial seizures. *Brain* (1999) **122**:1679–88. doi:10.1093/brain/122.9.1679
5. Lazeyras F, Blanke O, Perrig S, Zimine I, Golay X, Delavelle J, et al. EEG-triggered functional MRI in patients with pharmacoresistant epilepsy. *J Magn Reson Imaging* (2000) **12**:177–85. doi:10.1002/1522-2586(200007)12:1<177::AID-JMRI20>3.0.CO;2-3
6. Al-Asmi A, Bénar CG, Gross DW, Khani YA, Andermann F, Pike B, et al. fMRI activation in continuous and spike-triggered EEG-fMRI studies of epileptic spikes. *Epilepsia* (2003) **44**:1328–39. doi:10.1046/j.1528-1157.2003.01003.x
7. Bagshaw AP, Aghakhani Y, Bénar CG, Kobayashi E, Hawco C, Dubeau F, et al. EEG-fMRI of focal epileptic spikes: analysis with multiple haemodynamic functions and comparison with gadolinium-enhanced MR angiograms. *Hum Brain Mapp* (2004) **22**:179–92. doi:10.1002/hbm.20024
8. Bénar CG, Grova C, Kobayashi E, Bagshaw AP, Aghakhani Y, Dubeau F, et al. EEG-fMRI of epileptic spikes: concordance with EEG source localization and intracranial EEG. *Neuroimage* (2006) **30**:1161–70. doi:10.1016/j.neuroimage.2005.11.008
9. De Tiège X, Laufs H, Boyd SG, Harkness W, Allen PJ, Clark CA, et al. EEG-fMRI in children with pharmacoresistant focal epilepsy. *Epilepsia* (2007) **48**:385–9. doi:10.1111/j.1528-1167.2006.00951.x
10. Zijlmans M, Huiskamp G, Hersevoort M, Seppenwoolde JH, van Huffelen AC, Leijten FS. EEG-fMRI in the preoperative work-up for epilepsy surgery. *Brain* (2007) **130**:2343–53. doi:10.1093/brain/awm141
11. Tyvaert L, Hawco C, Kobayashi E, LeVan P, Dubeau F, Gotman J. Different structures involved during ictal and interictal epileptic activity in malformations of cortical development: an EEG-fMRI study. *Brain* (2008) **131**:2042–60. doi:10.1093/brain/awn145
12. Moeller F, Tyvaert L, Nguyen DK, LeVan P, Bouthillier A, Kobayashi E, et al. EEG-fMRI: adding to standard evaluations of patients with nonlesional frontal lobe epilepsy. *Neurology* (2009) **73**:2023–30. doi:10.1212/WNL.0b013e3181c55d17
13. Vulliemoz S, Rodionov R, Carmichael DW, Thornton R, Guye M, Lhatoo SD, et al. Continuous EEG source imaging enhances analysis of EEG-fMRI in focal epilepsy. *Neuroimage* (2010) **49**:3219–29. doi:10.1016/j.neuroimage.2009.11.055
14. Grouiller F, Thornton RC, Groening K, Spinelli L, Duncan JS, Schaller K, et al. With or without spikes: localization of focal epileptic activity by simultaneous electroencephalography and functional magnetic resonance imaging. *Brain* (2011) **134**:2867–86. doi:10.1093/brain/awr156
15. Zhang J, Liu W, Chen H, Xia H, Zhou Z, Wang L, et al. EEG-fMRI validation studies in comparison with icEEG: a review. *Int J Psychophysiol* (2012) **84**:233–9. doi:10.1016/j.ijpsycho.2012.01.021
16. Donaire A, Capdevila A, Carreño M, Setoain X, Rumià J, Aparicio J, et al. Identifying the cortical substrates of interictal epileptiform activity in patients with extratemporal epilepsy: an EEG-fMRI sequential analysis and FDG-PET study. *Epilepsia* (2013) **54**(4):678–90. doi:10.1111/epi.12091
17. van Houdt PJ, de Munck JC, Leijten FS, Huiskamp GJ, Colon AJ, Boon PA, et al. EEG-fMRI correlation patterns in the presurgical evaluation of focal epilepsy: a comparison with electrocorticographic data and surgical outcome measures. *Neuroimage* (2013) **75**:238–48. doi:10.1016/j.neuroimage.2013.02.033
18. Wang ZI, Jin K, Kakisaka Y, Mosher JC, Bingaman WE, Kotagal P, et al. Imag(in)ing seizure propagation: MEG-guided interpretation of epileptic activity from a deep source. *Hum Brain Mapp* (2012) **33**:2797–801. doi:10.1002/hbm.21401
19. Siegel AM, Roberts DW, Thadani VM, McInerney J, Jobst BC, Williamson PD. The role of intracranial electrode reevaluation in epilepsy patients after failed initial invasive monitoring. *Epilepsia* (2000) **41**:571–80. doi:10.1111/j.1528-1157.2000.tb00211.x
20. Kobayashi E, Bagshaw AP, Grova C, Gotman J, Dubeau F. Grey matter heterotopia: what EEG-fMRI can tell us about epileptogenicity of neuronal migration disorders. *Brain* (2006) **129**:366–74. doi:10.1093/brain/awh710
21. Thornton R, Vulliemoz S, Rodionov R, Carmichael DW, Chaudhary UJ, Diehl B, et al. Epileptic networks in focal cortical dysplasia revealed using electroencephalography-functional magnetic resonance imaging. *Ann Neurol* (2011) **70**:822–37. doi:10.1002/ana.22535
22. Pittau F, Dubeau F, Gotman J. Contribution of EEG/fMRI to the definition of the epileptic focus. *Neurology* (2012) **78**:1479–87. doi:10.1212/WNL.0b013e3182553bf7
23. van Houdt PJ, Ossenblok PP, Colon AJ, Boon PA, de Munck JC. A framework to integrate EEG-correlated fMRI and intracerebral recordings. *Neuroimage* (2012) **60**:2042–53. doi:10.1016/j.neuroimage.2012.02.023
24. Jann K, Wiest R, Hauf M, Meyer K, Boesch C, Mathis J, et al. BOLD correlates of continuously fluctuating epileptic activity isolated by independent component analysis. *Neuroimage* (2008) **42**:635–48. doi:10.1016/j.neuroimage.2008.05.001
25. Groening K, Brodbeck V, Moeller F, Wolff S, van Baalen A, Michel CM, et al. Combination of EEG-fMRI and EEG source analysis improves interpretation of spike-associated activation networks in paediatric pharmacoresistant focal epilepsies. *Neuroimage* (2009) **46**:827–33. doi:10.1016/j.neuroimage.2009.02.026
26. Elshoff L, Groening K, Grouiller F, Wiegand G, Wolff S, Michel C, et al. The value of EEG-fMRI and EEG source analysis in the presurgical setup of children with refractory focal epilepsy. *Epilepsia* (2012) **53**:1597–606. doi:10.1111/j.1528-1167.2012.03587.x
27. Dupont P, Van Paesschen W, Palmini A, Ambayi R, Van Loon J, Goffin J, et al. Ictal perfusion patterns associated with single MRI-visible focal dysplastic lesions: implications for the noninvasive delineation of the epileptogenic zone. *Epilepsia* (2006) **47**:1550–7. doi:10.1111/j.1528-1167.2006.00628.x
28. Huberfeld G, Habert MO, Clemenceau S, Maksud P, Baulac M, Adam C. Ictal brain hyperperfusion contralateral to seizure onset: the SPECT mirror image. *Epilepsia* (2006) **47**:123–33. doi:10.1111/j.1528-1167.2006.00378.x
29. Van Paesschen W, Dupont P, Sunaert S, Goffin K, Van Laere K. The use of SPECT and PET in routine clinical practice in epilepsy. *Curr Opin Neurol* (2007) **20**:194–202. doi:10.1097/WCO.0b013e328042baf6
30. Jacobs J, Dubeau F, Olivier A, Andermann F. Pathways of seizure propagation from the temporal to the occipital lobe. *Epileptic Disord* (2008) **10**:266–70. doi:10.1684/epd.2008.0217
31. Thornton R, Laufs H, Rodionov R, Cannadathu S, Carmichael DW, Vulliemoz S, et al. EEG correlated functional MRI and postoperative outcome in focal epilepsy. *J Neurol Neurosurg Psychiatry* (2010) **81**:922–7. doi:10.1136/jnnp.2009.196253
32. An D, Fahoum F, Hall J, Olivier A, Gotman J, Dubeau F. Electroencephalography/functional magnetic resonance imaging responses help predict surgical outcome in focal epilepsy. *Epilepsia* (2013) **54**(12):2184–94. doi:10.1111/epi.12434
33. Okonma SV, Blount JP, Gross RE. Planning extent of resection in epilepsy: limited versus large resections. *Epilepsy Behav* (2011) **20**:233–40. doi:10.1016/j.yebeh.2010.09.036
34. Chaudhary UJ, Rodionov R, Carmichael DW, Thornton RC, Duncan JS, Lemieux L. Improving the sensitivity of EEG-fMRI studies of epileptic activity by modelling eye blinks, swallowing and other video-EEG detected physiological confounds. *Neuroimage* (2012) **61**:1383–93. doi:10.1016/j.neuroimage.2012.03.028
35. Wieser HG, Blume WT, Fish D, Goldensohn E, Hufnagel A, King D, et al. ILAE Commission Report. Proposal for a new classification of outcome with respect to epileptic seizures following epilepsy surgery. *Epilepsia* (2001) **42**:282–6. doi:10.1046/j.1528-1157.2001.4220282.x
36. Newey CR, Wong C, Wang ZI, Wu G, Alexopoulos AV. Optimizing SPECT SISCOM analysis to localize seizure-onset zone by using varying z scores. *Epilepsia* (2013) **54**(4):793–800. doi:10.1111/epi.12139
37. Allen PJ, Josephs O, Turner R. A method for removing imaging artifact from continuous EEG recorded during functional MRI. *Neuroimage* (2000) **12**:230–9. doi:10.1006/nimg.2000.0599
38. Allen PJ, Polizzi G, Krakow K, Fish DR, Lemieux L. Identification of EEG events in the MR scanner: the problem of pulse artifact and a method for its subtraction. *Neuroimage* (1998) **8**:229–39. doi:10.1006/nimg.1998.0361
39. Fox MD, Snyder AZ, Vincent JL, Corbetta M, Van Essen DC, Raichle ME. The human brain is intrinsically organized into dynamic, anticorrelated functional networks. *Proc Natl Acad Sci U S A* (2005) **102**(27):9673–8. doi:10.1073/pnas.0504136102
40. Salek-Haddadi A, Dielh B, Hamandi K, Merschhemke M, Liston A, Friston K, et al. Hemodynamic correlates of epileptiform discharges: an EEG-fMRI study of 63 patients with focal epilepsy. *Brain Res* (2006) **1088**:148–66. doi:10.1016/j.brainres.2006.02.098

41. Lemieux L, Salek-Haddadi A, Lund TE, Laufs H, Carmichael D. Modelling large motion events in fMRI studies of patients with epilepsy. *Magn Reson Imaging* (2007) **25**:894–901. doi:10.1016/j.mri.2007.03.009
42. Spencer SS. Neural networks in human epilepsy: evidence of and implications for treatment. *Epilepsia* (2002) **43**:219–27. doi:10.1046/j.1528-1157.2002.26901.x
43. Laufs H. Functional imaging of seizures and epilepsy: evolution from zones to networks. *Curr Opin Neurol* (2012) **25**:194–200. doi:10.1097/WCO.0b013e3283515db9
44. Van Paesschen W. Qualitative and quantitative imaging of the hippocampus in mesial temporal lobe epilepsy with hippocampal sclerosis. *Neuroimaging Clin N Am* (2004) **14**:373–400. doi:10.1016/j.nic.2004.04.004
45. Liu Y, Yang T, Yang X, Liu I, Liao W, Lui S, et al. EEG-fMRI study of the interictal epileptic activity in patients with partial epilepsy. *J Neurol Sci* (2008) **268**:117–23. doi:10.1016/j.jns.2007.11.019
46. Hauf M, Jann K, Schindler K, Scheidegger O, Meyer K, Rummel C, et al. Localizing seizure-onset zones in presurgical evaluation of drug-resistant epilepsy by electroencephalography/fMRI: effectiveness of alternative thresholding strategies. *AJNR Am J Neuroradiol* (2012) **33**:1818–24. doi:10.3174/ajnr.A3052
47. Van Paesschen W. Ictal SPECT. *Epilepsia* (2004) **45**(Suppl 4):35–40. doi:10.1111/j.0013-9580.2004.04008.x
48. Salek-Haddadi A, Diehl B, Hamandi K, Merschhemke M, Liston A, Friston K, et al. Hemodynamic correlates of epileptiform discharges: an EEG-fMRI study of 63 patients with focal epilepsy. *Brain Res* (2006) **1088**:148–66. doi:10.1016/j.brainres.2006.02.098
49. Kobayashi E, Bagshaw AP, Bénar CG, Aghakhani Y, Andermann F, Dubeau F, et al. Temporal and extratemporal BOLD responses to temporal lobe interictal spikes. *Epilepsia* (2006) **47**:343–54. doi:10.1111/j.1528-1167.2006.00427.x
50. Richardson M. Current themes in neuroimaging of epilepsy: brain networks, dynamic phenomena, and clinical relevance. *Clin Neurophysiol* (2010) **121**:1153–75. doi:10.1016/j.clinph.2010.01.004
51. Flanagan D, Abbott DF, Jackson GD. How wrong can we be? The effect of inaccurate mark-up of EEG/fMRI studies in epilepsy. *Clin Neurophysiol* (2009) **120**:1637–47. doi:10.1016/j.clinph.2009.04.025
52. Burch J, Marson A, Beyer F, Soares M, Hinde S, Wieshmann U, et al. Dilemmas in the interpretation of diagnostic accuracy studies on presurgical workup for epilepsy surgery. *Epilepsia* (2012) **53**(8):1294–302. doi:10.1111/j.1528-1167.2012.03534.x
53. Pittau F, Fahoum F, Zelmann R, Dubeau F, Gotman J. Negative BOLD response to interictal epileptic discharges in focal epilepsy. *Brain Topogr* (2013) **26**(4):627–40. doi:10.1007/s10548-013-0302-1
54. Hamandi K, Powell HW, Laufs H, Symms MR, Barker GJ, Parker GJ, et al. Combined EEG-fMRI and tractography to visualise propagation of epileptic activity. *J Neurol Neurosurg Psychiatry* (2008) **79**:594–7. doi:10.1136/jnnp.2007.125401
55. Vulliemoz S, Thornton R, Rodionov R, Carmichael DW, Guye M, Lhatoo S, et al. The spatio-temporal mapping of epileptic networks: combination of EEG-fMRI and EEG source imaging. *Neuroimage* (2009) **46**:834–43. doi:10.1016/j.neuroimage.2009.01.070
56. So EL. Integration of EEG, MRI, and SPECT in localizing the seizure focus for epilepsy surgery. *Epilepsia* (2000) **41**(Suppl 3):S48–54. doi:10.1111/j.1528-1157.2000.tb01534.x
57. Labiner DM, Weinand ME, Brainerd CJ, Ahern GL, Herring AM, Melgar MA. Prognostic value of concordant seizure focus localizing data in the selection of temporal lobectomy candidates. *Neurol Res* (2002) **24**:747–55. doi:10.1179/016164102101200843
58. Kurian M, Spinelli L, Delavelle J, Willi JP, Velazquez M, Chaves V, et al. Multimodality imaging for focus localization in pediatric pharmacoresistant epilepsy. *Epileptic Disord* (2007) **9**:20–31. doi:10.1684/epd.2007.0070
59. Lee SK, Lee SY, Yun CH, Lee HY, Lee JS, Lee DS. Ictal SPECT in neocortical epilepsies: clinical usefulness and factors affecting the pattern of hyperperfusion. *Neuroradiology* (2006) **48**:678–84. doi:10.1007/s00234-006-0106-z
60. Blume WT, Borghesi JL, Lemieux JF. Interictal indices of temporal seizure origin. *Ann Neurol* (1993) **34**:703–9. doi:10.1002/ana.410340513
61. Jiang YJ, Ang LC, Blume WT. Extent of EEG epileptiform pattern distribution in "focal" cortical dysplasia. *J Clin Neurophysiol* (2010) **27**:309–11. doi:10.1097/WNP.0b013e3181f38693

15

Constructing carbon fiber motion-detection loops for simultaneous EEG–fMRI

David F. Abbott[1,2], Richard A. J. Masterton[1,2], John S. Archer[1,2,3], Steven W. Fleming[1], Aaron E. L. Warren[1,2] and Graeme D. Jackson[1,2,3]*

[1] The Florey Institute of Neuroscience and Mental Health, Austin Hospital, Melbourne, VIC, Australia
[2] The University of Melbourne, Melbourne, VIC, Australia
[3] Austin Hospital, Melbourne, VIC, Australia

***Correspondence:**
Graeme D. Jackson, Florey Institute of Neuroscience and Mental Health, Melbourne Brain Centre, 245 Burgundy Street, Heidelberg, VIC 3084, Australia
e-mail: BRI@brain.org.au

One of the most significant impediments to high-quality EEG recorded in an MRI scanner is subject motion. Availability of motion artifact sensors can substantially improve the quality of the recorded EEG. In the study of epilepsy, it can also dramatically increase the confidence that one has in discriminating true epileptiform activity from artifact. This is due both to the reduction in artifact and the ability to visually inspect the motion sensor signals when reading the EEG, revealing whether or not head motion is present. We have previously described the use of carbon fiber loops for detecting and correcting artifact in EEG acquired simultaneously with MRI. The loops, attached to the subject's head, are electrically insulated from the scalp. They provide a simple and direct measure of specific artifact that is contaminating the EEG, including both subject motion and residual artifact arising from magnetic field gradients applied during MRI. Our previous implementation was used together with a custom-built EEG–fMRI system that differs substantially from current commercially available EEG–fMRI systems. The present technical note extends this work, describing in more detail how to construct the carbon fiber motion-detection loops, and how to interface them with a commercially available simultaneous EEG–fMRI system. We hope that the information provided may help those wishing to utilize a motion-detection/correction solution to improve the quality of EEG recorded within an MRI scanner.

Keywords: EEG–fMRI, motion detection, cardioballistic artifact, cardioballistic artefact, gradient artifact, gradient artefact, artifact removal, artefact removal

SAFETY WARNING

This technical note describes construction and application of carbon fiber motion-detection leads. We have used these for simultaneous EEG–fMRI experiments, where a number of safety measures that are not detailed in this document have been taken to avoid inducing large currents causing injury. If you are considering use of similar equipment in an environment such as an MRI scanner then it is essential that you understand the safety implications. We recommend you to consult the literature for further information, for example, Ref. (1–3). We have used our leads with an EEG system that we developed in-house, and with commercially available systems. However, there is no guarantee that these leads will work properly with your EEG equipment. If you wish to use similar leads with a commercial EEG system then you should consult the manufacturer to ensure that there are no additional compatibility or safety issues. You should conduct your own testing to ensure the safety of the leads in your desired application.

DISCLAIMER

The authors do not warrant the quality, accuracy, completeness, or suitability of any information in this note. The information is provided "as is" without representations, warranties, or conditions of any kind, express, or implied. Your use of any information herein is entirely at your own risk. In no event shall we be liable for any damages whatsoever, including special, indirect, or consequential damages, arising out of or in connection with the use of information in this note.

INTRODUCTION

This technical note is provided to assist those wishing to construct carbon fiber motion-detection loops for use with simultaneous EEG–fMRI apparatus. Please read and understand both the safety warning and disclaimer above. Wires in an MRI scanner can be very dangerous if the proper precautions are not taken; these precautions are beyond the scope of this note.

Motion (including cardioballistic) artifact can be measured using insulated carbon fiber loops that are physically but not electrically attached to the subject's head. The signals generated by small movement of these wires in the magnetic field are then used to estimate and remove motion artifact from the EEG. We have already described, demonstrated, and validated the approach, elsewhere (4). The purpose of the current note is to assist those wishing to build their own motion detector loops as, at the time of writing, we are not aware of an equivalent commercially available product. We also describe how these motion loops can be used in conjunction with commercially available MRI-compatible EEG equipment. Adaption to a commercial system incorporates additional processing steps to minimize the impact of motion on gradient artifact reduction. These steps were not required for our custom EEG system as it avoids the gradient artifact during the EEG recording. In currently available commercial systems, the gradient artifact is fully recorded by the EEG system and the subsequent average-artifact correction techniques can be confounded by subject motion artifact.

Availability of direct motion artifact sensors can substantially improve the quality of the recorded EEG. In the application to which we most often use the system – the study of epilepsy, it can also dramatically increase the confidence that we have in discriminating true epileptiform activity from artifact. This is due both to the reduction in artifact and the ability to visually inspect the motion sensor signals when reading the EEG, revealing whether or not motion is present (5). Aside from motion-detection loops, other methods for microscopic subject motion detection may be suitable to reduce motion artifact in EEG acquired in an MRI scanner. For example, a promising optical moiré phase tracking method has recently been proposed (6). However, the carbon fiber loops that we describe herein confer the advantage of being a simple direct measure of specific artifact that is contaminating the EEG, including both subject motion and residual artifact arising from magnetic field gradients applied during MRI.

Carbon fiber electrodes have been constructed at our institute and used in-house with our 3 T MRI scanner since the year 2000 with no adverse effects; for example, Ref. (7–14). We have also used carbon fiber cables and electrodes for intracranial EEG in sheep (15). Subsequently, we developed motion detector loops (4), which are carbon fiber loops constructed in a similar manner to our electrode leads. We began using these loops in conjunction with our own in-house-built MRI-compatible EEG recording equipment, for example, Ref. (4, 5, 16–24) and more recently we adapted them for use with a commercially available MRI-compatible EEG recorder (BrainAmps, BrainProducts, Germany); it is these particular leads that we describe in this note.

METHODS (LOOP CONSTRUCTION)

The lead is constructed from bundles of carbon fiber thread (~1 mm bundles) enclosed in 2 mm diameter polyethylene tubing. At the amplifier end, the carbon fiber is crimped onto an appropriate connector to interface with the amplifier (e.g., a standard 1.5 mm touch-proof medical connector).

KEY COMPONENTS

Carbon fiber

This comes in many forms, but to make our "wire" we use weaved mats or tape, and small (1–2 mm diameter) bundles can be extracted from these. The length of the bundle used to make the wire will be determined by their intended use. We routinely constructed 2 m lengths of wire to reach from the back of our MRI scanner to the patient's head. We have managed to source long enough offcuts on eBay as needed (**Figure 1**).

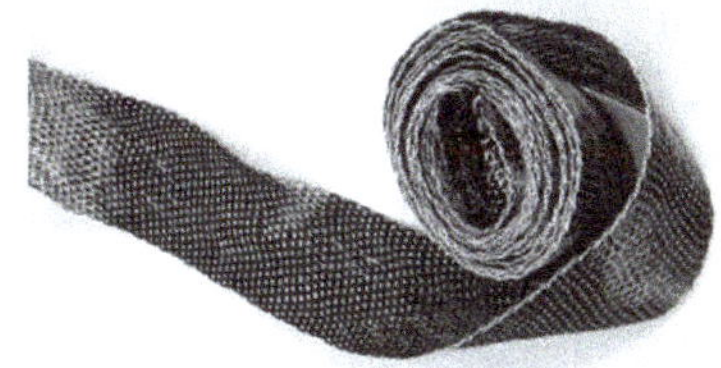

FIGURE 1 | Roll of carbon fiber tape from which bundles of "wire" can be extracted.

Polyethylene tubing

The carbon fiber will be threaded into lengths of PE tubing. We use 2 mm diameter tubing that we obtained from Microtube Extrusions Pty Ltd. in Australia [PE tubing 2.08 mm × 1.57 mm, rolls (30 m), Product Code PE208157][1].

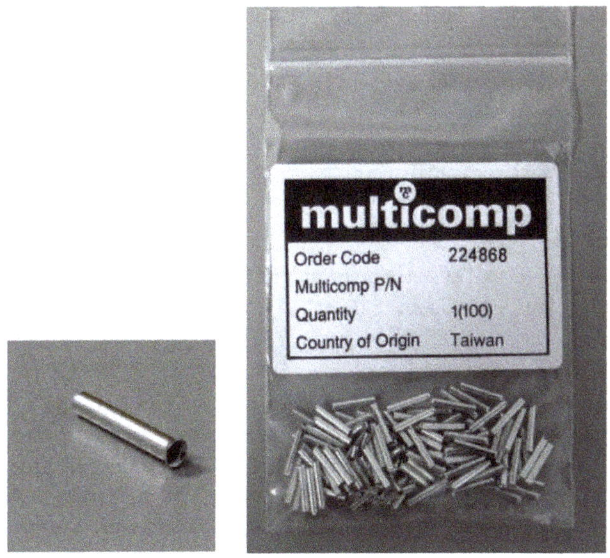

FIGURE 2 | Ferrules.

Ferrules

In order to make an electrical and physically robust connection between the carbon fiber and any metal components such as resistors, RF absorbers, or wire, we use ferrules (**Figure 2**) that can be fitted into the PE tubing and crimped down onto the carbon fiber and metal component. We obtain ferrules from element14 Pty. Ltd. in Australia [Ferrule, 1.0 mm (Packs of 100) Order Code: 224868][2].

RF absorber

In order to reduce radiofrequency contamination of the signal, we attach an RF absorber to the electrode at the amplifier end of each insulated carbon fiber wire (this is shown later in **Figure 10F**). We use a Chomerics CHO-DROP® EMI absorber (part number 80-10-9714-1000), which has a specified insertion loss of 15 dB at

[1] http://www.microtube.com.au/
[2] http://au.element14.com/

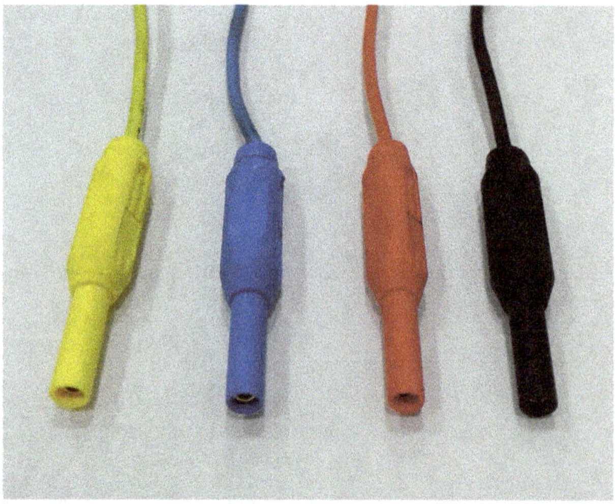

FIGURE 3 | Touch-proof safety connectors.

100 and 150 MHz. We obtain these from element14 Pty. Ltd. in Australia (Order Code: 152658)[2].

Resistors

We place a resistor of 32 kΩ in series with each motion loop. The value was chosen conservatively to be at least twice the measured DC resistance of a circuit consisting of two of the EEG electrodes supplied with the BrainAmps system. This resistor dominates the circuit, as the carbon fiber lead resistance is of the order of just a couple of 100 Ω.

Connectors

To connect the insulated carbon fiber wires to the amplifier, we use individual standard touch-proof safety connectors (**Figure 3**) sourced from element14 Pty. Ltd. in Australia [Touch-proof Plugs (typical EEG safety connectors); Pack Type: Black, Red (Packs of 4) Order Code: 41300, Pack Type: Multicolor (Packs of 6) Order Code: 1085511].

CONSTRUCTION

We first determine the length desired for the cables. We require different length wires for our different scanners; this depends on the room and scanner configuration. We then cut the carbon fiber tape and PE tubing to the appropriate length. We allow a little extra at this stage to allow for braiding of the cables later.

Making the cable

Carbon fiber tape often comes in a simple weave, and it is possible to extract the fiber in bundles, a millimeter or so in diameter (**Figure 4**). Inserting the fiber into the PE tubing is one of the more tedious parts of the job. We create a simple guide wire to help thread the carbon fiber (**Figure 5**). The guide wire is a long piece of thin, fairly stiff wire that can be threaded through the PE tubing. The wire must be longer than the PE tubing and much thinner than the diameter of the bore of the PE tubing. We bend a tight hook onto one end of the wire in order to catch the carbon fibers and drag them back through the PE tubing.

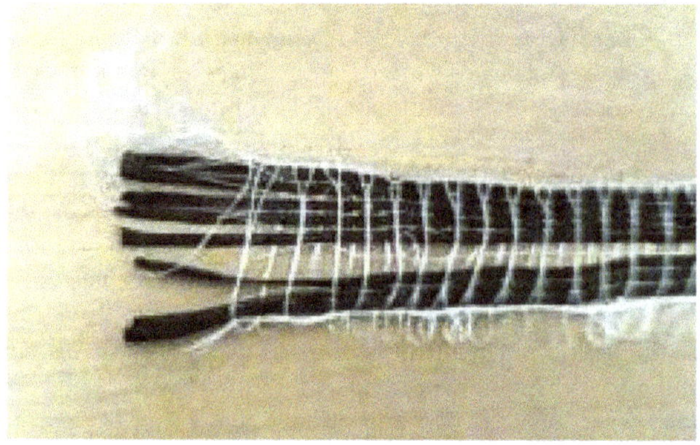

FIGURE 4 | Extracting carbon fiber bundles from woven tape.

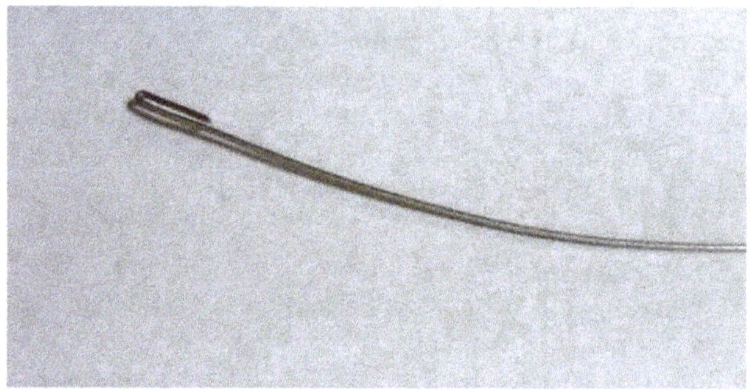

FIGURE 5 | Guide wire used to help thread carbon fiber through the PE tubing.

Since we need to pull the carbon fiber and wire back through the tubing, it works best if the wire is quite thin and has no kinks in it. Any kinks will increase the friction, and make the job a lot harder, and it may even result in perforation or tearing of the PE tubing. It is very important that the tubing has no holes in it where current may leak as that would be a significant patient safety problem.

We find the easiest way to thread the carbon fiber is to first lay out the length of PE tubing on a long table. It will work best if the table is longer than the intended cable. We tape the tubing in a straight line (**Figure 6A**), then carefully push the wire through the PE tubing until it comes out the other end (**Figures 6B,C**). Then, we catch the end of the length of carbon fiber with the wire hook and carefully pull the fiber all the way through the PE tubing (**Figures 6D,E**). Once we have an insulated carbon fiber cable (**Figure 7**), we visually check the cable closely to ensure that there are no tears or perforations.

Turning the insulated carbon fiber cable into movement detectors:

We use three movement detection loops to ensure artifact signal arising from movement in all three spatial dimensions can be captured. We have made them so that they can be individually

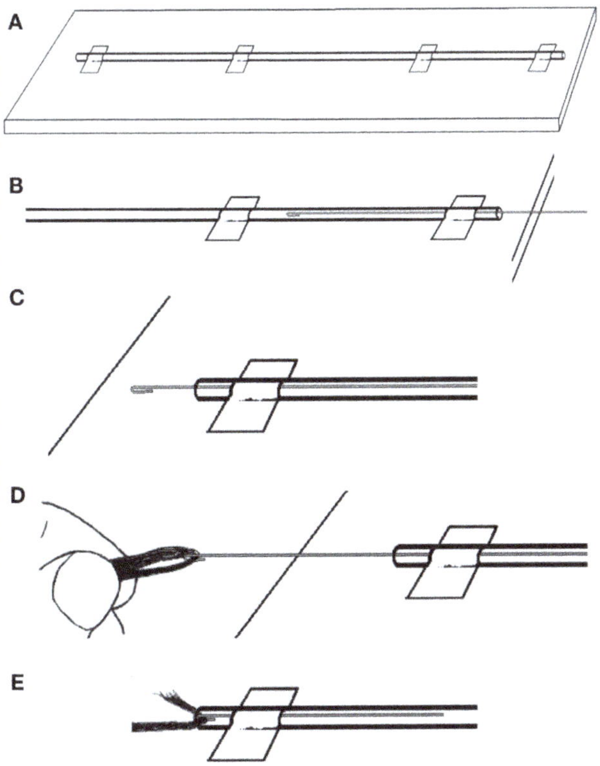

FIGURE 6 | To thread the guide wire through the PE tubing: (A) tape the tubing in a straight line then (B) carefully push the wire through the PE tubing until (C) it comes out the other end. Then **(D)** catch the end of the length of carbon fiber with the wire hook and **(E)** carefully pull the fiber into and then all the way through the PE tubing.

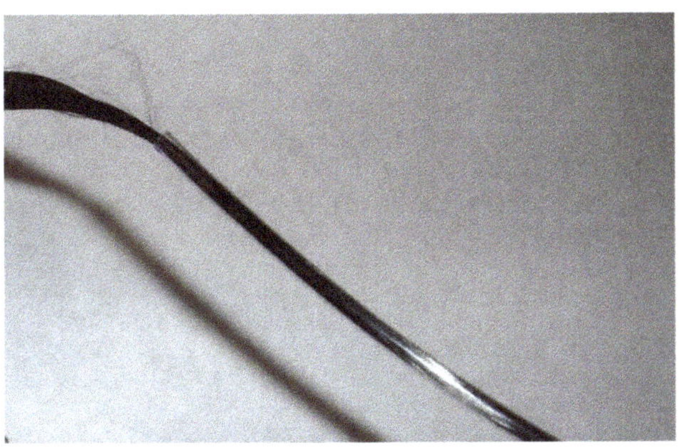

FIGURE 7 | Carbon fiber successfully threaded through PE tubing.

positioned on the patient's head in an approximately orthogonal spatial arrangement. To make the three movement sensors, four carbon fiber cables are used. Three (the sensors) have double loops introduced near the head end (with a diameter of around 5 cm) and the fourth (the ground) remains straight. After each movement sensor cable leaves the double loop, the exposed carbon fiber

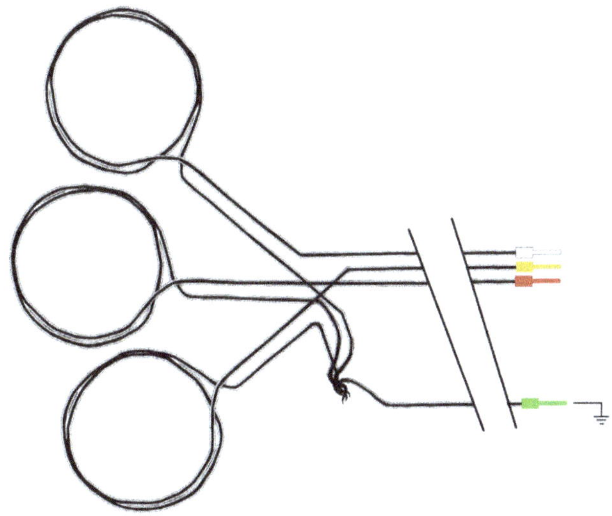

FIGURE 8 | Schematic diagram of carbon fiber movement loops. Each loop has a diameter of approximately 5 cm, and all three loops share a common ground carbon fiber wire.

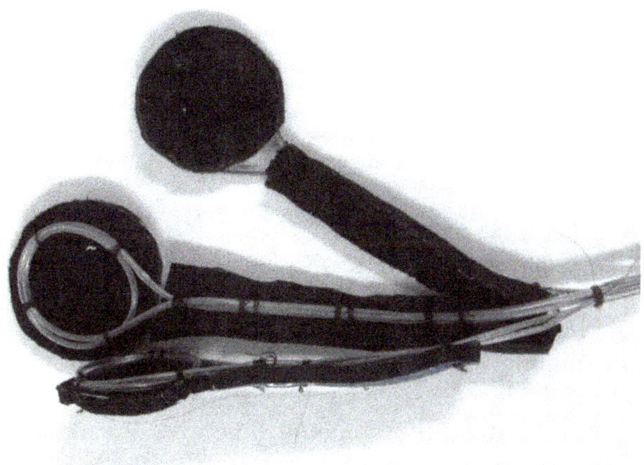

FIGURE 9 | Photograph of completed carbon fiber movement detection loops.

is twisted with the common ground fiber (**Figure 8**) and these are secured as best as possible and completely insulated with layers of heat-shrink tubing.

Due to the large loops of carbon fiber wire used in these motion detectors, there is an increased chance of heating or current leakage compared to conventional EEG electrodes. Therefore, we take an extra precaution and place the movement loops on a bed of neoprene of at least 4 mm thickness (4) (**Figure 9**).

Aside from the large intentional loops insulated on the bed of neoprene, it is important that we have no other loops near the patient that may compromise safety. Therefore, we construct a full lead set and adjust the length of each individual cable to minimize slack. We also plait the cables (this is critically important for EEG electrodes to reduce the gradient artifact as it minimizes loop area and provides some cancelation of currents that would otherwise arise from the remaining small loop area; it may be less important for motion loops since they are designed to measure artifact, however, it does help keep the cable organized). It is important to ensure that there is enough length of cable on each individual motion loop before plaiting starts to accommodate the largest of head sizes. We have studied over 250 people from 4 to 60 years of age with widely different head sizes and shapes with the same motion-loop set. Our plaiting starts a short distance (15–20 cm) from the vertex of the head with our current MRI head-coil configuration; the electrodes will leave the head from the vertex and travel down the bore of the magnet away from the patient. We use cotton thread to tie the cable bundle together at each end to stop the plaiting from unwinding, and also periodically along the length of the bundle to keep it tight.

Once all the cables are plaited and bundled together, they may end up having slightly different lengths. We trim some of the longer ones at this stage so that our final connections will be tidy. We also label each cable at each end to aid troubleshooting. We do this using printed paper labels that we slip under a section of clear heat-shrink tubing (these labels will survive our normal between-subject cleaning protocol). The labeling must be completed before the addition of components at the amplifier end of the cable. Applying the heat shrink can be tricky because the PE tubing will deform if it gets too warm. It can take a little practice to get this right, so we practice on some offcuts first until we are comfortable with the process.

Connecting to the amplifier

At the amplifier end of each cable, we attach an RF absorber to limit RF contamination of the signal of interest. This is particularly important for EEG electrodes as the absorber will filter noise from the EEG electronics escaping the EEG shielded box, and present high impedance to the patient. For the motion loops, we ideally want the artifact measured to be similar to that contaminating the recorded EEG, so we use a similar RF absorber. Note that the amplifier in our setup is sufficiently far from the head and outside the bore of the magnet so we can use a small amount of non-magnetic metal that will not compromise the imaging.

We also need to attach the carbon fiber to some sort of input plug for the amplifier. We do this by physically crimping the carbon fiber onto a ferrule threaded over the carbon fiber and inserted into the bore of the PE tubing. In order to make this connection more secure, we also fold the carbon fiber back on itself and hold it in place with some heat-shrink tubing. These steps are explained in more detail below.

First, we thread a small length of heat-shrink tubing onto the carbon fiber cable. Then, we draw the carbon fiber through the ferrule. While it might be possible to simply push the carbon fiber through the ferrule without a guide wire, we found this very difficult. Therefore, we again utilize the wire hook technique: for this purpose, we make another, smaller guide wire (**Figure 10A**). We thread the wire hook through the ferrule, and then catch the very end of the carbon fiber in the hook (**Figures 10B,C**). We then carefully pull the wire hook through the ferrule and the fiber comes with it (**Figure 10D**). We feed the carbon fiber through the ferrule until it is up against the PE tubing, and then push the ferrule into the PE tubing. If chosen appropriately, the ferrules fit snugly into the bore of the PE tubing (**Figure 10E**). Next, we fold the wire coming out of the RF absorber and push that into the ferrule (**Figures 10F,G**). We then use crimping pliers to firmly crimp the ferrule onto the carbon fiber/RF absorber wire (**Figure 10H**). Finally, we trim the excess carbon fiber and thread it back through the heat-shrink tubing that we put on the electrode cable earlier. We push this up to the RF absorber (**Figure 10I**) and then apply some heat to the heat-shrink tubing to hold the excess carbon fiber firmly. We make sure that there is no carbon fiber exposed outside of the heat-shrink, as this may cause the cable to short out if it touches any other conducting surface. We sometimes need to use another piece of heat-shrink to cover any loose ends.

We now have a piece of wire (the other end of the RF absorber) connected to the carbon fiber cable that we can solder things onto. We use short color coded wires, soldering one end to the RF absorber and the other end to the connector (**Figure 10J**). We also label the individual wires to help with troubleshooting and cover any exposed surfaces with heat-shrink tubing (remembering to slip the heat-shrink over the wire before soldering the final end of the wire on to the connector).

METHODS (APPLICATION)

We have previously described the principle of operation and validated the use of our motion loops for reduction of motion artifact when used with our in-house EEG–fMRI system (4). We take the opportunity in the present technical note to show that the system can also be successfully employed in conjunction with a commercially available fMRI-compatible EEG system: BrainAmp MR from Brain Products GmbH.

SUBJECTS

A healthy male subject aged 25 years and a female epilepsy patient aged 12 years, were studied. The patient had experienced seizure onset at the age of 3 years with electrographic diagnosis of continuous spikes and waves during sleep (CSWS) at age of 6 years. Ethical approval for this study was obtained from the Austin Hospital Human Research Ethics Committee. Written informed consent was obtained from the healthy subject and the father of the patient.

DATA ACQUISITION

Functional MRI of the healthy subject was acquired with a Siemens MAGNETOM TRIO MRI scanner (Siemens Medical Solutions, Erlangen, Germany) equipped with a Siemens Tx/Rx CP Head Coil. A gradient-echo echo-planar imaging (EPI) sequence was utilized with TR = 3 s; TE = 30 ms; flip angle = 85°; FOV = 216 mm × 216 mm; 72 × 72 matrix; voxel size 3 mm × 3 mm × 3 mm; 44 contiguous slices 3 mm thick, providing whole-brain coverage. Two hundred T2*-weighted whole-brain volumes were acquired in a 10 min scanning session.

Functional MRI of the patient was acquired with a Siemens MAGNETOM Skyra MRI scanner (Siemens Medical Solutions,

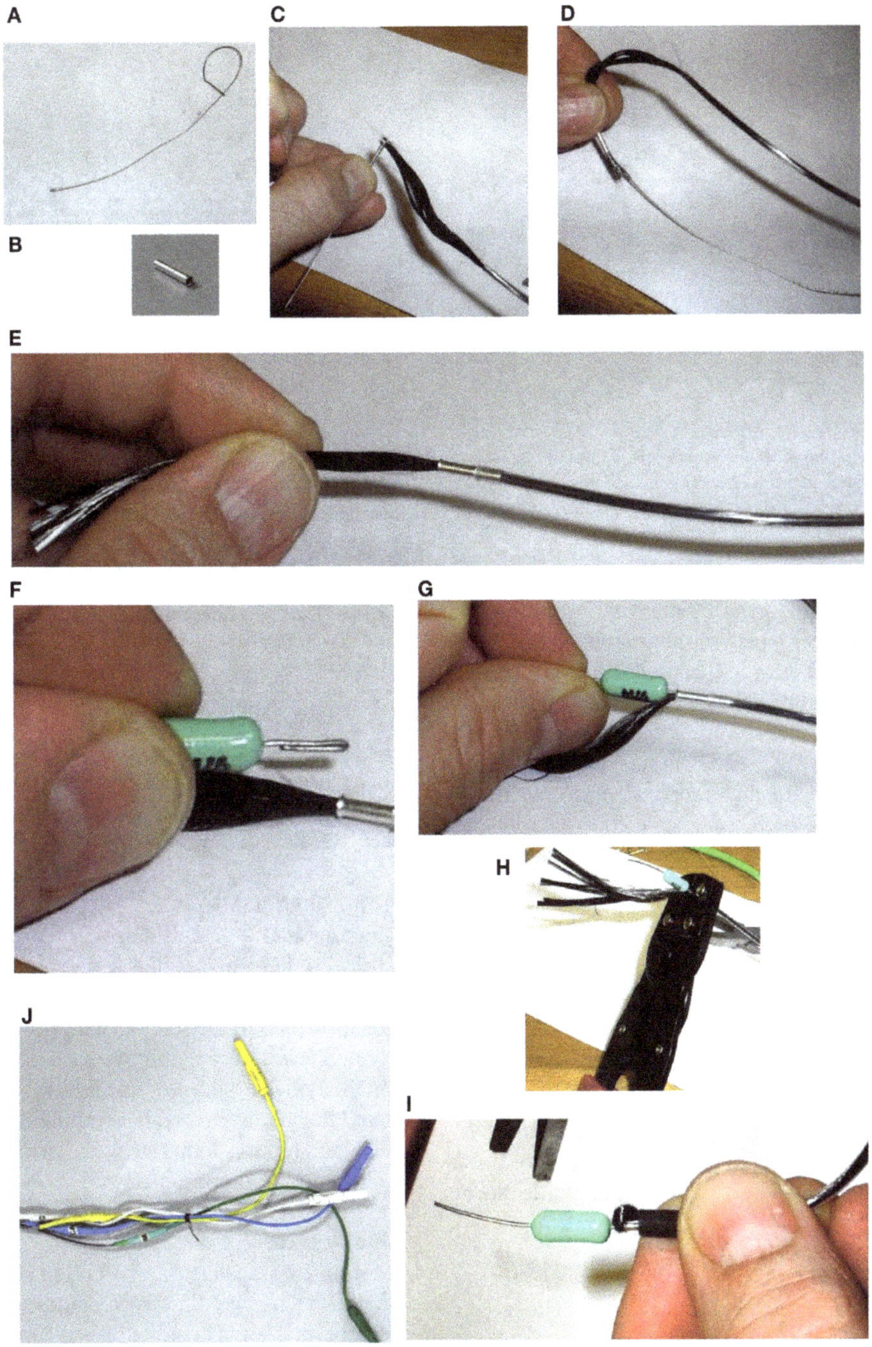

FIGURE 10 | Assembling the amplifier end of the carbon fiber cable. First, we thread a small length of heat shrink tubing onto the carbon fiber cable. Then a small guide wire **(A)**, is fashioned into a hook and used to thread the carbon fiber through a ferrule **(B)**, by catching the very end of the carbon fiber in the hook **(C)**, and carefully pulling the wire hook through the ferrule **(D)**. We feed the carbon fiber through the ferrule until it is up against the PE tubing, and then push the ferrule into the PE tubing **(E)**. Next, we fold the wire coming out of the RF Absorber and push that into the ferrule **(F,G)**. We then use crimping pliers to firmly crimp the ferrule onto the carbon fiber/RF Absorber wire **(H)**. We trim the excess carbon fiber and thread it back through the heat shrink tubing that we put on the electrode cable earlier. We push this up to the RF Absorber **(I)**, and then apply some heat to the heat shrink tubing to hold the excess carbon fiber firmly. Finally, we solder a short color-coded wire to the other end of the RF Absorber and connect the wire to a touch-proof connector **(J)**.

Erlangen, Germany) with an otherwise similar setup to that described above. Six hundred T2*-weighted whole-brain volumes were acquired in a 30 min scanning session.

EEG for both subjects was acquired using a Brain Products MR-compatible EEG system configured for 32-channel operation (BrainCap MR from EASYCAP GmbH). The cap is fitted with 32

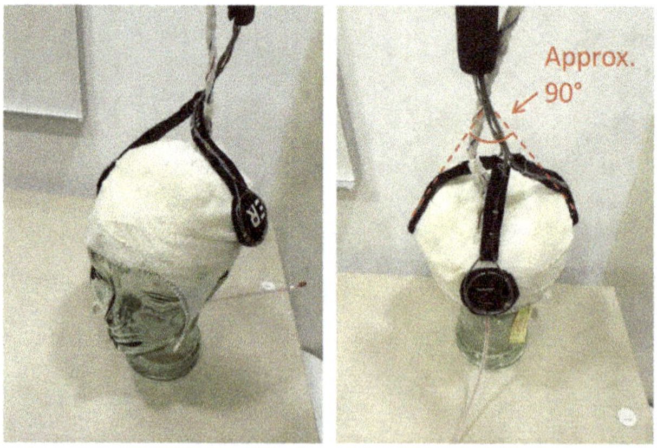

FIGURE 11 | Precise positioning of the motion loops is not critical; however, they should be placed on the head in an approximately orthogonal orientation, so they capture the effect of motion in any direction (i.e. no loop should be parallel to another).

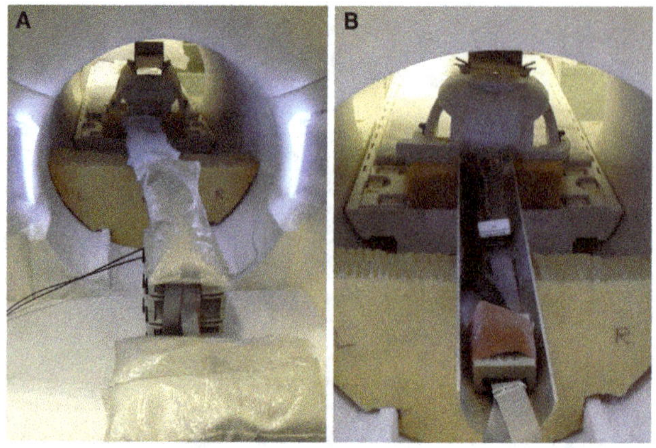

FIGURE 12 | Photographs of inside-MRI-scanner EEG equipment layout similar to that utilized in the present experiment. To obtain a clear view, these photographs were taken in our mock-scanner; in our real scanner, we use a head coil that permits entry of the cables directly from the rear. **(A)** The EEG amplifier and peripheral signal amplifier are both placed outside the scanner bore and the cable connecting the EEG cap to the amplifiers fixed in place in the center of the bore using plastic piping covered with sandbags, suspended on pieces of thick foam padding. **(B)** View of the cables with the sandbags removed.

electrodes (including the reference) with sintered Ag/AgCl sensors. Electrodes were arranged according to the international 10–20 system. Electrocardiogram was recorded using an electrode placed on the subject's back. Head movement detection loops (permanently attached to a bed of 4 mm thickness neoprene as shown in **Figure 9**) were placed on top of the EEG cap such that loop orientations were approximately mutually orthogonal. As a convenience measure, prior to placing the loops, we wrapped the electrode cap with a bandage to avoid getting surplus electrode gel on the motion loops (**Figure 11**). The loops were then affixed in place with further bandages. The EEG amplifier (BrainAmp MR, Brain Products GmbH) and peripheral signal amplifier used for the motion loops (BrainAmp ExG MR, Brain Products GmbH) were placed outside the scanner bore. The cables connecting the EEG cap and motion loops to the amplifiers were run down the center of the scanner bore, fixed in place using plastic piping and sandbags (**Figure 12**). The amplifiers were connected via fiber optic cabling to a computer outside the scanner room. The EEG clock was synchronized with the MRI scanner's clock using Brain Products' SyncBox. EEG was acquired using BrainVision Recorder using a sampling rate of 5000 Hz.

HEALTHY SUBJECT PARADIGM

EEG was first recorded for 10 min outside the scanner. The subject was verbally instructed to open and close eyes for alternating periods of 30 s. The subject was then moved to the MRI scanner where they were verbally instructed to open and close eyes for alternating periods of 30 s for the first 5 min of the fMRI scanning. For the next 5 min, the subject was instructed to keep their eyes closed. This 10 min paradigm was then repeated in a second study within the same scanning session, with the subject additionally instructed to occasionally move their head at random times of their choice throughout the scan.

EPILEPSY PATIENT PARADIGM

EEG was first recorded for 10 min outside the scanner to capture the morphology and distribution of epileptic discharges. The patient was instructed to keep their eyes closed for the duration of the recording. The patient was then moved to the MRI scanner where they were instructed to close their eyes during scanning, and encouraged to fall asleep.

OFFLINE EEG ANALYSIS

Offline analysis of the EEG data was performed using BrainVision Analyzer 2.0 software as follows:

1. Removal of MR gradient artifact from the EEG and motion-loop signals using a sliding average artifact template subtraction method. Twenty-one volume intervals (each corresponding to one TR = 3 s) were used to compute each average.
2. EEG and motion-loop signals downsampled to 250 Hz.
3. EEG and motion-loop signals low- and high-pass filtered at 70 and 0.5 Hz, respectively (Butterworth zero-phase filter, 48 dB/octave).
4. Motion/cardioballistic artifact (CBA) correction was then performed using two different methods, each in separate analysis streams that could be subsequently compared. The first method is a conventional method that does not utilise the motion loops. The second method utilises the motion loop signals. The methods are described below.

Method 1: cardioballistic artifact removal using BrainVision Analyzer algorithm. CBA removal was performed by identifying *R*-peak markers of each QRS complex from the ECG channel (*R*-peak search parameters: 60–100 pulses/min; average pulse length 800 ± 200 ms), and then performing a sliding average artifact template subtraction (25), with each subtraction template consisting of 21 *R*-peak intervals. The delay time (i.e., the time between the *R*-peak of the ECG and the CBA peak in the EEG trace) was computed across the whole EEG recording and used to center the artifact correction template to improve correction of each CBA episode (average delay time was 0.408 s for the healthy control, and 0.100 s for the patient).

Method 2: cardioballistic/motion artifact removal utilizing signals derived from the three motion loops. An estimate of the artifact contained in each recorded EEG channel was derived from the motion-loop signals and then subtracted from the EEG (4). In the present implementation, this was achieved using a multi-channel least squares algorithm implemented as an external custom MATLAB procedure called from BrainVision Analyzer (see Appendix).

We then took additional steps to check for and, if necessary, mitigate the effect of motion deleteriously affecting the average-gradient-artifact correction procedure. We first checked for the presence of large EEG signal likely due to motion so extreme that the motion-loop procedure was unable to remove it from the EEG. Specifically, we used the automated "raw data inspection" procedure available in BrainVision Analyzer software, applied to the motion-corrected EEG channels, to automatically search and mark periods of large EEG signal change as bad. Three criteria were used as follows: (i) "Check Gradient" was used to detect EEG signal amplitude steps >50 μV/ms and these were marked as bad commencing 200 ms before and concluding 200 ms after each instance; (ii) "check min/max amplitude" was used to mark as bad time intervals of 200 ms in which the maximum–minimum amplitude exceeded a threshold of 200 μV; (iii) "check minimum and maximum allowed amplitude" was used to mark as bad any instance of values lower than −200 μV or higher than +200 μV, with the excluded window commencing 200 ms prior and extending 200 ms after the deleterious event. If any epochs of large amplitude/change were identified, the gradient artifact subtraction was re-done as follows: the markers were upsampled to 5 kHz to match the original EEG acquisition. The gradient artifact correction steps 1–3 above were then re-done on the original uncorrected EEG and motion-loop signals, informing the procedure not to use the marked-as-bad epochs when generating average gradient correction templates. Finally, the (possibly improved) motion-loop signals were then inspected using the "raw data inspection" routine to detect significant motion (using a tighter constraint for "Check minimum and maximum allowed amplitude," marking as bad any instance of values lower than −100 μV or higher than +100 μV). If any was found in epochs not already marked as bad, the gradient artifact correction steps 1–3 above were re-done once more, this time excluding the expanded set of bad epochs. An estimate of the artifact contained in the newly processed EEG signals was then derived from the newly processed motion-loop signals and the artifact was subtracted as before.

Note that the voltage settings that we used in the "raw data inspection" step were chosen heuristically. Appropriate settings are likely to vary between systems. For example, the voltages returned by the motion loops will depend upon the area and number of turns of the constructed loops as well as the magnetic field strength of the MRI.

RESULTS

The measured resistance of a single electrode included with our BrainAmps system was 10 kΩ. Thus, a circuit consisting of two electrodes would be at least 20 kΩ. Allowing for scalp impedance (typically 8–10 kΩ as measured by the BrainAmps equipment at 15 Hz) and a comfortable margin, we selected a 32 kΩ resistor to use in series with each of our motion loops.

EPI image quality with the EEG leads and motion loops in place was acceptable (**Figure 13**). There were no adverse effects related to the use of the motion loops during this or any other study at our site. Segments of EEG demonstrating the performance of each motion removal method are displayed for the healthy subject in **Figure 14** and for the epilepsy patient in **Figure 15**. A particularly extreme motion event example from the second study undertaken by the healthy control is also shown in **Figure 16** to specifically demonstrate the ability of motion-loop correction to reduce propagated artifact related to motion contamination of the average-gradient-artifact correction template.

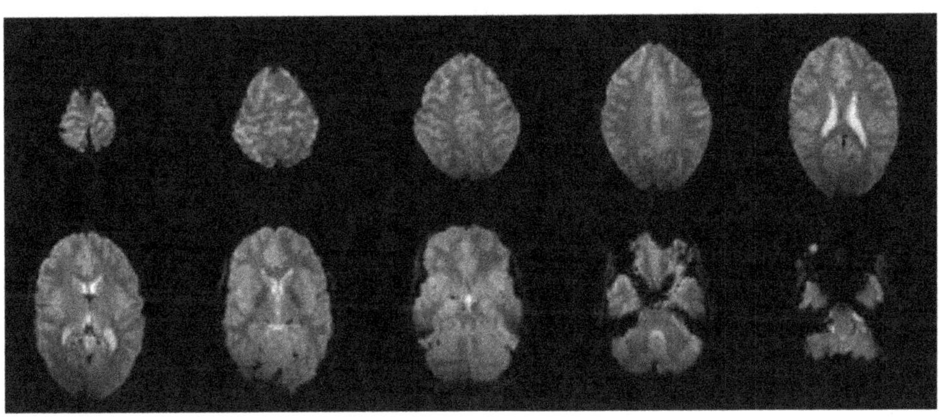

FIGURE 13 | Every fourth slice of an EPI volume acquired from the healthy subject while simultaneous EEG recording was in progress.

DISCUSSION

We have described the methods that we use to construct and utilize carbon fiber motion loops with a commercially available EEG–fMRI system. We observe that the quality of the EEG corrected by motion-loop signals is often superior to that of conventional software-only correction methods, especially in the presence of non-periodic motion. When applied in the study of epilepsy, the motion loops also confer the advantage of displaying a direct measure of artifact to the EEG reader, providing information that can increase confidence in EEG mark-up.

MITIGATING PROBLEMS WITH GRADIENT ARTIFACT CORRECTION

We have previously described the use of motion loops in conjunction with an EEG–fMRI system that we built in-house. In that EEG–fMRI system, gradient artifact was largely avoided during acquisition of the EEG, so average-gradient-artifact post-processing was not required. In current commercially available systems, a different approach is taken to gradient signals: the EEG including gradient artifact is measured in its entirety. A gradient-artifact-removal post-acquisition processing step is then performed – typically a gradient artifact waveform template of temporal length TR (the MRI repetition time) is determined by averaging the EEG over a number of successive time windows each of length TR. This can provide a good estimate of the gradient artifact, while the physiological signals of interest tend to average close to zero in the template. However, subject motion can contaminate the estimate of the average gradient artifact. This can then degrade the corrected EEG for the entire time period in which the affected average gradient template is used. A particularly severe example of this is shown in **Figure 16A** – gross motion has occurred to the extent that even the fraction 1/21 of the resultant artifact is substantial and this fraction has been propagated to surrounding epochs during the average template subtraction procedure (the template being an average of 21 epochs of length TR). This type of artifact also substantially affects gradient correction of the motion-loop signals, so it is difficult to be sure whether or not the motion-loop signals and EEG contain propagated or real motion or both. In the case of **Figure 16**, exclusion of the extreme epoch worked well to avoid large contamination of the average-gradient-artifact correction, as shown in **Figure 16B**. There are several methods available to help identify and remove such extreme epochs [for a comparison of several gradient-artifact-removal algorithms, see Ref. (26)]. However, the intent of this motion example is to illustrate that the motion loops alone can mitigate failures in gradient artifact removal, and assist with identification of real motion events. **Figure 16C** demonstrates that subtraction of the fitted motion-loop signals has alone almost completely removed the artifact that was propagated during gradient artifact pre-processing, even in this extreme example. The noise reduction benefits of the motion-loop subtraction method therefore include reduction of any directly measured motion artifact and reduction of artifact resulting from imperfect gradient artifact removal. In practice, we recommend an iterative procedure as this process yields the cleanest EEG (e.g., **Figure 16D**). The second iteration avoids average gradient template contamination by extreme events identified after the first iteration. This iterative process is more straightforward when motion loops are used because there can be a clearer distinction in the EEG between potential non-motion epochs and extreme real motion epochs (compare, for example, **Figures 16A,C**). The final iteration avoids average gradient template contamination by more subtle motion events that can now be identified from the improved motion-loop

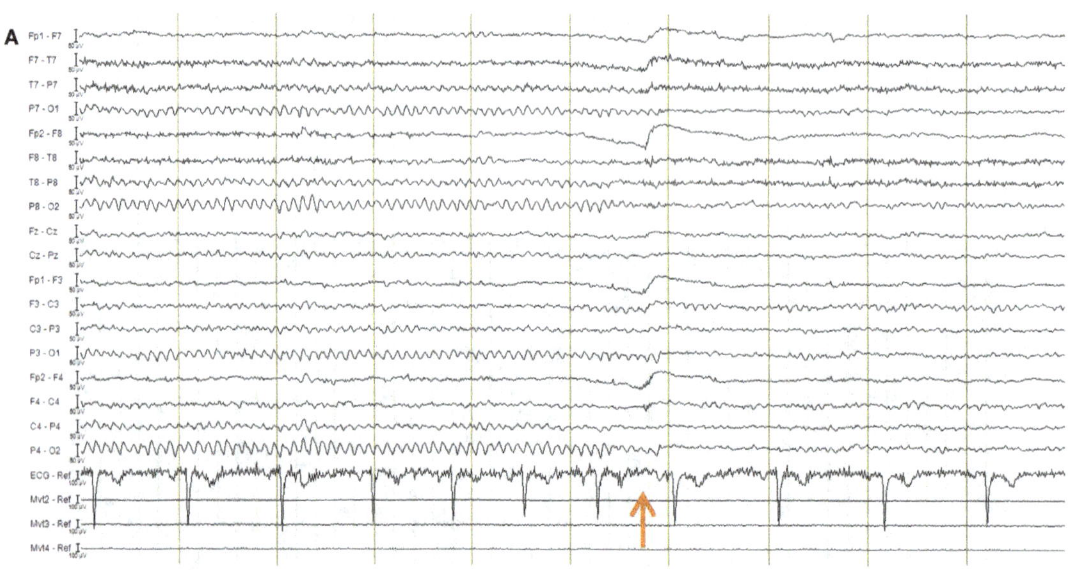

FIGURE 14 | EEG of the healthy subject shown in longitudinal bipolar ("double banana") montage. In every figure **(A–D)**, the lower three traces are motion-loop signals. **(A)** Ten second segment of EEG recorded outside the MRI scanner selected to show eyes closed then, following the time point indicated by the arrow, eyes open. Typical prominent alpha activity in the absence of MRI artifact is clearly evident while the subject's eyes are closed; a brief blink artifact is then evident as the subject opens their eyes at the time indicated by the arrow, followed by reduced alpha activity during the eyes open condition. Any motion of the subject is not detectable in the motion loops because they are not in a magnetic field.

(Continued)

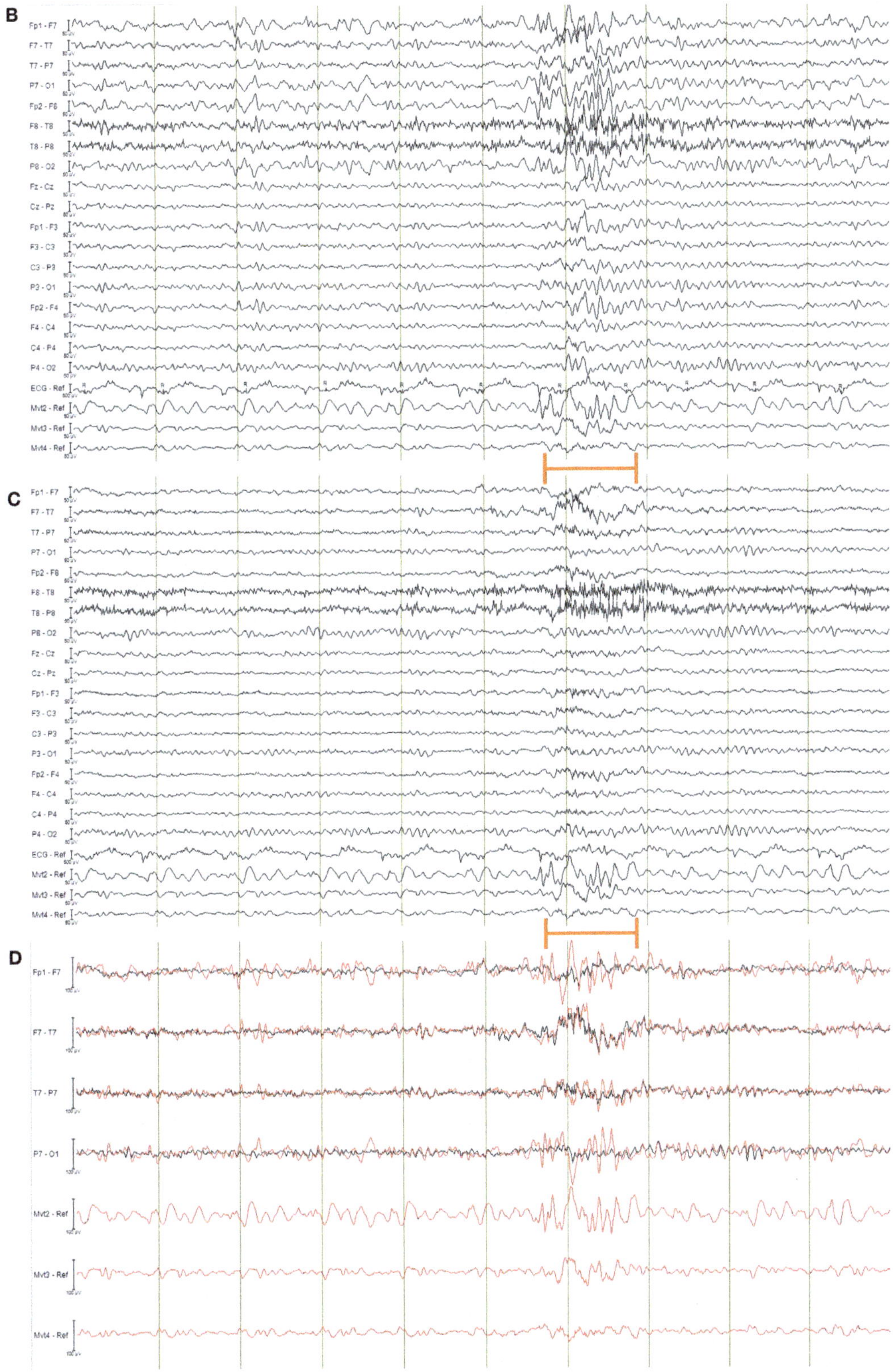

FIGURE 14 | Continued
(B–D) a 10 s segment of eyes-closed EEG recorded inside the scanner during fMRI acquisition, selected to include an obvious large movement event at the time indicated by the orange bar: **(B)** result when the EEG is corrected using conventional average-pulse-artifact subtraction; **(C)** result when motion-loop artifact removal is applied; **(D)** expanded overlay of four selected EEG channels more clearly demonstrating the superiority of the motion-loop artifact removal technique (black trace) compared to conventional pulse-artifact subtraction (red trace).

signals of the second iteration, because the motion loops are no longer substantially contaminated by propagated artifact from the more extreme events. The more subtle events may not have been detected in the EEG at the first iteration because they are more effectively removed by the motion-loop subtraction. Of course, the average gradient template subtraction procedure only needs to be re-run at each of these stages if additional bad epochs are actually detected.

Due to the high amplitude, high frequency, and highly consistent periodic nature of the gradient artifact, the procedure described above is substantially more effective than attempting to correct the entire gradient artifact by direct regression of the three motion-loop measurements. However, if residual gradient artifact is present in the EEG after this procedure (even if not as obvious as the extreme motion example presented in **Figure 16**), it will also be present in the motion-loop signals and so will be further attenuated by the subsequent motion-loop artifact regression procedure.

LIMITATIONS AND POTENTIAL TO DETECT RAPID MOTION THAT MAY ALSO AFFECT fMRI

We have previously shown that if motion artifact is too extreme, the motion-loop correction procedure is unable to effectively remove the contamination (although the motion loops do at least alert the user to the presence of motion in those circumstances) (4). **Figure 16** provides another demonstration of this limitation: while the propagated artifact could be removed, in this example, the epoch in which the actual motion event occurred could not be adequately corrected, suggesting substantial non-linear effects. We wondered how much motion had occurred during this epoch. It is not possible to determine the absolute amount of motion from our uncalibrated motion-loop signals. The magnitude of the artifact depends upon the rate of change of magnetic flux through the loop formed by the conductor, which in turn depends upon both the rate of movement and its direction with respect to the magnetic field. However, we can obtain a crude estimate of the actual motion from the fMRI acquisition. We determined the within-brain center of intensity change of the fMRI for the extreme motion epoch of **Figure 16** using iBrain software (27)[3]: the change in 2D center-of-mass (intensity) of each slice in the affected volume, compared to the same slice in the previous volume, ranged from 0.14 to 2.1 mm, while the change in 3D center-of-mass between volumes was 0.95 mm. We also estimated 3D shift and rotations using the rigid-body realignment procedure in SPM software[4]. The volume-to-volume change in displacement estimated this way was 0.76 mm accompanied by a change in pitch rotation of 0.68°. The peak motion detected in 2D slices in this example is thus considerably larger than volumetric parameters would suggest (i.e., motion was sufficiently rapid to affect slices within the volume differently, and this effect was partially averaged out in the rigid-body motion estimates across the entire volume). Given the relatively high temporal sampling rate of the EEG compared to the volume or slice acquisition time of fMRI, the motion-loop signals may have additional potential to be used to identify fMRI volumes that may be affected by rapid subject motion. For example, the inability of the motion loops to adequately remove motion artifact could be used as an indicator of the presence of motion severe enough to result in non-linear EEG artifact, and therefore, also likely to have a deleterious effect on the fMRI acquisition at that particular time. We recommend further work be undertaken to explore this potential.

[3] http://www.brain.org.au/software
[4] http://www.fil.ion.ucl.ac.uk/spm

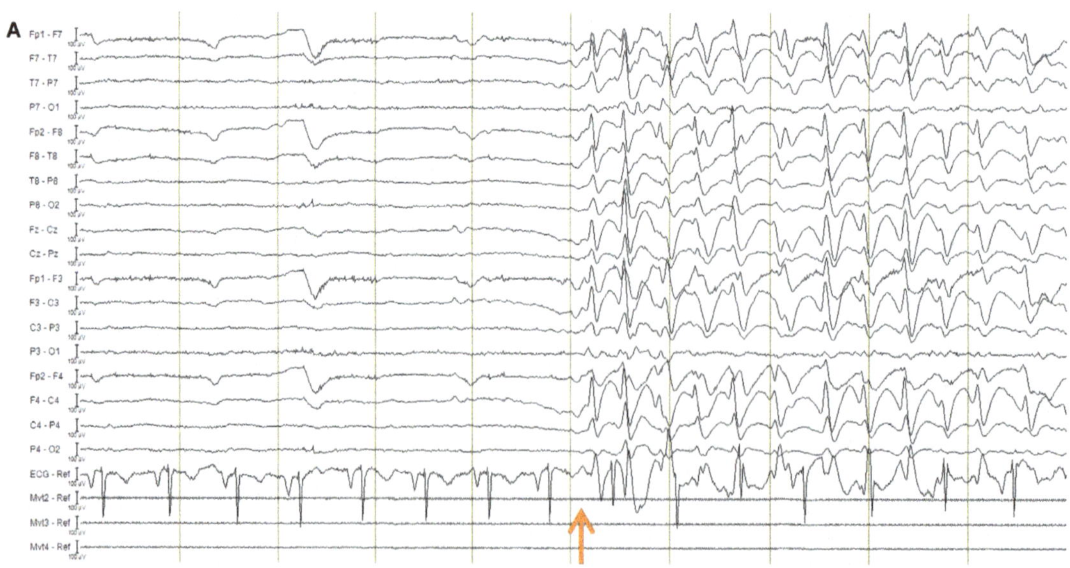

FIGURE 15 | EEG of the epilepsy patient shown in longitudinal bipolar ("double banana") montage. In every figure **(A–D)**, the lower three traces are motion-loop signals. **(A)** Ten second segment of EEG recorded outside the MRI scanner selected to show a typical epileptiform discharge of this patient (commencing at the time indicated by the arrow) in the absence of MRI artifact. Any motion of the subject is not detectable in the motion loops because they are not in a magnetic field.

(Continued)

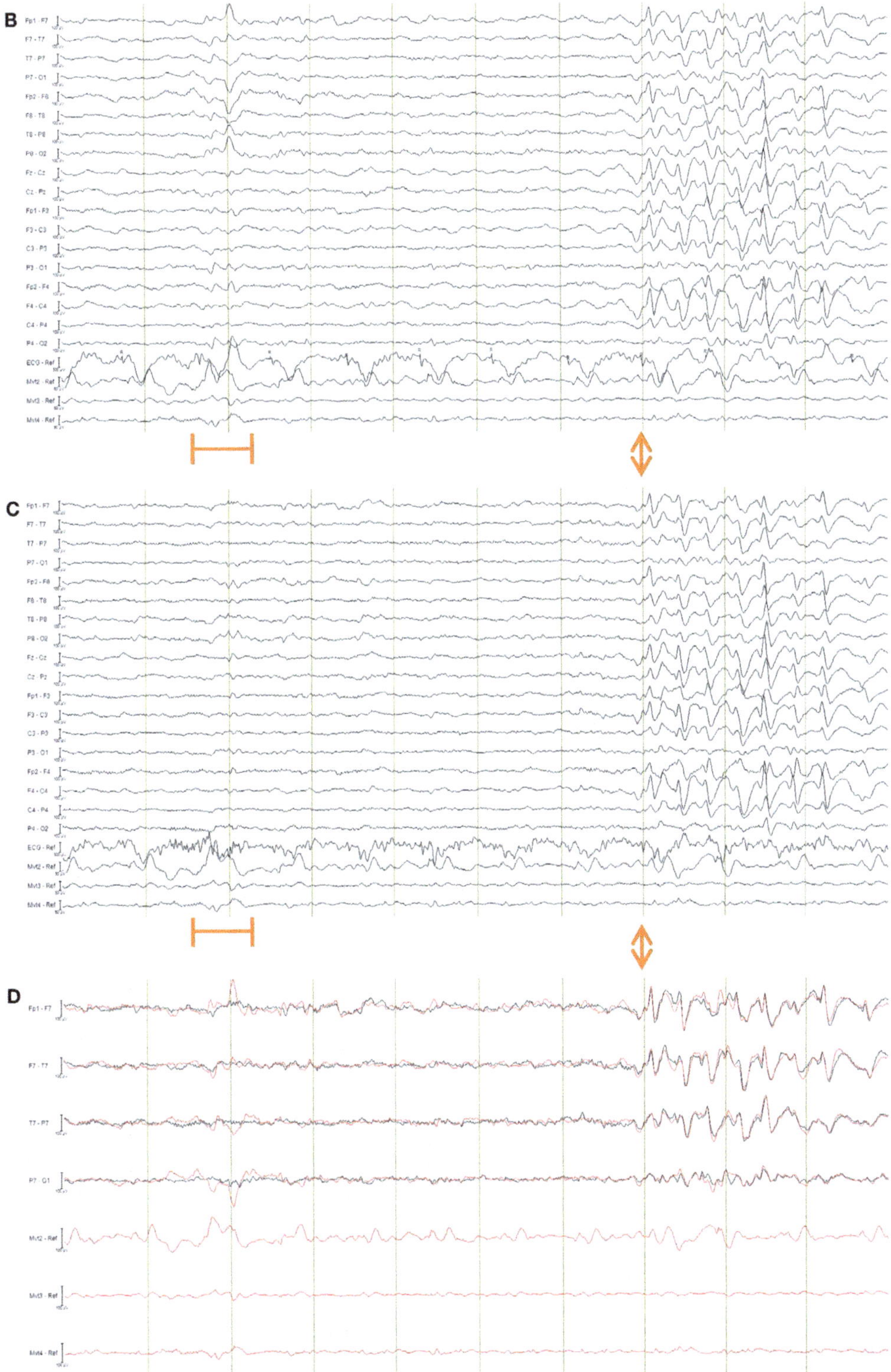

FIGURE 15 | Continued
(B–D) a 10 s segment of EEG recorded inside the scanner during fMRI acquisition, selected to include both a large movement event (at the time indicated by the orange bar) and a typical epileptiform discharge of this patient (commencing at the time indicated by the double arrows): **(B)** result when the EEG is corrected using conventional average-pulse-artifact subtraction; **(C)** result when motion-loop artifact removal is applied to the EEG – notice the large motion artifact early in the record is removed, as is cardioballistic artifact throughout the study, while epileptiform activity evident later is retained (the BrainAmps system also effectively removed the cardioballistic artifact in this example, however, it failed to remove the non-periodic motion event); **(D)** expanded overlay of four selected EEG channels more clearly demonstrating the superiority of the motion-loop artifact removal technique (black trace) compared to conventional pulse-artifact subtraction (red trace).

SAFETY

We remind the reader again that wires in an MRI scanner can be very dangerous if the proper precautions are not taken. For simultaneous EEG–fMRI experiments conducted with our leads, we have always used MRI head-coils that enable the EEG wires to leave at the vertex of the head and travel directly away from the

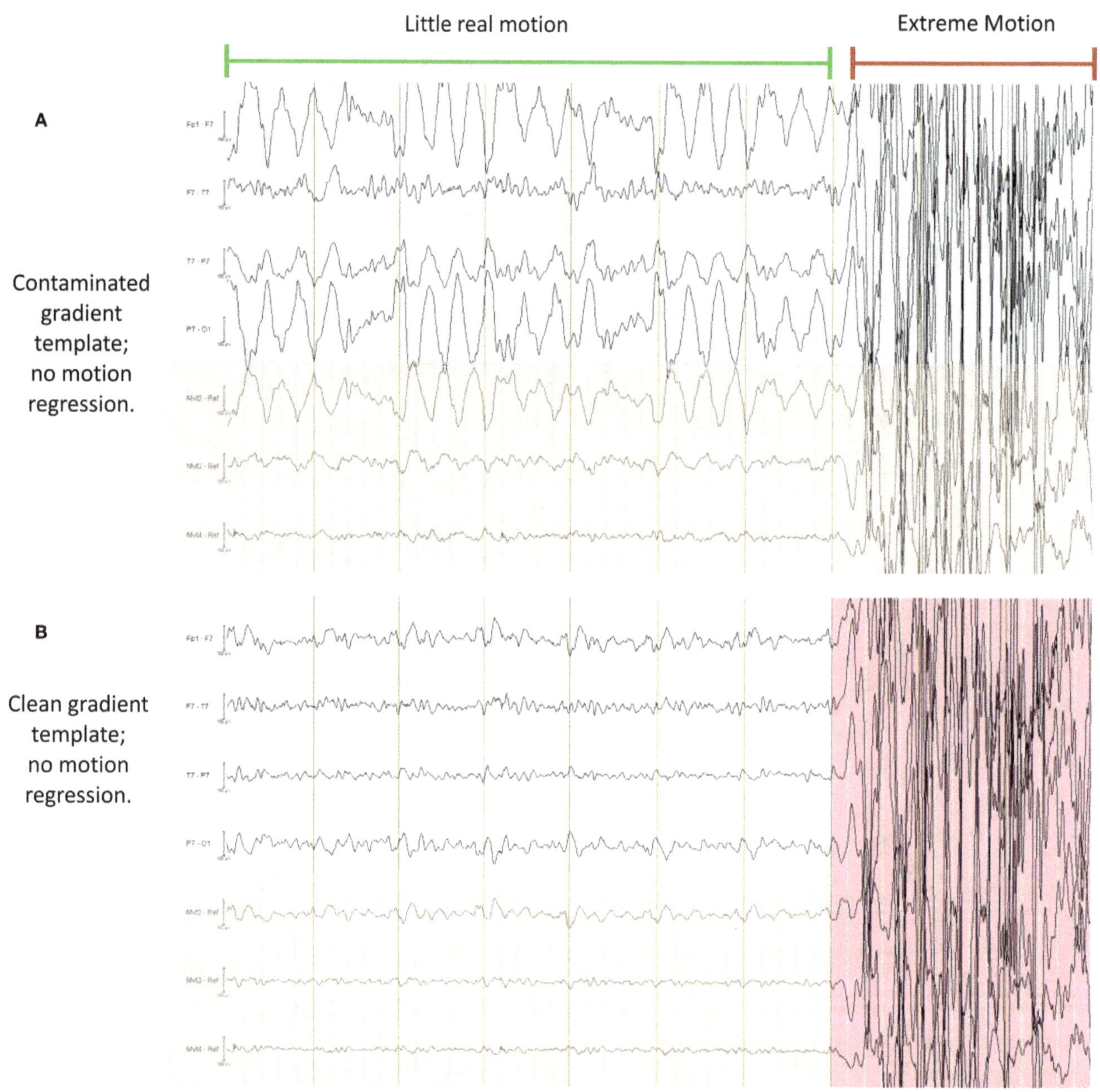

FIGURE 16 | This figure demonstrates a particularly severe example of deliberate motion contamination in the healthy control in which gross motion has occurred to such an extent that even the fraction 1/21 is substantial and has resulted in propagated artifact due to contamination of the average-gradient-artifact template (the template being an average of 21 epochs of length TR). In each of **(A)** through **(D)** the same 10 s period is shown with different processing applied; in each figure, the upper four traces are selected EEG traces, the lower three traces (with orange shading) are the corresponding motion-loop signals. The extreme motion event occurred during the time marked by the red indicator line. **(A)** is the conventional result without motion-loop subtraction. In this result, it appears as if there is also less intense yet still substantial motion contaminating the entire time shown prior to the extreme motion event (i.e., during the epoch indicated by the long green indicator line). In **(B)**, the gradient artifact correction has been re-run, excluding the use of the severe motion event from the gradient artifact correction template (i.e., the epoch highlighted in pink was excluded). This has substantially improved the remainder of the displayed EEG. Notice also that the motion-loop signals leading up to the extreme motion event no longer exhibit large motion signal, confirming the large apparent motion in the green epoch seen in **(A)** was actually due to a contaminated gradient correction template.

(Continued)

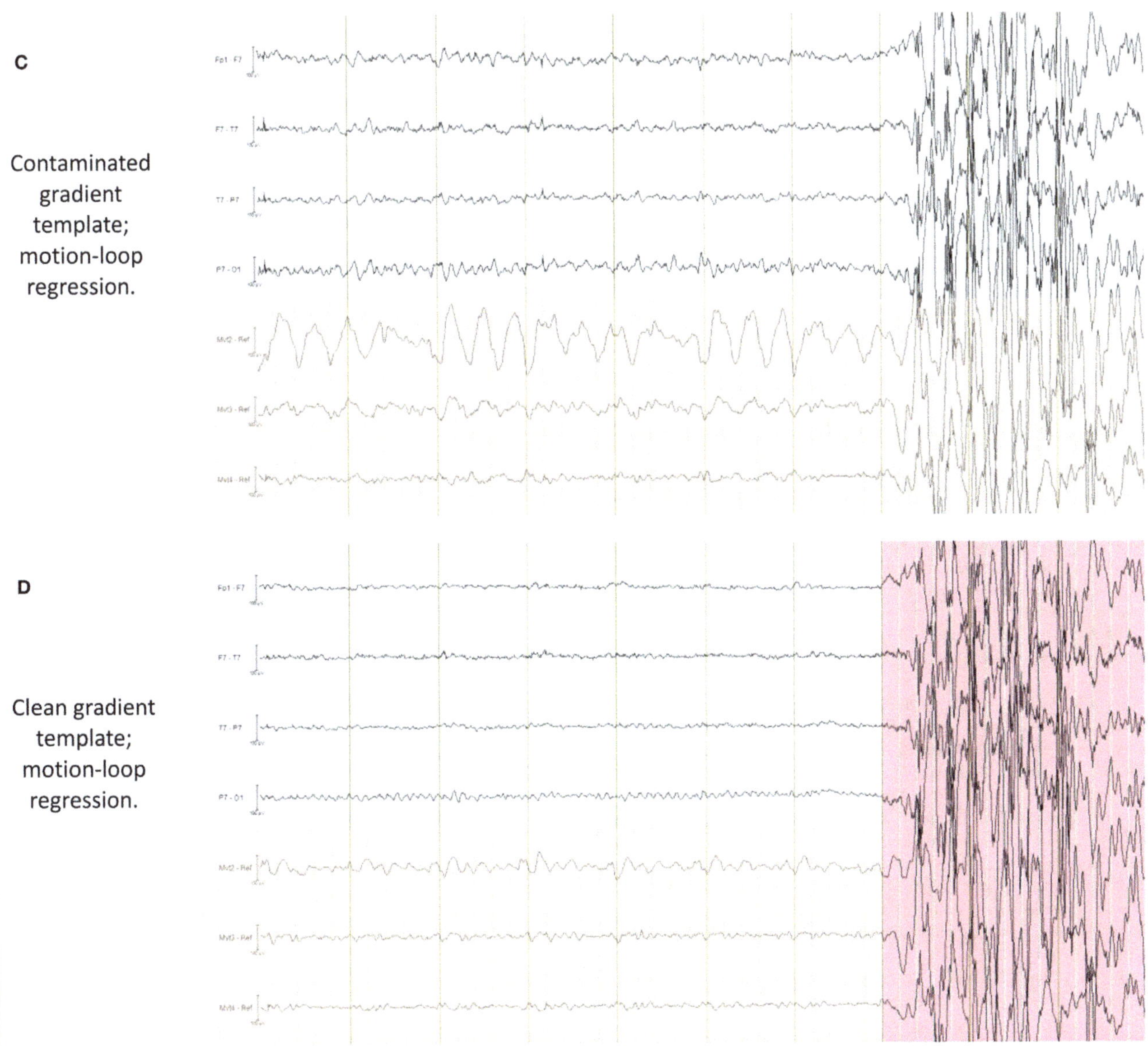

FIGURE 16 | Continued
(C) is the result of the first iteration of the motion-loop correction procedure, i.e., the same contaminated EEG shown in **(A)** has simply been subjected to motion-loop subtraction: the extreme motion event was too large to be completely removed (suggesting substantial non-linear effects); however, the smaller propagated artifact has been virtually eliminated from the EEG signal, and cardioballistic artifact is also reduced, so the EEG during the green labeled epoch is noticeably cleaner in **(C)** than in **(B)**, even though the gradient artifact correction template remains contaminated in **(C)**. Finally in **(D)**, the iterative process has been applied: the bad epoch was automatically identified from the result of the first iteration, then a second gradient artifact correction was applied to avoid motion contamination of the gradient artifact correction template, and finally motion-loop regression was applied to this improved data. This provides the cleanest EEG signal of all.

patient to the back of the scanner bore, rather than enclosed coils that would require leads to run back alongside the patient. It is likely that further insulating safety measures would be required to render these cables safe in the latter configuration.

ACKNOWLEDGMENTS

We thank Danny Flanagan for considerable work in documenting much of our existing loop assembly procedure, including creating the drawings and many of the photographs in this manuscript. We also thank Donna Parker and Mira Semmelroch for their assistance with EEG–fMRI studies and additional photographs. This work was supported in part by the National Health and Medical Research Council of Australia [project grant 318900 (John Stephen Archer), development grant 527825 (David F. Abbott), practitioner fellowship 527800 (Graeme D. Jackson)], the Australian Commonwealth Government via an Australian Postgraduate Award (Richard A. J. Masterton), and the Operational Infrastructure Support Program of the State Government of Victoria, Australia.

REFERENCES

1. Carmichael DW, Thornton JS, Rodionov R, Thornton R, McEvoy AW, Ordidge RJ, et al. Feasibility of simultaneous intracranial EEG-fMRI in humans: a safety study. *Neuroimage* (2010) **49**(1):379–90. doi:10.1016/j.neuroimage.2009.07.062
2. Lemieux L, Allen PJ, Franconi F, Symms MR, Fish DR. Recording of EEG during fMRI experiments: patient safety. *Magn Reson Med* (1997) **38**(6):943–52. doi:10.1002/mrm.1910380614
3. Lemieux L, Allen PJ, Krakow K, Symms MR, Fish DR. Methodological issues in EEG-correlated functional MRI experiments. *IJBEM* (1999) **1**(1):87–95.
4. Masterton RAJ, Abbott DF, Fleming SW, Jackson GD. Measurement and reduction of motion and ballistocardiogram artefacts from simultaneous EEG and fMRI recordings. *Neuroimage* (2007) **37**(1):202–11. doi:10.1016/j.neuroimage.2007.02.060
5. Flanagan D, Abbott DF, Jackson GD. How wrong can we be? The effect of inaccurate mark-up of EEG/fMRI studies in epilepsy. *Clin Neurophysiol* (2009) **120**(9):1637–47. doi:10.1016/j.clinph.2009.04.025
6. Maclaren J, Armstrong BS, Barrows RT, Danishad KA, Ernst T, Foster CL, et al. Measurement and correction of microscopic head motion during magnetic resonance imaging of the brain. *PLoS One* (2012) **7**(11):e48088. doi:10.1371/journal.pone.0048088
7. Briellmann RS, Little T, Harvey AS, Abbott DF, Jacobs R, Waites AB, et al. Pathologic and physiologic function in the subcortical band of double cortex. *Neurology* (2006) **67**(6):1090–3. doi:10.1212/01.wnl.0000237554.39283.6b
8. Waites AB, Shaw ME, Briellmann RS, Labate A, Abbott DF, Jackson GD. How reliable are fMRI-EEG studies of epilepsy? A nonparametric approach to analysis validation and optimization. *Neuroimage* (2005) **24**(1):192–9. doi:10.1016/j.neuroimage.2004.09.005
9. Labate A, Briellmann RS, Abbott DF, Waites AB, Jackson GD. Typical childhood absence seizures are associated with thalamic activation. *Epileptic Disord* (2005) **7**(4):373–7.
10. Federico P, Archer JS, Abbott DF, Jackson GD. Cortical/subcortical BOLD changes associated with epileptic discharges – an EEG-fMRI study at 3 T. *Neurology* (2005) **64**(7):1125–30. doi:10.1212/01.WNL.0000156358.72670.AD
11. Federico P, Abbott DF, Briellmann RS, Harvey AS, Jackson GD. Functional MRI of the pre-ictal state. *Brain* (2005) **128**:1811–7. doi:10.1093/brain/awh533
12. Archer JS, Briellmann RS, Syngeniotis A, Abbott DF, Jackson GD. Spike-triggered fMRI in reading epilepsy – involvement of left frontal cortex working memory area. *Neurology* (2003) **60**(3):415–21. doi:10.1212/WNL.60.3.415
13. Archer JS, Briellman RS, Abbott DF, Syngeniotis A, Wellard RM, Jackson GD. Benign epilepsy with centro-temporal spikes: spike triggered fMRI shows somato-sensory cortex activity. *Epilepsia* (2003) **44**(2):200–4. doi:10.1046/j.1528-1157.2003.02502.x
14. Archer JS, Abbott DF, Waites AB, Jackson GD. FMRI "deactivation" of the posterior cingulate during generalized spike and wave. *Neuroimage* (2003) **20**(4):1915–22. doi:10.1016/s0153-8119(03)00294-5
15. Opdam HI, Federico P, Jackson GD, Buchanan J, Abbott DF, Fabinyi GCA, et al. A sheep model for the study of focal epilepsy with concurrent intracranial EEG and functional MRI. *Epilepsia* (2002) **43**(8):779–87. doi:10.1046/j.1528-1157.2002.04202.x
16. Masterton RA, Carney PW, Abbott DF, Jackson GD. Absence epilepsy subnetworks revealed by event-related independent components analysis of functional magnetic resonance imaging. *Epilepsia* (2013) **54**(5):801–8. doi:10.1111/epi.12163
17. Masterton RA, Jackson GD, Abbott DF. Mapping brain activity using event-related independent components analysis (eICA): specific advantages for EEG-fMRI. *Neuroimage* (2012) **70C**:164–74. doi:10.1016/j.neuroimage.2012.12.025
18. Masterton RAJ, Harvey AS, Archer JS, Lillywhite LM, Abbott DF, Scheffer IE, et al. Focal epileptiform spikes do not show a canonical BOLD response in patients with benign rolandic epilepsy (BECTS). *Neuroimage* (2010) **51**(1):252–60. doi:10.1016/j.neuroimage.2010.01.109
19. Archer JS, Abbott DF, Masterton RA, Palmer SM, Jackson GD. Functional MRI interactions between dysplastic nodules and overlying cortex in periventricular nodular heterotopia. *Epilepsy Behav* (2010) **19**(4):631–4. doi:10.1016/j.yebeh.2010.09.018
20. Carney PW, Masterton RA, Flanagan D, Berkovic SF, Jackson GD. The frontal lobe in absence epilepsy: EEG-fMRI findings. *Neurology* (2012) **78**(15):1157–65. doi:10.1212/WNL.0b013e31824f801d
21. Carney PW, Masterton RA, Gill D, Jackson GD. Nodular heterotopia and absence seizures: fMRI evidence that they may be connected. *Epilepsy Res* (2013) **106**(3):451–5. doi:10.1016/j.eplepsyres.2013.07.005
22. Carney PW, Masterton RA, Harvey AS, Scheffer IE, Berkovic SF, Jackson GD. The core network in absence epilepsy. Differences in cortical and thalamic BOLD response. *Neurology* (2010) **75**(10):904–11. doi:10.1212/WNL.0b013e3181f11c06
23. Flanagan D, Badawy RA, Jackson GD. EEG-fMRI in focal epilepsy: local activation and regional networks. *Clin Neurophysiol* (2014) **125**(1):21–31. doi:10.1016/j.clinph.2013.06.182
24. Archer JS, Warren AE, Stagnitti MR, Masterton RA, Abbott DF, Jackson GD. Lennox-Gastaut syndrome and phenotype: secondary network epilepsies. *Epilepsia* (2014) **55**(8):1245–54. doi:10.1111/epi.12682
25. Allen PJ, Polizzi G, Krakow K, Fish DR, Lemieux L. Identification of EEG events in the MR scanner: the problem of pulse artifact and a method for its subtraction. *Neuroimage* (1998) **8**(3):229–39. doi:10.1006/nimg.1998.0361
26. Ritter P, Becker R, Graefe C, Villringer A. Evaluating gradient artifact correction of EEG data acquired simultaneously with fMRI. *Magn Reson Imaging* (2007) **25**(6):923–32. doi:10.1016/j.mri.2007.03.005
27. Abbott D, Jackson G. iBrain – software for analysis and visualisation of functional MR images. *Neuroimage* (2001) **13**(6):S59. doi:10.1016/S1053-8119(01)91402-8

16

Altered fMRI connectivity dynamics in temporal lobe epilepsy might explain seizure semiology

Helmut Laufs[1,2,3,4]*, Roman Rodionov[3,4], Rachel Thornton[3,4], John Sydney Duncan[3,4], Louis Lemieux[3,4] and Enzo Tagliazucchi[1]

[1] *Department of Neurology and Brain Imaging Center, Goethe-University Frankfurt am Main, Frankfurt am Main, Germany*
[2] *Department of Neurology, University Hospital Schleswig-Holstein, Christian-Albrechts-University Kiel, Kiel, Germany*
[3] *National Hospital for Neurology and Neurosurgery, University College London, London, UK*
[4] *The Epilepsy Society, Chalfont St. Peter, UK*

Correspondence:
Helmut Laufs, Theodor-Stern-Kai 7, 60590 Frankfurt am Main, Hessen, Germany
e-mail: h.laufs@em.uni-frankfurt.de

Temporal lobe epilepsy (TLE) can be conceptualized as a network disease. The network can be characterized by inter-regional functional connectivity, i.e., blood oxygen level-dependent (BOLD) signal correlations between any two regions. However, functional connectivity is not constant over time, thus computing correlation at a given time and then at some later time could give different results (non-stationarity). We hypothesized (1) that non-stationarities can be induced by epilepsy (e.g., interictal epileptic activity) increasing local signal variance and that (2) these transient events contribute to fluctuations in connectivity leading to pathological functioning, i.e., TLE semiology. We analyzed fMRI data from 27 patients with TLE and 22 healthy controls focusing on EEG-confirmed wake epochs only to protect against sleep-induced connectivity changes. Testing hypothesis (1), we identified brain regions where the BOLD signal variance was significantly greater in TLE than in controls: the temporal pole – including the hippocampus. Taking the latter as the seed region and testing hypothesis (2), we calculated the time-varying inter-regional correlation values (dynamic functional connectivity) to other brain regions and found greater connectivity variance in the TLE than the control group mainly in the precuneus, the supplementary and sensorimotor, and the frontal cortices. We conclude that the highest BOLD signal variance in the hippocampi is highly suggestive of a specific epilepsy-related effect. The altered connectivity dynamics in TLE patients might help to explain the hallmark semiological features of dyscognitive seizures including impaired consciousness (precuneus, frontal cortex), sensory disturbance, and motor automatisms (sensorimotor cortices, supplementary motor cortex). Accounting for the non-stationarity and state-dependence of functional connectivity are a prerequisite in the search for potential connectivity-derived biomarkers in TLE.

Keywords: functional connectivity, non-stationarity, temporal lobe epilepsy, biomarker, EEG-fMRI, interictal epileptiform discharges, semiology, seizure

INTRODUCTION

Epilepsy affects the brain both during seizures and interictally in the form of neurobehavioral problems. These are considered to be due to progressive structural and functional changes in the brain related to syndrome-specific "network" variations (1). In temporal lobe epilepsy (TLE), for example, interictal language and memory impairment are typical (2). In terms of seizure semiology, motor automatisms and consciousness impairment are characteristics of dyscognitive (complex partial) seizures typical for TLE. We hypothesized that, during seizure-free wakeful rest, brain activity is altered in syndrome-specific regions owing to so-called interictal epileptic activity – which may or may not be visible on scalp EEG (3) – and additionally any other sort of paroxysmal activity patterns differing from activity within a healthy brain, an "epileptic process." Hence, as a first step, we tested the basic assumption that in TLE patients any such paroxysmal process should induce bursts of the blood oxygen level-dependent (BOLD) signal leading to increased regional variance compared to healthy controls. Among the primary candidate regions, we expected either one or both of those contributing to "interictal" cognitive impairment and those functionally related to temporal lobe seizure semiology, i.e., not only temporal (e.g., hippocampal) but also extratemporal (consciousness subserving and motor) regions.

Temporal lobe epilepsy can be considered as a network disease (4, 5) because widespread anatomic abnormality exists outside the primary epileptic zone affecting inter-regional connectivity linked to distributed cognitive impairments (6). Hence, a natural second step is to explore to which other brain regions – exhibiting "normal" signal fluctuations – the locations of increased variance are more tightly connected in the epileptic condition than in the healthy control subjects. By always taking healthy brain activity as the reference, we ensured that the observed typical effects were specific for the epileptic condition, in particular TLE.

However, it has been shown that functional connectivity is not static (7–11) but differs between different stages of wakefulness (12), and in addition fluctuates within each stage over time. "Dynamic functional connectivity" is here understood in the context of fluctuating, non-constant coupling between brain areas when the coupling is computed over short temporal windows. In contrast with the traditional practice of assuming a steady correlation between regions, the study of dynamic connectivity aims to study how connectivity evolves in time, how stable connections are and what the possible short-term connectivity motifs are between regions. Assuming a paroxysmal pathological process influencing brain activity in TLE, it is conceivable that accounting for the non-stationarity of inter-regional BOLD signal correlations both between and within wake and other sleep stages is mandatory for obtaining specific results with high sensitivity. Because of this, we selected epochs of data recorded during epochs of wakefulness and within these based all inferences on dynamic functional connectivity measures as obtained by means of sliding window analysis. Then, the variability of dynamical functional connectivity was computed (as the variance of the functional connectivity time series), which represents the intensity of the temporal fluctuations in the connectivity of the regions. A low value of variance of the dynamic connectivity time series corresponds to stable connections, in which coupling does not deviate much from the average value. In contrast, large values of the variance correspond to widely fluctuating connectivity, i.e., switching over time between high and low values of the coupling between regions.

MATERIALS AND METHODS

All procedures were subject to the relevant local and national research ethics committees' approval.

SUBJECTS AND PATIENTS

Data from 22 healthy subjects (11 females) served as control in this study (age 35 ± 12 years), and data from 27 epilepsy patients [13 classified as left TLE (age 32 ± 9 years), 14 with right (age 33 ± 11 years); 16 females], who were selected from a larger dataset with the inclusion criteria of TLE based on electro-clinical information-informed expert classification (**Table 1**).

EEG-fMRI ACQUISITION

In this study, we assumed the presence of an "epileptic process" possibly reaching beyond epochs of interictal epileptic activity visible on scalp EEG. Accordingly, the EEG was not used for the detection of epileptiform EEG activity but to identify fMRI epochs of wakefulness in order to increase the sensitivity and specificity of our results (12).

EEG via a cap (modified Brain Cap MR, Easycap, Herrsching, Germany) was recorded continuously (sampling rate 5 kHz, low pass filter 1 kHz) during fMRI acquisition with an MRI-compatible EEG system (BrainAmp MR$^+$ and Brain Vision Analyzer; Brain Products GmbH, Gilching, Germany) yielding two 20-min sessions consisting of 404 T2*-weighted single-shot gradient-echo echo-planar images (EPIs; echo time/repetition time, 30/3000 ms; flip angle, 90°; 43 2.5 mm interleaved slices; FOV, 24 cm × 24 cm; matrix 64 × 64) acquired continuously on a 3T Signa Excite HDX MRI scanner (General Electric, Milwaukee, WI, USA).

EEG DATA PREPROCESSING

MRI and pulse artifact correction were performed based on the average artifact subtraction (AAS) method (13, 14) as implemented in Vision Analyzer 2 (BrainProducts, Germany) resulting in EEG with a sampling rate of 250 Hz. EEG was re-referenced to common average. Sleep stages were scored manually by an expert according to the AASM criteria (15). Epochs other than wakefulness were erased from the analysis (by excluding the corresponding BOLD time courses from both the variance and dynamic functional connectivity analyses). Epochs of wakefulness shorter than 2 min were not included in the analysis.

fMRI DATA PREPROCESSING

Using Statistical Parametric Mapping (SPM 8, http://www.fil.ion.ucl.ac.uk/spm), EPI data were realigned, normalized (MNI space), and spatially smoothed (Gaussian kernel, 5 mm^3 full width at half maximum). The time course of the average signal at the ventricles (CSF as given by FSL's Ventricle Mask standard image) as well as motion-induced noise was regressed out. We did not remove the global brain signal to avoid the issue of induced anti-correlations (16). Also, since there are direct electrophysiological correlates of the global resting-state signal (17), we believe that its removal is arbitrary and results in a loss of information. fMRI data was band pass filtered in the range 0.01–0.1 Hz using a sixth order Butterworth filter as described previously (8). In all cases, both 20 min fMRI sessions were analyzed and then the results were averaged within every subject (to guarantee the assumption of statistical independence) prior to statistical testing.

Subjects displayed similar degrees of head displacement across groups. Controls: 0.06 ± 0.02 mm, Left TLE: 0.08 ± 0.04 mm, Right TLE: 0.08 ± 0.05 mm. No significant differences ($p > 0.05$) between groups were found. As an additional control, we reproduced the results after erasing volumes associated with high (>0.3) head displacement amplitude (see Appendix).

DATA ANALYSIS

Computation of temporal variability

The temporal variability (variance) of BOLD signals carries important information about the brain state and also about task performance. An optimal value is typically observed during rest, which is decreased locally during task performance and increased in other brain states such as sleep (11, 18, 19). The possibility of interictal spikes occurring in TLE patient leads naturally to the hypothesis of locally increased variability (i.e., increased variance) of BOLD activity time courses. To quantify precisely the changes in variability observed in the patient vs. the control population, we use the traditional definition of variance in the time domain:

$$\sigma^2 = \langle (X - \langle X \rangle)^2 \rangle \quad (1)$$

where X is the BOLD signal, σ^2 the variance, and $\langle, \rangle$ denotes temporal averaging. This analysis is performed on a voxel-wise basis, resulting in spatial maps in which every voxel contains the variance of its associated time series. The procedure is summarized in **Figure 1A**.

Table 1 | Patient characteristics.

	Age (years)	Ictal	Interictal	Structural MRI	Seizure semiology included		VIQ	PIQ	Epilepsy duration (years)	Medication
		EEG changes			Reduced consciousness	Motor automatisms				
L1	49	Left	Left > right	Normal	Yes	Yes	84	99	Unknown	Unretrievable
L2	29	Initial left	Left	Normal	Yes	No	100	100	14	LTG
L3	28	Left (icEEG)	Left (icEEG)	Normal	Yes	Yes	87	100	18	LEV, VPA
L4	33	Left	Left	Left HS	Yes	Yes	71	81	28	Unretrievable
L5	27	Left	Left	Left HS	Yes	Yes	90	99	24	LEV, VPA, PGB
L6	30	Left (icEEG)	Left (icEEG)	Signal change in calcarine fissure	Yes	Yes	75	80	15	CBZ, LEV, CZ
L7	41	Left	Left	Left HS	Yes	Yes	80	93	Unknown	CBZ, LEV
L8	48	Left	Left > right	Normal	Yes	Yes	107	119	37	LEV, PHT
L9	19	Left	Left	Left HS	Uncertain	Yes	92	98	12	TPM, LTG
L10	26	Left	Left	Bilateral HS	Yes	Yes	99	106	19	LEV, LTG
L11	42	Left	Left	Left HS and parietal WML	Yes	Yes	97	99	33	LEV, PHT, PGB
L12	28	Left	Left (icEEG)	Left STG abnormality	Yes	Negative motor	102	106	Unknown	CBZ, LEV, LTG
L13	19	Left	Left, bilateral	Irregularly lobulated mass left temporal into frontal lobe	Yes	Yes	111	106	2	LTG
R1	25	Right	Right	Tumor right temporal lobe	Uncertain	Never observed	105	100	6	CBZ, LTG
R2	38	Bilateral	Right	Right HS	Yes	Yes	103	96	Unknown	CBZ, TPM
R3	20	Unretrievable	Unretrievable	Right HS	Uncertain	Never observed	80	73	4	CBZ, LEV
R4	23	No scalp discharges	Right	Right temporal gliosis	Yes	Yes	80	84	23	OXC, CZM, ACM
R5	25	Right (icEEG)	Right and independent left	Right HS, right temporal DNET	Yes	Yes	Unknown	Unknown	Unretrievable	Unretrievable
R6	40	Right temporal and left fronto -central	Right » left	Right HS	Yes	Yes	Unknown	Unknown	Unretrievable	TPM, PHB, PGB
R7	59	Right	Right	Bilateral WML	Uncertain	Yes	87	89	54	LEV
R8	30	Right	Right	Normal	Yes	Yes	80	80	13	OXC, GBP, CZM
R9	18	Right	Right	Right temporal DNET	Yes	Yes	101	110	11	OXC
R10	37	Right	Right	Normal	Yes	Yes	67	92	14	CBZ, LTG
R11	24	Right	Right > left	Normal	Yes	Yes	82	105	5	VPA, PGB, CZM
R12	41	Right	Right	Right HS	No	No	108	110	22	CBZ, LEV

(Continued)

Table 1 | Continued

	Age (years)	Ictal	Interictal	Structural MRI	Seizure semiology included		VIQ	PIQ	Epilepsy duration (years)	Medication
		EEG changes			Reduced consciousness	Motor automatisms				
R13	37	No scalp discharges	Right	Right HS	Yes	No	85	81	14	OXC, ZNS
R14	43	Right	Right	Normal	Yes	No	115	113	26	LTG, LCS

L[index], syndrome classified as left TLE, R[index], syndrome classified as right TLE; VIQ/PIQ, verbal/performance IQ (Wechsler D. WAIS III Administration and Scoring Manual, New York Psychological Corporation 1997); icEEG, intracranial EEG; HS, hippocampal sclerosis, DNET, dysembryoplastic neuroepithelial tumor; WML, white matter lesion(s); STG, superior temporal gyrus; ACT, acetazolamide; CBZ, carbamazepine; CZM, clobazam; LCS, lacosamide; LEV, levetiracetam; LTG, lamotrigine; OXC, oxcarbazepine; PGB, pregabalin; PHT, phenytoin; TPM, topiramate; VPA, valproate; ZNS, zonisamide.

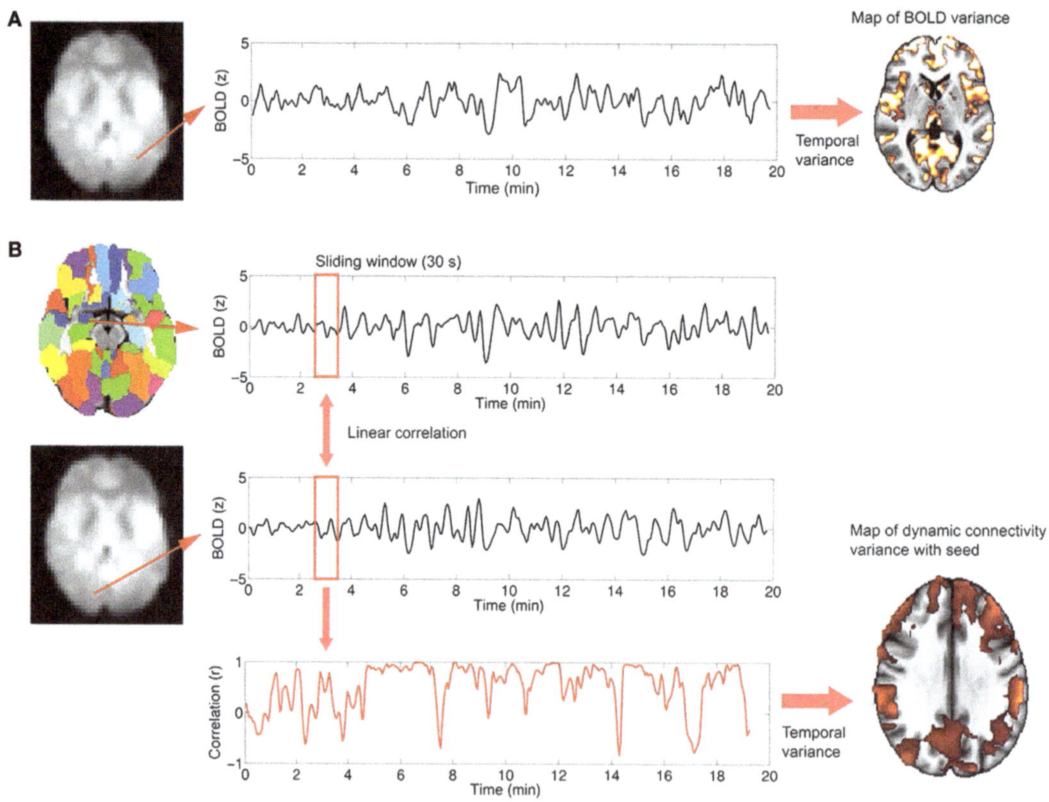

FIGURE 1 | Procedure to study BOLD signal and functional connectivity temporal variability. (A) To compute the voxel-wise map of BOLD signal variability, the time series for every voxel in the EPI data is first extracted. Then, the variance of the signal is computed, resulting in the required map. **(B)** To compute the voxel-wise map of BOLD functional connectivity temporal variability with a seed, a region in the AAL template is first selected (in this work, the left and right hippocampi are used as seeds) and the average signal in the region is computed. Then, for every voxel in the EPI data, correlations over time are obtained using a sliding window (30 s) and the temporal dynamics of functional connectivity are computed. Note that in this example the dynamics are non-constant with moments of drastic loss of connectivity between regions. Finally, the temporal variance of the functional connectivity time series is computed, resulting in a spatial map (see **Figure 4**) encoding the variability in the interaction between the seed region and every voxel.

Computation of functional connectivity variability

The study of functional connectivity between brain regions usually neglects the possibility of changes of connectivity occurring over time [*dynamical functional connectivity* (8)]. Not only functional connectivity values computed over extended periods of time characterize the healthy, resting brain but also a normal switching of connectivity values, representing the engagement and disengagement of different brain networks. At a first level, the normal level of this fluctuation in connectivity can be computed in two steps, which are also summarized graphically in **Figure 1B**:

(1) A temporal time course of functional connectivity is computed by means of a sliding window analysis. Inside each window, the normal correlation coefficient between the signal at a seed region and the signal at every voxel in the brain is computed. Then, the window is displaced one time step and the analysis repeated, obtaining one connectivity estimate per time unit. In this work, the sliding window length was set to 30 s, and the seed region to the left and right hippocampus [as defined in the automated anatomical labeling atlas (20)].
(2) Once the temporal time courses of functional connectivity are obtained, they are collapsed into a single spatial map by computing their temporal variability or variance (using Eq. 1). Thus, this results in a map in which every voxel has a value encoding how widely over time its connectivity with a seed region of interest is fluctuating.

STATISTICAL ANALYSIS

Both maps of temporal variability and of dynamical functional connectivity variability are compared between groups by means of mass univariate t-tests as implemented in the SPM8 software. All maps are reported at a level of $p < 0.001$ uncorrected with only clusters passing a threshold of $p < 0.05$ FWE corrected being shown.

RESULTS

On average, healthy controls slept more than left and right TLE patients (**Figure 2**). Controls were awake 71 ± 11% of the time, left TLE patients 85 ± 8%, and the right TLE patients 86 ± 9% of the time. This justifies the detection and deleting of BOLD data corresponding to sleep, considering the possibility of confounds due to comparing groups of subjects in different vigilance states (12).

The voxel-wise analysis of BOLD signal variance in TLE was greater than in controls in the anterior temporal lobe bilaterally (**Table 2**; **Figure 3**). Significantly reduced variance compared to controls was not found in any voxel. A significant difference between left TLE and right TLE was not observed.

Dynamic functional connectivity from the hippocampi in TLE (left and right TLE pooled) was greater than in controls in the supplementary motor area, the pre- and postcentral gyri, the (pre-)cuneus, the calcarine/middle occipital gyrus, and the superior frontal gyrus (**Tables 3** and **4**; **Figure 4**). A significant difference between left TLE and right TLE was not observed (compare **Tables 3** and **4** for seeding in the left and right hippocampus, respectively). Of the pooled analysis, only results for the left hippocampus as the seed region are displayed and differences between seeding in the left and the right hippocampus were not significant (compare **Tables 3** and **4**).

DISCUSSION

Interictally, compared to healthy controls and during wakefulness, in the TLE group we found increased BOLD signal variance in the anterior temporal lobe regions overlapping with the left and right hippocampi and that these regions showed increased dynamic functional connectivity most prominently to sensory motor structures, the precuneus, and superior frontal cortices.

Table 2 | Regions, hemisphere, and statistical significance of areas with increased BOLD signal variance in TLE patients compared to healthy controls (local maxima at least 8 mm apart).

Brain region	MNI coordinates (x, y, z)	Hemisphere	t-Value
Left + Right TLE > Healthy Controls			
Inferior temporal gyrus	(38, −4, −36)	Right	6.44
Temporal pole	(−38, 8, −30)	Left	5.30
Left TLE > Healthy Controls			
Temporal pole	(36, 0, −36)	Right	5.31
Right TLE > Healthy Controls			
Fusiform gyrus	(34, −8, −36)	Right	5.08
Inferior temporal gyrus	(−36, −4, −36)	Left	4.89

TLE, temporal lobe epilepsy.

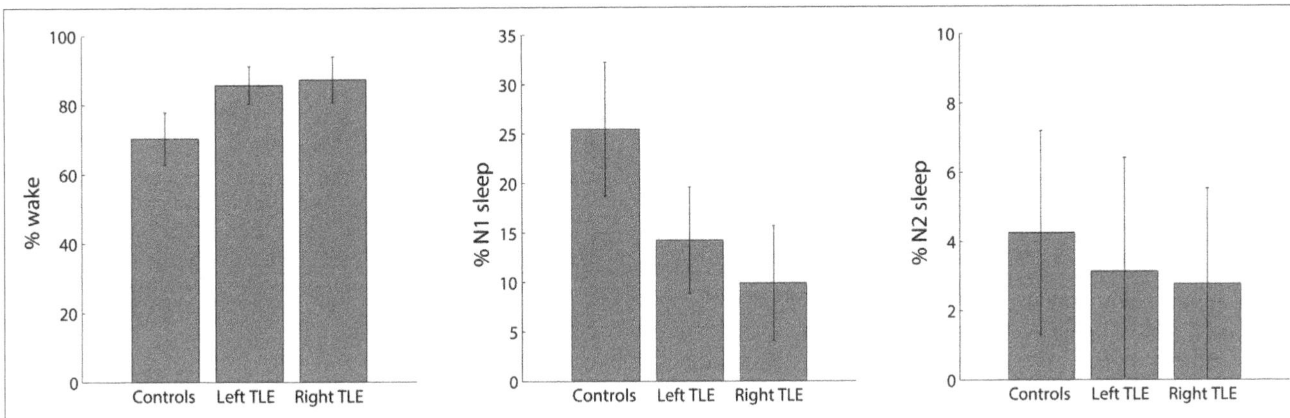

FIGURE 2 | Distribution of percent time spent in different sleep stages (wake, N1 and N2; no N3 sleep was observed) for healthy controls, left and right TLE patients (mean ± SEM).

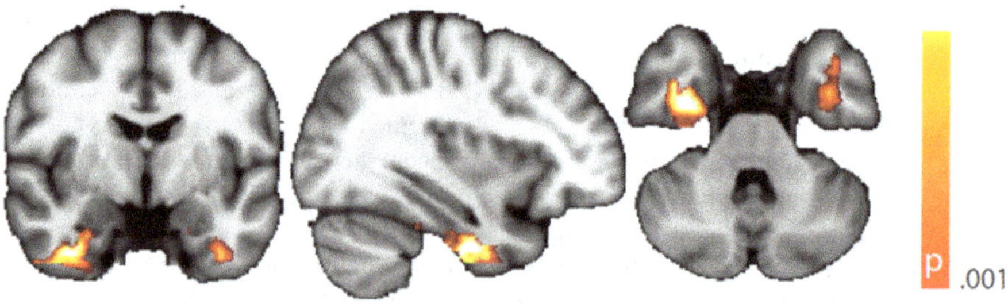

FIGURE 3 | Spatial map (coronal, sagittal, axial slices) of significantly greater variance of the blood oxygen level-dependent signal in patients with temporal lobe epilepsy (pooled right and left) than in healthy controls. Color bar indicates *p*-value (thresholded at $p < 0.001$ for display, cluster survives family-wise error correction at $p < 0.05$). Left on figure is right in the brain (coronal and axial slices).

Table 3 | Regions, hemisphere, and statistical significance of areas with increased variance of dynamic functional connectivity with the left hippocampus in patients compared to healthy controls.

Brain region	MNI coordinates (*x, y, z*)	Hemisphere	*t*-Value
Left + Right TLE > Healthy Controls			
Supp. motor area	(4, −12, 72)	Right	4.78
Postcentral gyrus	(−20, −24, 72)	Left	4.95
Precentral gyrus	(−44, 4, 52)	Left	4.81
Cuneus	(1, −76, 28)	Right	4.97
Calcarine	(1, −92, −8)	Right	4.66
Sup. frontal gyrus	(1, 76, 8)	Right	4.79
Middle frontal gyrus	(−12, 79, 24)	Left	3.74
Left TLE > Healthy Controls			
Paracentral lobule	(0, −28, 80)	Left/right	4.76
Postcentral gyrus	(36, −28, 60)	Right	4.56
Cuneus	(12, −76, 20)	Right	5.14
Sup. frontal gyrus	(−8, 24, −20)	Left	4.56
Parahippocampal gyrus	(−32, −24, −20)	Left	4.51
Middle frontal gyrus	(−12, 75, 22)	Left	3.64
Right TLE > Healthy Controls			
Supp. motor area	(0, −20, 64)	Left/right	4.57
Cuneus	(0, −80, 28)	Left/right	4.95
Middle cingulate gyrus	(−1, −24, 52)	Left	4.31
Sup. frontal gyrus	(0, 76, 8)	Left/right	4.33
Parahippocampal gyrus	(−32, −24, −21)	Left	4.15
Middle frontal gyrus	(−7, 83, 32)	Left	4.01

TLE, temporal lobe epilepsy, supp, supplementary, sup, superior.

Table 4 | Regions, hemisphere, and statistical significance of areas with increased variance of dynamic functional connectivity with the right hippocampus in patients compared to healthy controls.

Brain region	MNI coordinates (*x, y, z*)	Hemisphere	*t*-Value
Left + Right TLE > Healthy Controls			
Paracentral lobule	(0, −28, 80)	Left/right	5.10
Precuneus	(−8, −36, 60)	Left	4.35
Cuneus	(−12, −84, 40)	Left	4.82
Middle occipital gyrus	(28, −84, 28)	Right	4.84
Postcentral gyrus	(8, −40, 80)	Right	4.35
Sup. frontal gyrus	(0, 56, −20)	Left/right	4.12
Left TLE > Healthy Controls			
Paracentral lobule	(0, −24, 76)	Left/right	4.46
Precentral gyrus	(−40, −16, 64)	Left	4.06
Cuneus	(12, −96, 16)	Right	4.42
Fusiform gyrus	(−28, −24, −24)	Left	4.10
Middle frontal gyrus	(4, 84, −16)	Right	4.19
Right TLE > Healthy Controls			
Paracentral lobule	(0, −28, 80)	Left/right	4.26
Cuneus	(4, −80, 24)	Right	4.74
Middle frontal gyrus	(0, 60, 28)	Left/right	4.04
Inferior frontal gyrus	(48, 32, −16)	Right	4.15
Middle cingulate gyrus	(4, 36, 32)	Right	4.09

sup, superior.

The identification of anterior temporal lobe structures in particular including the hippocampi is highly suggestive of a syndrome-specific effect because these regions have long been known as crucial in TLE (21). The anterior hippocampus is thought to be highly epileptogenic (22). In the context of interictal neuropsychological dysfunction, it is essential for memory processes (23), and with respect to seizure control, its surgical removal has been shown to be associated with a good outcome (24). In addition, our study design in which we try to keep constant as many parameters as possible between the control and the patient group (including the state of wakefulness) ensures that any significant group differences are specific to the condition TLE. In particular, we can identify significant activity alterations in sets of brain regions constituting intrinsic connectivity networks, which can be present both in the patient and the control group and which might evade other analysis techniques such as independent component analysis or conventional seed region-based functional connectivity analysis.

INTERPRETATION OF INCREASED HIPPOCAMPAL BOLD SIGNAL VARIANCE

The first observation that in our group of TLE patients, we found the highest BOLD signal variance in the anterior temporal lobe

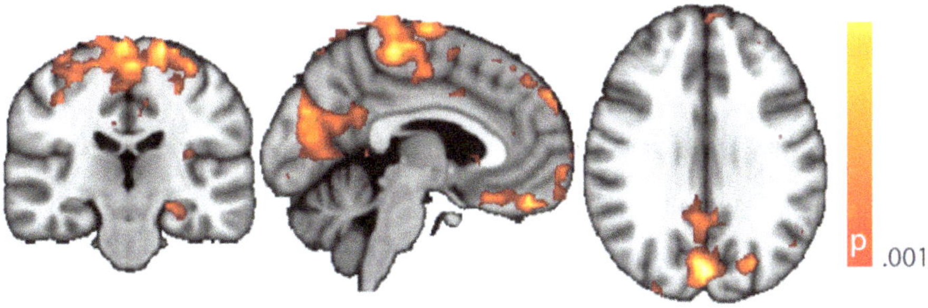

FIGURE 4 | Spatial map (coronal, sagittal, axial slices) of significantly greater variance of hippocampal dynamic functional connectivity in patients with temporal lobe epilepsy (here: seed in left hippocampus) than in healthy controls. For differences between seeding in the left hippocampus and in the right, see **Tables 3** and **4**, of the pooled analysis, only results for the left hippocampus as the seed region are displayed (seed in right hippocampus yielded most similar results). Color bar indicates *p*-value (thresholded at $p < 0.001$ for display, cluster survives family-wise error correction at $p < 0.05$). Left on figure is right in the brain (coronal and axial slices).

including, of note, the hippocampus supports our hypothesis of the presence of paroxysmal interictal activity resulting in regionally increased BOLD signal variance. It is well-established that local field potentials (LFP) explain the largest portion of this variance (25) and that interictal epileptic spikes in the anterior temporal lobe are reflected in LFP changes (26). We hence propose interictal epileptic activity ("epileptic process") as the most likely explanation for the high anterior temporal lobe variance common to our TLE group. Kobayashi and colleagues as well as ourselves previously identified hippocampal BOLD signal increases at the group level in TLE, when correlating by means of a general linear model (GLM) interictal scalp EEG activity with the BOLD signal (27, 28). For these GLM-based EEG-fMRI studies, the occurrence of a number of interictal spikes was essential, whereas in the present approach, we on purpose designed our analysis to be independent of scalp EEG interictal activity. We did this for two reasons: (1) the sensitivity of scalp EEG in TLE is compromised with respect to hippocampal interictal epileptic activity (3, 29), allowing the creation of a scalp EEG-based GLM with limited sensitivity only and (2) we sought to identify an fMRI marker for paroxysmal activity specific to the epileptic condition independently of the simultaneously recorded EEG. Such paroxysmal activity in addition to "true" interictal spikes (as can be demonstrated with intracranial EEG) might include other types of epileptic (neuronal) activity leading to bursts of energy consuming processes, e.g., owing to damaged cells in the hippocampus, alterations in the glial milieu, or pathology of blood flow parameters (30). The exclusive selection of epochs during which the patients and control subjects, respectively, were awake ensured increased sensitivity when comparing resting-state BOLD signal properties: it is well known that the functional architecture of the brain changes significantly depending on the level of wakefulness (12, 31) including the variance of the BOLD signal in different brain regions (11, 32), but also graph theoretical network measures (33, 34), and variance in the brain's functional connectivity structure (8).

We note that a very similar result (increased variance of BOLD signals in bilateral hippocampi) was recently found for subjects under the influence of a psychedelic substance (psilocybin) (35). Furthermore, a related result is discussed in the context of REM sleep (36), and in the psilocybin study the intensity of the "dream-like" experience, which was rated subjectively by the subjects, correlated positively with the magnitude of the hippocampal BOLD signal fluctuations. It can be speculated that subjective alterations in the conscious awareness of the patients – more subtle than full-blown seizures, but which can escalate into the former and also into auras – are shared in TLE and in the other altered states of consciousness mentioned above.

INTERPRETATION OF INCREASED HIPPOCAMPAL DYNAMIC FUNCTIONAL CONNECTIVITY

Increased variance of dynamic functional connectivity in TLE compared to healthy controls indicates region pairs, which exhibit stronger fluctuations of the correlation of their BOLD time series in the epileptic condition than in the healthy. While the measure does not assess an absolute difference in connectivity between the two cohorts, regions are identified, which link and unlink typically more in TLE than in the control group. Our study design motivates the hypothesis that the "epileptic process" is responsible for this coupling and uncoupling, possibly in the form of the interictal epileptiform activity in the hippocampus, which leads to increased functional connectivity variance. Further analyses should reveal whether such epileptic activity weakens or strengthens the functional connection between regions. It may even be that "erratic" hippocampal coupling (and uncoupling) with cortical regions disrupts the physiological interplay of the latter with yet further parts of the brain – including subcortical and that this eventually results in the observed dysfunctionality.

Van Paesschen and colleagues used single photon emission computed tomography (SPECT) to study patients with hippocampal sclerosis (HS) and observed both ictal hyper- and hypoperfusion in (lateralized) regions partly overlapping with those we describe here in our study, which also includes many cases of HS. Hyperperfusion was described in temporal lobe, middle frontal and central regions, and in the frontal lobes and the precuneus hypoperfusion was found (37). It hence appears that both a "gain" as well as a "loss of function" in different brain regions is linked with ictal dysfunctioning. For example, Chassagnon and colleagues studied patients with mesial TLE and found ictal–interictal hypoperfusion in the posterior cingulate and prefrontal regions, which might be interpreted as a loss of function in the sense of impaired consciousness (precuneus) and executive functioning (frontal regions) (38).

Looking at the particular brain regions in TLE with increased connectivity variance, we speculate that (1) the hippocampal activity interferes with language (39) and memory function (40), both interictally and ictally and that (2) the increased dynamic connectivity to the precuneus and frontal cortex is ictally associated with impaired consciousness (4, 41) and executive functioning (42). We also propose that (3) the increased dynamics in functional connectivity between the hippocampus and the sensorimotor cortices might pave the way for ictal sensory and motor dysfunction and – probably tightly related to the supplementary motor area – in particular motor automatisms (43). The superior frontal gyrus was also described relevant for introspection (44).

HOW ARE INTERICTAL CONNECTIVITY CHANGES LINKED WITH ICTAL SEMIOLOGY?

Our study does not offer any objective clues as to what the changes we describe in the TLE group interictally have to do with ictal changes in brain function. While it is well described that language and memory impairment are present interictally (45), sensorimotor dysfunction does not obviously occur interictally. One explanation could be that a qualitative difference between what is called interictal and ictal activity may not exist as such, but rather a quantitative one: Binnie a good decade ago pointed out that if only we tested carefully enough, transitory cognitive impairment could be related to "interictal" activity in many individuals (46). In our own EEG-fMRI study looking at BOLD signal changes related to formally interictal activity, we interpreted signal changes in regions of the so-called default mode network to explain reduced consciousness during dyscognitive seizures. However, we selected for the study cohort patients with very frequent interictal discharges on the EEG increasing the sensitivity of our discharge-correlated GLM analysis (27). With this in mind and taking Binnie's idea forward, it is conceivable that with so-called interictal activity vastly the same set of brain regions (network) is recruited as is ictally with the difference that when behavioral alterations become obvious they are called seizures and hence define "ictal activity." Of course, some additional features distinguish seizure from interictal activity going beyond "duration" alone but include spreading of epileptic activity. Still, such spreading of activity might occur along interictally pre-existing paths (47). Supporting our speculation further, in TLE, structural changes have been shown to progress over time and memory function was more closely related to structural hippocampal changes than the overt seizure frequency: the group of Bernasconi found neocortical thinning in TLE progressing over time in bilateral frontal (sensorimotor) and temporal (hippocampal, entorhinal, temporopolar) regions – overlapping with the regions we report here (48), and Pacagnella and colleagues most recently presented data proposing that memory impairment is more influenced by hippocampal damage than by seizure frequency (40). In our limited cohort, we failed to identify a correlation between epilepsy duration and BOLD signal variance or dynamic functional connectivity (analysis not shown).

UNIDIRECTIONAL DIFFERENCES AND LACK OF SIGNIFICANT LATERALIZATION OF OUR FINDINGS

We did not find any significantly lateralized or side-dependent results. Instead, significant differences between healthy subjects and controls were usually bilateral. This might be due to a lack of sensitivity of our analysis, which was not optimized for this purpose (balancing of handedness, type of left- and right-sided pathologies, and EEG abnormalities). We hence do not discuss our lateralized results. In general, however, on first sight, a lack of lateralized findings is surprising taking into account clinical practice and surgical success with unilateral resections and the efforts spent with non- and invasive video-EEG telemetry and imaging to identify in which temporal lobe (hippocampus) the epileptogenic zone is located (49). Although it is clinically not a contested issue that it is relevant indeed to operate on the correct side of the brain, we are not aware of any systematic review of epilepsy surgery cases in which – for whatever reason – retrospectively the wrong side was operated upon. It is likely that the vastly symmetrical results we present reflect secondary bilateral "network" effects of a lateralized primary cause.

It is equally interesting that we found exclusively variance increases – and not any decreases – of BOLD signal amplitude and hippocampal functional connectivity in patients with TLE compared to control subjects. However, we would like to note that this does not rule out the possibility of decreased absolute functional inter-regional connectivity in the epilepsy cohort, as this differs from the variance of functional connectivity, which we report in our study and the interpretation of which is discussed above. Still, a relationship between the two measures might exist because many of the regions in which we found altered dynamic functional connectivity were also reported by Haneef and colleagues. They compared TLE patients to controls and found that the classical measure of static hippocampal functional connectivity was greater to the bilateral temporal lobes, insula, fornix, frontal poles, angular gyrus, basal ganglia, thalamus, and cerebellum. They found reduced connectivity with the occipital pole, calcarine, lingual, precuneus, sensorimotor cortex, and parts of insula and frontal lobes as well as medial frontal areas (50). We report results of a "Standard Seed Correlation Analysis" of our data in the Appendix. Because we analyzed wakefulness epochs exclusively, comparability to other data remains limited.

LIMITATIONS

We are aware of the many factors influencing resting-state – and any other – fMRI studies (51) but not aware of any study formally assessing the order of relevance of the numerous confounding effects. We do know, though, from our own data (12, 31) that sleep alters the neuronal resting-state brain architecture significantly; and motion is known to introduce BOLD signal changes of several magnitudes the size of those commonly induced neuronally (52). In comparison, e.g., effects of sex and age are less pronounced both in terms of extent and intensity, and only optimized analysis methods will reveal such differences (53, 54). Nevertheless, we tried to match both gender and age as much as possible between the examined cohorts. We regressed rigid body motion from the data and in an additional analysis accounting for motion-induced variance in a very conservative way showed that our results were robust w.r.t.

motion-induced variance (see "Reproduction of Results Erasing High Amplitude Head Movements" in the Appendix; **Figures 5** and **6**).

Regarding confounding fluctuations in wakefulness, to our knowledge, this is the first "wakeful rest" functional connectivity study controlling for and restricting the analysis to true, EEG-defined, awake epochs only and in addition accounting for non-stationarity of the functional connectivity even within the awake state. We advocate both as a desirable standard. To demonstrate independence of our results to the length of the sliding window used in the dynamic functional connectivity analysis, we performed an additional analysis with a different (shorter) window length (see "Robustness against Changes in Sliding Window Length" in the Appendix, **Figure 7**).

We did not make a strong point about left TLE vs. right TLE comparisons, because we did not observe significant group differences. Evidently, absence of proof is not proof of absence but may be due to patient heterogeneity. Such is almost inevitable in patient studies like this one caused by a variety of factors, such as the range of dyscognitive seizure semiology (not any two patients have the same seizures), seizure frequency, and the potential occurrence of additional generalized tonic clonic seizures, type and location

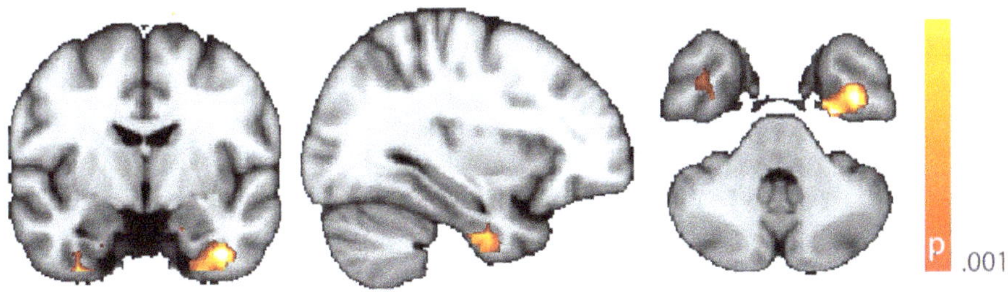

FIGURE 5 | Spatial map (coronal, sagittal, axial slices) of significantly greater variance of the blood oxygen level-dependent signal in patients with temporal lobe epilepsy (pooled right and left) than in healthy controls. An additional preprocessing step was performed by erasing volumes associated with large head displacements, as well as surrounding volumes. Color bar indicates p-value (thresholded at $p < 0.001$ for display, cluster survives family-wise error correction at $p < 0.05$). Left on figure is right in the brain (coronal and axial slices).

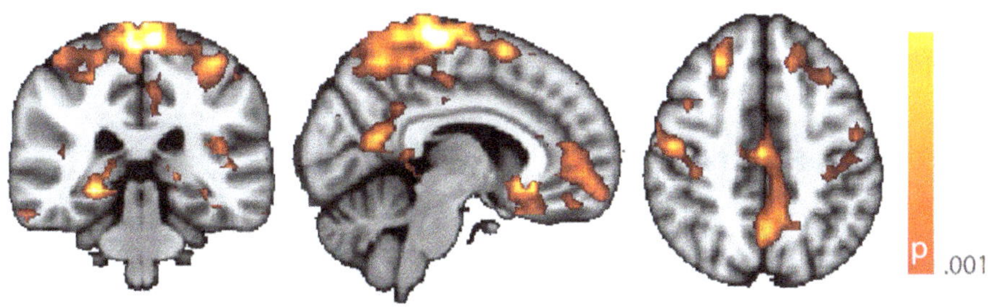

FIGURE 6 | Spatial map (coronal, sagittal, axial slices) of significantly greater variance of hippocampal dynamic functional connectivity in patients with temporal lobe epilepsy (here: seed in left hippocampus) than in healthy controls. An additional preprocessing step was performed by erasing volumes associated with large head displacements, as well as six surrounding volumes. Color bar indicates p-value (thresholded at $p < 0.001$ for display, cluster survives family-wise error correction at $p < 0.05$). Left on figure is right in the brain (coronal and axial slices).

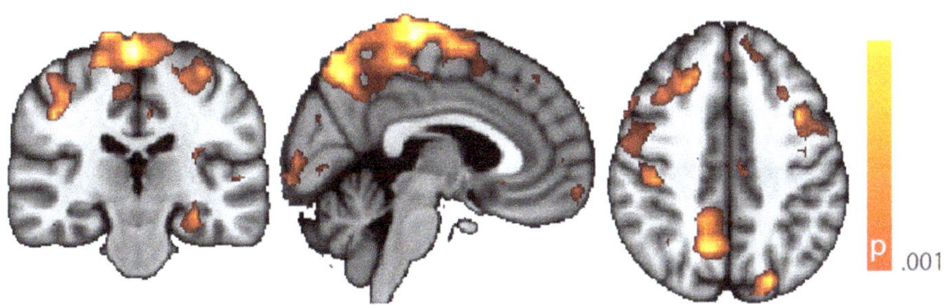

FIGURE 7 | Spatial map (coronal, sagittal, axial slices) of significantly greater variance of hippocampal dynamic functional connectivity in patients with temporal lobe epilepsy (here: seed in left hippocampus) than in healthy controls. A sliding window length of 15 s was used for the computation of dynamic functional connectivity time series. Color bar indicates p-value (thresholded at $p < 0.001$ for display, cluster survives family-wise error correction at $p < 0.05$). Left on figure is right in the brain (coronal and axial slices).

– or by current radiological standards even absence – of structural pathology visible on MRI, IQ, duration of epilepsy, and medication – just to name a few. Although epilepsy syndrome diagnosis relied on multidisciplinary experts reviewing extensive electro-clinical information, we cannot rule out classification errors. But differences within the TLE cohort between left and right TLE patients will not affect our main positive findings, i.e., the group differences between TLE and healthy controls. However, we note that any medication taken by the patients if systematically leading to, e.g., alterations of consciousness could have biased our results; but there is no evidence to date supporting this possibility for the specific patterns we observed.

In addition to these mere technical issues, like in any resting-state study, result interpretation conceptionally is limited given the absence of a task. We based the justification of the study design on the fact that interictal epileptic activity occurs spontaneously at rest as indicated by neuronal discharges measurable with EEG, although we assumed a more general "epileptic process" based on the well-established general clinical observation of interictal cognitive compromitation in TLE. In an attempt to tie our interpretation of our observations more closely to the results, we regressed IQ against BOLD signal variance and dynamic functional connectivity. We report this analysis only in "Correlations Between BOLD Signal Variance/Variance of Dynamic Connectivity Time Series with the Left Hippocampus and VIQ/PIQ" in the Appendix as it needs to be considered of anecdotal character owing to a lack of statistical significance. Causes of the latter include those discussed above.

CONCLUSION

We found evidence in support of our hypothesis that, interictally, brain activity is altered in syndrome-specific regions. Assuming that interictal processes like bursts of interictal epileptiform discharges will generate large changes in BOLD amplitude, we analyzed the variance of the BOLD signal and found this increased in anterior temporal regions, which suggest a TLE specific effect. Starting from the anterior temporal lobe, we found hippocampal dynamic connectivity increased in regions, which might explain the hallmark semiological features of complex partial seizures including impaired consciousness (precuneus, frontal cortex), sensory disturbance, and motor automatisms (sensorimotor cortices, supplementary motor area). Taking into account state of the art knowledge about the non-stationarity and state-dependence of functional connectivity, we sought to increase the sensitivity and specificity of our results. More generally, this work encourages the further development of connectivity-derived measures as potential functional imaging biomarkers in TLE.

ACKNOWLEDGMENTS

This work was funded by the Bundesministerium für Bildung und Forschung (grant 01 EV 0703), the Deutsche Forschungsgemeinschaft (grant LA 1452/3-1), and the LOEWE Neuronale Koordination Forschungsschwerpunkt Frankfurt (NeFF). We thank Verena Brodbeck, Astrid Morzelewski, and Sajitha Cannadathu for EEG processing including sleep scoring. We are indebted to Pam Thompson for neuropsychology assessments. We are grateful to the Wolfson Trust and the Epilepsy Society for supporting the Epilepsy Society MRI scanner. This work was undertaken at UCLH/UCL who received a proportion of funding from the Department of Health's NIHR UCLH Biomedical Research Centre funding scheme. We thank all participants of this study for their contribution.

REFERENCES

1. Hermann B, Seidenberg M, Jones J. The neurobehavioural comorbidities of epilepsy: can a natural history be developed? *Lancet Neurol* (2008) **7**:151–60. doi:10.1016/S1474-4422(08)70018-8
2. Sidhu MK, Stretton J, Winston GP, Bonelli S, Centeno M, Vollmar C, et al. A functional magnetic resonance imaging study mapping the episodic memory encoding network in temporal lobe epilepsy. *Brain* (2013) **136**:1868–88. doi:10.1093/brain/awt099
3. Pacia SV, Ebersole JS. Intracranial EEG substrates of scalp ictal patterns from temporal lobe foci. *Epilepsia* (1997) **38**:642–54. doi:10.1111/j.1528-1157.1997.tb01233.x
4. Laufs H. Functional imaging of seizures and epilepsy: evolution from zones to networks. *Curr Opin Neurol* (2012) **25**:194–200. doi:10.1097/WCO.0b013e3283515db9
5. Bernhardt BC, Hong S, Bernasconi A, Bernasconi N. Imaging structural and functional brain networks in temporal lobe epilepsy. *Front Hum Neurosci* (2013) **7**:624. doi:10.3389/fnhum.2013.00624
6. Bell B, Lin JJ, Seidenberg M, Hermann B. The neurobiology of cognitive disorders in temporal lobe epilepsy. *Nat Rev Neurol* (2011) **7**:154–64. doi:10.1038/nrneurol.2011.3
7. Chang C, Glover GH. Time-frequency dynamics of resting-state brain connectivity measured with fMRI. *Neuroimage* (2010) **50**:81–98. doi:10.1016/j.neuroimage.2009.12.011
8. Tagliazucchi E, Von Wegner F, Morzelewski A, Brodbeck V, Laufs H. Dynamic BOLD functional connectivity in humans and its electrophysiological correlates. *Front Hum Neurosci* (2012) **6**:339. doi:10.3389/fnhum.2012.00339
9. Chang C, Liu Z, Chen MC, Liu X, Duyn JH. EEG correlates of time-varying BOLD functional connectivity. *Neuroimage* (2013) **72**:227–36. doi:10.1016/j.neuroimage.2013.01.049
10. Hutchison RM, Womelsdorf T, Gati JS, Everling S, Menon RS. Resting-state networks show dynamic functional connectivity in awake humans and anesthetized macaques. *Hum Brain Mapp* (2013) **34**:2154–77. doi:10.1002/hbm.22058
11. Tagliazucchi E, Von Wegner F, Morzelewski A, Brodbeck V, Jahnke K, Laufs H. Breakdown of long-range temporal dependence in default mode and attention networks during deep sleep. *Proc Natl Acad Sci U S A* (2013) **110**:15419–24. doi:10.1073/pnas.1312848110
12. Tagliazucchi E, Laufs H. Decoding wakefulness levels from typical fMRI resting-state data reveals reliable drifts between wakefulness and sleep. *Neuron* (2014) **82**:695–708. doi:10.1016/j.neuron.2014.03.020
13. Allen PJ, Polizzi G, Krakow K, Fish DR, Lemieux L. Identification of EEG events in the MR scanner: the problem of pulse artifact and a method for its subtraction. *Neuroimage* (1998) **8**:229–39. doi:10.1006/nimg.1998.0361
14. Allen PJ, Josephs O, Turner R. A method for removing imaging artifact from continuous EEG recorded during functional MRI. *Neuroimage* (2000) **12**:230–9. doi:10.1006/nimg.2000.0599
15. AASM. *The AASM Manual for the Scoring of Sleep and Associated Events-Rules, Terminology and Technical Specifications.* Chicago: American Academy of Sleep Medicine (2007).
16. Murphy K, Birn RM, Handwerker DA, Jones TB, Bandettini PA. The impact of global signal regression on resting state correlations: are anti-correlated networks introduced? *Neuroimage* (2009) **44**:893–905. doi:10.1016/j.neuroimage.2008.09.036
17. Scholvinck ML, Maier A, Ye FQ, Duyn JH, Leopold DA. Neural basis of global resting-state fMRI activity. *Proc Natl Acad Sci USA* (2010) **107**:10238–43. doi:10.1073/pnas.0913110107
18. Garrett DD, Kovacevic N, Mcintosh AR, Grady CL. The importance of being variable. *J Neurosci* (2011) **31**:4496–503. doi:10.1523/JNEUROSCI.5641-10.2011
19. He BJ. Scale-free properties of the functional magnetic resonance imaging signal during rest and task. *J Neurosci* (2011) **31**:13786–95. doi:10.1523/JNEUROSCI.2111-11.2011
20. Tzourio-Mazoyer N, Landeau B, Papathanassiou D, Crivello F, Etard O, Delcroix N, et al. Automated anatomical labeling of activations in SPM using a

macroscopic anatomical parcellation of the MNI MRI single-subject brain. *Neuroimage* (2002) **15**:273–89. doi:10.1006/nimg.2001.0978
21. Engel J Jr. Surgery for seizures. *N Engl J Med* (1996) **334**:647–52. doi:10.1056/NEJM199603073341008
22. Bartolomei F, Chauvel P, Wendling F. Epileptogenicity of brain structures in human temporal lobe epilepsy: a quantified study from intracerebral EEG. *Brain* (2008) **131**:1818–30. doi:10.1093/brain/awn111
23. Bonelli SB, Powell RH, Yogarajah M, Samson RS, Symms MR, Thompson PJ, et al. Imaging memory in temporal lobe epilepsy: predicting the effects of temporal lobe resection. *Brain* (2010) **133**:1186–99. doi:10.1093/brain/awq006
24. Wyler AR, Hermann BP, Richey ET. Results of reoperation for failed epilepsy surgery. *J Neurosurg* (1989) **71**:815–9. doi:10.3171/jns.1989.71.6.0815
25. Goense JB, Logothetis NK. Neurophysiology of the BOLD fMRI signal in awake monkeys. *Curr Biol* (2008) **18**:631–40. doi:10.1016/j.cub.2008.03.054
26. Demont-Guignard S, Benquet P, Gerber U, Wendling F. Analysis of intracerebral EEG recordings of epileptic spikes: insights from a neural network model. *IEEE Trans Biomed Eng* (2009) **56**:2782–95. doi:10.1109/TBME.2009.2028015
27. Laufs H, Hamandi K, Salek-Haddadi A, Kleinschmidt AK, Duncan JS, Lemieux L. Temporal lobe interictal epileptic discharges affect cerebral activity in "default mode" brain regions. *Hum Brain Mapp* (2007) **28**:1023–32. doi:10.1002/hbm.20323
28. Kobayashi E, Grova C, Tyvaert L, Dubeau F, Gotman J. Structures involved at the time of temporal lobe spikes revealed by interindividual group analysis of EEG/fMRI data. *Epilepsia* (2009) **50**:2549–56. doi:10.1111/j.1528-1167.2009.02180.x
29. Bettus G, Ranjeva JP, Wendling F, Benar CG, Confort-Gouny S, Regis J, et al. Interictal functional connectivity of human epileptic networks assessed by intracerebral EEG and BOLD signal fluctuations. *PLoS One* (2011) **6**:e20071. doi:10.1371/journal.pone.0020071
30. Amzica F. Physiology of sleep and wakefulness as it relates to the physiology of epilepsy. *J Clin Neurophysiol* (2002) **19**:488–503. doi:10.1097/00004691-200212000-00002
31. Tagliazucchi E, Von Wegner F, Morzelewski A, Borisov S, Jahnke K, Laufs H. Automatic sleep staging using fMRI functional connectivity data. *Neuroimage* (2012) **63**:63–71. doi:10.1016/j.neuroimage.2012.06.036
32. Fukunaga M, Horovitz SG, Van Gelderen P, De Zwart JA, Jansma JM, Ikonomidou VN, et al. Large-amplitude, spatially correlated fluctuations in BOLD fMRI signals during extended rest and early sleep stages. *Magn Reson Imaging* (2006) **24**:979–92. doi:10.1016/j.mri.2006.04.018
33. Spoormaker VI, Schroter MS, Gleiser PM, Andrade KC, Dresler M, Wehrle R, et al. Development of a large-scale functional brain network during human non-rapid eye movement sleep. *J Neurosci* (2010) **30**:11379–87. doi:10.1523/JNEUROSCI.2015-10.2010
34. Tagliazucchi E, Von Wegner F, Morzelewski A, Brodbeck V, Borisov S, Jahnke K, et al. Large-scale brain functional modularity is reflected in slow electroencephalographic rhythms across the human non-rapid eye movement sleep cycle. *Neuroimage* (2013) **70**:327–39. doi:10.1016/j.neuroimage.2012.12.073
35. Tagliazucchi E, Carhart-Harris R, Leech R, Nutt D, Chialvo DR. Enhanced repertoire of brain dynamical states during the psychedelic experience. *Hum Brain Mapp* (2014). doi:10.1002/hbm.22562
36. Cantero JL, Atienza M, Stickgold R, Kahana MJ, Madsen JR, Kocsis B. Sleep-dependent theta oscillations in the human hippocampus and neocortex. *J Neurosci* (2003) **23**:10897–903.
37. Van Paesschen W, Dupont P, Van Driel G, Van Billoen H, Maes A. SPECT perfusion changes during complex partial seizures in patients with hippocampal sclerosis. *Brain* (2003) **126**:1103–11. doi:10.1093/brain/awg108
38. Chassagnon S, Namer IJ, Armspach JP, Nehlig A, Kahane P, Kehrli P, et al. SPM analysis of ictal-interictal SPECT in mesial temporal lobe epilepsy: relationships between ictal semiology and perfusion changes. *Epilepsy Res* (2009) **85**:252–60. doi:10.1016/j.eplepsyres.2009.03.020
39. Dupont S. Investigating temporal pole function by functional imaging. *Epileptic Disord* (2002) **4**(Suppl 1):S17–22.
40. Pacagnella D, Lopes TM, Morita ME, Yasuda CL, Cappabianco FA, Bergo F, et al. Memory impairment is not necessarily related to seizure frequency in mesial temporal lobe epilepsy with hippocampal sclerosis. *Epilepsia* (2014) **55**:1197–204. doi:10.1111/epi.12691
41. Blumenfeld H. Impaired consciousness in epilepsy. *Lancet Neurol* (2012) **11**:814–26. doi:10.1016/S1474-4422(12)70188-6
42. Stretton J, Thompson PJ. Frontal lobe function in temporal lobe epilepsy. *Epilepsy Res* (2012) **98**:1–13. doi:10.1016/j.eplepsyres.2011.10.009
43. Baumgartner C, Flint R, Tuxhorn I, Van Ness PC, Kosalko J, Olbrich A, et al. Supplementary motor area seizures: propagation pathways as studied with invasive recordings. *Neurology* (1996) **46**:508–14. doi:10.1212/WNL.46.2.508
44. Goldberg II, Harel M, Malach R. When the brain loses its self: prefrontal inactivation during sensorimotor processing. *Neuron* (2006) **50**:329–39. doi:10.1016/j.neuron.2006.03.015
45. Powell HW, Duncan JS. Functional magnetic resonance imaging for assessment of language and memory in clinical practice. *Curr Opin Neurol* (2005) **18**:161–6. doi:10.1097/01.wco.0000162858.60144.ca
46. Binnie CD. Cognitive impairment during epileptiform discharges: is it ever justifiable to treat the EEG? *Lancet Neurol* (2003) **2**:725–30. doi:10.1016/S1474-4422(03)00584-2
47. Vulliemoz S, Lemieux L, Daunizeau J, Michel CM, Duncan JS. The combination of EEG source imaging and EEG-correlated functional MRI to map epileptic networks. *Epilepsia* (2010) **51**:491–505. doi:10.1111/j.1528-1167.2009.02342.x
48. Bernhardt BC, Bernasconi N, Concha L, Bernasconi A. Cortical thickness analysis in temporal lobe epilepsy: reproducibility and relation to outcome. *Neurology* (2010) **74**:1776–84. doi:10.1212/WNL.0b013e3181e0f80a
49. Rosenow F, Lüders H. Presurgical evaluation of epilepsy. *Brain* (2001) **124**:1683–700. doi:10.1093/brain/124.9.1683
50. Haneef Z, Lenartowicz A, Yeh HJ, Levin HS, Engel J Jr., Stern JM. Functional connectivity of hippocampal networks in temporal lobe epilepsy. *Epilepsia* (2014) **55**:137–45. doi:10.1111/epi.12476
51. Duncan NW, Northoff G. Overview of potential procedural and participant-related confounds for neuroimaging of the resting state. *J Psychiatry Neurosci* (2013) **38**:84–96. doi:10.1503/jpn.120059
52. Friston KJ, Williams S, Howard R, Frackowiak RS, Turner R. Movement-related effects in fMRI time-series. *Magn Reson Med* (1996) **35**:346–55. doi:10.1002/mrm.1910350312
53. Mowinckel AM, Espeseth T, Westlye LT. Network-specific effects of age and in-scanner subject motion: a resting-state fMRI study of 238 healthy adults. *Neuroimage* (2012) **63**:1364–73. doi:10.1016/j.neuroimage.2012.08.004
54. Smith DV, Utevsky AV, Bland AR, Clement N, Clithero JA, Harsch AE, et al. Characterizing individual differences in functional connectivity using dual-regression and seed-based approaches. *Neuroimage* (2014) **95**:1–12. doi:10.1016/j.neuroimage.2014.03.042
55. Lemieux L, Salek-Haddadi A, Lund TE, Laufs H, Carmichael D. Modelling large motion events in fMRI studies of patients with epilepsy. *Magn Reson Imaging* (2007) **25**:894–901. doi:10.1016/j.mri.2007.03.009
56. Power JD, Mitra A, Laumann TO, Snyder AZ, Schlaggar BL, Petersen SE. Methods to detect, characterize, and remove motion artifact in resting state fMRI. *Neuroimage* (2014) **84**:320–41. doi:10.1016/j.neuroimage.2013.08.048
57. Wong C, Gallate J. The function of the anterior temporal lobe: a review of the empirical evidence. *Brain Res* (2012) **1449**:94–116. doi:10.1016/j.brainres.2012.02.017
58. Simmons WK, Martin A. The anterior temporal lobes and the functional architecture of semantic memory. *J Int Neuropsychol Soc* (2009) **15**:645–9. doi:10.1017/S1355617709990348

APPENDIX

REPRODUCTION OF RESULTS ERASING HIGH AMPLITUDE HEAD MOVEMENTS

Following the work of Lemieux et al. and Power et al. (55, 56), we have scanned the time course of estimated head movement and erased those volumes associated with a displacement larger than 0.3 mm, as well as the three previous and following volumes. We then reproduced **Figures 3** and **4** using this alternative preprocessing. Results are shown in **Figure 5** (voxel-wise variance, controls vs. TLE) and **Figure 6** (hippocampus-based dynamic functional connectivity variance, controls vs. TLE). It can be appreciated from both figures that the general composition of the patterns discussed in the main text is preserved.

ROBUSTNESS AGAINST CHANGES IN SLIDING WINDOW LENGTH

The computation of dynamic functional connectivity time series requires the specification of a sliding window length, which can be seen as a free parameter (even though its correct choice bears an obvious relationship with the time scale where the changes occur). We demonstrate that results are robust against a chance of this parameter by reproducing **Figure 4** using a different, shorter window length (15 s). Results are shown in **Figure 7**. From this figure, it is evident that the main differences between controls and TLE patients still hold using this different window length.

STANDARD SEED CORRELATION ANALYSIS

We performed a standard "static" linear correlation analysis seeded in the left hippocampus. Results of the controls vs. TLE comparison are presented in **Figure A1**. A decrease in seed connectivity was observed in the patient group relative to the control group in brain areas including visual cortex, precuneus, and sensorimotor cortex. Compared to the regions in which a change in dynamic connectivity variance was observed (**Figure 4**), these regions overlap but also include a less extended network than that observed in

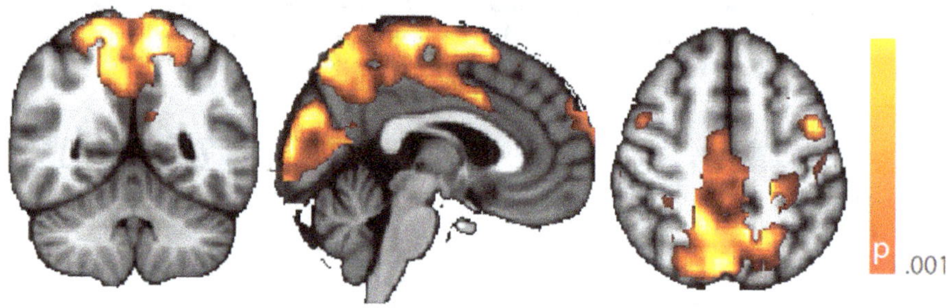

FIGURE A1 | Spatial map (coronal, sagittal, axial slices) of significantly decreased hippocampal signal linear correlation in patients with temporal lobe epilepsy (here: seed in left hippocampus) than in healthy controls. Color bar indicates *p*-value (thresholded at $p < 0.001$ for display, cluster survives family-wise error correction at $p < 0.05$). Left on figure is right in the brain (coronal and axial slices).

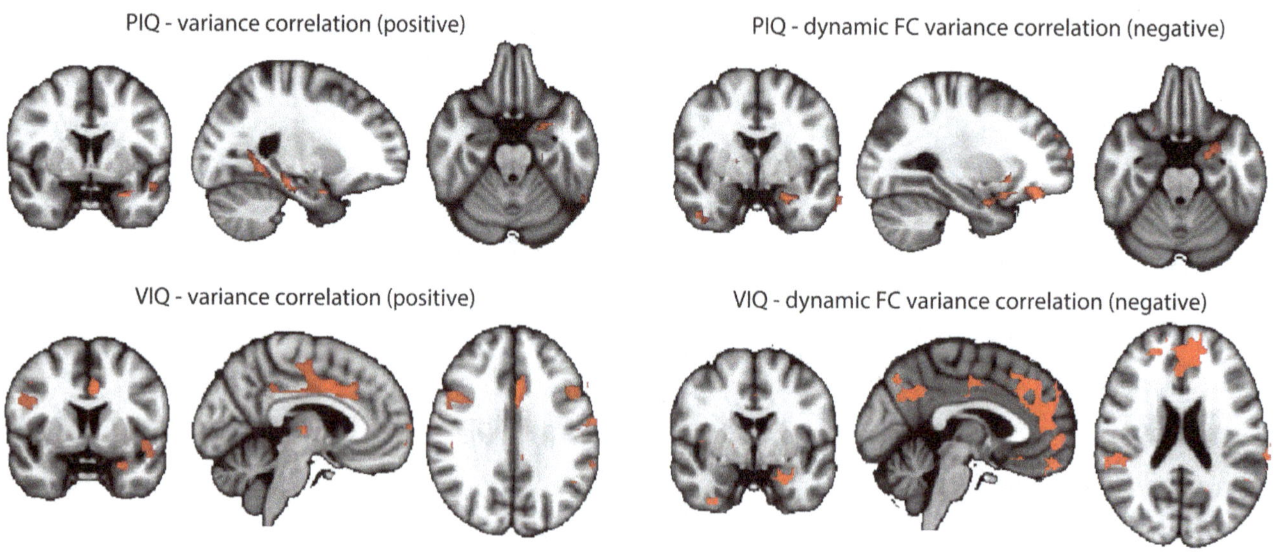

FIGURE A2 | Correlations between BOLD signal variance/variance of dynamic connectivity time series with the left hippocampus and VIQ/PIQ scores for the TLE group (left + right). Statistical significance was determined at $p < 0.05$ with a cluster threshold of 10 voxels. Maps were masked with the regions where the metrics were significantly different between controls and TLE patients. Left: results for PIQ and VIQ correlation with variance. In all cases positive correlations were found. Right: results for PIQ and VIQ correlation with variance of connectivity time series with the left hippocampus. In all cases negative correlations were found.

the dynamic analysis; in particular, frontal regions do not appear. To a large extent, for regions having strong baseline connectivity, increased variance of the dynamic connectivity time series implies decreased "static" correlation. The opposite, however, is not true. This points to an origin of the decreased "static" correlation that can be traced to a dynamic transient phenomenon, which we hypothesize corresponds to paroxysmal events.

CORRELATIONS BETWEEN BOLD SIGNAL VARIANCE/VARIANCE OF DYNAMIC CONNECTIVITY TIME SERIES WITH THE LEFT HIPPOCAMPUS AND VIQ/PIQ

In an attempt to link the results derived from resting-state data more tightly to our interpretation, we performed a correlation analysis of the behavioral measures PIQ/VIQ (obtained close in time to the fMRI experiment) and fMRI signal changes in the regions of increased BOLD signal variance and increased dynamic functional connectivity, respectively (**Figure A2**). We found positive correlations between the IQ measures and the BOLD signal variance, and negative correlations with the dynamic BOLD functional connectivity. With the caveat of uncorrected significance values – possibly a power or, alternatively, a conceptual problem – this argues for a relationship of our findings obtained at rest with these psychological measures, i.e., a connection between interictal cognitive impairment and the observed changes between the TLE and the control cohorts. That a lower IQ score is linked to higher functional connectivity could be interpreted as paroxysmal interference of the "epileptic process" with normally required and less pronounced variations in functional connectivity. Why at the same time an impaired IQ is associated with reduced variance in the BOLD signal time series in regions characterized by an overall increase in BOLD signal variance in TLE compared to controls – admittedly – is difficult to interpret. Although the functional role of anterior temporal lobe is still debated (57), it might be possible that increased "inertia" (i.e., reduced BOLD signal variance) of the anterior temporal lobe reflects deficits in semantic memory (58).

17

Functional network alterations and their structural substrate in drug-resistant epilepsy

Lorenzo Caciagli, Boris C. Bernhardt, Seok-Jun Hong, Andrea Bernasconi and Neda Bernasconi*

Neuroimaging of Epilepsy Laboratory, McConnell Brain Imaging Center, Montreal Neurological Institute and Hospital, McGill University, Montreal, QC, Canada

***Correspondence:**
Neda Bernasconi, Montreal Neurological Institute, 3801 University Street, Montreal, QC H3A 2B4, Canada
e-mail: neda@bic.mni.mcgill.ca

The advent of MRI has revolutionized the evaluation and management of drug-resistant epilepsy by allowing the detection of the lesion associated with the region that gives rise to seizures. Recent evidence indicates marked chronic alterations in the functional organization of lesional tissue and large-scale cortico-subcortical networks. In this review, we focus on recent methodological developments in functional MRI (fMRI) analysis techniques and their application to the two most common drug-resistant focal epilepsies, i.e., temporal lobe epilepsy related to mesial temporal sclerosis and extra-temporal lobe epilepsy related to focal cortical dysplasia. We put particular emphasis on methodological developments in the analysis of task-free or "resting-state" fMRI to probe the integrity of intrinsic networks on a regional, inter-regional, and connectome-wide level. In temporal lobe epilepsy, these techniques have revealed disrupted connectivity of the ipsilateral mesiotemporal lobe, together with contralateral compensatory reorganization and striking reconfigurations of large-scale networks. In cortical dysplasia, initial observations indicate functional alterations in lesional, peri-lesional, and remote neocortical regions. While future research is needed to critically evaluate the reliability, sensitivity, and specificity, fMRI mapping promises to lend distinct biomarkers for diagnosis, presurgical planning, and outcome prediction.

Keywords: epilepsy, connectivity, resting-state, graph-theory

INTRODUCTION

About 50 million people worldwide suffer from epilepsy (Kwan and Brodie, 2000). This condition is one of the most prevalent chronic neurological disorders, affecting about 1% of the general population (Leonardi and Ustun, 2002). Epilepsy is broadly characterized by recurrent spontaneous seizures resulting from an altered balance between excitation and inhibition in brain networks (Scharfman, 2007). Approximately one third of epileptic patients suffer from intractable seizures despite adequate medical treatment (Kwan et al., 2010). Patients with drug-resistant epilepsy should be promptly identified and successfully managed, as refractory seizures are associated with progressive brain damage (Cascino, 2009), devastating cognitive and socio-economic consequences (Pugliatti et al., 2007), as well as an increased risk of mortality (Mohanraj et al., 2006). The most frequent drug-resistant epilepsy syndromes are temporal lobe epilepsy (TLE) related to hippocampal sclerosis, and extra-temporal lobe epilepsy related to focal cortical dysplasia (FCD). Epilepsy surgery is recognized as the most effective treatment strategy to ensure seizure freedom (Engel et al., 2012).

The advent of structural Magnetic Resonance Imaging (MRI) has revolutionized the preoperative workup in intractable epilepsy (Koepp and Woermann, 2005; Duncan, 2010; Bernasconi et al., 2011). Furthermore, by allowing a reliable identification of the lesion giving rise to the seizures, MRI quantitative analysis lends non-invasive markers that have substantially increased the success rate of epilepsy surgery (Duncan, 2010; Bernasconi et al., 2011; Engel et al., 2013). Nevertheless, despite constant improvements in MRI acquisition and analysis technology, up to 50% of operated patients continue having seizures (McIntosh et al., 2004; Tellez-Zenteno et al., 2005; De Tisi et al., 2011). Although reasons for unfavorable results are not fully understood, emerging imaging data suggest that anomalies extending beyond the lesion may negatively impact outcome (Keller et al., 2007; Bernhardt et al., 2010, 2011; Voets et al., 2011; Bonilha et al., 2013). These observations challenge the conventional model of "focal epilepsy" and revive the concept of distributed neural networks (Spencer, 2002; Richardson, 2012).

Advances in non-invasive neuroimaging techniques allow probing connectivity *in vivo*. While physical properties of structural brain networks can be derived from diffusion MRI, functional techniques (such as functional MRI and magnetoencephalography) model connectivity as statistical dependencies of neurophysiological time series (Biswal et al., 1995; Srinivasan et al., 2007; Friston, 2011). Functional MRI (fMRI) utilizes changes in blood oxygen level-dependent (BOLD) signal to infer neuronal activity (Logothetis et al., 2001). The link is understood under a neurovascular coupling model: neuronal activity in a region leads to increased blood flow to supply oxygen and nutrients. The vascular response leads to a biomagnetic perturbation of susceptibility, which is detected by T2* sequence used for BOLD fMRI. Conventionally, fMRI has a relatively coarse time-resolution (order of seconds; but see Feinberg et al., 2010), but good spatial-resolution and whole-brain coverage. In drug-resistant epilepsy, most earlier studies have used task-related fMRI to map brain activation of eloquent areas, mainly those subserving language, memory (Berl et al., 2005; Janszky et al., 2005; Voets et al., 2009), and sensory-motor function (Janszky et al., 2003; Jirsch et al., 2006; Dumoulin et al., 2007; Sommer et al., 2013). Recent advances focus on spontaneous modulations in BOLD signal that occur during "resting" (i.e., task-free) conditions (**Figure 1**) (Fox and Raichle, 2007; Van Essen et al., 2012; Cabral et al., 2014). Advantages over task-related paradigms include the possibility to examine multiple cortical areas in one session, minimal demands on patients with reduced ability to perform tasks, and the possibility to aggregate data across sites. Resting-state networks are highly reproducible across subjects (Damoiseaux et al., 2006; Biswal et al., 2010; Cabral et al., 2014) and have been shown to correspond closely to brain systems engaging in specific tasks (Greicius et al., 2003; Fox et al., 2006; Smith et al., 2009).

In this review, we will principally focus on TLE, and outline the available evidence of functional anomalies spanning from limbic circuits to whole-brain networks. We will also detail preliminary findings on functional disruptions in FCD, although studies on patients with this condition are relatively sparse and cohorts often inhomogeneous. We will discuss how functional alterations could be related to those observed in structural MRI. Finally, we will critically evaluate whether and how fMRI measures could serve as effective biomarkers for the pre-surgical workup in drug-resistant epilepsy. **Figure 1** provides a schematic overview of the methods to assess resting-state brain function and **Figure 2** summarizes findings in TLE.

THE STUDY OF FUNCTIONAL NETWORKS USING RESTING-STATE FMRI

Recent years have witnessed a dramatic increase in resting-state fMRI analyses to probe intrinsic functional networks in healthy and diseased populations (Biswal et al., 1995, 2010; Greicius et al., 2003; Smith et al., 2009). In most studies, the participant lies still in the scanner for 5–7 min, a scan-time that was previously shown to deliver stable connectivity measures (Van Dijk et al., 2010). More recent work suggests that reliability can be further improved when with longer duration scans of 9–12 min (Birn et al., 2013), and work focusing on individual subject classification suggests even longer acquisitions (Anderson et al., 2011). There is some evidence for variable effects of eye opening (with or without fixation) or closure on connectivity measures, possibly hampering replication of findings (Yan et al., 2009; Patriat et al., 2013).

Reflecting the growing importance of resting-state acquisitions, numerous software packages have been developed for automatic data processing (e.g., Yan and Zang, 2010). Conventional processing includes the discarding of a few time points at the onset of the recording to ensure steady-state magnetization, followed by correction for subject motion through linear registration of individual time points to a reference time point, as well as co-registration between structural and functional images. These basic operations are often followed by statistical correction for subject-motion and average signal from the white matter and cerebro-spinal fluid as a proxy for physiological activity. While most early resting-state studies corrected for global signal, the validity of this preprocessing step is currently controversially discussed (Fox et al., 2009; Murphy et al., 2009). More

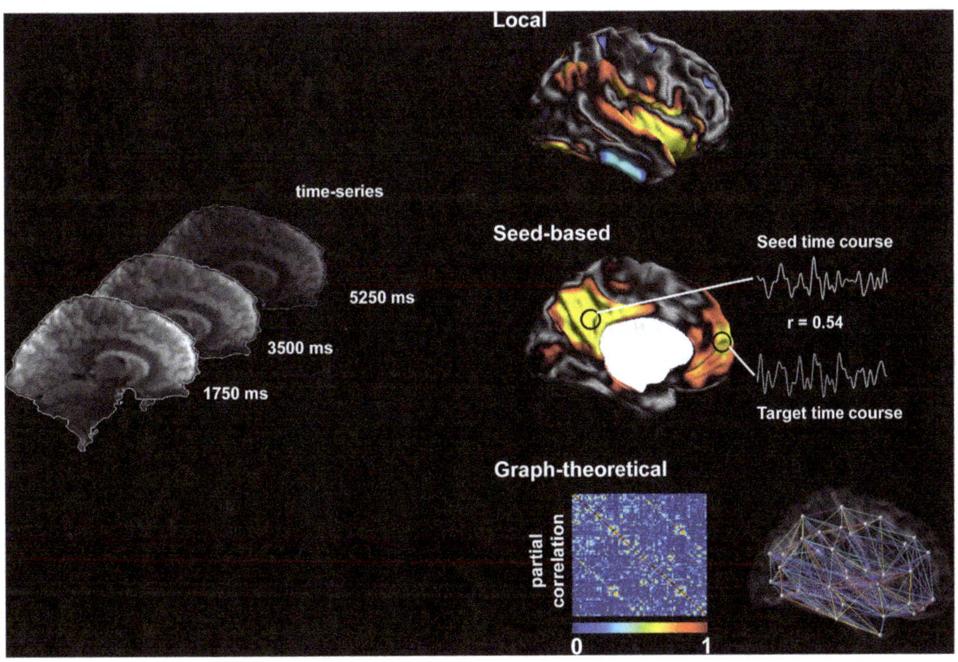

FIGURE 1 | Methods to assess resting-state brain function. Resting-state fMRI time series allow the description of functional networks at multiple levels. Local markers of functional integrity can be derived from the amplitude of low-frequency fluctuations. Seed-based analysis of connectivity relies on cross-correlations between time-series of seed and target regions. Systematic seeding across multiple regions allows for the generation of connectivity matrices and equivalent connectivity graphs; these can, in turn, be analyzed using graph-theory to address large-scale network topology.

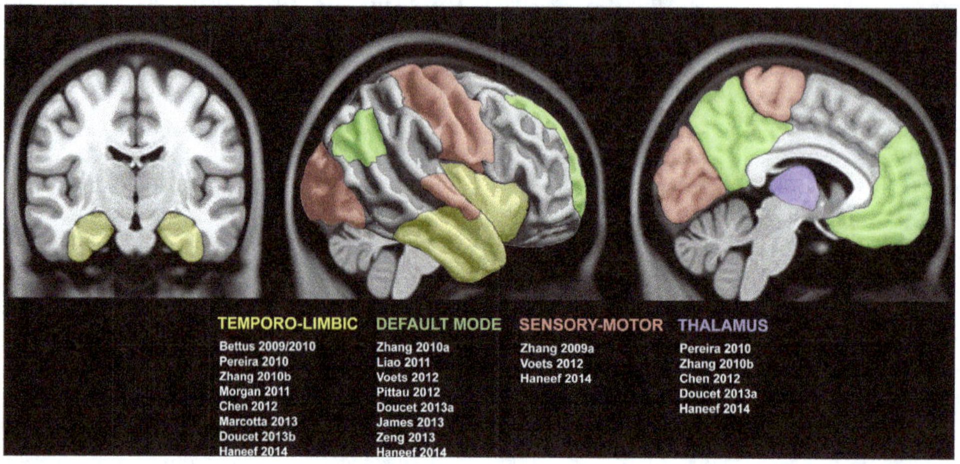

FIGURE 2 | Summary of studies reporting functional connectivity anomalies in temporal lobe epilepsy. Cortical and subcortical regions displaying functional alterations are color-coded with respect to the associated network. See text for details.

recent work invokes *scrubbing*, an approach that models time points affected by heavy motion as additional nuisance regressors (Power et al., 2012). Corrected time-series are filtered, mostly to a pass-band close to 0.1–0.01 Hz, and often subsequently mapped to individual cortical surface models and/or a standard stereotaxic space for group-level inference. Analytical approaches include seed-based functional connectivity assessments, data-driven approaches that cluster the brain into regional assemblies showing similar functional activations such as independent component analysis (ICA), the extraction of voxel-based regional markers, and graph theoretical assessments to study topology at large scale.

Previous work in healthy individuals has shown that resting-state fMRI networks are generally reproducible across subjects (Damoiseaux et al., 2006), show appropriate test-retest reliability (Shehzad et al., 2009), and may closely correspond to brain systems engaging in specific tasks (Biswal et al., 1995; Smith et al., 2009; Laird et al., 2011; Tusche et al., 2014). Studies in primates have suggested a close correspondence between intrinsic functional connections and anatomical pathways derived from tract tracing (Margulies et al., 2009; Mantini et al., 2011; Shen et al., 2012). Analysis of resting-state patterns may furthermore help to subdivide specific anatomical regions (Margulies et al., 2007; Mars et al., 2011; Steinbeis et al., 2014). Finally, resting-state connectivity may be altered in disease conditions (Greicius, 2008; Fox and Greicius, 2010; Kelly et al., 2012).

FUNCTIONAL NETWORK DISRUPTIONS IN TLE: LIMBIC AND PERI-LIMBIC CONNECTIVITY

The majority of resting-state fMRI work in TLE addressed the functional connectivity of limbic structures through seed-based analysis. Impaired connectivity has been consistently detected within mesiotemporal structures ipsilateral to the seizure focus; the most prominent local alterations involve the links between rostral and caudal hippocampus, and between the rostral hippocampus and the enthorinal cortex (Bettus et al., 2009, 2010). Reduced functional connectivity is observed between ipsilateral and contralateral hippocampi (Pereira et al., 2010; Morgan et al., 2011; Maccotta et al., 2013), as well as between the epileptogenic mesial temporal structures and bilateral lateral temporal neocortices (Pereira et al., 2010; Maccotta et al., 2013; Doucet et al., 2013a). Left TLE patients seem to display more marked connectivity alterations than those with right TLE, both in the epileptogenic hemisphere and in contralateral limbic areas (Pereira et al., 2010). Breakdowns in ipsilateral functional connectivity may co-occur with connectivity increases in contralateral mesiotemporal networks, which have been shown to positively correlate with working memory performance (Bettus et al., 2009, 2010). Such increases may reflect reorganization of limbic networks. Supporting evidence for abnormal local functional connectivity within peri-limbic regions comes from a preliminary observation of enhanced amplitude of the low-frequency fluctuations of BOLD signal, a local functional marker possibly reflective of long-range neuronal synchronization (Balduzzi et al., 2008), in the ipsilateral mesiotemporal structures and lateral temporal neocortex (Zhang et al., 2010b).

The spatial patterns of resting-state functional alterations seem to parallel the structural damage identified by quantitative MRI analysis. In agreement with histopathological studies, atrophy has been confirmed beyond the hippocampus to include the enthorinal cortex and the amygdala complex (Bernasconi et al., 1999, 2001b, 2003; Salmenperä et al., 2000; Bartolomei et al., 2005), with evidence for subregional disease progression (Briellmann et al., 2002; Fuerst et al., 2003; Bernasconi et al., 2005; Bernhardt et al., 2013b). Besides, morphological disruptions have been identified in the perirhinal, temporo-polar, and lateral temporal neocortices ipsilateral to the focus (Jutila et al., 2001; Moran et al., 2001; Coste et al., 2002; Bernasconi et al., 2004; Sankar et al., 2008; Voets et al., 2011). Interestingly, we detected increased cortical folding complexity, which involved the contralateral temporo-polar region in right TLE (Voets et al., 2011). Differently from the cognitively adaptive functional reorganization (Bettus et al., 2009, 2010), the contralateral increase in cortical folding predicted unfavorable post-surgical outcome (Voets et al., 2011).

Further evidence for limbic and peri-limbic disruptions comes from structural connectivity studies, which have employed either diffusion imaging or structural MRI covariance (Bernhardt et al., 2013a). Diffusion imaging constitutes a versatile tool to assess the microstructural integrity of the white matter, and to investigate its architecture through the reconstruction of fiber pathways. Fractional anisotropy, indicating the extent to which water diffusion deviates from a random spherical model, is consistently decreased in temporo-limbic tracts, such as the fornix, the cingulum (Ahmadi et al., 2009; Concha et al., 2009), and the uncinate fasciculus (Rodrigo et al., 2007; Diehl et al., 2008; McDonald et al., 2008). Mean diffusivity, a scalar measure of overall diffusivity, appears markedly altered in the proximity of the epileptogenic zone (Focke et al., 2008; Concha et al., 2009, 2012). Structural MRI covariance analysis relies instead on inter-regional correlations of structural markers, such as cortical thickness or gray matter volume, to infer network properties (Alexander-Bloch et al., 2013). We and others (Bonilha et al., 2007; Bernhardt et al., 2008) have shown decreased structural coordination between mesiotemporal regions and lateral temporal neocortices. These results parallel functional connectivity derangement within the temporo-limbic circuits (Maccotta et al., 2013).

FUNCTIONAL DISRUPTIONS IN TLE: INVOLVEMENT OF WIDESPREAD BRAIN NETWORKS

Several studies have identified abnormal connectivity patterns between seeds placed within the epileptogenic mesiotemporal region and bilateral clusters in the posterior cingulate cortices, precuneus, inferior parietal lobules and mesial prefrontal cortices (Pittau et al., 2012; James et al., 2013; Doucet et al., 2013b; Haneef et al., 2014). Along with the hippocampi and the parahippocampal gyri, this set of regions constitutes the default mode network (DMN), a system putatively involved in internally-focused activities including memory retrieval, mind wandering and envisioning the future (Buckner et al., 2008; Christoff et al., 2009). Functional connectivity disruptions in the DMN have been elucidated in TLE patients also by studies extracting resting-state networks via ICA (Zhang et al., 2010a; Liao et al., 2011; Voets et al., 2012), placing seeds in non-temporal DMN areas (Haneef et al., 2012), or assessing regional homogeneity of resting fMRI time-courses (Zeng et al., 2013). Prominent DMN alterations in TLE could be explained in view of the relevance of the hippocampi in this resting-state network (Buckner et al., 2008). As a complementary finding, EEG-fMRI analyses have also shown dysfunction in relation to epileptic spikes in areas pertaining to the DMN (Kobayashi et al., 2006; Laufs et al., 2007). The extent to which left and right TLE patients differ with respect to DMN connectivity is not clear: some studies did not identify substantial differences (Pittau et al., 2012), while others reported greater functional disconnectivity in left (James et al., 2013; Doucet et al., 2013b; Haneef et al., 2014) or right TLE (Zhang et al., 2010a; Haneef et al., 2012; Voets et al., 2012). Inconsistencies regarding the extent of DMN abnormalities and divergences with regard to seizure focus could be ascribed to methodological discrepancies among studies, such as procedures involved in network extraction (e.g., seed-based vs. ICA-based approaches), statistical thresholding and differences across patient cohorts, particularly in relation to pharmaco-response. Resting-state fMRI analyses, both ICA and seed-based, have also detected connectional disruptions in areas involved in primary sensory processing (Zhang et al., 2009a; Voets et al., 2012; Haneef et al., 2014) and attention (Zhang et al., 2009b). Furthermore, impaired functional interactions are reported between the epileptogenic mesiotemporal lobes and subcortical areas, including the thalamus and the brainstem (Pereira et al., 2010; Pittau et al., 2012; Doucet et al., 2013b; Haneef et al., 2014).

Addressing the relationship between connectivity and cognitive performance, Waites et al. (2006) described altered functional signaling at rest in middle and inferior frontal as well as cingulate regions in patients with left TLE (Waites et al., 2006). Their findings might represent an intrinsic functional correlate of the subtle language disturbances often identified in this group (Hermann et al., 1997). In left TLE, increased functional interactions between epileptogenic mesial temporal structures and the ipsilateral posterior DMN appear to be associated with poorer verbal memory abilities (Doucet et al., 2013a; Holmes et al., 2014), while increased coupling between the ipsilateral hippocampus and contralateral posterior DMN shows a positive relation with improved verbal memory (Holmes et al., 2014). In right TLE, strengthening of connections between the left mesial temporal lobe and ROIs in the ipsilateral mesial prefrontal cortex predicted better non-verbal memory (Doucet et al., 2013a). This suggests that functional reorganization involving the recruitment of contralateral areas might represent a compensatory phenomenon favoring cognitive performance.

A number of seed-based studies have sought for possible functional correlates of psychiatric comorbidities in relation to depression. Derangements in functional connectivity between mesiotemporal lobes and prefrontal cortices might occur in depressed TLE patients (Chen et al., 2012; Kemmotsu et al., 2013). Compared to non-depressed subjects, depressed patients seem also to exhibit increased functional coupling between the limbic system and the angular gyrus, possibly suggestive of an intensified susceptibility to environmental cues (Chen et al., 2012). Furthermore, there is preliminary evidence that maladaptive reorganizations of functional connections between bilateral amygdalae and prefrontal (Kemmotsu et al., 2013), lateral temporal cortex and the cuneus (Doucet et al., 2013b) might relate to depressive and anxiety symptoms.

Evidence for functional disruptions in multiple brain networks in TLE confirms and expands the literature on extra-temporal structural abnormalities. Extensive neocortical anomalies have been pinpointed in several volumetric and cortical thickness analyses (Bernasconi et al., 2004; Lin et al., 2007; Bernhardt et al., 2008, 2009b; Keller and Roberts, 2008; Mueller et al., 2009), and gray matter loss has been observed in subcortical structures, including the thalamus and basal ganglia (Dreifuss et al., 2001; Natsume et al., 2003; Bernhardt et al., 2012). Structural connectivity studies employing diffusion imaging have demonstrated decreased fractional anisotropy in a consistent set of white matter tracts, including the inferior and superior longitudinal fascicles (Focke et al., 2008; Lin et al., 2008; Ahmadi et al., 2009), the internal and external capsule, and the corpus callosum (Arfanakis et al., 2002; Gross et al., 2006; Concha et al.,

2009). On the other hand, disruptions in mean diffusivity seem to be relatively less extended (Concha et al., 2005; Focke et al., 2008). Our group has recently shown that diffusivity values normalize as a function of the anatomical distance from the seizure focus (Concha et al., 2012). Structural covariance analyses have described abnormal correlations between mesiotemporal regions and a variety of areas, including pre-frontal, fronto-central, cingulate and occipito-temporal neocortices (Bonilha et al., 2007; Bernhardt et al., 2008; Mueller et al., 2009). We demonstrated that thalamic atrophy co-varies with cortical thickness of mesiotemporal, fronto-central and lateral temporal cortices (Bernhardt et al., 2012).

Although there are similarities in the location of functional and structural abnormalities, systematic assessments of the relationship between changes in both domains are scarce. On the one hand, it is not very well understood whether more gray matter in a certain region relates to stronger functional activation, or changes in functional connectivity. On the other hand, patients may express significantly higher structural variability of certain brain regions than controls. This may possibly impact the quality of across-subjects alignment during preprocessing differentially in both groups, particularly when conventional group-level analyses are carried out in a standard voxel space. Functional analysis in subject-specific space, ideally on anatomy-informed models of the cortex, may control for some of these confounds. While multimodal imaging could shed light on structure-function relationships in epilepsy, few studies have directly addressed this question. For instance, a study showed that impaired functional connectivity between mesial temporal lobes and posterior cingulate cortex correlated with reduced white matter density of bundles connecting the two regions (Liao et al., 2011). Using whole-brain analysis, our group found disruptions in functional connectivity between mesiotemporal regions and neocortical areas, including regions in the DMN and sensory-motor networks. Importantly, functional connectivity changes of the hippocampus were partially explained by gray matter density estimates of this region, suggesting that altered signal coupling may reflect hippocampal damage. Moreover, functional connectivity changes outside of mesiotemporal region correlated with diffusion parameters interconnecting fiber tracts (Voets et al., 2012). This lead us postulate that morphological and architectural derangements account for alterations in intrinsic functional connectivity in TLE.

EVIDENCE OF DISRUPTED NETWORK TOPOLOGY IN TLE: INSIGHTS FROM GRAPH THEORY

Although there is significant support for local and inter-regional connectivity disruptions in TLE, the above-discussed analyses have not characterized organizational properties of brain networks. In this context, graph theoretical analysis provides a unique framework to quantify whole-brain network topology (Bullmore and Sporns, 2009; Bassett and Gazzaniga, 2011). Networks can be modeled as collections of nodes, corresponding to brain regions, which are interconnected via links (or edges). Nodal selection exerts a crucial influence on graph-theoretical parameters (Zalesky et al., 2010), and several investigations have aimed at improving the reliability of parcellation techniques (Geyer et al., 2011; Glasser and Van Essen, 2011). Network edges can be derived from both structural and functional connectivity datasets, as shown by the variety of graph-theoretical analyses relying on electrophysiology (Ponten et al., 2007), fMRI (Salvador et al., 2005), diffusion MRI (Gong et al., 2009), and structural MRI covariance (He et al., 2007). While segregation measures refer to the existence of tightly interconnected nodes within the network, known as *clusters* or *modules*, their integration is mediated via interconnecting *paths* (Bullmore and Sporns, 2009). Centrality measures are employed to identify *hubs*, i.e., nodes with a high degree of connections (Van Den Heuvel and Sporns, 2011). The global topology of brain networks in healthy individuals exhibits a *small-world* organization (Bullmore and Sporns, 2009). This architecture, which has been consistently shown across various imaging modalities, enables both segregation and integration of information processing while being maximally efficient in terms of wiring costs.

In TLE, only a few studies performed graph-theoretical analyses on functional (Liao et al., 2010; Wang et al., 2014) or structural (Bernhardt et al., 2011; Bonilha et al., 2012; Liu et al., 2014) MRI datasets. Deriving brain networks from resting-state fMRI measures, a study reported decreased clustering and path length, and disruptions in the distribution of network hubs, in favor of a random network topology (Liao et al., 2010). Conversely, a more recent study showed increased clustering and path length, a finding rather typical of a regularized topology (Wang et al., 2014). Interestingly, the latter findings are in line with our graph-theory analysis of structural networks constructed from cortical thickness correlations (Bernhardt et al., 2011), with graph-theoretical studies on diffusion MRI data (Bonilha et al., 2012; Liu et al., 2014) and with electrophysiology-derived network analyses (Bartolomei et al., 2013). Preliminary evidence suggests that alterations in brain structural (Bernhardt et al., 2011) and functional (Wang et al., 2014) networks intensify over time. We have shown that patients with a poor outcome after surgery exhibit more pronounced network disruptions compared to those who achieved seizure freedom. These findings suggest that whole-brain network analysis might be a valuable asset for clinical decision-making (Bernhardt et al., 2011).

FOCAL CORTICAL DYSPLASIA: EVIDENCE FOR WIDESPREAD EXTRA-LESIONAL ABNORMALITIES

Focal cortical dysplasia (FCD) is an epileptogenic malformation of cortical development resulting from localized abnormalities in neuronal migration and organization (Barkovich et al., 2012). Neocortical epilepsy secondary to FCD accounts for approximately half of pediatric patients and a quarter of adult subjects (Lerner et al., 2009; Bernasconi et al., 2011). Cortical dysplasias encompass a wide spectrum of histopathological changes related to cortical disorganization, including isolated dyslamination typical of FCD type I, and more severe lesions characterized by dyslamination and cytological abnormalities such as dysmorphic cells or balloon cells in FCD type II (Blumcke et al., 2011). Associated alterations in the subcortical white matter adjacent to the lesion are also frequently observed in pathological specimens (Andres et al., 2005; Sisodiya et al., 2009). The degree of histopathological disruptions influences lesional visibility on structural MRI (Lerner et al., 2009; Bernasconi et al., 2011). In this regard, patients with FCD type II display a significantly wider spectrum of MRI abnormalities compared to those with FCD type I, of whom the vast majority shows unremarkable routine MRI (Tassi et al., 2002; Krsek et al., 2008).

In recent years, MRI processing has allowed for an increased detection of subtle dysplasias (Bernasconi et al., 2001a; Antel et al., 2003; Wilke et al., 2003; Huppertz et al., 2005; Srivastava et al., 2005; Colliot et al., 2006a; Besson et al., 2008; Hong et al., 2014). Morphological anomalies, including increased gray matter density and sulcal depth may be found in areas remote from the dysplastic cortex (Bonilha et al., 2006; Colliot et al., 2006b; Besson et al., 2008). We recently employed surface-based multivariate pattern recognition to automatically detect FCD type II, and showed that 50% of patients presented at least one extralesional cluster characterized by abnormal sulcal morphology (Hong et al., 2014). Whole-brain diffusion imaging studies have shown evidence for peri-lesional abnormalities in the subcortical white matter contiguous to the dysplastic cortex (Lee et al., 2004; Gross et al., 2005; Widjaja et al., 2007, 2009; Diehl et al., 2010) and at distance (Eriksson et al., 2001; Guye et al., 2007; Fonseca Vde et al., 2012).

To date, relatively few fMRI studies have probed the integrity of functional networks in FCD. Assessing various malformations of cortical development, a study reported impaired activation of dysplasias located in language areas (Vitali et al., 2008). Other task-related fMRI studies assessing language in a variety of cortical malformations, have shown that disruptions may not be limited to the lesional cortex, with evidence for intra- and interhemispheric redistribution of function (Janszky et al., 2003; Yuan et al., 2006; Gaillard et al., 2007; Mbwana et al., 2009). Location of the lesions may have a differential impact on the expression of language dominance (Duke et al., 2012). In heterogeneous populations of non-operated adults and children with focal epilepsy and presumed dysplasia, functional connectivity disruptions have been detailed in language networks (Vlooswijk et al., 2010) and in a wide set of intrinsic functional networks (Luo et al., 2011; Widjaja et al., 2013). Additional indications of widespread functional disruptions may come from EEG-fMRI studies, which showed that spike-related BOLD signal changes occur in brain areas distant from the putative seizure onset zone, suggestive of diffuse epileptogenic networks (Federico et al., 2005; Tyvaert et al., 2008; Thornton et al., 2011). A graph-theoretical study in adults with MRI-negative focal epilepsy reported decreased global network efficiency, together with reductions in network clustering, indicative of a reorganized topology relative to controls (Vlooswijk et al., 2011). In more recent work in children with non-lesional frontal lobe epilepsy, the same group has suggested that patients present with a more regular global topology than typically developing children (Vaessen et al., 2013, 2014). It is tempting to interpret these findings in light of the fine-tuning in global network properties taking place during brain maturation (Fair et al., 2009; Dosenbach et al., 2010), which could account for shifts in brain topology across lifespan.

CONCLUSIONS

The advent of functional mapping techniques has substantially advanced our knowledge of brain connectivity in drug-resistant epilepsy. In TLE, a growing body of evidence indicates marked connectional derangements primarily in limbic circuits, but also across multiple networks, together with profound shifts in global network topology. FCD may also be associated with complex connectional reconfigurations, both locally and at a whole-brain level, although the literature is rather sparse and patient groups are frequently inhomogeneous. On the whole, current findings suggest that these focal epilepsy syndromes may be interpreted as disorders of distributed networks in both structural and functional domains.

An important avenue for future research will be to advance our understanding of how functional connectivity relates to brain structure. Studies in healthy controls have provided evidence for substantial overlap (Honey et al., 2007; Skudlarski et al., 2008; Greicius et al., 2009). In focal epilepsy, although impairments in resting-state functional coupling seem to parallel morphological disruptions unveiled by structural MRI, very few multi-modal imaging studies specifically addressed this issue so far (Liao et al., 2011; Voets et al., 2012). Importantly, causal links between changes in both domains have not been addressed. The putative polysynaptic features of functional coupling across the brain occasionally allow for the detection of functional connectivity in the absence of direct structural connections (Uddin et al., 2008; Honey et al., 2009; Lu et al., 2011), and this complicates the interpretation and the evaluation of accuracy. Another avenue for future research is the assessment of possible variations in intrinsic connectivity over time. So far, despite ample evidence for progressive structural damage (Bernasconi and Bernhardt, 2009; Cascino, 2009; Bernhardt et al., 2009a), the ability of functional markers to track disease progression is unclear. A first assessment suggested that ipsilateral and contralateral hippocampal functional connectivity alterations might undergo variable trajectories throughout the course of the disease (Morgan et al., 2011). Combined longitudinal analysis of structure and function in clinically well characterized groups of newly diagnosed patients, particularly those with acquired conditions such as post-traumatic epilepsy may shed light on seizure-related alterations vs. those related to the epileptogenic process.

Due to their relative accessibility and ability in unveiling functional disruptions, resting-state fMRI has strongly impacted the neuroimaging community. In epilepsy, preliminary results suggest a promising role for this technique to provide biomarkers for the diagnosis, pre-surgical planning, and prediction of surgical outcome (Bettus et al., 2010; Negishi et al., 2011; Castellanos et al., 2013). Despite some evidence in psychiatric conditions for medication affecting intrinsic networks, both in the context of treatment (Schmidt et al., 2013) drug abuse (Kelly et al., 2011), there are currently no reliable predictors of drug-response and monitoring of drug-related side effects in epilepsy (Koepp, 2014). A number of caveats need to be addressed. Firstly, it is paramount to evaluate and likely improve the reliability (Castellanos et al., 2013; Fiecas et al., 2013) and validity of functional markers, given potentially profound influences of artifacts and preprocessing choices on results (Birn et al., 2006; Niazy et al., 2011; Power et al., 2012; Buckner et al., 2013). A further prerequisite will be the evaluation of sensitivity and specificity; only few studies have systematically addressed this issue in patients in the context of focus

(Bettus et al., 2010; Zhang et al., 2010b; Chiang et al., 2014) and language lateralization based on resting-state fMRI data (Doucet et al., 2014). Analyzing clinically well-defined patient cohorts and cross-site assessment of reproducibility will be important to determine the clinical applicability of resting fMRI. To address the complex pathophysiology and individual susceptibilities future approaches will likely require a combination of quantitative functional and structural imaging modalities to generate biomarkers that operate at various stages of the epileptogenic process.

ACKNOWLEDGMENTS

This work was funded by the Canadian Institutes of Health Research (MOP-57840 and MOP-235790). Lorenzo Caciagli was supported by a scholarship of the Scuola Superiore Sant'Anna, Pisa, Italy. Boris C. Bernhardt was supported by CIHR and a Jeanne Timmins Costello Fellowship of the Montreal Neurological Institute.

REFERENCES

1. Ahmadi, M. E., Hagler, D. J. Jr., McDonald, C. R., Tecoma, E. S., Iragui, V. J., Dale, A. M., et al. (2009). Side matters: diffusion tensor imaging tractography in left and right temporal lobe epilepsy. *AJNR Am. J. Neuroradiol.* 30, 1740–1747. doi: 10.3174/ajnr.A1650
2. Alexander-Bloch, A., Giedd, J. N., and Bullmore, E. (2013). Imaging structural co- variance between human brain regions. *Nat. Rev. Neurosci.* 14, 322–336. doi: 10.1038/nrn3465
3. Anderson, J. S., Ferguson, M. A., Lopez-Larson, M., and Yurgelun-Todd, D. (2011). Reproducibility of single-subject functional connectivity measurements. *AJNR Am. J. Neuroradiol.* 32, 548–555. doi: 10.3174/ajnr.A2330
4. Andres, M., Andre, V. M., Nguyen, S., Salamon, N., Cepeda, C., Levine, M. S., et al. (2005). Human cortical dysplasia and epilepsy: an ontogenetic hypothesis based on volumetric mri and neun neuronal density and size measurements. *Cereb. Cortex* 15, 194–210. doi: 10.1093/cercor/bhh122
5. Antel, S. B., Collins, D. L., Bernasconi, N., Andermann, F., Shinghal, R., Kearney, R. E., et al. (2003). Automated detection of focal cortical dysplasia lesions using computational models of their MRI characteristics and texture analysis. *Neuroimage* 19, 1748–1759. doi: 10.1016/S1053-8119(03)00226-X
6. Arfanakis, K., Hermann, B. P., Rogers, B. P., Carew, J. D., Seidenberg, M., and Meyerand, M. E. (2002). Diffusion tensor MRI in temporal lobe epilepsy. *Magn. Reson. Imaging* 20, 511–519. doi: 10.1016/S0730-725X(02)00509-X
7. Balduzzi, D., Riedner, B. A., and Tononi, G. (2008). A BOLD window into brain waves. *Proc. Natl. Acad. Sci. U.S.A.* 105, 15641–15642. doi: 10.1073/pnas.0808310105
8. Barkovich, A. J., Guerrini, R., Kuzniecky, R. I., Jackson, G. D., and Dobyns, W. B. (2012). A developmental and genetic classification for malformations of cortical development: update 2012. *Brain* 135, 1348–1369. doi: 10.1093/brain/aws019
9. Bartolomei, F., Bettus, G., Stam, C. J., and Guye, M. (2013). Interictal net- work properties in mesial temporal lobe epilepsy: a graph theoretical study from intracerebral recordings. *Clin. Neurophysiol.* 124, 2345–2353. doi: 10.1016/j.clinph.2013.06.003
10. Bartolomei, F., Khalil, M., Wendling, F., Sontheimer, A., Regis, J., Ranjeva, J. P., et al. (2005). Entorhinal cortex involvement in human mesial temporal lobe epilepsy: an electrophysiologic and volumetric study. *Epilepsia* 46, 677–687. doi: 10.1111/j.1528-1167.2005.43804.x
11. Bassett, D. S., and Gazzaniga, M. S. (2011). Understanding complexity in the human brain. *Trends Cogn. Sci.* 15, 200–209. doi: 10.1016/j.tics.2011.03.006 Berl, M. M., Balsamo, L. M., Xu, B., Moore, E. N., Weinstein, S. L., Conry, J. A., et al. (2005). Seizure focus affects regional language networks assessed by fMRI. *Neurology* 65, 1604–1611. doi: 10.1212/01.wnl.0000184502.06647.28
12. Bernasconi, A., Antel, S. B., Collins, D. L., Bernasconi, N., Olivier, A., Dubeau, F., et al. (2001a). Texture analysis and morphological processing of magnetic resonance imaging assist detection of focal cortical dysplasia in extra-temporal partial epilepsy. *Ann. Neurol.* 49, 770–775. doi: 10.1002/ana.1013
13. Bernasconi, A., Bernasconi, N., Bernhardt, B. C., and Schrader, D. (2011). Advances in MRI for 'cryptogenic' epilepsies. *Nat. Rev. Neurol.* 7, 99–108. doi: 10.1038/nrneurol.2010.199
14. Bernasconi, N., Bernasconi, A., Andermann, F., Dubeau, F., Feindel, W., and Reutens, D. C. (1999). Entorhinal cortex in temporal lobe epilepsy: a quantitative MRI study. *Neurology* 52, 1870–1876. doi: 10.1212/WNL.52.9.1870
15. Bernasconi, N., Bernasconi, A., Caramanos, Z., Antel, S. B., Andermann, F., and Arnold, D. L. (2003). Mesial temporal damage in temporal lobe epilepsy: a volu- metric MRI study of the hippocampus, amygdala and parahippocampal region. *Brain* 126, 462–469. doi: 10.1093/brain/awg034
16. Bernasconi, N., Bernasconi, A., Caramanos, Z., Dubeau, F., Richardson, J., Andermann, F., et al. (2001b). Entorhinal cortex atrophy in epilepsy patients exhibiting normal hippocampal volumes. *Neurology* 56, 1335–1339. doi: 10.1212/WNL.56.10.1335
17. Bernasconi, N., and Bernhardt, B. C. (2009). Temporal lobe epilepsy is a progressive disorder. *Nat. Rev. Neurol.* 6, 1. doi: 10.1038/nrneurol.2009.82-c1
18. Bernasconi, N., Duchesne, S., Janke, A., Lerch, J., Collins, D. L., and Bernasconi, A. (2004). Whole-brain voxel-based statistical analysis of gray matter and white matter in temporal lobe epilepsy. *Neuroimage* 23, 717–723. doi: 10.1016/j.neuroimage.2004.06.015
19. Bernasconi, N., Natsume, J., and Bernasconi, A. (2005). Progression in temporal lobe epilepsy: differential atrophy in mesial temporal structures. *Neurology* 65, 223–228. doi: 10.1212/01.wnl.0000169066.46912.fa
20. Bernhardt, B. C., Bernasconi, N., Concha, L., and Bernasconi, A. (2010). Cortical thickness analysis in temporal lobe epilepsy: reproducibility and relation to outcome. *Neurology* 74, 1776–1784. doi: 10.1212/WNL.0b013e3181e0f80a
21. Bernhardt, B. C., Bernasconi, N., Kim, H., and Bernasconi, A. (2012). Mapping thalamocortical network pathology in temporal lobe epilepsy. *Neurology* 78, 129–136. doi: 10.1212/WNL.0b013e31823efd0d
22. Bernhardt, B. C., Chen, Z., He, Y., Evans, A. C., and Bernasconi, N. (2011). Graph-theoretical analysis reveals disrupted small-world organization of cor- tical thickness correlation networks in temporal lobe epilepsy. *Cereb. Cortex* 21, 2147–2157. doi: 10.1093/cercor/bhq291
23. Bernhardt, B. C., Hong, S., Bernasconi, A., and Bernasconi, N. (2013a). Imaging structural and functional brain networks in temporal lobe epilepsy. *Front. Hum. Neurosci.* 7:624. doi: 10.3389/fnhum.2013.00624
24. Bernhardt, B. C., Kim, H., and Bernasconi, N. (2013b). Patterns of subregional mesiotemporal disease progression in temporal lobe epilepsy. *Neurology* 81, 1840–1847. doi: 10.1212/01.wnl.0000436069.20513.92
25. Bernhardt, B. C., Rozen, D. A., Worsley, K. J., Evans, A. C., Bernasconi, N., and Bernasconi, A. (2009a). Thalamo-cortical network pathology in idiopathic gen- eralized epilepsy: insights from MRI-based morphometric correlation analysis. *Neuroimage* 46, 373–381. doi: 10.1016/j.neuroimage.2009.01.055
26. Bernhardt, B. C., Worsley, K. J., Besson, P., Concha, L., Lerch, J. P., Evans, A. C., et al. (2008). Mapping limbic network organization in temporal lobe epilepsy using morphometric correlations: insights on the relation between mesiotemporal connectivity and cortical atrophy. *Neuroimage* 42, 515–524. doi: 10.1016/j.neuroimage.2008.04.261
27. Bernhardt, B. C., Worsley, K. J., Kim, H., Evans, A. C., Bernasconi, A., and Bernasconi, N. (2009b). Longitudinal and cross-sectional analysis of atrophy in pharmacoresistant temporal lobe epilepsy. *Neurology* 72, 1747–1754. doi: 10.1212/01.wnl.0000345969.57574.f5
28. Besson, P., Andermann, F., Dubeau, F., and Bernasconi, A. (2008). Small focal cor- tical dysplasia lesions are located at the bottom of a deep sulcus. *Brain* 131, 3246–3255. doi: 10.1093/brain/awn224
29. Bettus, G., Bartolomei, F., Confort-Gouny, S., Guedj, E., Chauvel, P., Cozzone, P. J., et al. (2010). Role of resting state functional connectivity MRI in presurgical investigation of mesial temporal lobe epilepsy. *J. Neurol. Neurosurg. Psychiatr.* 81, 1147–1154. doi: 10.1136/jnnp.2009.191460
30. Bettus, G., Guedj, E., Joyeux, F., Confort-Gouny, S., Soulier, E., Laguitton, V., et al. (2009). Decreased basal fMRI functional connectivity in epileptogenic networks and contralateral compensatory mechanisms. *Hum. Brain Mapp.* 30, 1580–1591. doi: 10.1002/hbm.20625
31. Birn, R. M., Diamond, J. B., Smith, M. A., and Bandettini, P. A. (2006). Separating respiratory-variation-related fluctuations from neuronal-activity-related fluctuations in fMRI. *Neuroimage* 31, 1536–1548. doi: 10.1016/j.neuroimage.2006.02.048
32. Birn, R. M., Molloy, E. K., Patriat, R., Parker, T., Meier, T. B.,

Kirk, G. R., et al. (2013). The effect of scan length on the reliability of resting-state fMRI connectivity estimates. *Neuroimage* 83, 550–558. doi: 10.1016/j.neuroimage.2013.05.099

33. Biswal, B. B., Mennes, M., Zuo, X. N., Gohel, S., Kelly, C., Smith, S. M., et al. (2010). Toward discovery science of human brain function. *Proc. Natl. Acad. Sci. U.S.A.* 107, 4734–4739. doi: 10.1073/pnas.0911855107
34. Biswal, B., Yetkin, F. Z., Haughton, V. M., and Hyde, J. S. (1995). Functional con- nectivity in the motor cortex of resting human brain using echo-planar MRI. *Magn. Reson. Med.* 34, 537–541. doi: 10.1002/mrm.1910340409
35. Blumcke, I., Thom, M., Aronica, E., Armstrong, D. D., Vinters, H. V., Palmini, A., et al. (2011). The clinicopathologic spectrum of focal cortical dysplasias: a consensus classification proposed by an ad hoc Task Force of the ILAE Diagnostic Methods Commission. *Epilepsia* 52, 158–174. doi: 10.1111/j.1528- 1167.2010.02777.x
36. Bonilha, L., Helpern, J. A., Sainju, R., Nesland, T., Edwards, J. C., Glazier, S. S., et al. (2013). Presurgical connectome and postsurgical seizure control in temporal lobe epilepsy. *Neurology* 81, 1704–1710. doi: 10.1212/01.wnl.0000435306.95271.5f
37. Bonilha, L., Montenegro, M. A., Rorden, C., Castellano, G., Guerreiro, M. M., Cendes, F., et al. (2006). Voxel-based morphometry reveals excess gray matter concentration in patients with focal cortical dysplasia. *Epilepsia* 47, 908–915. doi: 10.1111/j.1528-1167.2006.00548.x
38. Bonilha, L., Nesland, T., Martz, G. U., Joseph, J. E., Spampinato, M. V., Edwards, J. C., et al. (2012). Medial temporal lobe epilepsy is associated with neuronal fibre loss and paradoxical increase in structural connectivity of limbic structures. *J. Neurol. Neurosurg. Psychiatr.* 83, 903–909. doi: 10.1136/jnnp-2012-302476
39. Bonilha, L., Rorden, C., Halford, J. J., Eckert, M., Appenzeller, S., Cendes, F., et al. (2007). Asymmetrical extra-hippocampal grey matter loss related to hippocam- pal atrophy in patients with medial temporal lobe epilepsy. *J. Neurol. Neurosurg. Psychiatr.* 78, 286–294. doi: 10.1136/jnnp.2006.103994
40. Briellmann, R. S., Berkovic, S. F., Syngeniotis, A., King, M. A., and Jackson, G. D. (2002). Seizure-associated hippocampal volume loss: a longitudinal mag- netic resonance study of temporal lobe epilepsy. *Ann. Neurol.* 51, 641–644. doi: 10.1002/ana.10171
41. Buckner, R. L., Andrews-Hanna, J. R., and Schacter, D. L. (2008). The brain's default network: anatomy, function, and relevance to disease. *Ann. N.Y. Acad. Sci.* 1124, 1–38. doi: 10.1196/annals.1440.011
42. Buckner, R. L., Krienen, F. M., and Yeo, B. T. (2013). Opportunities and limita- tions of intrinsic functional connectivity MRI. *Nat. Neurosci.* 16, 832–837. doi: 10.1038/nn.3423
43. Bullmore, E., and Sporns, O. (2009). Complex brain networks: graph theoretical analysis of structural and functional systems. *Nat. Rev. Neurosci.* 10, 186–198. doi: 10.1038/nrn2575
44. Cabral, J., Kringelbach, M. L., and Deco, G. (2014). Exploring the network dynam- ics underlying brain activity during rest. *Prog. neurobiol.* 114C, 102–131. doi: 10.1016/j.pneurobio.2013.12.005
45. Cascino, G. D. (2009). Temporal lobe epilepsy is a progressive neuro- logic disorder: time means neurons! *Neurology* 72, 1718–1719. doi: 10.1212/WNL.0b013e3181a4e465
46. Castellanos, F. X., Di Martino, A., Craddock, R. C., Mehta, A. D., and Milham, M. P. (2013). Clinical applications of the functional connectome. *Neuroimage* 80, 527–540. doi: 10.1016/j.neuroimage.2013.04.083
47. Chen, S., Wu, X., Lui, S., Wu, Q., Yao, Z., Li, Q., et al. (2012). Resting-state fMRI study of treatment-naive temporal lobe epilepsy patients with depressive symptoms. *Neuroimage* 60, 299–304. doi: 10.1016/j.neuroimage.2011.11.092
48. Chiang, S., Levin, H. S., and Haneef, Z. (2014). Computer-automated focus later- alization of temporal lobe epilepsy using fMRI. *J. Magn. Reson. Imaging*. doi: 10.1002/jmri.24696. [Epub ahead of print].
49. Christoff, K., Gordon, A. M., Smallwood, J., Smith, R., and Schooler, J. W. (2009). Experience sampling during fMRI reveals default network and executive system contributions to mind wandering. *Proc. Natl. Acad. Sci. U.S.A.* 106, 8719–8724. doi: 10.1073/pnas.0900234106
50. Colliot, O., Antel, S. B., Naessens, V. B., Bernasconi, N., and Bernasconi, A. (2006a). *In vivo* profiling of focal cortical dysplasia on high-resolution MRI with compu- tational models. *Epilepsia* 47, 134–142. doi: 10.1111/j.1528-1167.2006.00379.x
51. Colliot, O., Bernasconi, N., Khalili, N., Antel, S. B., Naessens, V., and Bernasconi, A. (2006b). Individual voxel-based analysis of gray matter in focal cortical dysplasia. *Neuroimage* 29, 162–171. doi: 10.1016/j.neuroimage.2005.07.021
52. Concha, L., Beaulieu, C., Collins, D. L., and Gross, D. W. (2009). White-matter diffusion abnormalities in temporal-lobe epilepsy with and without mesial temporal sclerosis. *J. Neurol. Neurosurg. Psychiatr.* 80, 312–319. doi: 10.1136/jnnp.2007.139287
53. Concha, L., Beaulieu, C., and Gross, D. W. (2005). Bilateral limbic diffusion abnor- malities in unilateral temporal lobe epilepsy. *Ann. Neurol.* 57, 188–196. doi: 10.1002/ana.20334
54. Concha, L., Kim, H., Bernasconi, A., Bernhardt, B. C., and Bernasconi, N. (2012). Spatial patterns of water diffusion along white matter tracts in temporal lobe epilepsy. *Neurology* 79, 455–462. doi: 10.1212/WNL.0b013e31826170b6
55. Coste, S., Ryvlin, P., Hermier, M., Ostrowsky, K., Adeleine, P., Froment, J. C., et al. (2002). Temporopolar changes in temporal lobe epilepsy: a quantitative MRI- based study. *Neurology* 59, 855–861. doi: 10.1212/WNL.59.6.855
56. Damoiseaux, J. S., Rombouts, S. A., Barkhof, F., Scheltens, P., Stam, C. J., Smith, S. M., et al. (2006). Consistent resting-state networks across healthy subjects. *Proc. Natl. Acad. Sci. U.S.A.* 103, 13848–13853. doi: 10.1073/pnas.0601417103
57. De Tisi, J., Bell, G. S., Peacock, J. L., McEvoy, A. W., Harkness, W. F., Sander, J. W., et al. (2011). The long-term outcome of adult epilepsy surgery, patterns of seizure remission, and relapse: a cohort study. *Lancet* 378, 1388–1395. doi: 10.1016/S0140-6736(11)60890-8
58. Diehl, B., Busch, R. M., Duncan, J. S., Piao, Z., Tkach, J., and Luders, H. O. (2008). Abnormalities in diffusion tensor imaging of the uncinate fasciculus relate to reduced memory in temporal lobe epilepsy. *Epilepsia* 49, 1409–1418. doi: 10.1111/j.1528-1167.2008.01596.x
59. Diehl, B., Tkach, J., Piao, Z., Ruggieri, P., Lapresto, E., Liu, P., et al. (2010). Diffusion tensor imaging in patients with focal epilepsy due to cortical dys- plasia in the temporo-occipital region: electro-clinico-pathological correlations. *Epilepsy Res.* 90, 178–187. doi: 10.1016/j.eplepsyres.2010.03.006
60. Dosenbach, N. U., Nardos, B., Cohen, A. L., Fair, D. A., Power, J. D., Church, J. A., et al. (2010). Prediction of individual brain maturity using fMRI. *Science* 329, 1358–1361. doi: 10.1126/science.1194144
61. Doucet, G. E., Pustina, D., Skidmore, C., Sharan, A., Sperling, M. R., and Tracy, J. I. (2014). Resting-state functional connectivity predicts the strength of hemi- spheric lateralization for language processing in temporal lobe epilepsy and normals. *Hum. Brain Mapp.* doi: 10.1002/hbm.22628. [Epub ahead of print].
62. Doucet, G. E., Skidmore, C., Sharan, A. D., Sperling, M. R., and Tracy, J. I. (2013b). Functional connectivity abnormalities vary by amygdala subdivision and are associated with psychiatric symptoms in unilateral temporal epilepsy. *Brain Cogn.* 83, 171–182. doi: 10.1016/j.bandc.2013.08.001
63. Doucet, G., Osipowicz, K., Sharan, A., Sperling, M. R., and Tracy, J. I. (2013a). Extratemporal functional connectivity impairments at rest are related to mem- ory performance in mesial temporal epilepsy. *Hum. Brain Mapp.* 34, 2202–2216. doi: 10.1002/hbm.22059
64. Dreifuss, S., Vingerhoets, F. J., Lazeyras, F., Andino, S. G., Spinelli, L., Delavelle, J., et al. (2001). Volumetric measurements of subcortical nuclei in patients with temporal lobe epilepsy. *Neurology* 57, 1636–1641. doi: 10.1212/WNL.57.9.1636 Duke, E. S., Tesfaye, M., Berl, M. M., Walker, J. E., Ritzl, E. K., Fasano, R. E., et al. (2012). The effect of seizure focus on regional language processing areas. *Epilepsia* 53, 1044–1050. doi: 10.1111/j.1528-1167.2012.03490.x
65. Dumoulin, S. O., Jirsch, J. D., and Bernasconi, A. (2007). Functional organiza- tion of human visual cortex in occipital polymicrogyria. *Hum. Brain Mapp.* 28, 1302–1312. doi: 10.1002/hbm.20370
66. Duncan, J. S. (2010). Imaging in the surgical treatment of epilepsy. *Nat. Rev. Neurol.* 6, 537–550. doi: 10.1038/nrneurol.2010.131
67. Engel, J. Jr., McDermott, M. P., Wiebe, S., Langfitt, J. T., Stern, J. M., Dewar, S., et al. (2012). Early surgical therapy for drug-resistant temporal lobe epilepsy: a randomized trial. *JAMA* 307, 922–930. doi: 10.1001/jama.2012.220
68. Engel, J. Jr., Pitkanen, A., Loeb, J. A., Dudek, F. E., Bertram, E. H. 3rd., Cole, A. J., et al. (2013). Epilepsy biomarkers. *Epilepsia* 54(Suppl. 4), 61–69. doi: 10.1111/epi.12299
69. Eriksson, S. H., Rugg-Gunn, F. J., Symms, M. R., Barker, G. J., and Duncan, J. S. (2001). Diffusion tensor imaging in patients with epilepsy and malformations of cortical development. *Brain* 124, 617–626. doi: 10.1093/brain/124.3.617
70. Fair, D. A., Cohen, A. L., Power, J. D., Dosenbach, N. U., Church, J. A., Miezin, F. M., et al. (2009). Functional brain networks develop from a

"local to distributed" organization. *PLoS Comput. Biol.* 5:e1000381. doi: 10.1371/jour- nal.pcbi.1000381

71. Federico, P., Archer, J. S., Abbott, D. F., and Jackson, G. D. (2005). Cortical/ subcortical BOLD changes associated with epileptic dis- charges: an EEG-fMRI study at 3 T. *Neurology* 64, 1125–1130. doi: 10.1212/01. WNL.0000156358.72670.AD
72. Feinberg, D. A., Moeller, S., Smith, S. M., Auerbach, E., Ramanna, S., Gunther, M., et al. (2010). Multiplexed echo planar imaging for sub-second whole brain
73. FMRI and fast diffusion imaging. *PLoS ONE* 5:e15710. doi: 10.1371/ jour- nal.pone.0015710
74. Fiecas, M., Ombao, H., Van Lunen, D., Baumgartner, R., Coimbra, A., and Feng, D. (2013). Quantifying temporal correlations: a test-retest evaluation of functional connectivity in resting-state fMRI. *Neuroimage* 65, 231–241. doi: 10.1016/j.neuroimage.2012.09.052
75. Focke, N. K., Yogarajah, M., Bonelli, S. B., Bartlett, P. A., Symms, M. R., and Duncan, J. S. (2008). Voxel-based diffusion tensor imaging in patients with mesial temporal lobe epilepsy and hippocampal sclerosis. *Neuroimage* 40, 728–737. doi: 10.1016/j.neuroimage.2007.12.031
76. Fonseca Vde, C., Yasuda, C. L., Tedeschi, G. G., Betting, L. E., and Cendes, F. (2012). White matter abnormalities in patients with focal cortical dysplasia revealed by diffusion tensor imaging analysis in a voxelwise approach. *Front. Neurol.* 3:121. doi: 10.3389/fneur.2012.00121
77. Fox, M. D., Corbetta, M., Snyder, A. Z., Vincent, J. L., and Raichle, M. E. (2006). Spontaneous neuronal activity distinguishes human dorsal and ven- tral attention systems. *Proc. Natl. Acad. Sci. U.S.A.* 103, 10046–10051. doi: 10.1073/pnas.0604187103
78. Fox, M. D., and Greicius, M. (2010). Clinical applications of resting state functional connectivity. *Front. Syst. Neurosci.* 4:19. doi: 10.3389/ fnsys.2010.00019
79. Fox, M. D., and Raichle, M. E. (2007). Spontaneous fluctuations in brain activity observed with functional magnetic resonance imaging. *Nat. Rev. Neurosci.* 8, 700–711. doi: 10.1038/nrn2201
80. Fox, M. D., Zhang, D., Snyder, A. Z., and Raichle, M. E. (2009). The global signal and observed anticorrelated resting state brain networks. *J. Neurophysiol.* 101, 3270–3283. doi: 10.1152/jn.90777.2008
81. Friston, K. J. (2011). Functional and effective connectivity: a review. *Brain Connect.* 1, 13–36. doi: 10.1089/brain.2011.0008
82. Fuerst, D., Shah, J., Shah, A., and Watson, C. (2003). Hippocampal sclerosis is a progressive disorder: a longitudinal volumetric MRI study. *Ann. Neurol.* 53, 413–416. doi: 10.1002/ana.10509
83. Gaillard, W. D., Berl, M. M., Moore, E. N., Ritzl, E. K., Rosenberger, R., Weinstein, S. L., et al. (2007). Atypical language in lesional and nonlesional complex partial epilepsy. *Neurology* 69, 1761–1771. doi: 10.1212/01.wnl.0000289650.48830.1a
84. Geyer, S., Weiss, M., Reimann, K., Lohmann, G., and Turner, R. (2011). Microstructural parcellation of the human cerebral cortex - from brodmann's post-mortem map to *in vivo* mapping with high-field magnetic resonance imaging. *Front. Hum. Neurosci.* 5:19. doi: 10.3389/ fnhum.2011.00019
85. Glasser, M. F., and Van Essen, D. C. (2011). Mapping human cortical areas *in vivo* based on myelin content as revealed by T1- and T2-weighted MRI. *J. Neurosci.* 31, 11597–11616. doi: 10.1523/JNEUROSCI.2180-11.2011
86. Gong, G., He, Y., Concha, L., Lebel, C., Gross, D. W., Evans, A. C., et al. (2009). Mapping anatomical connectivity patterns of human cerebral cortex using *in vivo* diffusion tensor imaging tractography. *Cereb. Cortex* 19, 524–536. doi: 10.1093/cercor/bhn102
87. Greicius, M. (2008). Resting-state functional connectivity in neuropsychiatric disorders. *Curr. Opin. Neurol.* 21, 424–430. doi: 10.1097/ WCO.0b013e328306f2c5 Greicius, M. D., Krasnow, B., Reiss, A. L., and Menon, V. (2003). Functional con- nectivity in the resting brain: a network analysis of the default mode hypothesis. *Proc. Natl. Acad. Sci. U.S.A.* 100, 253–258. doi: 10.1073/pnas.0135058100
88. Greicius, M. D., Supekar, K., Menon, V., and Dougherty, R. F. (2009). Resting- state functional connectivity reflects structural connectivity in the default mode network. *Cereb. Cortex* 19, 72–78. doi: 10.1093/cercor/bhn059
89. Gross, D. W., Bastos, A., and Beaulieu, C. (2005). Diffusion tensor imaging abnormalities in focal cortical dysplasia. *Can. J. Neurol. Sci.* 32, 477–482.
90. Gross, D. W., Concha, L., and Beaulieu, C. (2006). Extratemporal white matter abnormalities in mesial temporal lobe epilepsy demonstrated with diffusion tensor imaging. *Epilepsia* 47, 1360–1363. doi: 10.1111/j.1528-1167.2006.00603.x Guye, M., Ranjeva, J. P., Bartolomei, F., Confort-Gouny, S., McGonigal, A., Regis, J., et al. (2007). What is the significance of interictal water dif- fusion changes in frontal lobe epilepsies? *Neuroimage* 35, 28–37. doi: 10.1016/j.neuroimage.2006.11.049
91. Haneef, Z., Lenartowicz, A., Yeh, H. J., Engel, J. Jr., and Stern, J. M. (2012). Effect of lateralized temporal lobe epilepsy on the default mode network. *Epilepsy Behav.* 25, 350–357. doi: 10.1016/j.yebeh.2012.07.019
92. Haneef, Z., Lenartowicz, A., Yeh, H. J., Levin, H. S., Engel, J. Jr., and Stern, J. (2014). Functional connectivity of hippocampal networks in temporal lobe epilepsy. *Epilepsia* 55, 137–145. doi: 10.1111/epi.12476
93. He, Y., Chen, Z. J., and Evans, A. C. (2007). Small-world anatomical networks in the human brain revealed by cortical thickness from MRI. *Cereb. Cortex* 17, 2407–2419. doi: 10.1093/cercor/bhl149
94. Hermann, B. P., Seidenberg, M., Schoenfeld, J., and Davies, K. (1997). Neuropsychological characteristics of the syndrome of mesial temporal lobe epilepsy. *Arch. Neurol.* 54, 369–376. doi: 10.1001/ archneur.1997.00550160019010
95. Holmes, M., Folley, B. S., Sonmezturk, H. H., Gore, J. C., Kang, H., Abou-Khalil, B., et al. (2014). Resting state functional connectivity of the hippocampus asso- ciated with neurocognitive function in left temporal lobe epilepsy. *Hum. Brain Mapp.* 35, 735–744. doi: 10.1002/hbm.22210
96. Honey, C. J., Kotter, R., Breakspear, M., and Sporns, O. (2007). Network structure of cerebral cortex shapes functional connectivity on multiple time scales. *Proc. Natl. Acad. Sci. U.S.A.* 104, 10240–10245. doi: 10.1073/ pnas.0701519104
97. Honey, C. J., Sporns, O., Cammoun, L., Gigandet, X., Thiran, J. P., Meuli, R., et al. (2009). Predicting human resting-state functional connectivity from structural connectivity. *Proc. Natl. Acad. Sci. U.S.A.* 106, 2035–2040. doi: 10.1073/pnas.0811168106
98. Hong, S., Kim, H., Bernasconi, N., Bernhardt, B. C., and Bernasconi, A. (2014). Automated detection of cortical dysplasia type II in MRI-negative epilepsy. *Neurology* 83, 48–55. doi: 10.1212/WNL.0000000000000543
99. Huppertz, H. J., Grimm, C., Fauser, S., Kassubek, J., Mader, I., Hochmuth, A., et al. (2005). Enhanced visualization of blurred gray-white matter junctions in focal cortical dysplasia by voxel-based 3D MRI analysis. *Epilepsy Res.* 67, 35–50. doi: 10.1016/j.eplepsyres.2005.07.009
100. James, G. A., Tripathi, S. P., Ojemann, J. G., Gross, R. E., and Drane, D. L. (2013). Diminished default mode network recruitment of the hippocampus and parahippocampus in temporal lobe epilepsy. *J. Neurosurg.* 119, 288–300. doi: 10.3171/2013.3.JNS121041
101. Janszky, J., Ebner, A., Kruse, B., Mertens, M., Jokeit, H., Seitz, R. J., et al. (2003). Functional organization of the brain with malformations of cortical develop- ment. *Ann. Neurol.* 53, 759–767. doi: 10.1002/ana.10545
102. Janszky, J., Jokeit, H., Kontopoulou, K., Mertens, M., Ebner, A., Pohlmann-Eden, B., et al. (2005). Functional MRI predicts memory performance after right mesiotemporal epilepsy surgery. *Epilepsia* 46, 244–250. doi: 10.1111/j.0013- 9580.2005.10804.x
103. Jirsch, J. D., Bernasconi, N., Villani, F., Vitali, P., Avanzini, G., and Bernasconi, A. (2006). Sensorimotor organization in double cortex syndrome. *Hum. Brain Mapp.* 27, 535–543. doi: 10.1002/hbm.20197
104. Jutila, L., Ylinen, A., Partanen, K., Alafuzoff, I., Mervaala, E., Partanen, J., et al. (2001). MR volumetry of the entorhinal, perirhinal, and temporopolar cor- tices in drug-refractory temporal lobe epilepsy. *AJNR Am. J. Neuroradiol.* 22, 1490–1501.
105. Keller, S. S., Cresswell, P., Denby, C., Wieshmann, U., Eldridge, P., Baker, G., et al. (2007). Persistent seizures following left temporal lobe surgery are associated with posterior and bilateral structural and functional brain abnormalities. *Epilepsy Res.* 74, 131–139. doi: 10.1016/j. eplepsyres.2007. 02.005
106. Keller, S. S., and Roberts, N. (2008). Voxel-based morphometry of temporal lobe epilepsy: an introduction and review of the literature. *Epilepsia* 49, 741–757. doi: 10.1111/j.1528-1167.2007.01485.x
107. Kelly, C., Biswal, B. B., Craddock, R. C., Castellanos, F. X., and Milham, M. P. (2012). Characterizing variation in the functional connectome: promise and pitfalls. *Trends Cogn. Sci.* 16, 181–188. doi: 10.1016/j.tics.2012.02.001
108. Kelly, C., Zuo, X. N., Gotimer, K., Cox, C. L., Lynch, L., Brock, D., et al. (2011). Reduced interhemispheric resting state functional connectivity in cocaine addiction. *Biol. Psychiatry* 69, 684–692. doi: 10.1016/j.biopsych.2010. 11.022
109. Kemmotsu, N., Kucukboyaci, N. E., Cheng, C. E., Girard, H. M., Tecoma, E. S., Iragui, V. J., et al. (2013). Alterations in functional connectivity between the hippocampus and prefrontal cortex as a correlate of depres-

sive symptoms in temporal lobe epilepsy. *Epilepsy Behav.* 29, 552–559. doi: 10.1016/j.yebeh.2013.09.039

110. Kobayashi, E., Bagshaw, A. P., Benar, C. G., Aghakhani, Y., Andermann, F., Dubeau, F., et al. (2006). Temporal and extratemporal BOLD responses to temporal lobe interictal spikes. *Epilepsia* 47, 343–354. doi: 10.1111/j.1528-1167.2006.0 0427.x
111. Koepp, M. J. (2014). Neuroimaging of drug resistance in epilepsy. *Curr. Opin. Neurol.* 27, 192–198. doi: 10.1097/WCO.0000000000000072
112. Koepp, M. J., and Woermann, F. G. (2005). Imaging structure and function in refractory focal epilepsy. *Lancet Neurol.* 4, 42–53. doi: 10.1016/S1474- 4422(04)00965-2
113. Krsek, P., Maton, B., Korman, B., Pacheco-Jacome, E., Jayakar, P., Dunoyer, C., et al. (2008). Different features of histopathological subtypes of pediatric focal cortical dysplasia. *Ann. Neurol.* 63, 758–769. doi: 10.1002/ana.21398
114. Kwan, P., Arzimanoglou, A., Berg, A. T., Brodie, M. J., Allen Hauser, W., Mathern, G., et al. (2010). Definition of drug resistant epilepsy: consensus proposal by the ad hoc Task Force of the ILAE commission on therapeutic strategies. *Epilepsia* 51, 1069–1077. doi: 10.1111/j.1528-1167.2009.02397.x
115. Kwan, P., and Brodie, M. J. (2000). Early identification of refractory epilepsy. *N. Engl. J. Med.* 342, 314–319. doi: 10.1056/NEJM200002033420503
116. Laird, A. R., Fox, P. M., Eickhoff, S. B., Turner, J. A., Ray, K. L., McKay, D. R., et al. (2011). Behavioral interpretations of intrinsic connectivity networks. *J. Cogn. Neurosci.* 23, 4022–4037. doi: 10.1162/jocn_a_00077
117. Laufs, H., Hamandi, K., Salek-Haddadi, A., Kleinschmidt, A. K., Duncan, J. S., and Lemieux, L. (2007). Temporal lobe interictal epileptic discharges affect cerebral activity in "default mode" brain regions. *Hum. Brain Mapp.* 28, 1023–1032. doi: 10.1002/hbm.20323
118. Lee, S. K., Kim, D. I., Mori, S., Kim, J., Kim, H. D., Heo, K., et al. (2004). Diffusion tensor MRI visualizes decreased subcortical fiber connectivity in focal cortical dysplasia. *Neuroimage* 22, 1826–1829. doi: 10.1016/j.neuroimage.2004.04.028
119. Leonardi, M., and Ustun, T. B. (2002). The global burden of epilepsy. *Epilepsia* 43(Suppl. 6), 21–25. doi: 10.1046/j.1528-1157.43.s.6.11.x
120. Lerner, J. T., Salamon, N., Hauptman, J. S., Velasco, T. R., Hemb, M., Wu, J. Y., et al. (2009). Assessment and surgical outcomes for mild type I and severe type II cortical dysplasia: a critical review and the UCLA experience. *Epilepsia* 50, 1310–1335. doi: 10.1111/j.1528-1167.2008.01998.x
121. Liao, W., Zhang, Z., Pan, Z., Mantini, D., Ding, J., Duan, X., et al. (2010). Altered functional connectivity and small-world in mesial temporal lobe epilepsy. *PLoS ONE* 5:e8525. doi: 10.1371/journal.pone.0008525
122. Liao, W., Zhang, Z., Pan, Z., Mantini, D., Ding, J., Duan, X., et al. (2011). Default mode network abnormalities in mesial temporal lobe epilepsy: a study combin- ing fMRI and DTI. *Hum. Brain Mapp.* 32, 883–895 doi: 10.1002/hbm.21076
123. Lin, J. J., Riley, J. D., Juranek, J., and Cramer, S. C. (2008). Vulnerability of the frontal-temporal connections in temporal lobe epilepsy. *Epilepsy Res.* 82, 162–170. doi: 10.1016/j.eplepsyres.2008.07.020
124. Lin, J. J., Salamon, N., Lee, A. D., Dutton, R. A., Geaga, J. A., Hayashi, K. M., et al. (2007). Reduced neocortical thickness and complexity mapped in mesial tem- poral lobe epilepsy with hippocampal sclerosis. *Cereb. Cortex* 17, 2007–2018. doi: 10.1093/cercor/bhl109
125. Liu, M., Chen, Z., Beaulieu, C., and Gross, D. W. (2014). Disrupted anatomic white matter network in left mesial temporal lobe epilepsy. *Epilepsia* 55, 674–682. doi: 10.1111/epi.12581
126. Logothetis, N. K., Pauls, J., Augath, M., Trinath, T., and Oeltermann, A. (2001). Neurophysiological investigation of the basis of the fMRI signal. *Nature* 412, 150–157. doi: 10.1038/35084005
127. Lu, J., Liu, H., Zhang, M., Wang, D., Cao, Y., Ma, Q., et al. (2011). Focal pontine lesions provide evidence that intrinsic functional connectivity reflects polysynaptic anatomical pathways. *J. Neurosci.* 31, 15065–15071. doi: 10.1523/JNEUROSCI.2364-11.2011
128. Luo, C., Qiu, C., Guo, Z., Fang, J., Li, Q., Lei, X., et al. (2011). Disrupted func tional brain connectivity in partial epilepsy: a resting-state fMRI study. *PLoS ONE* 7:e28196. doi: 10.1371/journal.pone.0028196
129. Maccotta, L., He, B. J., Snyder, A. Z., Eisenman, L. N., Benzinger, T. L., Ances, B. M., et al. (2013). Impaired and facilitated functional networks in temporal lobe epilepsy. *Neuroimage Clin.* 2, 862–872. doi: 10.1016/j.nicl.2013.06.011
130. Mantini, D., Gerits, A., Nelissen, K., Durand, J. B., Joly, O., Simone, L., et al. (2011). Default mode of brain function in monkeys. *J. Neurosci.* 31, 12954–12962. doi: 10.1523/JNEUROSCI.2318-11.2011
131. Margulies, D. S., Kelly, A. M., Uddin, L. Q., Biswal, B. B., Castellanos, F. X., and Milham, M. P. (2007). Mapping the functional connectivity of anterior cingulate cortex. *Neuroimage* 37, 579–588. doi: 10.1016/j.neuroimage.2007.05.019
132. Margulies, D. S., Vincent, J. L., Kelly, C., Lohmann, G., Uddin, L. Q., Biswal, B. B., et al. (2009). Precuneus shares intrinsic functional architecture in humans and monkeys. *Proc. Natl. Acad. Sci. U.S.A.* 106, 20069–20074. doi: 10.1073/pnas.0905314106
133. Mars, R. B., Sallet, J., Schuffelgen, U., Jbabdi, S., Toni, I., and Rushworth, M. F. (2011). Connectivity-based subdivisions of the human right "temporoparietal junction area": evidence for different areas participating in different cortical networks. *Cereb. Cortex* 22, 1894–1903. doi: 10.1093/cercor/bhr268
134. Mbwana, J., Berl, M. M., Ritzl, E. K., Rosenberger, L., Mayo, J., Weinstein, S., et al. (2009). Limitations to plasticity of language network reorganization in localization related epilepsy. *Brain* 132, 347–356. doi: 10.1093/brain/awn329
135. McDonald, C. R., Ahmadi, M. E., Hagler, D. J., Tecoma, E. S., Iragui, V. J., Gharapetian, L., et al. (2008). Diffusion tensor imaging correlates of memory and language impairments in temporal lobe epilepsy. *Neurology* 71, 1869–1876. doi: 10.1212/01.wnl.0000327824.05348.3b
136. McIntosh, A. M., Kalnins, R. M., Mitchell, L. A., Fabinyi, G. C., Briellmann, R. S., and Berkovic, S. F. (2004). Temporal lobectomy: long-term seizure outcome, late recurrence and risks for seizure recurrence. *Brain* 127, 2018–2030. doi: 10.1093/brain/awh221
137. Mohanraj, R., Norrie, J., Stephen, L. J., Kelly, K., Hitiris, N., and Brodie, M. J. (2006). Mortality in adults with newly diagnosed and chronic epilepsy: a retrospective comparative study. *Lancet Neurol.* 5, 481–487. doi: 10.1016/S1474- 4422(06)70448-3
138. Moran, N. F., Lemieux, L., Kitchen, N. D., Fish, D. R., and Shorvon, S. D. (2001). Extrahippocampal temporal lobe atrophy in temporal lobe epilepsy and mesial temporal sclerosis. *Brain* 124, 167–175. doi: 10.1093/brain/124.1.167
139. Morgan, V. L., Rogers, B. P., Sonmezturk, H. H., Gore, J. C., and Abou-Khalil, B. (2011). Cross hippocampal influence in mesial temporal lobe epilepsy measured with high temporal resolution functional magnetic resonance imaging. *Epilepsia* 52, 1741–1749. doi: 10.1111/j.1528-1167.2011.03196.x
140. Mueller, S. G., Laxer, K. D., Barakos, J., Ian, C., Garcia, P., and Weiner, M. W. (2009). Widespread neocortical abnormalities in temporal lobe epilepsy with and without mesial sclerosis. *Neuroimage* 46, 353–359. doi: 10.1016/j.neuroimage.2009.02.020
141. Murphy, K., Birn, R. M., Handwerker, D. A., Jones, T. B., and Bandettini, P. A. (2009). The impact of global signal regression on resting state correla- tions: are anti-correlated networks introduced? *Neuroimage* 44, 893–905. doi: 10.1016/j.neuroimage.2008.09.036
142. Natsume, J., Bernasconi, N., Andermann, F., and Bernasconi, A. (2003). MRI volumetry of the thalamus in temporal, extratemporal, and idiopathic gener- alized epilepsy. *Neurology* 60, 1296–1300. doi: 10.1212/01.WNL.0000058764.34 968.C2
143. Negishi, M., Martuzzi, R., Novotny, E. J., Spencer, D. D., and Constable, R. T. (2011). Functional MRI connectivity as a predictor of the surgical outcome of epilepsy. *Epilepsia* 52, 1733–1740. doi: 10.1111/j.1528-1167.2011.03191.x
144. Niazy, R. K., Xie, J., Miller, K., Beckmann, C. F., and Smith, S. M. (2011). Spectral characteristics of resting state networks. *Prog. Brain Res.* 193, 259–276. doi: 10.1016/B978-0-444-53839-0.00017-X
145. Patriat, R., Molloy, E. K., Meier, T. B., Kirk, G. R., Nair, V. A., Meyerand, M. E., et al. (2013). The effect of resting condition on resting-state fMRI reliability and consistency: a comparison between resting with eyes open, closed, and fixated. *Neuroimage* 78, 463–473. doi: 10.1016/j.neuroimage.2013. 04.013
146. Pereira, F. R., Alessio, A., Sercheli, M. S., Pedro, T., Bilevicius, E., Rondina, J. M., et al. (2010). Asymmetrical hippocampal connectivity in mesial tempo- ral lobe epilepsy: evidence from resting state fMRI. *BMC Neurosci.* 11:66. doi: 10.1186/1471-2202-11-66
147. Pittau, F., Grova, C., Moeller, F., Dubeau, F., and Gotman, J. (2012). Patterns of altered functional connectivity in mesial temporal lobe epilepsy. *Epilepsia* 53, 1013–1023. doi: 10.1111/j.1528-1167.2012.03464.x
148. Ponten, S. C., Bartolomei, F., and Stam, C. J. (2007). Small-world networks and epilepsy: graph theoretical analysis of intracerebrally recorded mesial temporal lobe seizures. *Clin. Neurophysiol.* 118, 918–927. doi: 10.1016/j.clinph.2006.12.002
149. Power, J. D., Barnes, K. A., Snyder, A. Z., Schlaggar, B. L., and Petersen, S. E. (2012). Spurious but systematic correlations in functional

connectivity MRI networks arise from subject motion. *Neuroimage* 59, 2142–2152. doi: 10.1016/j.neuroimage.2011.10.018

150. Pugliatti, M., Beghi, E., Forsgren, L., Ekman, M., and Sobocki, P. (2007). Estimating the cost of epilepsy in Europe: a review with economic modeling. *Epilepsia* 48, 2224–2233. doi: 10.1111/j.1528-1167.2007.01251.x

151. Richardson, M. P. (2012). Large scale brain models of epilepsy: dynamics meets connectomics. *J. Neurol. Neurosurg. Psychiatr.* 83, 1238–1248. doi: 10.1136/jnnp-2011-301944

152. Rodrigo, S., Oppenheim, C., Chassoux, F., Golestani, N., Cointepas, Y., Poupon, C., et al. (2007). Uncinate fasciculus fiber tracking in mesial temporal lobe epilepsy. Initial findings. *Eur. Radiol.* 17, 1663–1668. doi: 10.1007/s00330-006-0558-x

153. Salmenperä, T., Kälviäinen, R., Partanen, K., and Pitkänen, A. (2000). Quantitative MRI volumetry of the entorhinal cortex in temporal lobe epilepsy. *Seizure* 9, 208–215. doi: 10.1053/seiz.1999.0373

154. Salvador, R., Suckling, J., Schwarzbauer, C., and Bullmore, E. (2005). Undirected graphs of frequency-dependent functional connectivity in whole brain networks. *Philos. Trans. R. Soc. Lond. B Biol. Sci.* 360, 937–946. doi: 10.1098/rstb.2005.1645

155. Sankar, T., Bernasconi, N., Kim, H., and Bernasconi, A. (2008). Temporal lobe epilepsy: differential pattern of damage in temporopolar cortex and white matter. *Hum. Brain Mapp.* 29, 931–944. doi: 10.1002/hbm.20437

156. Scharfman, H. E. (2007). The neurobiology of epilepsy. *Curr. Neurol. Neurosci. Rep.* 7, 348–354. doi: 10.1007/s11910-007-0053-z

157. Schmidt, A., Smieskova, R., Aston, J., Simon, A., Allen, P., Fusar-Poli, P., et al. (2013). Brain connectivity abnormalities predating the onset of psychosis: cor- relation with the effect of medication. *JAMA Psychiatry* 70, 903–912. doi: 10.1001/jamapsychiatry.2013.117

158. Shehzad, Z., Kelly, A. M., Reiss, P. T., Gee, D. G., Gotimer, K., Uddin, L. Q., et al. (2009). The resting brain: unconstrained yet reliable. *Cereb. Cortex* 19, 2209–2229. doi: 10.1093/cercor/bhn256

159. Shen, K., Bezgin, G., Hutchison, R. M., Gati, J. S., Menon, R. S., Everling, S., et al. (2012). Information processing architecture of functionally defined clusters in the macaque cortex. *J. Neurosci.* 32, 17465–17476. doi: 10.1523/JNEUROSCI.2709-12.2012

160. Sisodiya, S. M., Fauser, S., Cross, J. H., and Thom, M. (2009). Focal cortical dysplasia type II: biological features and clinical perspectives. *Lancet Neurol.* 8, 830–843. doi: 10.1016/S1474-4422(09)70201-7

161. Skudlarski, P., Jagannathan, K., Calhoun, V. D., Hampson, M., Skudlarska, B. A., and Pearlson, G. (2008). Measuring brain connectivity: diffusion tensor imag- ing validates resting state temporal correlations. *Neuroimage* 43, 554–561. doi: 10.1016/j.neuroimage.2008.07.063

162. Smith, S. M., Fox, P. T., Miller, K. L., Glahn, D. C., Fox, P. M., Mackay, C. E., et al. (2009). Correspondence of the brain's functional architecture dur- ing activation and rest. *Proc. Natl. Acad. Sci. U.S.A.* 106, 13040–13045. doi: 10.1073/pnas.0905267106

163. Sommer, B., Grummich, P., Coras, R., Kasper, B. S., Blumcke, I., Hamer, H. M., et al. (2013). Integration of functional neuronavigation and intraoperative MRI in surgery for drug-resistant extratemporal epilepsy close to eloquent brain areas. *Neurosurg. Focus* 34, E4. doi: 10.3171/2013.2.FOCUS12397

164. Spencer, S. S. (2002). Neural networks in human epilepsy: evidence of and implications for treatment. *Epilepsia* 43, 219–227. doi: 10.1046/j.1528- 1157.2002.26901.x

165. Srinivasan, R., Winter, W. R., Ding, J., and Nunez, P. L. (2007). EEG and MEG coherence: measures of functional connectivity at distinct spa- tial scales of neocortical dynamics. *J. Neurosci. Methods* 166, 41–52. doi: 10.1016/j.jneumeth.2007.06.026

166. Srivastava, S., Maes, F., Vandermeulen, D., Van Paesschen, W., Dupont, P., and Suetens, P. (2005). Feature-based statistical analysis of structural MR data for automatic detection of focal cortical dysplastic lesions. *Neuroimage* 27, 253–266. doi: 10.1016/j.neuroimage.2005.03.045

167. Steinbeis, N., Bernhardt, B. C., and Singer, T. (2014). Age-related differences in function and structure of rSMG and reduced functional connectivity with DLPFC explains heightened emotional egocentricity bias in childhood. *Soc. Cogn. Affect. Neurosci.* doi: 10.1093/scan/nsu057. [Epub ahead of print].

168. Tassi, L., Colombo, N., Garbelli, R., Francione, S., Lo, R. G., Mai, R., et al. (2002). Focal cortical dysplasia: neuropathological subtypes, EEG, neuroimaging and surgical outcome. *Brain* 125, 1719–1732. doi: 10.1093/brain/awf175

169. Tellez-Zenteno, J. F., Dhar, R., and Wiebe, S. (2005). Long-term seizure outcomes following epilepsy surgery: a systematic review and meta-analysis. *Brain* 128, 1188–1198. doi: 10.1093/brain/awh449

170. Thornton, R., Vulliemoz, S., Rodionov, R., Carmichael, D. W., Chaudhary, U. J., Diehl, B., et al. (2011). Epileptic networks in focal cortical dysplasia revealed using electroencephalography-functional magnetic resonance imaging. *Ann. Neurol.* 70, 822–837. doi: 10.1002/ana.22535

171. Tusche, A., Smallwood, J., Bernhardt, B. C., and Singer, T. (2014). Classifying the wandering mind: revealing the affective content of thoughts during task-free rest periods. *Neuroimage* 97, 107–116. doi: 10.1016/j.neuroimage.2014.03.076

172. Tyvaert, L., Hawco, C., Kobayashi, E., Levan, P., Dubeau, F., and Gotman, J. (2008). Different structures involved during ictal and interictal epileptic activity in mal- formations of cortical development: an EEG-fMRI study. *Brain* 131, 2042–2060. doi: 10.1093/brain/awn145

173. Uddin, L. Q., Mooshagian, E., Zaidel, E., Scheres, A., Margulies, D. S., Kelly, A. M., et al. (2008). Residual functional connectivity in the split-brain revealed with resting-state functional MRI. *Neuroreport* 19, 703–709. doi: 10.1097/WNR.0b013e3282fb8203

174. Vaessen, M. J., Braakman, H. M., Heerink, J. S., Jansen, J. F., Debeij-Van Hall, M. H., Hofman, P. A., et al. (2013). Abnormal modular organization of functional net- works in cognitively impaired children with frontal lobe epilepsy. *Cereb. Cortex* 23, 1997–2006. doi: 10.1093/cercor/bhs186

175. Vaessen, M. J., Jansen, J. F., Braakman, H. M., Hofman, P. A., De Louw, A., Aldenkamp, A. P., et al. (2014). Functional and structural network impairment in childhood frontal lobe epilepsy. *PLoS ONE* 9:e90068. doi: 10.1371/jour- nal.pone.0090068

176. Van Den Heuvel, M. P., and Sporns, O. (2011). Rich-club organization of the human connectome. *J. Neurosci.* 31, 15775–15786. doi: 10.1523/JNEUROSCI.3539-11.2011

177. Van Dijk, K. R., Hedden, T., Venkataraman, A., Evans, K. C., Lazar, S. W., and Buckner, R. L. (2010). Intrinsic functional connectivity as a tool for human con- nectomics: theory, properties, and optimization. *J. Neurophysiol.* 103, 297–321. doi: 10.1152/jn.00783.2009

178. Van Essen, D. C., Ugurbil, K., Auerbach, E., Barch, D., Behrens, T. E., Bucholz, R., et al. (2012). The Human Connectome Project: a data acquisition perspective. *Neuroimage* 62, 2222–2231. doi: 10.1016/j.neuroimage.2012.02.018

179. Vitali, P., Minati, L., D'incerti, L., Maccagnano, E., Mavilio, N., Capello, D., et al. (2008). Functional MRI in malformations of cortical development: activation of dysplastic tissue and functional reorganization. *J. Neuroimaging* 18, 296–305. doi: 10.1111/j.1552-6569.2007.00164.x

180. Vlooswijk, M. C., Jansen, J. F., Majoie, H. J., Hofman, P. A., De Krom, M. C., Aldenkamp, A. P., et al. (2010). Functional connectivity and language impair- ment in cryptogenic localization-related epilepsy. *Neurology* 75, 395–402. doi: 10.1212/WNL.0b013e3181ebdd3e

181. Vlooswijk, M. C., Vaessen, M. J., Jansen, J. F., De Krom, M. C., Majoie, H. J., Hofman, P. A., et al. (2011). Loss of network efficiency associ- ated with cognitive decline in chronic epilepsy. *Neurology* 77, 938–944. doi: 10.1212/WNL.0b013e31822cfc2f

182. Voets, N. L., Adcock, J. E., Stacey, R., Hart, Y., Carpenter, K., Matthews, P. M., et al. (2009). Functional and structural changes in the memory network asso- ciated with left temporal lobe epilepsy. *Hum. Brain Mapp.* 30, 4070–4081. doi: 10.1002/hbm.20830

183. Voets, N. L., Beckmann, C. F., Cole, D. M., Hong, S., Bernasconi, A., and Bernasconi, N. (2012). Structural substrates for resting network disruption in temporal lobe epilepsy. *Brain* 135, 2350–2357. doi: 10.1093/brain/aws137

184. Voets, N. L., Bernhardt, B. C., Kim, H., Yoon, U., and Bernasconi, N. (2011). Increased temporolimbic cortical folding complexity in temporal lobe epilepsy. *Neurology* 76, 138–144. doi: 10.1212/WNL.0b013e318205d521

185. Waites, A. B., Briellmann, R. S., Saling, M. M., Abbott, D. F., and Jackson, G. D. (2006). Functional connectivity networks are disrupted in left temporal lobe epilepsy. *Ann. Neurol.* 59, 335–343. doi: 10.1002/ana.20733

186. Wang, J., Qiu, S., Xu, Y., Liu, Z., Wen, X., Hu, X., et al. (2014). Graph theoretical analysis reveals disrupted topological properties of whole brain functional networks in temporal lobe epilepsy. *Clin. Neurophysiol.* 125, 1744–1756. doi: 10.1016/j.clinph.2013.12.120

187. Widjaja, E., Blaser, S., Miller, E., Kassner, A., Shannon, P., Chuang, S. H., et al. (2007). Evaluation of subcortical white matter and deep white matter tracts in malformations of cortical development. *Epilepsia* 48, 1460–1469. doi: 10.1111/j.1528-1167.2007.01105.x

188. Widjaja, E., Zamyadi, M., Raybaud, C., Snead, O. C., and Smith, M. L.

(2013). Abnormal functional network connectivity among resting-state networks in children with frontal lobe epilepsy. *AJNR Am. J. Neuroradiol.* 34, 2386–2392. doi: 10.3174/ajnr.A3608

189. Widjaja, E., Zarei Mahmoodabadi, S., Otsubo, H., Snead, O. C., Holowka, S., Bells, S., et al. (2009). Subcortical alterations in tis- sue microstructure adjacent to focal cortical dysplasia: detection at diffusion-tensor MR imaging by using magnetoencephalographic dipole cluster localization. *Radiology* 251, 206–215. doi: 10.1148/radiol.25110 81092

190. Wilke, M., Kassubek, J., Ziyeh, S., Schulze-Bonhage, A., and Huppertz, H. J. (2003). Automated detection of gray matter malformations using optimized voxel- based morphometry: a systematic approach. *Neuroimage* 20, 330–343. doi: 10.1016/S1053-8119(03)00296-9

191. Yan, C., Liu, D., He, Y., Zou, Q., Zhu, C., Zuo, X., et al. (2009). Spontaneous brain activity in the default mode network is sensitive to different resting-state conditions with limited cognitive load. *PLoS ONE* 4:e5743. doi: 10.1371/jour- nal.pone.0005743

192. Yan, C., and Zang, Y. (2010). DPARSF: a MATLAB toolbox for "pipeline" data analysis of resting-state fMRI. *Front. Syst. Neurosci.* 4:13. doi: 10.3389/fnsys.2010.00013

193. Yuan, W., Szaflarski, J. P., Schmithorst, V. J., Schapiro, M., Byars, A. W., Strawsburg, R. H., et al. (2006). fMRI shows atypical language lateralization in pedi- atric epilepsy patients. *Epilepsia* 47, 593–600. doi: 10.1111/j.1528-1167.2006.0 0474.x

194. Zalesky, A., Fornito, A., Harding, I. H., Cocchi, L., Yucel, M., Pantelis, C., et al. (2010). Whole-brain anatomical networks: does the choice of nodes matter? *Neuroimage* 50, 970–983. doi: 10.1016/j.neuroimage.2009.12.027

195. Zeng, H., Pizarro, R., Nair, V. A., La, C., and Prabhakaran, V. (2013). Alterations in regional homogeneity of resting-state brain activity in mesial temporal lobe epilepsy. *Epilepsia* 54, 658–666. doi: 10.1111/epi.12066

196. Zhang, Z., Lu, G., Zhong, Y., Tan, Q., Liao, W., Chen, Z., et al. (2009a). Impaired perceptual networks in temporal lobe epilepsy revealed by resting fMRI. *J. Neurol.* 256, 1705–1713. doi: 10.1007/s00415-009- 5187-2

197. Zhang, Z., Lu, G., Zhong, Y., Tan, Q., Liao, W., Wang, Z., et al. (2010a). Altered spontaneous neuronal activity of the default-mode network in mesial temporal lobe epilepsy. *Brain Res.* 1323, 152–160. doi: 10.1016/j. brainres.2010. 01.042

198. Zhang, Z., Lu, G., Zhong, Y., Tan, Q., Yang, Z., Liao, W., et al. (2009b). Impaired attention network in temporal lobe epilepsy: a resting FMRI study. *Neurosci. Lett.* 458, 97–101. doi: 10.1016/j.neulet.2009.04.040

199. Zhang, Z. Q., Lu, G. M., Zhong, Y., Tan, Q. F., Chen, Z. L., Liao, W., et al. (2010b). MRI study of mesial temporal lobe epilepsy using amplitude of low-frequency fluctuation analysis. *Hum. Brain Mapp.* 31, 1851–1861. doi: 10.1002/hbm.20982

18

Conceptualizing Lennox–Gastaut syndrome as a secondary network epilepsy

John S. Archer[1,2,3]*, Aaron E. L. Warren[1], Graeme D. Jackson[1,2,3] and David F. Abbott[1,2]

[1] Department of Medicine, Austin Health, The University of Melbourne, Heidelberg, VIC, Australia
[2] Florey Institute of Neuroscience and Mental Health, Heidelberg, VIC, Australia
[3] Department Neurology, Austin Health, Heidelberg, VIC, Australia

***Correspondence:**
John S. Archer, Melbourne Brain Centre, 245 Burgundy Street, Heidelberg, VIC 3084, Australia
e-mail: jarcher@unimelb.edu.au

Lennox–Gastaut Syndrome (LGS) is a category of severe, disabling epilepsy, characterized by frequent, treatment-resistant seizures, and cognitive impairment. Electroencephalography (EEG) shows characteristic generalized epileptic activity that is similar in those with lesional, genetic, or unknown causes, suggesting a common underlying mechanism. The condition typically begins in young children, leaving many severely disabled with recurring seizures throughout their adult life. Scalp EEG of the tonic seizures of LGS is characterized by a diffuse high-voltage slow transient evolving into generalized low-voltage fast activity, likely reflecting sustained fast neuronal firing over a wide cortical area. The typical interictal discharges (runs of slow spike-and-wave and bursts of generalized paroxysmal fast activity) also have a "generalized" electrical field, suggesting widespread cortical involvement. Recent brain mapping studies have begun to reveal which cortical and subcortical regions are active during these "generalized" discharges. In this critical review, we examine findings from neuroimaging studies of LGS and place these in the context of the electrical and clinical features of the syndrome. We suggest that LGS can be conceptualized as "secondary network epilepsy," where the epileptic activity is expressed through large-scale brain networks, particularly the attention and default-mode networks. Cortical lesions, when present, appear to chronically interact with these networks to produce network instability rather than triggering each individual epileptic discharge. LGS can be considered as "secondary" network epilepsy because the epileptic manifestations of the disorder reflect the networks being driven, rather than the specific initiating process. In this review, we begin with a summation of the clinical manifestations of LGS and what this has revealed about the underlying etiology of the condition. We then undertake a systematic review of the functional neuroimaging literature in LGS, which leads us to conclude that LGS can best be conceptualized as "secondary network epilepsy."

Keywords: Lennox–Gastaut syndrome, generalized epilepsy, tonic seizure, EEG–fMRI, default-mode network, attention network, paroxysmal fast activity, slow spike and wave

LENNOX–GASTAUT SYNDROME – DEFINITION AND CLINICAL FEATURES

Lennox–Gastaut Syndrome (LGS) is a severe epilepsy phenotype, usually beginning in childhood, and commonly associated with intellectual disability. Onset of LGS is typically before the age of 8 years (1–3), with peak onset age between 3 and 5 years (4). Once established, 80% of LGS patients will continue to have seizures into adulthood (5, 6). Individual patients may have a variety of genetic abnormalities or cortical lesions (7), and in a significant proportion of patients, perhaps 25% (8, 9), the underlying cause is unknown.

The core features of LGS were described by Henri Gastaut in 1966 (10). Patients may have a variety of seizure types, often with multiple daily attacks, but tonic seizures, which cause patients to suddenly and unpredictably stiffen and drop to the ground, are a key diagnostic feature (11). On electroencephalography (EEG), tonic seizures are characterized by a diffuse high-voltage slow wave followed by generalized low-voltage fast activity (LVFA) (**Figure 1A**), likely reflecting sustained fast neuronal firing over a wide cortical area (12). The interictal EEG shows frequent runs of pseudo-rhythmic 1.5–2.5 Hz diffuse slow spike-and-wave (SSW), and intermittent bursts of generalized paroxysmal fast activity (GPFA), particularly in sleep (4). The electrical features of GPFA show similarity to the LVFA of tonic seizures, suggesting that they probably recruit similar brain networks.

Although LGS is relatively uncommon [0.24–0.28 per 1,000 births; (14, 15)], the persistent nature of seizures results in a relatively high prevalence, estimated at 1–10% of all children with epilepsy (8, 16–21), and 3–17% of patients with epilepsy and intellectual disability (22–24). LGS patients are not uncommon in epilepsy clinics.

LENNOX–GASTAUT "PHENOTYPE"

Patients with some, but not all, the features of LGS, were previously classified as having "secondary generalized epilepsy" (6, 25, 26). This term was removed from the 2010 International League

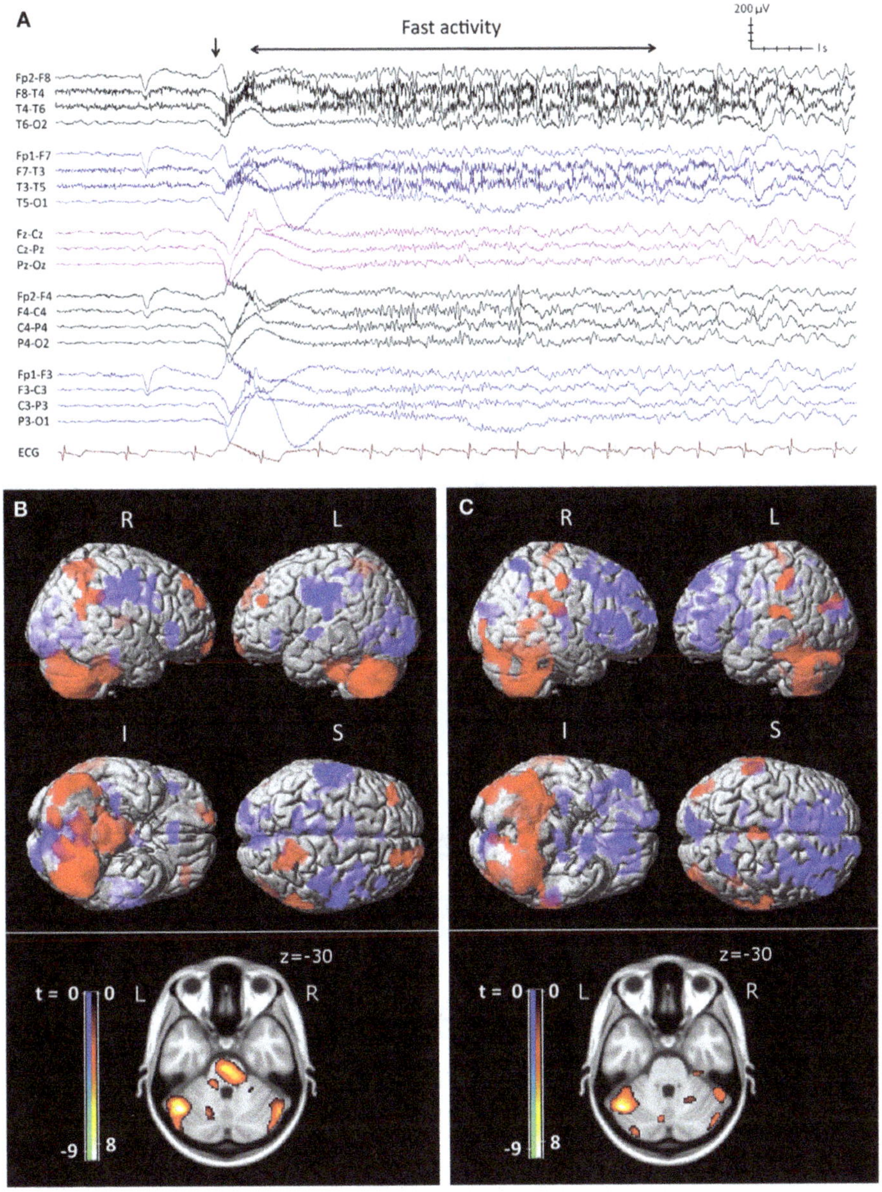

FIGURE 1 | Ictal EEG features and peri-ictal SPECT of tonic seizures in LGS. **(A)** Clinical onset of seizure corresponds with a high-voltage slow transient (vertical arrow) followed by apparent diffuse attenuation, evolving into low-voltage fast activity (LVFA) and later a run of slow spike-and-wave mixed with notched delta. **(B)** Early radiotracer injection (<10 s after offset of LVFA) and subsequent SPECT shows an early pattern of increased (red) cerebral blood flow in frontal and parietal "attention" areas, pons, and cerebellum, and decreased (blue) CBF in primary cortical areas. **(C)** Late radiotracer injection (>10 s after offset of LVFA) and subsequent SPECT shows an evolution toward a pattern of increased CBF over lateral parietal cortex and cerebellum, and decreased CBF bi-frontally, while the pons is no longer involved. **(B,C)** Top: surface renderings displayed at $p < 0.02$ (uncorrected), extent $k > 125$ voxels. Below: overlay onto axial slice of MNI T1 152 average brain displayed at $p < 0.05$ [cluster-corrected for family-wise error (FWE)]. R = right, L = left, I = inferior, S = superior. Adapted and re-printed with permission from Intusoma and colleagues (13).

Against Epilepsy (ILAE) updated classification of the epilepsies (11), as it was felt the diagnostic category had become an unhelpful "dumping ground" for poorly defined cases of severe epilepsy. It is clear that many recent advances in understanding disease mechanisms in epilepsy have come from genetic discoveries, derived from careful electroclinical phenotyping (27, 28). Unfortunately, in clinical practice, this has meant patients who manifest most of the electrical features of LGS (tonic seizures, SSW, and GPFA), but who might have an older than usual age of onset, minimal EEG background slowing, or mild intellectual disability, are no longer easily classified. We have begun using the term "Lennox–Gastaut Phenotype" (LGP) to describe these patients (29), as we believe the similarities in electroclinical expression likely reflect similarities in the neural networks being driven by epileptic activity.

EPILEPTIC ENCEPHALOPATHY

Lennox–Gastaut Syndrome is classified as one of the epileptic encephalopathies (11), as it seems likely that the epileptic process pervasively inhibits cognition and cognitive development. Patients with LGS frequently show cognitive regression around the time of diagnosis, while established LGS is almost always associated with moderate to severe cognitive impairment. Twenty to sixty percent of patients show intellectual disability at the time of diagnosis, increasing to 75–95% within 5 years of the syndrome's onset (4). Fifty-five percent of LGS patients have an IQ under 50 (30), and impairment is often global. On continuous performance tasks, children and adolescents with LGS show impaired information processing with marked slowing of reaction times to cognitive and motor stimuli (31). Behavioral and psychiatric disturbances are frequent in LGS, compounding the burden of care. Common problems include aggressiveness, hyperactivity, and autistic traits (32–38). Long-term outcomes are typically very poor, with the majority of patients remaining under home-care or institutionalization (2, 39), and some needing to wear a helmet to prevent seizure-related head and face injuries (40).

Cognitive impairment in LGS appears related to the age of onset and persistence of seizures. An earlier age of seizure onset (<5 years) has been associated with more severe cognitive impairment, while patients who develop LGS later in life (>9 years) follow a more favorable cognitive course (3, 30, 32, 41–43). In a group of patients with normal mental development before the onset of LGS, Ohtsuka (44) found that 95.7% (22/23) of patients with persistent seizures showed cognitive impairment after a follow-up period of at least 5 years compared with 12.5% (1/8) of patients who had been seizure free for at least 1 year.

If seizures remain poorly controlled, there appears to be progressive cognitive impairment over time. Oguni (1) followed 72 patients for a mean of 17 years and found a decrease of at least 15 IQ points from onset of diagnosis to end of follow-up in around 80% of patients with LGS. In contrast, there are a number of case reports of improved cognitive trajectory in patients with LGS due to a lesion, who become seizure free following resective surgery (45, 46).

VARIABLE CAUSES, COMMON ELECTROCLINICAL FEATURES

No single pathophysiology underlies the development of LGS (25), although the age-dependent expression implies that there is something about the immature brain that renders it susceptible to development of the LGS phenotype (47). Approximately 10–30% of patients have an epileptogenic abnormality visible on structural MRI (3, 48), with focal, multifocal, or diffuse structural abnormalities described. Etiologies include focal cortical dysplasia, perinatal anoxia, ischemic stroke, intracranial hemorrhage, and encephalitis (7, 49). A variety of genetic factors, particularly *de novo* mutations, have been implicated in some patients (7, 50). However, approximately 25% of patients with LGS (8, 9) have no obvious structural brain abnormalities and no confirmed genetic abnormalities. These cases may be considered LGS of unknown cause (11). It is notable that the electroclinical features of tonic seizures and interictal discharges in LGS are remarkably similar whether or not there is a causative lesion, and independent of lesion location or pathology. Conversely, the same etiology may lead to LGS or a more benign epilepsy phenotype. For example, tuberous sclerosis is a condition, in which inherited or spontaneous mutations of the TSC1 or TSC2 gene lead to a failure of inhibition of the mTOR (mammalian target of rapamycin) pathway, causing abnormal cell proliferation. In this condition, defects in the same molecular pathway, and at times the same genetic abnormality, may produce epileptic spasms, an LGS phenotype, or focal epilepsy (51, 52). Hence, there are factors other than the specific molecular mechanism that determine whether a patient will express the LGS phenotype.

POTENTIALLY REVERSIBLE

Seizures and developmental delay are not necessarily permanent in LGS. With regards to seizures, as early as 1979 it was shown that surgical removal of a parietotemporal neoplasm in a child with LGS led to a complete remission of seizures and SSW patterns on EEG (53). We recently showed similar improvements in three patients who had their lesions removed (29) (**Figure 2**), consistent with other reports of seizure freedom following focal or lobar resections in LGS patients with parietal, frontal, temporal, and hypothalamic lesions on MRI (45, 46, 54–62). Following successful epilepsy surgery, some LGS patients show an initial persistence of seizures or "generalized" epileptic discharges, which subsequently resolve ("winding down"; **Figure 2**) (29, 45, 46, 54, 56). This demonstrates that although lesions can cause the LGS phenotype, at least in some patients the lesions themselves are not triggering each individual epileptic discharge ("secondary bi-synchrony"). It suggests instead that lesions are interacting with key networks to create an unstable mode of network behavior (29). Once the destabilizing influence is removed, in this case the cortical lesion, cerebral networks are able to gradually return to a more stable (non-epileptic) state.

In addition to reductions in seizure frequency and normalization of EEG abnormalities, there are several reports of post-operative cognitive gains (45, 46, 54, 55, 57–60), supporting the notion that intellectual deterioration may in part be due to seizures and interictal discharges (63, 64). For example, Liu (59) performed comprehensive pre- and post-operative neuropsychological assessment in 15 patients with LGS who underwent single-lobe/lesionectomy or multi-lobe resection, and found a significant mean IQ increase from 56.1 to 67.4 after surgery. These benefits become less certain as duration of LGS prior to surgery increases (59, 65), a trend found in other severe childhood epilepsies (66–69). Hence, there appears to be a time window in which the epileptic brain is both vulnerable to irreversible cognitive decline and amenable to treatments that restore normal development.

INVOLVEMENT OF SUBCORTICAL STRUCTURES

THALAMUS

The generalized nature of epileptic discharges and seizures has led many to postulate that the thalamus may be a key initiator of epileptic activity in LGS. Recordings from the thalamus during generalized epileptic discharges of LGS confirm that the thalamus is involved (70, 71). EEG–functional magnetic resonance imaging (fMRI) studies have shown thalamic involvement during SSW (29, 72, 73) and generalized spike-and-wave (74, 75). High-frequency electrical deep brain stimulation (DBS) of the thalamic centromedian nucleus has been reported to reduce generalized seizures by 80% in a group of 13 LGS patients (76). However,

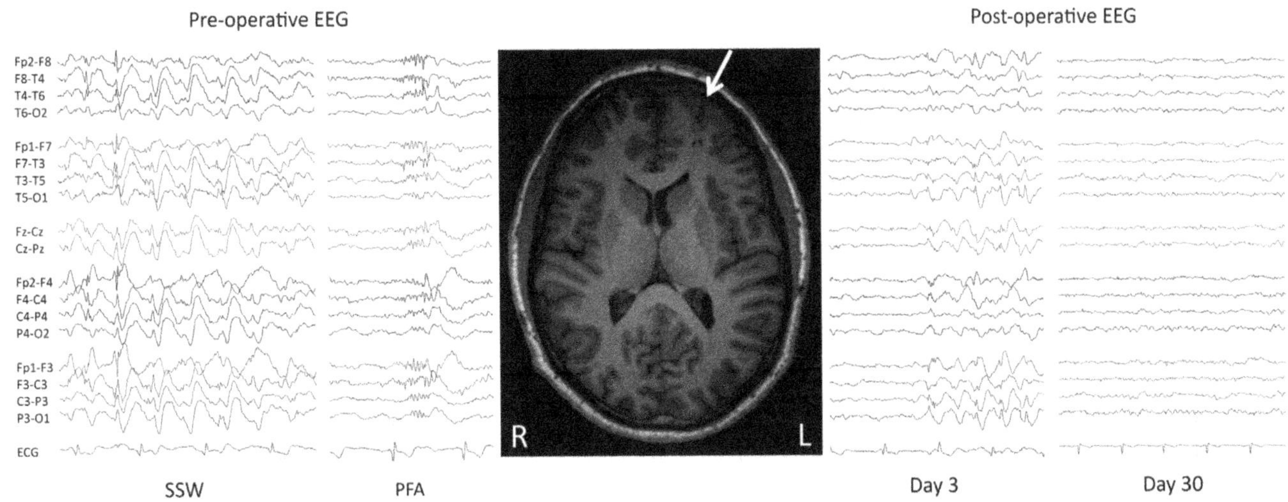

FIGURE 2 | Pre- and post-operative EEG. Pre- and post-operative EEG in a 38-year-old male with LGS, a lesion, and intractable seizures since childhood. Prior to resection of a left frontal cortical dysplasia (arrowed), the patient suffered daily seizures. Pre-operative interictal EEG showed bursts of slow spike-and-wave (SSW) and generalized paroxysmal fast activity (GPFA). Day 3 post-operative EEG showed persistence of SSW, while day 30 EEG showed complete normalization, consistent with a winding down of the epileptic process. The patient is 2 years seizure free, consistent with LGS being potentially reversible. Re-printed with permission from Archer and colleagues (29).

given that cortical lesions can cause LGS, and their removal can lead to abolition of the epileptic process, it seems likely in this case that the thalamus is probably acting as a synchronizer and amplifier, rather than initiator.

PONS

The pons appears involved in tonic seizures. Direct electrical stimulation of pons in animals reproduces posturing similar to a tonic seizure, with predominant axial muscle involvement (77). Auditory stimulation of the brainstem in a rat model of generalized epilepsy causes animals to have convulsive attacks with electrophysiological evidence of excessive brainstem firing, but no evidence of cortical involvement (78). We have shown increased blood flow in the pons during tonic seizures in humans, consistent with increased pontine neuronal activity (13). However, as noted above, cortical lesions can cause LGS, and their removal can lead to abolition of the epileptic process. Hence, although the pons is involved in seizure expression, it does not appear to be the initiator of epileptic activity and seizures (79).

A NETWORK DISORDER

The shared electroclinical and cognitive features of LGS suggest that common cerebral networks are involved. Epilepsy is increasingly being recognized as a disorder of cerebral networks (29, 72, 74, 80–84). The electroclinical features of an epilepsy syndrome can be considered as reflecting the specific cerebral networks being recruited. In this context, a neural network comprises anatomically and functionally connected cortical and subcortical brain structures, where activity in any one part of the network may affect activity in all the others (80). Network-based considerations of epilepsy are useful and clinically relevant because they can help explain seizure semiology can suggest which cerebral networks may be dysfunctional in the interictal state, and can help guide medical and surgical management directions. For example, the diagnosis of temporal lobe epilepsy (TLE), reflecting seizures predominantly expressed in the limbic system, makes sense of the memory, olfactory, and other symptoms the patient may experience during an "aura." It permits interpretation of ictal features, including spread patterns. It suggests particular imaging and genetic studies directed at epilepsy involving this region, while leaving open the idea that seizure activity could have started elsewhere (e.g., occipital lobe) but be maximally expressed through the temporal lobe. Finally, the label of TLE helps interpretation of memory deficits, which are associated with dysfunction of this particular network. The neuroimaging evidence for network involvement in LGS is reviewed below.

EPILEPSY NETWORKS OF LGS: A SYSTEMATIC REVIEW OF THE FUNCTIONAL NEUROIMAGING LITERATURE

In this section, we review the functional neuroimaging studies in LGS, in particular, positron emission tomography (PET), interictal and peri-ictal single-photon-emission computed tomography (SPECT), and combined electroencephalography (EEG) and functional magnetic resonance imaging (EEG–fMRI).

SEARCH STRATEGY

A literature search in the bibliographic database PubMed (1982 to April 2014) was undertaken. Search terms were restricted to articles' titles and abstracts. A combination of the following search terms was used: LGS AND PET OR positron OR SPECT OR photon OR fMRI OR EEG–fMRI OR neuroimaging. Furthermore, we examined each article's reference list and used Google to search for websites that might provide additional references. This effort resulted in 95 citations that were selected for review. Included articles were limited to studies reporting primary data; review articles were read but are excluded here. A total of 70 citations were excluded as irrelevant, with 25 remaining for review.

POSITRON EMISSION TOMOGRAPHY

The most common radio-ligand is fluoro-2-deoxy-D-glucose (FDG-PET), which images glucose uptake, to display average cerebral metabolism over the course of the image acquisition, usually 30–60 min in duration (85). Several interictal PET studies with small numbers of LGS patients have shown unilateral focal or multifocal hypometabolic abnormalities, predominantly in frontal and temporal regions, that tend to correlate with structural abnormalities observed on structural imaging or epileptic foci determined by EEG (86–89). Others have observed more diffuse abnormalities, including generalized bilateral hypometabolism, most prominent fronto-temporally (90). Some patients show normal cerebral glucose metabolism (91). The variability in these results was recapitulated in a larger series of 15 children with LGS (92), where four major metabolic subtypes were identified: unilateral focal hypometabolism in frontal or temporal regions; unilateral diffuse hypometabolism; bilateral diffuse hypometabolism; and normal metabolic patterns. Ferrie (93) aimed to establish whether PET would reveal focal abnormalities in a group of LGS patients who had no localizing features evident on clinical examination, EEG, or high resolution MRI. Using asymmetry indices for patients' own homologous cortical regions to detect metabolic defects, no focal abnormalities were found in patients with *de novo* LGS, while LGS cases following West syndrome more commonly showed unilateral focal hypometabolism in temporal, frontal, or parietal regions. Repeat PET performed 1 year later in a subset of patients with focal abnormalities showed that hypometabolic defects were stable over time (94). In a further semi-quantitative analysis comparing metabolic rates in LGS to age-matched controls, Ferrie (95) observed widespread, generalized hypometabolism in cortical and thalamic regions in LGS patients with and without previously reported focal abnormalities (93). The degree of hypometabolism in the frontal lobes was later reported to be inversely correlated with measures of patients' adaptive behavior (96).

Taken together, these results agree with the clinical impression that LGS is a disorder of heterogeneous etiologies. However, they add further evidence that, in some cases at least, generalized epileptic activity in LGS may be caused by focal cortical abnormalities. This notion is supported by more recent uses of PET in the identification of metabolic defects in LGS patients who undergo resective surgery and subsequently show seizure improvement (57, 58, 60). An additional observation across these studies is that in patients who do show aberrant metabolic activity, whether focal, multifocal, or diffuse, the abnormality appears largely confined to association cortex (involving frontal, temporal, and parietal lobes), typically sparing primary cortical areas (e.g., primary visual and motor cortex). This pattern of common cerebral network involvement has been observed in other functional neuroimaging modalities, which are discussed below.

SINGLE-PHOTON-EMISSION COMPUTED TOMOGRAPHY

Single-photon-emission computed tomography is able to image regional cerebral blood flow (CBF) to identify brain regions that are active during a seizure (97, 98). To date, very few studies have been performed in LGS patients. A small number of case reports have found diffuse foci of reduced CBF in frontal, temporal, or parietal regions (99–103); however, their interpretation is limited because studies were only performed interictally, making it difficult to differentiate normal from epileptogenic tissue (104). To address this gap in the literature, we recently performed a voxel-wise comparison of ictal and interictal SPECT in a group of 10 scan pairs from 7 LGS patients who were studied during video EEG-confirmed tonic seizures (13). Five patients had focal structural abnormalities on MRI. Across the whole group, tonic seizures were associated with increased CBF in the lateral parietal lobe and cerebellum, and reduced CBF bilaterally in frontal and occipital regions. The evolution of CBF changes was also explored by examining patient subgroups who were injected with a radiotracer early (<10 s) or late (>10 s) after the offset of EEG LVFA (**Figure 1**). The early injection group showed increased CBF in the pons, cerebellum, and bilateral fronto-parietal regions, and reduced CBF in primary cortical areas, including pericentral and occipital cortex. The late injection group showed an evolution of this pattern toward increased CBF over lateral parietal cortex and the cerebellum, and reduced CBF frontally. Despite some of these patients having a focal cortical lesion in different locations, we observed a common pattern of early association cortex involvement and reduced activity in primary cortical areas. We postulated that tonic seizures in LGS reflect activity in a corticopontine pathway, arising in a network of bilateral frontal and parietal association cortices before projecting via cortico-reticular pathways to the pons, and from there via reticulo-spinal pathways to spinal motor neurons (**Figure 3**).

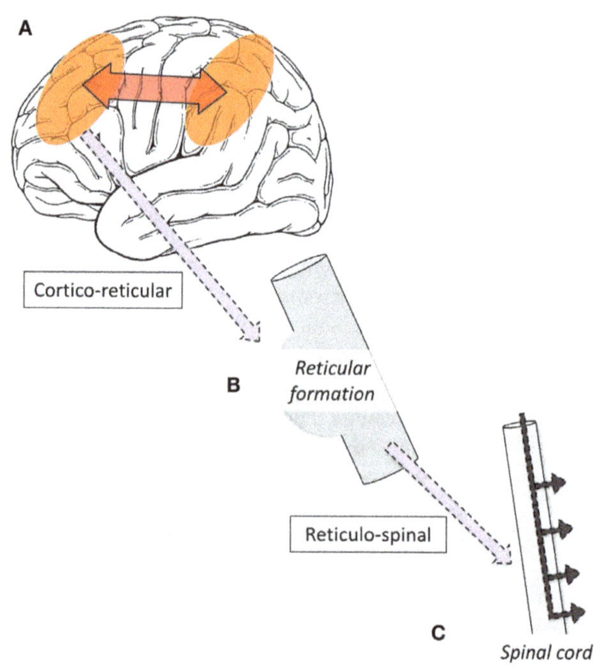

FIGURE 3 | Schematic illustration of proposed mechanism of tonic seizures in LGS is shown. **(A)** Epileptiform activity initiated in cortex, and rapidly amplified within intrinsic attention and default-mode networks. **(B)** Epileptiform activity projects via cortico-reticular pathway – Brodmann area 6 (premotor cortex) to ponto-medullary reticular formation (105, 106). **(C)** Epileptiform activity projects via the reticulo-spinal pathway to motor neurons innervating proximal muscles at multiple levels (107).

EEG–fMRI

An understanding of the importance of cerebral networks in epilepsy has been driven by insights gained through combined EEG and functional MRI (EEG–fMRI) studies, including key publications from our laboratory (29, 72, 74, 75, 108–114). Recording low-voltage scalp EEG signals in the MR environment poses a number of challenges (115–117), but these can be largely overcome (118, 119).

Electroencephalography–functional magnetic resonance imaging utilizes the blood–oxygen-level-dependent (BOLD) response (120) to visualize activity changes associated with epileptiform discharges across the whole brain. Functional MRI activity represents summed local field potentials across time [fMRI volume acquisition time (TR) is typically 2–3 s] and space (voxel size is typically 3–5 mm^3) (121). Hence, EEG–fMRI provides an overview of cerebral network behavior during epileptic discharges. Indeed, because fMRI is sensitive to brain activity that is not necessarily hypersynchronized, it can do more than simply map the brain regions active at the time of the spike; it can also map brain activity time-locked to but preceding the EEG spike (113, 122), thus providing a more complete picture of the brain networks associated with epileptic discharges.

A relatively small number of EEG–fMRI papers have examined LGS. One study of spike-and-wave activity in 16 subjects with "secondary generalized epilepsy" who were scanned at 1.5 T showed thalamic activation in addition to widespread cortical changes that included variable activation and deactivation in frontal and parietal regions (123). Similar results were observed in two of these patients who were studied again at 3 T using simultaneous EEG with BOLD and arterial spin label (ASL) fMRI (124). BOLD activation and deactivation during spike-and-wave observed in frontal and parietal regions corresponded, respectively, with CBF increases and decreases recorded with ASL. A group analysis of 11 children with LGS, with EEG–fMRI performed under chloral hydrate sedation, found BOLD increases in the thalamus and brainstem (73). These changes were found on an analysis that combined all discharges, including SSW and "polyspike" discharges, potentially diluting the differential effects of SSW and GPFA on cortical activity.

We have recently shown that GPFA and SSW, the two pathognomonic interictal discharges of LGS, are associated with quite different changes in neuronal activity (29, 72). GPFA is associated with diffuse association network activation (**Figure 4**), consistent with the GPFA EEG signature of widespread fast activity. Association cortex contains two dominant cognitive systems: the attention network, which modulates focused attention to task across a range of cognitive domains; and the default-mode network (DMN), that engages during quiet reflection, reminiscing, and internal thinking. Neural activity in these two networks is normally anticorrelated, consistent with their diametrically opposed cognitive functions (125–128). Epileptiform activity in LGS appears to be associated with a highly unusual pattern of co-activation of attention networks and the DMN. Furthermore, there is a very similar pattern of network activation in LGS whether or not there is

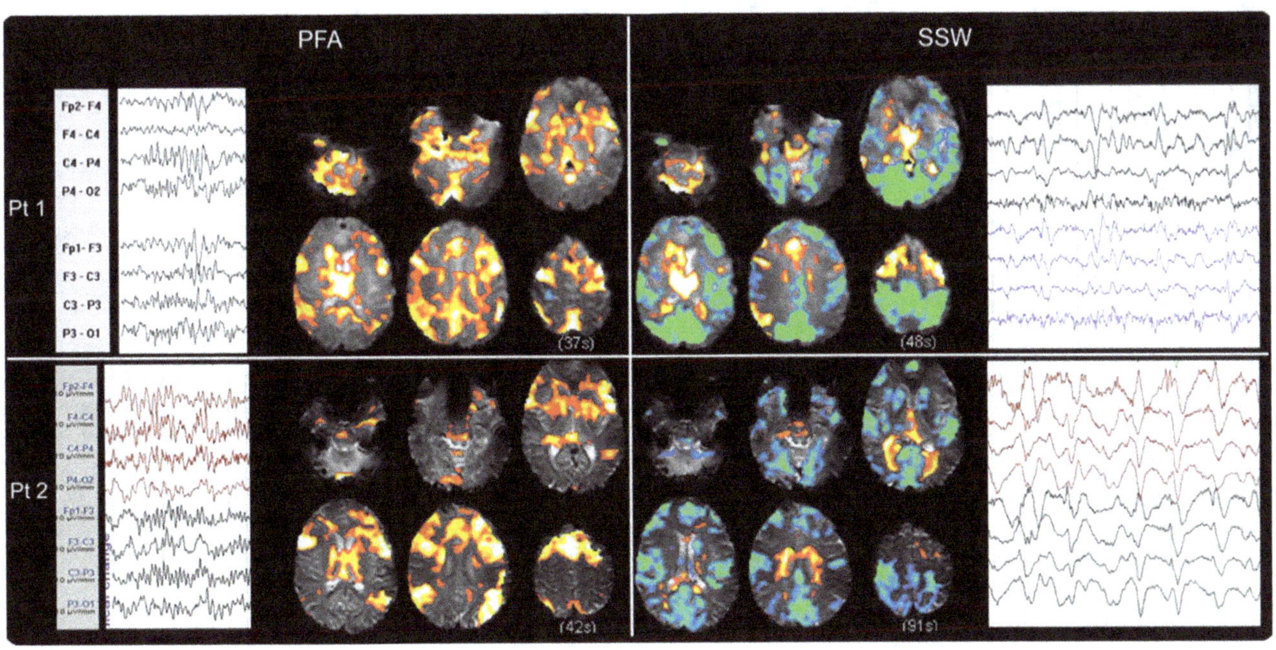

FIGURE 4 | Electroencephalography–functional magnetic resonance imaging of generalized paroxysmal fast activity (GPFA) and slow spike-and-wave (SSW) in individual LGS patients is shown. In individual patients, GPFA and SSW produce different blood–oxygen-level-dependent (BOLD) response patterns. GPFA shows increased BOLD in diffuse association network regions, as well as brainstem, basal ganglia, and thalamus. SSW shows a different pattern, with decreased BOLD signal in primary cortical areas. The number of events in seconds, at the bottom of each panel, is the sum of the length of all individual epileptiform events recorded during the EEG for each patient. Pt, patient. Re-printed with permission from Pillay and colleagues (72).

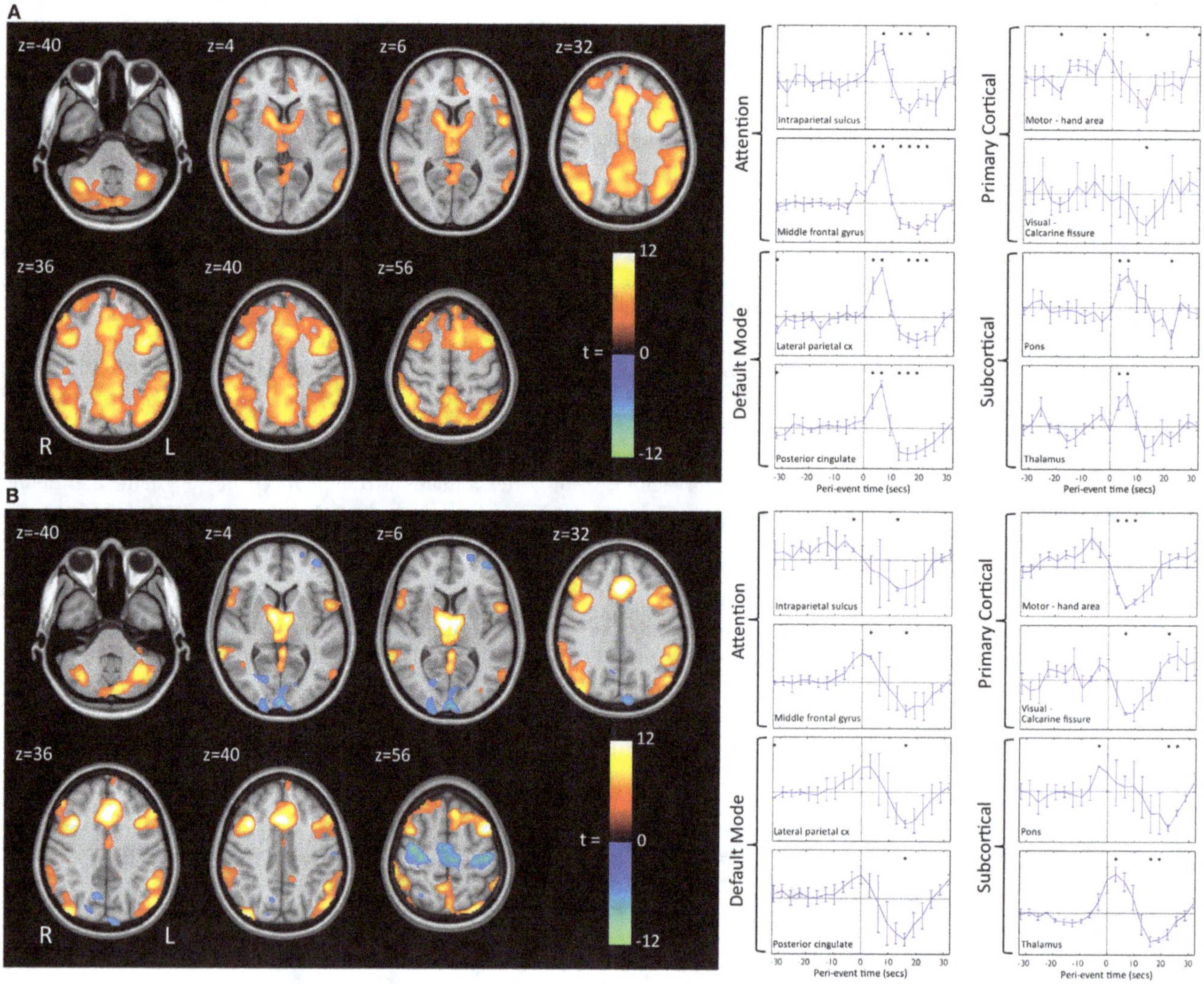

FIGURE 5 | Group-level EEG–fMRI activation maps and peri-event BOLD signal time-courses in LGS patients with epileptogenic lesions in different cortical locations are shown. (A) Generalized paroxysmal fast activity (GPFA). *Left*: fixed-effects whole-brain group EEG–fMRI analysis in six patients with cortical lesions in different locations showing co-activation of two normally anti-correlated cognitive systems in diffuse association cortex: the attention and default-mode networks. Activations are displayed as two-tailed *t*-statistics thresholded at $p < 0.05$ (corrected for FWE) and overlaid on axial slices of the MNI T1 152 average brain. *Right*: random-effects peri-event time-course analysis showing GPFA group mean BOLD signal change from regions of interest. Time-courses are displayed in 3.2 s time-bins, from 32 s before to 32 s after event onset (indicated by vertical line). Error bars indicate standard errors. Asterisks indicate time-bins of significant mean BOLD signal change (two-tailed single sample *t*-tests, $p < 0.05$, uncorrected). Time-course analysis confirms simultaneous BOLD signal increases in frontal and parietal association cortical areas, thalamus, and pons, and reduced signal in primary cortical areas. **(B)** Slow spike-and-wave (SSW). *Left*: fixed-effects whole-brain group EEG–fMRI analysis in three subjects with cortical lesions in different locations showing mixed increased and decreased BOLD signal, including activation in thalamus and lateral frontal and parietal areas, and deactivation in primary cortex including pericentral and occipital regions. Activations are displayed as per **(A)**. *Right*: random-effects peri-event time-course analysis showing SSW group mean BOLD signal change from regions of interest, as displayed in **(A)**. Time-course analysis shows a complex set of activity changes that are only partially captured by the whole-brain maps. Attention and default-mode networks are being driven simultaneously, but with a steady "pre-spike" increase in activity followed by a decrease in signal at the time of scalp-detected SSW. Primary cortical regions show signal decreases. Adapted and re-printed with permission from Archer and colleagues (29).

an underlying epileptogenic lesion, and independent of lesion location (**Figure 5**), supporting our hypothesis that the shared electroclinical features of LGS reflect underlying similarities in the recruited brain networks.

Slow spike-and-wave also appears to simultaneously recruit the attention and DMNs, but with a more complex pattern (**Figure 4**). SSW shows a steady upward drift of activity for more than 6 s prior to scalp-detected activity, followed by an abrupt fall in activity with the appearance of SSW on the scalp (**Figure 5**). The curious phenomenon of "pre-spike" fMRI activity changes has been observed in generalized spike-and-wave of genetic generalized epilepsy (74, 129–131), and may reflect the need of the brain to be in a specific state for spike-and-wave discharges to occur. The shape of the hemodynamic changes around the time of SSW is a poor fit for the canonical hemodynamic response function (HRF) that is typically used in event-related analyses to generate maps of activity changes (132). This may explain the variability seen with our EEG–fMRI maps of SSW. EEG–fMRI studies of epileptic discharges in other epilepsy syndromes have also observed that BOLD responses to discharges show differences to the canonical HRF (113, 114, 133–135).

We and others have observed reduced activity in primary cortical regions during interictal discharges (GPFA and SSW; **Figures 4** and **5**) (29, 73). This is consistent with our observation of reduced blood flow in sensorimotor cortex during tonic seizures (13). Hence, it appears that epileptic activity in LGS is not predominantly expressed through primary cortical regions. This suggests that an alternate pathway generates the axial predominant movements of tonic seizures, perhaps cortico-reticular pathways (105, 106), driving the pontine reticular formation, with outflow via reticulo-spinal projections, which innervate predominately axial muscles at multiple spinal levels (107) (**Figure 3**).

CONCLUSION

Patients with LGS have a similar electroclinical phenotype, despite varying etiologies, consistent with a common underlying mechanism. The EEG features suggest that there is widespread cortical recruitment during epileptic activity. Functional neuroimaging has confirmed that epileptic activity in LGS recruits widespread areas of association cortex (diffuse association network activity), and spares primary cortical regions. Hence, LGS appears to be a network epilepsy, where the epileptic discharges and seizures reflect abnormal neuronal firing within intrinsic cognitive brain networks, specifically the attention and DMNs. Furthermore, epileptic activity in LGS appears to be characterized by a fundamental breakdown in normal brain network behavior, with co-activation of attention networks and the DMN. However, it is not yet clear whether it is the attention network, the DMN, or both that are key to the LGS phenotype.

The epileptic process in LGS appears to be initiated from the cortex. Cortical lesions can cause LGS, and their removal can abolish seizures. Some patients show "winding down" of interictal discharges following removal of an epileptogenic lesion. This strongly suggests that cortical lesions, when present, chronically interact with these networks to produce network instability rather than triggering each individual epileptic discharge. Presumably, a wide range of molecular and neuronal mechanisms could produce a similar pattern of network instability. In patients without an obvious cortical lesion, therapies that seek to reduce network instability, such as "generalized" anti-convulsants, are likely to be beneficial (4). Preliminary evidence suggests that thalamic DBS may also be beneficial (76), possibly by modulating network excitability. Although the epileptic process is driven from the cortex, it appears that tonic seizures are expressed through the reticular formation of the pons. We propose that when epileptic activity in the cognitive networks reaches a particular threshold, it triggers cortico-reticular pathways, which connect premotor cortex (Brodmann area 6) to the pontine reticular formation. Trunkal predominant movement is likely generated via reticulo-spinal pathways, which innervate axial muscles at multiple levels. These primitive pathways are normally responsible for postural control and orienting behavior, such as turning to visual, auditory, or tactile stimuli (105, 106), but in LGS are being driven by epileptic outflow from the cortex.

Lennox–Gastaut syndrome can be conceptualized as secondary network epilepsy, where the epileptic discharges and seizures reflect epileptic activity being amplified through intrinsic cognitive brain networks. The epileptic features of LGS reflect activity in these networks, rather than the specific lesional, genetic, or other cause. We believe that the label of "secondary network epilepsy" is useful as it captures and explains the key electroclinical features, including tonic seizures, SSW, and GPFA. The label allows initial management decisions to be made, including consideration of "generalized" drug therapies, while acting as a reminder to continue to search for specific underlying causes. Finally, the label reminds us that the process is potentially reversible, if an underlying treatable cause such as a lesion can be identified early.

ACKNOWLEDGMENTS

We acknowledge financial support from the National Health and Medical Research Council (NHMRC) of Australia, specifically project grant no. 628725 (John S. Archer and David F. Abbott) and practitioner fellowship no. 1060312 (Graeme D. Jackson). Aaron E. L. Warren is supported by an Australian Postgraduate Award from the Commonwealth Government of Australia. The Florey Institute of Neuroscience and Mental Health also acknowledges the strong support from the Victorian Government and in particular the funding from the Operational Infrastructure Support Grant.

REFERENCES

1. Oguni H, Hayashi K, Osawa M. Long-term prognosis of Lennox-Gastaut syndrome. *Epilepsia* (1996) **37**(s3):44–7. doi:10.1111/j.1528-1157.1996.tb01820.x
2. Yagi K. Evolution of Lennox-Gastaut syndrome: a long-term longitudinal study. *Epilepsia* (1996) **37**(s3):48–51. doi:10.1111/j.1528-1157.1996.tb01821.x
3. Goldsmith IL, Zupanc ML, Buchhalter JR. Long-term seizure outcome in 74 patients with Lennox–Gastaut syndrome: effects of incorporating MRI head imaging in defining the cryptogenic subgroup. *Epilepsia* (2000) **41**(4):395–9. doi:10.1111/j.1528-1157.2000.tb00179.x
4. Arzimanoglou A, French J, Blume WT, Cross JH, Ernst J-P, Feucht M, et al. Lennox-Gastaut syndrome: a consensus approach on diagnosis, assessment, management, and trial methodology. *Lancet Neurol* (2009) **8**(1):82–93. doi:10.1016/S1474-4422(08)70292-8
5. Crumrine PK. Lennox-Gastaut syndrome. *J Child Neurol* (2002) **17**(1 Suppl):S70–5. doi:10.1177/08830738020170011001
6. Van Rijckevorsel K. Treatment of Lennox-Gastaut syndrome: overview and recent findings. *Neuropsychiatr Dis Treat* (2008) **4**(6):1001. doi:10.2147/NDT.S1668
7. Blume WT. Pathogenesis of Lennox-Gastaut syndrome: considerations and hypotheses. *Epileptic Disord* (2001) **3**(4):183–96.
8. Hancock EC, Cross JH. Treatment of Lennox-Gastaut syndrome. *Cochrane Database Syst Rev* (2013) (2):CD003277. doi:10.1002/14651858.CD003277.pub3
9. Widdess-Walsh P, Dlugos D, Fahlstrom R, Joshi S, Shellhaas R, Boro A, et al. Lennox-Gastaut syndrome of unknown cause: phenotypic characteristics of patients in the Epilepsy Phenome/Genome Project. *Epilepsia* (2013) **54**(11):1898–904. doi:10.1111/epi.12395
10. Gastaut H, Roger J, Soulayrol R, Tassinari C, Regis H, Dravet C, et al. Childhood epileptic encephalopathy with diffuse slow spike-waves (otherwise known as "Petit Mal Variant") or Lennox syndrome. *Epilepsia* (1966) **7**(2):139–79. doi:10.1111/j.1528-1167.1966.tb06263.x
11. Berg AT, Berkovic SF, Brodie MJ, Buchhalter J, Cross JH, Van Emde Boas W, et al. Revised terminology and concepts for organization of seizures and epilepsies:

report of the ILAE commission on classification and terminology, 2005–2009. *Epilepsia* (2010) **51**(4):676–85. doi:10.1111/j.1528-1167.2010.02522.x

12. Tao JX, Ray A, Hawes-Ebersole S, Ebersole JS. Intracranial EEG substrates of scalp EEG interictal spikes. *Epilepsia* (2005) **46**(5):669–76. doi:10.1111/j.1528-1167.2005.11404.x
13. Intusoma U, Abbott DF, Masterton RA, Stagnitti MR, Newton MR, Jackson GD, et al. Tonic seizures of Lennox-Gastaut syndrome: periictal single-photon emission computed tomography suggests a corticopontine network. *Epilepsia* (2013) **54**(12):2151–7. doi:10.1111/epi.12398
14. Heiskala H. Community-based study of Lennox-Gastaut syndrome. *Epilepsia* (1997) **38**(5):526–31. doi:10.1111/j.1528-1157.1997.tb01136.x
15. Rantala H, Putkonen T. Occurrence, outcome, and prognostic factors of infantile spasms and Lennox-Gastaut syndrome. *Epilepsia* (1999) **40**(3):286–9. doi:10.1111/j.1528-1157.1999.tb00705.x
16. Aicardi J. *Epilepsy in Children.* New York: Raven Press (1986).
17. Cowan LD, Bodensteiner JB, Leviton A, Doherty L. Prevalence of the epilepsies in children and adolescents. *Epilepsia* (1989) **30**(1):94–106. doi:10.1111/j.1528-1157.1989.tb05289.x
18. Sidenvall R, Forsgren L, Heijbel J. Prevalence and characteristics of epilepsy in children in northern Sweden. *Seizure* (1996) **5**(2):139–46. doi:10.1016/S1059-1311(96)80108-7
19. Eriksson K, Koivikko M. Prevalence, classification, and severity of epilepsy and epileptic syndromes in children. *Epilepsia* (1997) **38**(12):1275–82. doi:10.1111/j.1528-1157.1997.tb00064.x
20. Kramer U, Nevo Y, Neufeld MY, Fatal A, Leitner Y, Harel S. Epidemiology of epilepsy in childhood: a cohort of 440 consecutive patients. *Pediatr Neurol* (1998) **18**(1):46–50. doi:10.1016/S0887-8994(97)00154-9
21. Waaler P, Blom B, Skeidsvoll H, Mykletum A. Prevalence, classification, and severity of epilepsy in children in western Norway. *Epilepsia* (2000) **41**(7):802–10. doi:10.1111/j.1528-1157.2000.tb00246.x
22. Forsgren L, Edvinsson S-O, Heijbel J, Sidenvall R. Epilepsy in a population of mentally retarded children and adults. *Epilepsy Res* (1990) **6**(3):234–48. doi:10.1016/0920-1211(90)90079-B
23. Trevathan E, Murphy CC, Yeargin-Allsopp M. Prevalence and descriptive epidemiology of Lennox-Gastaut syndrome among Atlanta children. *Epilepsia* (1997) **38**(12):1283–8. doi:10.1111/j.1528-1157.1997.tb00065.x
24. Steffenburg U, Hedström A, Lindroth A, Wiklund LM, Hagberg G, Kyllerman M. Intractable epilepsy in a population-based series of mentally retarded children. *Epilepsia* (1998) **39**(7):767–75. doi:10.1111/j.1528-1157.1998.tb01163.x
25. Dulac O, N'guyen T. The Lennox-Gastaut Syndrome. *Epilepsia* (1993) **34**(s7):S7–17. doi:10.1111/j.1528-1157.1993.tb04593.x
26. Camfield PR. Definition and natural history of Lennox-Gastaut syndrome. *Epilepsia* (2011) **52**(s5):3–9. doi:10.1111/j.1528-1167.2011.03177.x
27. Scheffer IE, Mullen SA. Epilepsy in 2012: advances in epilepsy shed light on key questions. *Nat Rev Neurol* (2013) **9**(2):66–8. doi:10.1038/nrneurol.2012.272
28. Jensen FE. Epilepsy in 2013: progress across the spectrum of epilepsy research. *Nat Rev Neurol* (2014) **10**(2):63–4. doi:10.1038/nrneurol.2013.277
29. Archer JS, Warren AEL, Stagnitti MR, Masterton R, Abbott DF, Jackson G. Lennox-Gastaut syndrome and phenotype: secondary network epilepsies. *Epilepsia* (2014) **55**(8):1245–54. doi:10.1111/epi.12682
30. Chevrie J, Aicardi J. Childhood epileptic encephalopathy with slow spike-wave a statistical study of 80 cases. *Epilepsia* (1972) **13**(2):259–71. doi:10.1111/j.1528-1157.1972.tb05260.x
31. Erba G, Cavazzuti V. Ictal and interictal response-latency in Lennox-Gastaut syndrome. *Electroencephalogr Clin Neurophysiol* (1977) **42**(5):717.
32. Markand ON. Slow spike-wave activity in EEG and associated clinical features: often called 'Lennox' or 'Lennox-Gastaut' syndrome. *Neurology* (1977) **27**(8):746. doi:10.1212/WNL.27.8.746
33. Boyer J, Deschatrette A, Delwarde M. [Convulsive autism? apropos of 9 cases of primary autism associated with the Lennox-Gastaut syndrome]. *Pediatrie* (1980) **36**(5):353–68.
34. Roger J, Remy C, Bureau M, Oller-Daurella L, Beaumanoir A, Favel P, et al. [Lennox-Gastaut syndrome in the adult]. *Rev Neurol* (1986) **143**(5):401–5.
35. Besag F. Behavioral aspects of pediatric epilepsy syndromes. *Epilepsy Behav* (2004) **5**:3–13. doi:10.1016/j.yebeh.2003.11.002
36. Boel MJ. Behavioural and neuropsychological problems in refractory paediatric epilepsies. *Eur J Paediatr Neurol* (2004) **8**(6):291–7. doi:10.1016/j.ejpn.2004.08.002
37. Pellock JM. Defining the problem: psychiatric and behavioral comorbidity in children and adolescents with epilepsy. *Epilepsy Behav* (2004) **5**:3–9. doi:10.1016/j.yebeh.2004.06.010
38. Rocha J, Guerra C, Oliveira R, Dória S, Rego R, Rosas MJ. Late-onset Lennox-Gastaut syndrome as a phenotype of 15q11. 1q13. 3 duplication. *Epileptic Disord* (2012) **14**(2):159–62. doi:10.1684/epd.2012.0502
39. Camfield C, Camfield P. Twenty years after childhood-onset symptomatic generalized epilepsy the social outcome is usually dependency or death: a population-based study. *Dev Med Child Neurol* (2008) **50**(11):859–63. doi:10.1111/j.1469-8749.2008.03165.x
40. Schmidt D, Bourgeois B. A risk-benefit assessment of therapies for Lennox-Gastaut syndrome. *Drug Safety* (2000) **22**(6):467–77. doi:10.2165/00002018-200022060-00005
41. Blume WT, David RB, Gomez MR. Generalized sharp and slow wave complexes associated clinical features and long-term follow-up. *Brain* (1973) **96**(2):289–306. doi:10.1093/brain/96.2.289
42. Hoffmann-Riem M, Diener W, Benninger C, Unnebrink K, Stephani U, Ernst H-P, et al. Nonconvulsive status epilepticus-a possible cause of mental retardation in patients with Lennox-Gastaut syndrome. *Neuropediatrics* (2000) **31**(04):169–74. doi:10.1055/s-2000-7456
43. Shyu H-Y, Lin J-H, Chen C, Kwan S-Y, Yiu C-H. An atypical case of Lennox-Gastaut syndrome not associated with mental retardation: a nosological issue. *Seizure* (2011) **20**(10):820–3. doi:10.1016/j.seizure.2011.08.001
44. Ohtsuka Y, Amano R, Mizukawa M, Ohtahara S. Long-term prognosis of the Lennox-Gastaut syndrome. *Psychiatry Clin Neurosci* (1990) **44**(2):257–64. doi:10.1111/j.1440-1819.1990.tb01404.x
45. Quarato PP, Gennaro GD, Manfredi M, Esposito V. Atypical Lennox–Gastaut syndrome successfully treated with removal of a parietal dysembryoplastic tumour. *Seizure* (2002) **11**(5):325–9. doi:10.1053/seiz.2001.0609
46. Freeman J, Harvey A, Rosenfeld J, Wrennall J, Bailey C, Berkovic S. Generalized epilepsy in hypothalamic hamartoma evolution and postoperative resolution. *Neurology* (2003) **60**(5):762–7. doi:10.1212/01.WNL.0000049457.05670.7D
47. Ohtahara S, Ohtsuka Y, Tyoshinga H, Iyoda K, Amano R, Yamatogi Y, et al. Lennox-Gastaut syndrome: etiological considerations. In: Niedermeyer E, Degen R editors. *The Lennox-Gastaut Syndrome.* New York: Alan R. Liss (1988). p. 47–63.
48. Li L, Fish D, Sisodiya S, Shorvon S, Alsanjari N, Stevens J. High resolution magnetic resonance imaging in adults with partial or secondary generalised epilepsy attending a tertiary referral unit. *J Neurol Neurosurg Psychiatry* (1995) **59**(4):384–7. doi:10.1136/jnnp.59.4.384
49. Farrell K, Tatum W. Encephalopathic generalized epilepsy and Lennox-Gastaut syndrome. 4th ed. In: Wyllie E editor. *The Treatment of Epilepsy: Practice and Principals.* Baltimore: Lippincott, Williams & Williams (2006). p. 429–40.
50. Project EPG, Consortium EK. De novo mutations in epileptic encephalopathies. *Nature* (2013) **501**(7466):217–21. doi:10.1038/nature12439
51. Wong M. Mechanisms of epileptogenesis in tuberous sclerosis complex and related malformations of cortical development with abnormal glioneuronal proliferation. *Epilepsia* (2008) **49**(1):8–21. doi:10.1111/j.1528-1167.2007.01270.x
52. Holmes GL, Stafstrom CE. Tuberous sclerosis complex and epilepsy: recent developments and future challenges. *Epilepsia* (2007) **48**(4):617–30. doi:10.1111/j.1528-1167.2007.01035.x
53. Angelini L, Broggi G, Riva D, Solero CLA. Case of Lennox-Gastaut syndrome successfully treated by removal of a parietotemporal astrocytoma. *Epilepsia* (1979) **20**(6):665–9. doi:10.1111/j.1528-1157.1979.tb04850.x
54. Gupta A, Chirla A, Wyllie E, Lachhwani DK, Kotagal P, Bingaman WE. Pediatric epilepsy surgery in focal lesions and generalized electroencephalogram abnormalities. *Pediatr Neurol* (2007) **37**(1):8–15. doi:10.1016/j.pediatrneurol.2007.03.004
55. Liu S, An N, Yang H, Yang M, Hou Z, Liu L, et al. Pediatric intractable epilepsy syndromes: reason for early surgical intervention. *Brain Dev* (2007) **29**(2):69–78. doi:10.1016/j.braindev.2006.06.009
56. Wyllie E, Lachhwani D, Gupta A, Chirla A, Cosmo G, Worley S, et al. Successful surgery for epilepsy due to early brain lesions despite generalized EEG findings. *Neurology* (2007) **69**(4):389–97. doi:10.1212/01.wnl.0000266386.55715.3f
57. You SJ, Lee J-K, Ko T-S. Epilepsy surgery in a patient with Lennox–Gastaut syndrome and cortical dysplasia. *Brain Dev* (2007) **29**(3):167–70. doi:10.1016/j.braindev.2006.07.013

58. Lee YJ, Kang H-C, Lee JS, Kim SH, Kim D-S, Shim K-W, et al. Resective pediatric epilepsy surgery in Lennox-Gastaut syndrome. *Pediatrics* (2010) **125**(1):e58–66. doi:10.1542/peds.2009-0566
59. Liu S-Y, An N, Fang X, Singh P, Oommen J, Yin Q, et al. Surgical treatment of patients with Lennox-Gastaut syndrome phenotype. *Scientific World Journal* (2012) **2012**:614263. doi:10.1100/2012/614263
60. Lee YJ, Lee JS, Kang HC, Kim DS, Shim KW, Eom S, et al. Outcomes of epilepsy surgery in childhood-onset epileptic encephalopathy. *Brain Dev* (2014) **36**(6):496–504. doi:10.1016/j.braindev.2013.06.010
61. Park SY, Kwon HE, Kang H-C, Lee JS, Kim DS, Kim HD. Epilepsy surgery in pediatric intractable epilepsy with destructive encephalopathy. *J Epilepsy Res* (2013) **3**(2):48. doi:10.14581/jer.13010
62. Pati S, Deep A, Troester MM, Kossoff EH, Ng Y-T. Lennox-Gastaut syndrome symptomatic to hypothalamic hamartoma: evolution and long-term outcome following surgery. *Pediatr Neurol* (2013) **49**(1):25–30. doi:10.1016/j.pediatrneurol.2013.03.016
63. Aldenkamp AP. Effect of seizures and epileptiform discharges on cognitive function. *Epilepsia* (1997) **38**(s1):S52–5. doi:10.1111/j.1528-1157.1997.tb04520.x
64. Helmstaedter C. Neuropsychological aspects of epilepsy surgery. *Epilepsy Behav* (2004) **5**:45–55. doi:10.1016/j.yebeh.2003.11.006
65. Bladin P. Adult Lennox Gastaut syndrome: patients with large focal structural lesions. *Clin Exp Neurol* (1985) **21**:105–14.
66. Asarnow R, LoPresti C, Guthrie D, Elliott T, Cynn V, Shields WD, et al. Developmental outcomes in children receiving resection surgery for medically intractable infantile spasms. *Dev Med Child Neurol* (1997) **39**(7):430–40. doi:10.1111/j.1469-8749.1997.tb07462.x
67. Bourgeois M, Sainte-Rose C, Lellouch-Tubiana A, Malucci C, Brunelle F, Maixner W, et al. Surgery of epilepsy associated with focal lesions in childhood. *J Neurosurg* (1999) **90**(5):833–42. doi:10.3171/jns.1999.90.5.0833
68. Freitag H, Tuxhorn I. Cognitive function in preschool children after epilepsy surgery: rationale for early intervention. *Epilepsia* (2005) **46**(4):561–7. doi:10.1111/j.0013-9580.2005.03504.x
69. Loddenkemper T, Holland KD, Stanford LD, Kotagal P, Bingaman W, Wyllie E. Developmental outcome after epilepsy surgery in infancy. *Pediatrics* (2007) **119**(5):930–5. doi:10.1542/peds.2006-2530
70. Velasco M, Velasco F, Alcalá H, Dávila G, Díaz-de-León AE. Epileptiform EEG Activity of the centromedian thalamic nuclei in children with intractable generalized seizures of the Lennox-Gastaut syndrome. *Epilepsia* (1991) **32**(3):310–21. doi:10.1111/j.1528-1157.1991.tb04657.x
71. Velasco M, Velasco F, Velasco AL. Temporo-spatial correlations between cortical and subcortical EEG spike-wave complexes of the Idiopathic Lennox-Gastaut syndrome. *Stereotact Funct Neurosurg* (1997) **69**(1–4 Pt 2):216–20. doi:10.1159/000099877
72. Pillay N, Archer JS, Badawy RA, Flanagan DF, Berkovic SF, Jackson G. Networks underlying paroxysmal fast activity and slow spike and wave in Lennox-Gastaut syndrome. *Neurology* (2013) **81**(7):665–73. doi:10.1212/WNL.0b013e3182a08f6a
73. Siniatchkin M, Coropceanu D, Moeller F, Boor R, Stephani U. EEG-fMRI reveals activation of brainstem and thalamus in patients with Lennox-Gastaut syndrome. *Epilepsia* (2011) **52**(4):766–74. doi:10.1111/j.1528-1167.2010.02948.x
74. Carney P, Masterton R, Harvey A, Scheffer I, Berkovic S, Jackson G. The core network in absence epilepsy differences in cortical and thalamic BOLD response. *Neurology* (2010) **75**(10):904–11. doi:10.1212/WNL.0b013e3181f11c06
75. Labate A, Briellmann RS, Abbott DF, Waites AB, Jackson GD. Typical childhood absence seizures are associated with thalamic activation. *Epileptic Disord* (2005) **7**(4):373–7.
76. Velasco AL, Velasco F, Jiménez F, Velasco M, Castro G, Carrillo-Ruiz JD, et al. Neuromodulation of the centromedian thalamic nuclei in the treatment of generalized seizures and the improvement of the quality of life in patients with Lennox–Gastaut syndrome. *Epilepsia* (2006) **47**(7):1203–12. doi:10.1111/j.1528-1167.2006.00593.x
77. Burnham W. Electrical stimulation studies: generalised convulsions triggered from the brain-stem. In: Fromm G, Faingold C, Browning R, Burnham W editors. *Epilepsy and the Reticular Formation; The Role of the Reticular Core in Convulsive Seizures.* New York: Alan R. Liss, Inc (1987). p. 25–38.
78. Faingold CL. Brainstem networks: reticulo-cortical synchronization in generalized convulsive seizures. 4th ed. In: Noebels JL, Avoli M, Rogawski MA, Olsen RW, Delgado-Escueta AV editors. *Jasper's Basic Mechanisms of the Epilepsies.* Bethesda (MD): National Center for Biotechnology Information (US) (2012). p. 257–71.
79. Fromm GH. The role of the reticular formation in the pathogenesis of seizures. *Psychiatry Clin Neurosci* (1991) **45**(2):229–34. doi:10.1111/j.1440-1819.1991.tb02462.x
80. Spencer SS. Neural networks in human epilepsy: evidence of and implications for treatment. *Epilepsia* (2002) **43**(3):219–27. doi:10.1046/j.1528-1157.2002.26901.x
81. Laufs H. Functional imaging of seizures and epilepsy: evolution from zones to networks. *Curr Opin Neurol* (2012) **25**(2):194–200. doi:10.1097/WCO.0b013e3283515db9
82. Richardson MP. Large scale brain models of epilepsy: dynamics meets connectomics. *J Neurol, Neurosurg Psychiatry* (2012) **83**(12):1238–48. doi:10.1136/jnnp-2011-301944
83. Diessen E, Diederen SJ, Braun KP, Jansen FE, Stam CJ. Functional and structural brain networks in epilepsy: what have we learned? *Epilepsia* (2013) **54**(11):1855–65. doi:10.1111/epi.12350
84. Engel J, Thompson PM, Stern JM, Staba RJ, Bragin A, Mody I. Connectomics and epilepsy. *Curr Opin Neurol* (2013) **26**(2):186–94. doi:10.1097/WCO.0b013e32835ee5b8
85. Reivich M, Kuhl D, Wolf A, Greenberg J, Phelps M, Ido T, et al. The [18F] fluorodeoxyglucose method for the measurement of local cerebral glucose utilization in man. *Circ Res* (1979) **44**(1):127–37. doi:10.1161/01.RES.44.1.127
86. Gur RC, Sussman NM, Alavi A, Gur RE, Rosen AD, O'Connor M, et al. Positron emission tomography in two cases of childhood epileptic encephalopathy (Lennox-Gastaut syndrome). *Neurology* (1982) **32**(10):1191. doi:10.1212/WNL.32.10.1191
87. Iinuma K, Yanai K, Yanagisawa T, Fueki N, Tada K, Ito M, et al. Cerebral glucose metabolism in five patients with Lennox-Gastaut syndrome. *Pediatr Neurol* (1987) **3**(1):12–8. doi:10.1016/0887-8994(87)90047-6
88. Yanai K, Iinuma K, Matsuzawa T, Ito M, Miyabayashi S, Narisawa K, et al. Cerebral glucose utilization in pediatric neurological disorders determined by positron emission tomography. *Eur J Nucl Med* (1987) **13**(6):292–6. doi:10.1007/BF00256553
89. Miyauchi T, Nomura Y, Ohno S, Kishimoto H, Matsushita M. Positron emission tomography in three cases of Lennox-Gastaut syndrome. *Psychiatry Clin Neurosci* (1988) **42**(4):795–804. doi:10.1111/j.1440-1819.1988.tb01168.x
90. Theodore WH, Rose D, Patronas N, Sato S, Holmes M, Bairamian D, et al. Cerebral glucose metabolism in the Lennox-Gastaut syndrome. *Ann Neurol* (1987) **21**(1):14–21. doi:10.1002/ana.410210105
91. Theodore W, Brooks R, Patronas N, Rose D, Sato S, Bairamian D, et al. Positron emission tomography in the Lennox-Gastaut syndrome. *Neurology* (1984) **34**(Suppl 1):106–7.
92. Chugani HT, Mazziotta JC, Engel J, Phelps ME. The Lennox-Gastaut syndrome: metabolic subtypes determined by 2-deoxy-2 [18F] fluoro-d-glucose positron emission tomography. *Ann Neurol* (1987) **21**(1):4–13. doi:10.1002/ana.410210104
93. Ferrie CD, Maisey M, Cox T, Polkey C, Barrington SF, Panayiotopoulos C, et al. Focal abnormalities detected by 18FDG PET in epileptic encephalopathies. *Arch Dis Child* (1996) **75**(2):102–7. doi:10.1136/adc.75.2.102
94. Parker AP, Ferrie CD, Keevil S, Newbold M, Cox T, Maisey M, et al. Neuroimaging and spectroscopy in children with epileptic encephalopathies. *Arch Dis Child* (1998) **79**(1):39–43. doi:10.1136/adc.79.1.39
95. Ferrie C, Marsden P, Maisey M, Robinson R. Cortical and subcortical glucose metabolism in childhood epileptic encephalopathies. *J Neurol Neurosurg Psychiatry* (1997) **63**(2):181–7. doi:10.1136/jnnp.63.2.181
96. Ferrie C, Madigan C, Tilling K, Maisey M, Marsden PK, Robinson RO. Adaptive and maladaptive behaviour in children with epileptic encephalopathies: correlation with cerebral glucose metabolism. *Dev Med Child Neurol* (1997) **39**(9):588–95. doi:10.1111/j.1469-8749.1997.tb07494.x
97. Newton MR, Berkovic SF, Austin MC, Reutens DC, McKay WJ, Bladin PF. Dystonia, clinical lateralization, and regional blood flow changes in temporal lobe seizures. *Neurology* (1992) **42**(2):371–7. doi:10.1212/WNL.42.2.371
98. Newton MR, Berkovic SF, Austin MC, Rowe CC, McKay WJ, Bladin PF. Postictal switch in blood flow distribution and temporal lobe seizures. *J Neurol Neurosurg Psychiatry* (1992) **55**(10):891–4. doi:10.1136/jnnp.55.10.891

99. Iivanainen M, Launes J, Pihko H, Nikkinen P, Lindroth L. Single-photon emission computed tomography of brain perfusion: analysis of 60 paediatric cases. *Dev Med Child Neurol* (1990) **32**(1):63–8. doi:10.1111/j.1469-8749.1990.tb08468.x
100. Heiskala H, Launes J, Pihko H, Nikkinen P, Santavuori P. Brain perfusion SPECT in children with frequent fits. *Brain Dev* (1993) **15**(3):214–8. doi:10.1016/0387-7604(93)90067-I
101. Buoni S, Zannolli R, Macucci F, Pieri S, Galluzzi P, Mariottini A, et al. Delayed response of seizures with vagus nerve stimulation in Lennox–Gastaut syndrome. *Neurology* (2004) **63**(8):1539–40. doi:10.1212/01.WNL.0000141854.58301.4C
102. Hur YJ, Kang H-C, Kim DS, Choi SR, Kim HD, Lee JS. Uncovered primary seizure foci in Lennox–Gastaut syndrome after corpus callosotomy. *Brain Dev* (2011) **33**(8):672–7. doi:10.1016/j.braindev.2010.11.005
103. Sueda K, Takeuchi F, Shiraishi H, Nakane S, Sakurai K, Yagyu K, et al. Magnetoencephalographic analysis of paroxysmal fast activity in patients with epileptic spasms. *Epilepsy Res* (2013) **104**(1):68–77. doi:10.1016/j.eplepsyres.2012.09.001
104. Rowe CC, Berkovic SF, Austin MC, Saling M, Kalnins RM, McKay WJ, et al. Visual and quantitative analysis of interictal SPECT with technetium-99m-HMPAO in temporal lobe epilepsy. *J Nucl Med* (1991) **32**(9):1688–94.
105. Kuypers HG, Fleming WR, Farinholt JW. Subcorticospinal projections in the rhesus monkey. *J Comp Neurol* (1962) **118**:107–37. doi:10.1002/cne.901180109
106. Matsuyama K, Mori F, Nakajima K, Drew T, Aoki M, Mori S. Locomotor role of the corticoreticular-reticulospinal-spinal interneuronal system. *Prog Brain Res* (2004) **143**:239–49. doi:10.1016/S0079-6123(03)43024-0
107. Lemon RN, Landau W, Tutssel D, Lawrence DG. Lawrence and Kuypers (1968a, b) revisited: copies of the original filmed material from their classic papers in Brain. *Brain* (2012) **135**(Pt 7):2290–5. doi:10.1093/brain/aws037
108. Archer JS, Abbott DF, Waites AB, Jackson GD. fMRI "deactivation" of the posterior cingulate during generalized spike and wave. *Neuroimage* (2003) **20**(4):1915–22. doi:10.1016/S1053-8119(03)00294-5
109. Archer J, Briellmann R, Syngeniotis A, Abbott D, Jackson G. Spike triggered fMRI in reading epilepsy: involvement of left frontal cortex working memory area. *Neurology* (2003) **60**:415–21. doi:10.1212/WNL.60.3.415
110. Archer JS, Briellman RS, Abbott DF, Syngeniotis A, Wellard RM, Jackson GD. Benign epilepsy with centro-temporal spikes: spike triggered fMRI shows somato-sensory cortex activity. *Epilepsia* (2003) **44**(2):200–4. doi:10.1046/j.1528-1157.2003.02502.x
111. Federico P, Archer JS, Abbott DF, Jackson GD. Cortical/subcortical BOLD changes associated with epileptic discharges An EEG-fMRI study at 3 T. *Neurology* (2005) **64**(7):1125–30. doi:10.1212/01.WNL.0000156358.72670.AD
112. Federico P, Abbott DF, Briellmann RS, Harvey AS, Jackson GD. Functional MRI of the pre-ictal state. *Brain* (2005) **128**(8):1811–7. doi:10.1093/brain/awh533
113. Archer JS, Abbott DF, Masterton RA, Palmer SM, Jackson GD. Functional MRI interactions between dysplastic nodules and overlying cortex in periventricular nodular heterotopia. *Epilepsy Behav* (2010) **19**(4):631–4. doi:10.1016/j.yebeh.2010.09.018
114. Masterton RA, Carney PW, Abbott DF, Jackson GD. Absence epilepsy subnetworks revealed by event-related independent components analysis of functional magnetic resonance imaging. *Epilepsia* (2013) **54**(5):801–8. doi:10.1111/epi.12163
115. Lemieux L, Allen PJ, Franconi F, Symms MR, Fish DK. Recording of EEG during fMRI experiments: patient safety. *Magn Reson Med* (1997) **38**(6):943–52. doi:10.1002/mrm.1910380614
116. Waites AB, Shaw ME, Briellmann RS, Labate A, Abbott DF, Jackson GD. How reliable are fMRI-EEG studies of epilepsy? A nonparametric approach to analysis validation and optimization. *Neuroimage* (2005) **24**(1):192–9. doi:10.1016/j.neuroimage.2004.09.005
117. Flanagan D, Abbott DF, Jackson GD. How wrong can we be? The effect of inaccurate mark-up of EEG/fMRI studies in epilepsy. *Neurophysiol Clin* (2009) **120**(9):1637–47. doi:10.1016/j.clinph.2009.04.025
118. Allen PJ, Polizzi G, Krakow K, Fish DR, Lemieux L. Identification of EEG events in the MR scanner: the problem of pulse artifact and a method for its subtraction. *Neuroimage* (1998) **8**:229–39. doi:10.1006/nimg.1998.0361
119. Masterton RA, Abbott DF, Fleming SW, Jackson GD. Measurement and reduction of motion and ballistocardiogram artefacts from simultaneous EEG and fMRI recordings. *Neuroimage* (2007) **37**(1):202–11. doi:10.1016/j.neuroimage.2007.02.060
120. Ogawa S, Lee T, Kay A, Tank D. Brain magnetic resonance imaging with contrast dependent on blood oxygenation. *Proc Natl Acad Sci U S A* (1990) **87**(24):9868–72. doi:10.1073/pnas.87.24.9868
121. Logothetis NK, Wandell BA. Interpreting the BOLD signal. *Annu Rev Physiol* (2004) **66**:735–69. doi:10.1146/annurev.physiol.66.082602.092845
122. Masterton RA, Jackson GD, Abbott DF. Mapping brain activity using event-related independent components analysis (eICA): specific advantages for EEG-fMRI. *Neuroimage* (2013) **70**:164–74. doi:10.1016/j.neuroimage.2012.12.025
123. Hamandi K, Salek-Haddadi A, Laufs H, Liston A, Friston K, Fish DR, et al. EEG–fMRI of idiopathic and secondarily generalized epilepsies. *Neuroimage* (2006) **31**(4):1700–10. doi:10.1016/j.neuroimage.2006.02.016
124. Hamandi K, Laufs H, Nöth U, Carmichael DW, Duncan JS, Lemieux L. BOLD and perfusion changes during epileptic generalised spike wave activity. *Neuroimage* (2008) **39**(2):608–18. doi:10.1016/j.neuroimage.2007.07.009
125. Raichle ME, MacLeod AM, Snyder AZ, Powers WJ, Gusnard DA, Shulman GL. A default mode of brain function. *Proc Natl Acad Sci U S A* (2001) **98**(2):676–82. doi:10.1073/pnas.98.2.676
126. Greicius MD, Krasnow B, Reiss AL, Menon V. Functional connectivity in the resting brain: a network analysis of the default mode hypothesis. *Proc Natl Acad Sci U S A* (2003) **100**(1):253–8. doi:10.1073/pnas.0135058100
127. Fox MD, Snyder AZ, Vincent JL, Corbetta M, Van Essen DC, Raichle ME. The human brain is intrinsically organized into dynamic, anticorrelated functional networks. *Proc Natl Acad Sci U S A* (2005) **102**(27):9673–8. doi:10.1073/pnas.0504136102
128. Fransson P. Spontaneous low-frequency BOLD signal fluctuations: an fMRI investigation of the resting-state default mode of brain function hypothesis. *Hum Brain Mapp* (2005) **26**(1):15–29. doi:10.1002/hbm.20113
129. Hawco CS, Bagshaw AP, Lu Y, Dubeau F, Gotman J. BOLD changes occur prior to epileptic spikes seen on scalp EEG. *Neuroimage* (2007) **35**(4):1450–8. doi:10.1016/j.neuroimage.2006.12.042
130. Moeller F, Siebner HR, Wolff S, Muhle H, Boor R, Granert O, et al. Changes in activity of striato-thalamo-cortical network precede generalized spike wave discharges. *Neuroimage* (2008) **39**(4):1839–49. doi:10.1016/j.neuroimage.2007.10.058
131. Bai X, Vestal M, Berman R, Negishi M, Spann M, Vega C, et al. Dynamic time course of typical childhood absence seizures: EEG, behavior, and functional magnetic resonance imaging. *J Neurosci* (2010) **30**(17):5884–93. doi:10.1523/JNEUROSCI.5101-09.2010
132. Lemieux L, Salek-Haddadi A, Josephs O, Allen P, Toms N, Scott C, et al. Event-related fMRI with simultaneous and continuous EEG: description of the method and initial case report. *Neuroimage* (2001) **14**(3):780–7. doi:10.1006/nimg.2001.0853
133. Kang JK, Bénar C-G, Al-Asmi A, Khani YA, Pike GB, Dubeau F, et al. Using patient-specific hemodynamic response functions in combined EEG-fMRI studies in epilepsy. *Neuroimage* (2003) **20**(2):1162–70. doi:10.1016/S1053-8119(03)00290-8
134. Bénar C-G, Gross DW, Wang Y, Petre V, Pike B, Dubeau F, et al. The BOLD response to interictal epileptiform discharges. *Neuroimage* (2002) **17**(3):1182–92. doi:10.1006/nimg.2002.1164
135. Jacobs J, Hawco C, Kobayashi E, Boor R, LeVan P, Stephani U, et al. Variability of the hemodynamic response as a function of age and frequency of epileptic discharge in children with epilepsy. *Neuroimage* (2008) **40**(2):601–14. doi:10.1016/j.neuroimage.2007.11.056

Permissions

All chapters in this book were first published by Frontiers; hereby published with permission under the Creative Commons Attribution License or equivalent. Every chapter published in this book has been scrutinized by our experts. Their significance has been extensively debated. The topics covered herein carry significant findings which will fuel the growth of the discipline. They may even be implemented as practical applications or may be referred to as a beginning point for another development.

The contributors of this book come from diverse backgrounds, making this book a truly international effort. This book will bring forth new frontiers with its revolutionizing research information and detailed analysis of the nascent developments around the world.

We would like to thank all the contributing authors for lending their expertise to make the book truly unique. They have played a crucial role in the development of this book. Without their invaluable contributions this book wouldn't have been possible. They have made vital efforts to compile up to date information on the varied aspects of this subject to make this book a valuable addition to the collection of many professionals and students.

This book was conceptualized with the vision of imparting up-to-date information and advanced data in this field. To ensure the same, a matchless editorial board was set up. Every individual on the board went through rigorous rounds of assessment to prove their worth. After which they invested a large part of their time researching and compiling the most relevant data for our readers.

The editorial board has been involved in producing this book since its inception. They have spent rigorous hours researching and exploring the diverse topics which have resulted in the successful publishing of this book. They have passed on their knowledge of decades through this book. To expedite this challenging task, the publisher supported the team at every step. A small team of assistant editors was also appointed to further simplify the editing procedure and attain best results for the readers.

Apart from the editorial board, the designing team has also invested a significant amount of their time in understanding the subject and creating the most relevant covers. They scrutinized every image to scout for the most suitable representation of the subject and create an appropriate cover for the book.

The publishing team has been an ardent support to the editorial, designing and production team. Their endless efforts to recruit the best for this project, has resulted in the accomplishment of this book. They are a veteran in the field of academics and their pool of knowledge is as vast as their experience in printing. Their expertise and guidance has proved useful at every step. Their uncompromising quality standards have made this book an exceptional effort. Their encouragement from time to time has been an inspiration for everyone.

The publisher and the editorial board hope that this book will prove to be a valuable piece of knowledge for researchers, students, practitioners and scholars across the globe.

List of Contributors

Patrick W. Carney
The Florey Institute for Neuroscience and Mental Health, Heidelberg, VIC, Australia
The University of Melbourne, Parkville, VIC, Australia
Austin Health, Heidelberg, VIC, Australia

Graeme D. Jackson
The Florey Institute for Neuroscience and Mental Health, Heidelberg, VIC, Australia
The University of Melbourne, Parkville, VIC, Australia
Austin Health, Heidelberg, VIC, Australia
Department of Neurology, Austin Health, Heidelberg, VIC, Australia
Department of Medicine, University of Melbourne, Melbourne, VIC, Australia
The Florey Institute of Neuroscience and Mental Health, Austin Hospital, Melbourne, VIC, Australia
Department of Medicine, Austin Health, The University of Melbourne, Heidelberg, VIC, Australia

Renaud Lopes and Xavier Leclerc
UMR 1046, University of Lille 2, Lille, France
In vivo Imaging Core Facility, IMPRT-IFR114, Lille University Medical Center, Lille, France

Friederike Moeller and Michael Siniatchkin
Department of Neuropaediatrics, Christian-Albrechts-University, Kiel, Germany

Pierre Besson, William Szurhaj, Philippe Derambure and Louise Tyvaert
UMR 1046, University of Lille 2, Lille, France
Department of Clinical Neurophysiology, Lille University Medical Center, Lille, France

François Ogez
UMR 1046, University of Lille 2, Lille, France

Mathilde Chipaux
Department of Pediatric Neurosurgery, Fondation Ophtalmologique A. de Rothschild, Paris, France

Nahla L. Faizo, Marcus Gray and Graham Galloway
Centre for Advanced Imaging, University of Queensland, Brisbane, QLD, Australia

Hana Burianová
Centre for Advanced Imaging, University of Queensland, Brisbane, QLD, Australia
ARC Centre of Excellence in Cognition and its Disorders, Macquarie University, Sydney, NSW, Australia

Julia Hocking
Centre for Advanced Imaging, University of Queensland, Brisbane, QLD, Australia
School of Psychology and Counseling, Queensland University of Technology, Brisbane, QLD, Australia

David Reutens
Centre for Advanced Imaging, University of Queensland, Brisbane, QLD, Australia
Royal Brisbane and Women's Hospital, Brisbane, QLD, Australia

Laurent Spinelli, Margitta Seeck and Serge Vulliemoz
EEG and Epilepsy Unit, Neurology Department, University Hospitals and Faculty of Medicine of Geneva, Geneva, Switzerland

Francesca Pittau
EEG and Epilepsy Unit, Neurology Department, University Hospitals and Faculty of Medicine of Geneva, Geneva, Switzerland
Neurology and Neurosurgery Department, Montreal Neurological Institute, McGill University, Montreal, QC, Canada

Pierre Mégevand
Laboratory for Multimodal Human Brain Mapping, Hofstra North Shore LIJ School of Medicine, Manhasset, NY, USA

Laurent Sheybani and Christoph M. Michel
Functional Brain Mapping Laboratory, Department of Fundamental Neurosciences, University of Geneva, Geneva, Switzerland

Eugenio Abela
Support Center of Advanced Neuroimaging (SCAN), Institute for Diagnostic and Interventional Neuroradiology, University Hospital Inselspital, Bern, Switzerland

Frédéric Grouiller
Radiology Department, University Hospitals and Faculty of Medicine of Geneva, Geneva, Switzerland

Chong H. Wong and Andrew F. Bleasel
Sydney Medical School, University of Sydney, Sydney, NSW, Australia
Department of Neurology, Westmead Hospital, Westmead, NSW, Australia

Armin Mohamed and Michael Fulham
Sydney Medical School, University of Sydney, Sydney, NSW, Australia
Department of PET and Nuclear Medicine, Royal Prince Alfred Hospital, Camperdown, NSW, Australia

Lingfeng Wen and Stefan Eberl
Department of PET and Nuclear Medicine, Royal Prince Alfred Hospital, Camperdown, NSW, Australia
School of Information Technologies, University of Sydney, Sydney, NSW, Australia

Ernest Somerville
Department of Neurology, Westmead Hospital, Westmead, NSW, Australia
Institute of Neurological Sciences, Prince of Wales Hospital, Randwick, NSW, Australia

Mark J. Cook
Department of Medicine, St. Vincent's Hospital, University of Melbourne, Fitzroy, VIC, Australia

Andrea Varsavsky and Iven Mareels
Department of Electrical and Electronic Engineering, University of Melbourne, Fitzroy, VIC, Australia

David Himes and Kent Leyde
Neurovista Corporation, Seattle, WA, USA

Samuel Frank Berkovic
Department of Medicine, Austin and Repatriation Medical Centre, University of Melbourne, Fitzroy, VIC, Australia

Terence O'Brien
Department of Medicine, Royal Melbourne Hospital, University of Melbourne, Fitzroy, VIC, Australia

David N. Vaughan
Florey Institute of Neuroscience and Mental Health, Heidelberg, VIC, Australia
Department of Neurology, Austin Health, Heidelberg, VIC, Australia

Gaelle Eve Doucet
Department of Neurology, Thomas Jefferson University, Philadelphia, PA, USA
Department of Neurosurgery, Thomas Jefferson University, Philadelphia, PA, USA

Christopher Skidmore
Department of Neurology, Thomas Jefferson University, Philadelphia, PA, USA

James Evans and Ashwini Sharan
Department of Neurosurgery, Thomas Jefferson University, Philadelphia, PA, USA

Michael R. Sperling, Dorian Pustina and Joseph I. Tracy
Department of Neurology, Thomas Jefferson University, Philadelphia, PA, USA

Stephen E. Jones, Erik B. Beall, Imad Najm, Ken E. Sakaie, Michael D. Phillips and Jorge A. Gonzalez-Martinez
Cleveland Clinic, Cleveland, OH, USA

Myron Zhang
Ohio State University College of Medicine, Columbus, OH, USA

George Petkov, Marc Goodfellow and John R. Terry
College of Engineering, Mathematics and Physical Sciences, University of Exeter, Exeter, UK

Mark P. Richardson
Institute of Psychiatry, King's College London, London, UK

Mona Maneshi and Firas Fahoum
Montreal Neurological Institute and Hospital, McGill University, Montreal, QC, Canada

Christophe Grova
Montreal Neurological Institute and Hospital, McGill University, Montreal, QC, Canada
Multimodal Functional Imaging Laboratory, Department of Biomedical Engineering, McGill University, Montreal, QC, Canada
Neurology and Neurosurgery Department, Montreal Neurological Institute, McGill University, Montreal, QC, Canada
Physics Department, PERFORM Center, Concordia University, Montreal, QC, Canada

Christian L. Dansereau
Multimodal Functional Imaging Lab, Biomedical Engineering Department, McGill University, Montreal, QC, Canada
Neurology and Neurosurgery Department, Montreal Neurological Institute, McGill University, Montreal, QC, Canada
Centre de Recherche de l'Institut Universitaire de Gériatrie de Montréal, Functional Neuroimaging Unit, Université de Montréal, Montreal, QC, Canada

Pierre Bellec
Centre de Recherche de l'Institut Universitaire de Gériatrie de Montréal, Functional Neuroimaging Unit, Université de Montréal, Montreal, QC, Canada
Department of Computer Science and Operations Research, University of Montreal, Montreal, Quebec, Canada

Shahabeddin Vahdat
Functional Neuroimaging Unit, Centre de Recherche de l'Institut Universitaire de Gériatrie de Montréal, Montreal, QC, Canada

Kangjoo Lee
Multimodal Functional Imaging Lab, Biomedical Engineering Department, McGill University, Montreal, QC, Canada
Neurology and Neurosurgery Department, Montreal Neurological Institute, McGill University, Montreal, QC, Canada

Jean Gotman
Neurology and Neurosurgery Department, Montreal Neurological Institute, McGill University, Montreal, QC, Canada
Montreal Neurological Institute and Hospital, McGill University, Montreal, QC, Canada

Julia Jacobs
Department of Neuropediatrics and Muscular Diseases, University Medical Center Freiburg, Freiburg, Germany
Epilepsy Center, University Medical Center Freiburg, Freiburg, Germany

Antonia Menzel and Katharina Körbl
Department of Neuropediatrics and Muscular Diseases, University Medical Center Freiburg, Freiburg, Germany

Georgia Ramantani and Andreas Schulze-Bonhage
Epilepsy Center, University Medical Center Freiburg, Freiburg, Germany

Jakob Assländer, Jürgen Hennig and Pierre LeVan
Medical Physics, Freiburg, Germany

Simon Tousseyn and Wim Van Paesschen
Laboratory for Epilepsy Research, UZ Leuven and KU Leuven, Leuven, Belgium
Medical Imaging Research Center, UZ Leuven and KU Leuven, Leuven, Belgium

Patrick Dupont
Laboratory for Epilepsy Research, UZ Leuven and KU Leuven, Leuven, Belgium
Medical Imaging Research Center, UZ Leuven and KU Leuven, Leuven, Belgium
Laboratory for Cognitive Neurology, UZ Leuven and KU Leuven, Leuven, Belgium

Lorenzo Caciagli, Boris C. Bernhardt, Seok-Jun Hong, Andrea Bernasconi and Neda Bernasconi
Neuroimaging of Epilepsy Laboratory, McConnell Brain Imaging Center, Montreal Neurological Institute and Hospital, McGill University, Montreal, QC, Canada

Stefan Sunaert
Medical Imaging Research Center, UZ Leuven and KU Leuven, Leuven, Belgium
Radiology Department, UZ Leuven and KU Leuven, Leuven, Belgium

Karolien Goffin
Department of Nuclear Medicine, UZ Leuven and KU Leuven, Leuven, Belgium

Richard A. J. Masterton
The Florey Institute of Neuroscience and Mental Health, Austin Hospital, Melbourne, VIC, Australia
The University of Melbourne, Melbourne, VIC, Australia

John S. Archer
The Florey Institute of Neuroscience and Mental Health, Austin Hospital, Melbourne, VIC, Australia
The University of Melbourne, Melbourne, VIC, Australia
Austin Hospital, Melbourne, VIC, Australia
Department of Medicine, Austin Health, The University of Melbourne, Heidelberg, VIC, Australia
Florey Institute of Neuroscience and Mental Health, Heidelberg, VIC, Australia
Department Neurology, Austin Health, Heidelberg, VIC, Australia

Steven W. Fleming
The Florey Institute of Neuroscience and Mental Health, Austin Hospital, Melbourne, VIC, Australia

Helmut Laufs
Department of Neurology and Brain Imaging Center, Goethe-University Frankfurt am Main, Frankfurt am Main, Germany
Department of Neurology, University Hospital Schleswig-Holstein, Christian-Albrechts-University Kiel, Kiel, Germany
National Hospital for Neurology and Neurosurgery, University College London, London, UK
The Epilepsy Society, Chalfont St. Peter, UK

Roman Rodionov, Rachel Thornton, John Sydney Duncan and Louis Lemieux
National Hospital for Neurology and Neurosurgery, University College London, London, UK
The Epilepsy Society, Chalfont St. Peter, UK

Aaron E. L. Warren
Department of Medicine, Austin Health, The University of Melbourne, Heidelberg, VIC, Australia
The Florey Institute of Neuroscience and Mental Health, Austin Hospital, Melbourne, VIC, Australia
The University of Melbourne, Melbourne, VIC, Australia

David F. Abbott
Department of Medicine, Austin Health, The University of Melbourne, Heidelberg, VIC, Australia
Florey Institute of Neuroscience and Mental Health, Heidelberg, VIC, Australia
The Florey Institute of Neuroscience and Mental Health, Austin Hospital, Melbourne, VIC, Australia
The University of Melbourne, Melbourne, VIC, Australia

Enzo Tagliazucchi
Department of Neurology and Brain Imaging Center, Goethe-University Frankfurt am Main, Frankfurt am Main, Germany

Index

www.ingramcontent.com/pod-product-compliance
Lightning Source LLC
LaVergne TN
LVHW060059220926
848484LV00008BA/2261
9798887403014